Oh! 1001 Homemade Turkey Recipes

(Oh! 1001 Homemade Turkey Recipes - Volume 1)

Carrie Milian

Copyright: Published in the United States by Carrie Milian/ © CARRIE MILIAN

Published on October, 09 2020

All rights reserved. No part of this publication may be reproduced, stored in retrieval system, copied in any form or by any means, electronic, mechanical, photocopying, recording or otherwise transmitted without written permission from the publisher. Please do not participate in or encourage piracy of this material in any way. You must not circulate this book in any format. CARRIE MILIAN does not control or direct users' actions and is not responsible for the information or content shared, harm and/or actions of the book readers.

In accordance with the U.S. Copyright Act of 1976, the scanning, uploading and electronic sharing of any part of this book without the permission of the publisher constitute unlawful piracy and theft of the author's intellectual property. If you would like to use material from the book (other than just simply for reviewing the book), prior permission must be obtained by contacting the author at author@tempehrecipes.com

Thank you for your support of the author's rights.

Content

CHAPTER 1: GROUND TURKEY RECIPES 15

1. 'Unstuffed' Cabbage With A Kick 15
2. 30 Minute White Bean Chili 15
3. Actually Delicious Buffalo Turkey Burgers 16
4. Actually Delicious Turkey Burgers 16
5. All White Meat Meatloaf 17
6. Allie's BIL's Thanksgiving Or Celebration Ground Turkey Meatloaf 17
7. Amazing Ground Turkey Tomato Sauce ..18
8. Amazing Turkey Jerky 18
9. Amy's Delicious Turkey Burgers 19
10. Ang's Turkey Burritos 19
11. Asian Turkey Sliders 20
12. Awesome Sausage, Apple And Cranberry Stuffing 20
13. Bab's Turkey Mushroom Lasagna Rolls 21
14. Bacon Mushroom Turkey Burger 22
15. Baked Turkey Meatballs 22
16. Basil Turkey Burgers 23
17. Best Turkey Meatloaf 23
18. Big Game Sunday Chili Dip 24
19. Breakfast Meatloaf 24
20. Breakfast For Dinner Casserole 24
21. Brittany's Turkey Burgers 25
22. Buffalo Turkey Meatballs 25
23. Buffalo Turkey Meatloaf 26
24. Buttermilk Turkey Meatloaf Muffins 27
25. Butternut Squash And Turkey Chili 27
26. California Turkey Burger 28
27. Cameron's Ground Turkey Salsa Ranchera For Tacos And Burritos 28
28. Carrot, Tomato, And Spinach Quinoa Pilaf With Ground Turkey 28
29. Cheese Stuffed Turkey Meat Loaf 29
30. Chef John's Turkey Burger 30
31. Chicken & Quinoa Stuffed Peppers 30
32. Chili With Turkey And Beans 31
33. Chinese Firecrackers 31
34. Chipotle Fiesta Chili 32
35. Chris's Incredible Italian Turkey Meatloaf 32
36. Christine's Meat Loaf 33
37. Cilantro Turkey Burgers 34
38. Cocktail Turkey Meatballs 34
39. Colorful Garlic Orzo 35
40. Coriander, Barley, Leek Soup 35
41. Corn Noodle Casserole 36
42. Country Casserole 36
43. Crazy Delicious Turkey Meatloaf 37
44. Cream Of Mushroom, Turkey, And Potato Soup 37
45. Crispy Ground Turkey Tostadas 38
46. Cumin Turkey Burgers 39
47. Curried Fowl Balls 39
48. Curried Turkey Meatballs 40
49. Dana's Taco Salad 40
50. DannyZ's Turkey Pumpkin Chili 41
51. David's Favorite Football Dip 41
52. Delicious Spinach And Turkey Lasagna 42
53. Delicious Turkey Burgers 42
54. Deluxe Egg Rolls 43
55. Easiest Turkey Loaf 43
56. Easy Easy Casserole 44
57. Easy Gluten Free Turkey Burgers 44
58. Easy Personal Turkey Pot Pies 45
59. Easy Slow Cooker Enchiladas 45
60. Easy Turkey Chili 46
61. Easy Turkey Meatballs 47
62. Easy Turkey Taco Soup 47
63. Egg, Cheese, And Turkey Breakfast Burritos 48
64. Eggless Organic Turkey Meatballs For Baby 48
65. Elimination Meatballs With Zucchini 49
66. Enchilada Lasagna 49
67. Enoki Protein Egg Bakes 50
68. Fabulous Ground Turkey Meatloaf 50
69. Fairuzah's Chili 51
70. Fajita Chili Con Carne 52
71. Family Favorite Slow Cooker Turkey Chili 52
72. Famous Turkey Burgers 53
73. Fantastic Black Bean Chili 53
74. Fast Turkey Bolognese 53
75. Fast And Friendly Meatballs 54
76. Feta Cheese Turkey Burgers 54
77. Feta And Turkey Stuffed Green Peppers ..55
78. Fiesta Chili 55
79. Fiesta Stuffed Turkey Burgers 56

80. Fiesta Turkey Tavern 56
81. Frank's Famous Spaghetti Sauce 57
82. French Burgers 58
83. Fried Pot Stickers 58
84. Gail's Turkey Lentil Stew 59
85. Garlic And Ranch Turkey Burgers 59
86. Gary's Turkey Burritos 60
87. Glazed Tofu Meatloaf 60
88. Gluten Free South Of The Border Spaghetti 61
89. Gluten Free Casserole 61
90. Gluten Free Stuffing 62
91. Gluten Free Turkey Meatballs 63
92. Goat Cheese And Spinach Turkey Burgers 63
93. Grandma Gladys's Zucchini Soup 64
94. Grandma's Easy Turkey Taco Salad 64
95. Granny's Easy Turkey Pie 65
96. Greek Turkey Burgers 65
97. Grilled Turkey Burgers With Cranberry Horseradish Dressing 66
98. Ground Turkey Burritos 66
99. Ground Turkey Burritos That Will Fool Your Kids 67
100. Ground Turkey Enchilada Stew With Quinoa 67
101. Ground Turkey Noodle Bake 68
102. Ground Turkey Taco Meat 68
103. Ground Turkey Tacos 69
104. Ground Turkey Zucchini Boats 69
105. Ground Turkey, Black Bean, And Kale Soup 70
106. Guacamole Turkey Burger 70
107. Hawaiian Stuffed Peppers 71
108. Healthier World's Best Lasagna 72
109. Healthy Turkey Loaf 73
110. Healthy Turkey Tex Mex Chili 73
111. Healthy And Savory Turkey Meatballs 74
112. Hearty Meatball Soup I 74
113. Herb & Garlic Turkey Burgers 75
114. Hidden Veggie Meatloaf 75
115. Hill Country Turkey Chili With Beans 76
116. Homemade BBQ Meatballs 76
117. Homemade Dog Food 77
118. Homemade Sausage 77
119. Homemade Turkey Breakfast Sausage 78
120. Homemade Turkey Chorizo 78
121. Idahoan Mexican Casserole 79
122. Italian Style Turkey Meatloaf 79
123. Italian Turkey Meatloaf 80
124. Jan's Yummy Spaghetti 80
125. Jay's Spicy Slow Cooker Turkey Chili 81
126. Jesse's Spicy Veggie And Turkey Meatball Stew 81
127. Jive Turkey Burgers 82
128. Joy's Lebanese Stuffed Zucchini 82
129. Kate's Turkey Meatballs 83
130. Ke's Cajun (Dirty) Rice 83
131. Kelly's Enchiladas 84
132. Kelly's Hot Hash 85
133. Kickin' Spicy Turkey Beer Chili 85
134. King Of The Hill Frito® Pie 86
135. Kristin's Turkey Butternut Squash Casserole 86
136. Larb Gai Nikki Style 87
137. Laura's Quick Slow Cooker Turkey Chili .. 87
138. Lazygirl's Ground Turkey Stroganoff 88
139. Lee's Taco Salad 88
140. Light And Delicious Lasagna 89
141. Lighter Cretons 90
142. Lighter Simple Lasagna Roll Ups 90
143. Low Cholesterol Turkey Tacos 91
144. Low Fat Turkey Burgers 91
145. Low Carb Turkey Quinoa Lasagna 92
146. Low Carb, Low Fat Turkey Goulash 92
147. Low Fat Mexican Turkey Casserole 93
148. M's Sloppy Joe Sauce 94
149. Maple Apple Turkey Sausage 94
150. Mexican Black Bean And Turkey Wraps ... 95
151. Mexican Corn Bread Casserole With Turkey 95
152. Mexican Enchilada Casserole 96
153. Mexican Ground Turkey Dip 96
154. Mexican Spaghetti Squash Stir Fry 97
155. Mexican Stuffed Shells 98
156. Mexican Turkey Burgers 98
157. Mexican Turkey Burgers With Pico De Gallo 99
158. Mexican Turkey Corn Bread Casserole 99
159. Mexican Turkey Dip 100
160. Mexican Style Spaghetti And Meatballs ... 100
161. Mexican Style Taco Salad 101
162. Miami Street Style Turkey Tacos 102
163. Middle Eastern Rice With Black Beans And

Chickpeas 102
164. Middle Eastern Turkey Dogs 103
165. Mild Mannered Chili 103
166. Moist Spicy Turkey Burgers 104
167. Moist Turkey Burgers 104
168. Momma's Sloppy Joes 105
169. Mozzarella Stuffed Pesto Turkey Meatballs 105
170. Mum's Dairy Free Stroganoff 106
171. Mushroom Blue Cheese Turkey Burgers 106
172. My Italian Turkey Meatballs 107
173. New York Turkey Meatball 107
174. Non Dairy Baked Penne Pasta 108
175. One Pot Ground Turkey Black Bean Taco Soup 109
176. Paleo Turkey Sweet Potato Casserole With Eggplant And Tomato 109
177. Paleo Turkey Cashew Chili 110
178. Peachy Turkey Burger Over Greens With Endive, Bacon, Avocado, And Gorgonzola 111
179. Perfect Healthy Meatloaf 111
180. Polynesian Meatballs 112
181. Popa's Simple White Chili 113
182. Pumpkin Turkey Chili 113
183. Quick Bean And Turkey Italian Meatballs 114
184. Quinoa With Ground Turkey 114
185. Quinoa, Bean, And Ground Turkey Chili 115
186. Rachel's Turkey Loaf 115
187. Robert's Homemade Italian Sausage 116
188. Rosemary Turkey Meatloaf 116
189. S.O.B. (South Of The Border) Casserole 117
190. Sarah's Incredible Turkey Chili 117
191. Seasoned Turkey Burgers 118
192. Seattle Style Turkey Lettuce Wraps 118
193. Shannon's Stuffed Delicata Squash 119
194. Shepherd's Pie III 120
195. Shepherd's Turkey Pie 120
196. Simple Scandinavian Turkey Chili 121
197. Sloppy Joe With Ground Turkey 122
198. Slow Cooker 3 Bean Chili 122
199. Slow Cooker Pumpkin Turkey Chili 123
200. Slow Cooker Sauce With Meatballs 123
201. Slow Cooker Turkey Chili With Kidney Beans 124
202. Smothered Mexican Lasagna 125
203. Sophia's Spicy Sriracha Meatballs 125
204. Southwest Stuffed Zucchini 126
205. Southwestern Macaroni And Cheese With Ground Turkey 126
206. Southwestern Mini Turkey Meatballs 127
207. Spaghetti Casserole I 127
208. Spanish Rice Soup 128
209. Spicy Bacon Cheeseburger Turkey Wraps 128
210. Spicy Breakfast Meatballs 129
211. Spicy Chipotle Turkey Burgers 129
212. Spicy Turkey Burgers 130
213. Spicy Turkey Four Bean Chili 130
214. Spicy Turkey Sloppy Joes 131
215. Spicy And Thick Turkey Chili 131
216. Spinach And Feta Turkey Burgers 132
217. Spinach, Turkey, And Mushroom Lasagna 132
218. Spooky Slow Cooker Turkey Lentil Chili 133
219. Strange But True Casserole 134
220. Stroganoff Casserole 134
221. Stuffed Orange Peppers 135
222. Stuffed Peppers With Turkey And Vegetables 135
223. Stuffed Red Peppers With Quinoa, Mushrooms, And Turkey 136
224. Stuffed Shells IV 136
225. Swedish Turkey Meatballs 137
226. Swedish Turkey Meatballs With Cream Of Mushroom Soup 138
227. Sweet Potato Chili 138
228. Sweet Potato And Turkey Shepherd's Pie 139
229. Sweet Potato Turkey Meatloaf 140
230. Sweet Turkey Chili From RED GOLD® 141
231. Sweet And Spicy Pumpkin Turkey Pasta 141
232. Taco Stuffed Zucchini Boats 142
233. Tarragon Turkey Soup 142
234. Tastes Like Beef Turkey Burgers 143
235. Tasty Ground Turkey Tacos 143
236. Tasty Shepherd's Pie With Mashed Cauliflower And Ground Turkey 144
237. Tasty Turkey Meatloaf With Sauce 144
238. Tequila Meatballs 145
239. Teriyaki Meatballs From Reynolds Wrap® 146

240. Teriyaki Pineapple Turkey Burgers 146
241. Terrific Turkey Chili 147
242. Tex Mex Turkey Chili With Black Beans, Corn And Butternut Squash 147
243. Texas Ground Turkey Burrito 148
244. Thai Style Turkey Burgers 148
245. Thanksgiving Flavored Turkey Burgers .. 149
246. Thanksgiving Style Turkey Meatloaf 149
247. The Best Turkey Chili 150
248. Three Meat Meatloaf 151
249. Tim's Turkey Tortilla Soup 151
250. Travis's Turkey Burgers With A Bite 152
251. Turffaloaf 152
252. Turkey Bolognese Recipe 153
253. Turkey Bolognese Sauce 153
254. Turkey Bolognese With Penne 154
255. Turkey Burgers With Brie, Cranberries, And Fresh Rosemary 154
256. Turkey Cheeseburger Meatloaf 155
257. Turkey Chorizo Burger 156
258. Turkey Garbanzo Bean And Kale Soup With Pasta 156
259. Turkey Goulash With Penne 157
260. Turkey Joes 157
261. Turkey Kofta Kabobs 158
262. Turkey Lasagna With Butternut Squash, Zucchini, And Spinach 158
263. Turkey Lettuce Wraps With Shiitake Mushrooms 159
264. Turkey Loaf 160
265. Turkey Meatballs 160
266. Turkey Meatloaf And Gravy 161
267. Turkey Meatloaf With Kale And Tomatoes 162
268. Turkey Mushroom Stew 162
269. Turkey Mustard Burgers 163
270. Turkey Nacho Bake 163
271. Turkey Pasta Sauce 164
272. Turkey Patties 164
273. Turkey Patties With Cranberry Cream Sauce 165
274. Turkey Picadillo 165
275. Turkey Picadillo II 166
276. Turkey Pinwheel 166
277. Turkey Portobello Pizza 167
278. Turkey Ragu With Fontina And Parmesan 168
279. Turkey Reuben Burgers 168
280. Turkey Salisbury Steak 169
281. Turkey Salisbury Steak With Cranberry Orange Gravy 169
282. Turkey Sausage Patties 170
283. Turkey Shepherd's Pie 171
284. Turkey Sloppy Joes 171
285. Turkey Soft Tacos 172
286. Turkey Spaghetti Zoodles 172
287. Turkey Spinach Crispy Baked Egg Rolls .172
288. Turkey Taco Soup 173
289. Turkey Vegetable Soup With Red Potatoes 174
290. Turkey Veggie Meatloaf Cups 174
291. Turkey Zucchini Meatballs 175
292. Turkey And Couscous Stuffed Peppers With Feta 176
293. Turkey And Potato Pockets 176
294. Turkey And Quinoa Meatballs 177
295. Turkey And Quinoa Meatloaf 178
296. Turkey And Rice Meatballs (Albondigas)178
297. Turkey And Veggie Nachos 179
298. Turkey And Yam Spicy Tacos 180
299. Turkey Zucchini Enchilada Meatballs 180
300. Veggie Sneak In Meatballs 181
301. Vietnamese Kabocha Squash Soup 181
302. Waistline Friendly Turkey Chili 182
303. Weeknight Crack Slaw 182
304. White Chili With Ground Turkey 183
305. Yummy White Bean Chili 183
306. Zesty Turkey Burgers 184
307. Zucchini Boats With Ground Turkey 184

CHAPTER 2: TURKEY SAUSAGE RECIPES 185

308. Acorn Squash With Sweet Spicy Sausage 185
309. Apple Sausage Wagon Wheel 186
310. Bean And Sausage Soup 186
311. Breaklava 187
312. Butternut Squash And Spicy Sausage Soup 187
313. Caroline And Brian's Stuffed Mushrooms 188
314. Cheesy Sausage Lasagna Soup 189
315. Chicken And Sausage With Bowties 189
316. Chicken With Sausage And Dried Fruit ..190
317. Classic Smoked Sausage Mac And Cheese

190
318. Drunk Turkey Bites 191
319. Healthier Baked Ziti 191
320. Hot Italian Turkey Sausage Spread 192
321. Italian Hot Turkey Sausage And Black Eyed Peas 192
322. Italian Sausage And Bean Soup 193
323. Italian Sausage And Tomato Soup 193
324. Jenny's Jambalaya 194
325. Loaded Stuffed Jalapeno Poppers 194
326. Mushroom St. Thomas 195
327. Omelet Muffins With Sausage And Cheese 195
328. Pasta Primavera With Italian Turkey Sausage 196
329. Pasta With Roasted Butternut Squash And Sage 197
330. Penne With Peppers And Sausage 197
331. Potato, Sausage And Egg Breakfast Casserole 198
332. Pressure Cooker Italian Chicken Soup 198
333. Red Rice And Sausage 199
334. Rice Dressing 199
335. Sausage With Mango Salsa 200
336. Sausage, Mushroom And Cranberry Tart 200
337. Sheet Pan Baked Seville Chicken, Sausage, And Vegetables 201
338. Slow Cooker Kosher Autumn Mashup ... 202
339. Smoked Sausage Frittata 202
340. Smoked Turkey Sausage Tex Mex Style Pizza 203
341. Southwestern Breakfast Tacos 203
342. Spicy Sausage And Peppers Over Rice 204
343. Spicy Turkey Sweet Potato Gumbo 204
344. Stoplight Sausage Pasta 205
345. Sunchoke And Sausage Soup 206
346. Ten Bean Soup II 206
347. Toscano Soup 207
348. Turkey Sausage Barley Soup 207
349. Turkey Sausage Breakfast 208
350. Turkey Sausage Noodles 208
351. Turkey Sausage Pie 209
352. Turkey Sausage Sauce 209
353. Turkey Sausage And Egg Pie 210
354. Turkey Spinach Sweet Potato Breakfast Casserole 210
355. Turkey Spinach Sweet Potato Casserole . 211

356. Turkey Lentil Chili 211
357. Uptown Red Beans And Rice 212
358. Yam Sausage Spread 212

CHAPTER 3: TURKEY DINNER RECIPES 213

359. Apple Almond Stuffed Turkey 213
360. Apricot Stuffed Turkey Breast 214
361. Arkansas Travelers 214
362. Baked Deli Focaccia Sandwich 215
363. Barbecue Turkey Wings 215
364. Barley Wraps 216
365. Big Sandwich 216
366. Breaded Turkey Breasts 217
367. Butter & Herb Turkey 217
368. Cashew Turkey Salad Sandwiches 218
369. Cassoulet For Today 218
370. Champagne Basted Turkey 219
371. Chili Stuffed Poblano Peppers 219
372. Citrus Herb Turkey 220
373. Classic Stuffed Turkey 221
374. Cranberry Turkey Loaf 221
375. Creamy Turkey Tetrazzini 222
376. Creole Stuffed Turkey 222
377. Deli Club Sandwich 223
378. Effortless Alfredo Pizza 223
379. Fiesta Fry Pan Dinner 224
380. Garlic Rosemary Turkey 224
381. Garlic Ginger Turkey Tenderloins 225
382. Golden Roasted Turkey 225
383. Gourmet Deli Turkey Wraps 226
384. Great Grandma's Italian Meatballs 227
385. Grilled Turkey Tenderloin 227
386. Ground Turkey Stroganoff 228
387. Ground Turkey And Hominy 228
388. Hearty Chicken Club 229
389. Herb Glazed Turkey 229
390. Herb Glazed Turkey Slices 230
391. Herb Roasted Turkey 230
392. Herbed Roast Turkey Breast 231
393. Herbed Rubbed Turkey 231
394. Herbed Stuffed Green Peppers 232
395. Herbed Turkey Breast 232
396. Herbed Turkey Tetrazzini 233
397. Herbed Turkey And Dressing 234
398. Hickory Turkey 235
399. Honey Glazed Turkey 235

400. Hot Brown Turkey Casserole..................236
401. Italian Sausage Orzo.................................237
402. Italian Turkey Meatballs.............................237
403. Juicy Roast Turkey......................................238
404. Leftover Turkey Croquettes.....................238
405. Lemon Garlic Turkey Breast....................239
406. Low Sodium Herb Rubbed Turkey..........239
407. Make Ahead Turkey And Gravy..............240
408. Maple Butter Turkey With Gravy............241
409. Maple Sage Brined Turkey.......................242
410. Marinated Thanksgiving Turkey...............243
411. Marinated Turkey.......................................243
412. Marinated Turkey For Two......................244
413. Meaty Spanish Rice...................................244
414. Mock Monte Cristos..................................245
415. Moist & Tender Turkey Breast.................245
416. Moist Italian Turkey Breast......................246
417. Moist Turkey Breast..................................246
418. Mushroom Meat Loaf...............................247
419. Mushroom Turkey Tetrazzini...................247
420. Mushroom Onion Stuffed Turkey...........248
421. Nutty Turkey Slices...................................249
422. Orange Barbecued Turkey.......................249
423. Orange Roasted Turkey...........................250
424. Orange Turkey Croissants.......................251
425. Orange Turkey Stir Fry............................251
426. Orange Glazed Turkey..............................251
427. Peanutty Asian Lettuce Wraps.................252
428. Pepper Lover's BLT..................................253
429. Pepperoni Pizza Casserole........................253
430. Posse Stew..254
431. Pronto Pita Pizzas......................................254
432. Quick And Easy Stromboli......................254
433. Raspberry Turkey Tenderloins.................255
434. Red Beans And Rice With Turkey Sausage 256
435. Roasted Citrus & Herb Turkey................256
436. Roasted Turkey Breast Tenderloins & Vegetables...257
437. Roasted Turkey With Cornbread Dressing 258
438. Roasted Wild Turkey.................................258
439. Romano Basil Turkey Breast....................259
440. Rosemary Turkey Breast..........................259
441. Sausage & Rice Stew.................................260
442. Sausage And Pumpkin Pasta....................260
443. Sesame Turkey Stir Fry.............................261
444. Skillet Tacos..262
445. Slow Cooker Turkey Breast......................262
446. Slow Cooker Turkey Pesto Lasagna.........262
447. Slow Cooker Turkey Stuffed Peppers.....263
448. Slow Cooked Turkey With Berry Compote 264
449. Slow Cooked Turkey With Herbed Stuffing 264
450. Southern Barbecue Spaghetti Sauce.........265
451. Spaghetti With Homemade Turkey Sausage 266
452. Spatchcocked Herb Roasted Turkey........266
453. Special Roast Turkey.................................267
454. Spicy Chili Mac..267
455. Spicy Skillet Supper...................................268
456. Spinach Turkey Meatballs.........................268
457. Spinach And Turkey Pinwheels................269
458. Stuffing Crust Turkey Potpie....................269
459. Super Italian Sub..270
460. Super Supper Hero....................................270
461. Sweet And Sour Turkey Meat Loaf.........271
462. Taco Skillet Supper....................................271
463. Tasty Turkey Sub..272
464. Tasty Turkey And Mushrooms.................272
465. Terrific Turkey Enchiladas........................273
466. Thanksgiving Sandwiches.........................273
467. Toasted Turkey Sandwiches.....................274
468. Tropical Turkey Meat Loaf......................274
469. Turkey & Cornbread Stuffing Rellenos...275
470. Turkey 'N' Beef Loaf.................................276
471. Turkey 'n' Stuffing Pie...............................276
472. Turkey Asparagus Casserole.....................277
473. Turkey BLT..277
474. Turkey Biscuit Stew...................................278
475. Turkey Bow Tie Skillet..............................278
476. Turkey Burger Pie......................................279
477. Turkey Burritos..279
478. Turkey Cranwich..280
479. Turkey Day Bake..280
480. Turkey Dressing Pie..................................281
481. Turkey Dumpling Stew.............................281
482. Turkey Hero..282
483. Turkey Lasagna Roll Ups..........................282
484. Turkey Legs With Mushroom Gravy........283
485. Turkey Lime Kabobs.................................283
486. Turkey Linguine...284
487. Turkey Manicotti..285

488. Turkey Meat Loaf 285
489. Turkey Minute Steaks 286
490. Turkey Mushroom Tetrazzini 286
491. Turkey Noodle Casserole 287
492. Turkey Pasta Primavera 287
493. Turkey Penne With Lemon Cream Sauce 288
494. Turkey Piccata 288
495. Turkey Pita Tacos 289
496. Turkey Pitas With Creamy Slaw 290
497. Turkey Potato Meatballs 290
498. Turkey Potato Pancakes............................291
499. Turkey Primavera........................291
500. Turkey Ranch Wraps 292
501. Turkey Ravioli Lasagna 292
502. Turkey Sausage Stew 293
503. Turkey Sausage Stuffed Acorn Squash 293
504. Turkey Scallopini........................294
505. Turkey Scallopini With Marsala Sauce.....294
506. Turkey Stew With Dumplings...................295
507. Turkey Stir Fry............................296
508. Turkey Stir Fry Supper 296
509. Turkey Stroganoff With Spaghetti Squash 297
510. Turkey Stuffing Roll Ups...........................297
511. Turkey Tenderloins With Shallot Berry Sauce 298
512. Turkey Thyme Risotto 298
513. Turkey Turnovers 299
514. Turkey Vegetable Skillet............................300
515. Turkey Wafflewiches 300
516. Turkey With Rye Dressing 300
517. Turkey A La King With Rice 301
518. Turkey And Mushroom Potpies................302
519. Turkey In Cream Sauce..............................302
520. Turkey In Mushroom Sauce......................303
521. Turkey In The Strawganoff........................303
522. Turkey With Cornbread Dressing.............304
523. Turkey With Country Ham Stuffing 304
524. Turkey With Cranberry Sauce...................305
525. Turkey With Herbed Rice Dressing..........306
526. Turkey With Mushroom Sauce 306
527. Turkey With Sausage Stuffing...................307
528. Turkey With Sausage Pecan Stuffing 307
529. Turkey Stuffed Peppers..............................308
530. Upside Down Frito Pie 309
531. Waffle Monte Cristos 309
532. Waldorf Turkey Sandwiches.....................310
533. Zesty Turkey...............................310
534. Zippy Turkey Tortilla Bake 311

CHAPTER 4: TURKEY APPETIZER RECIPES 311

535. After Christmas Empanadas 311
536. Appetizer Roll Ups 312
537. Asparagus Pepperoni Triangles 313
538. BBQ Turkey Meatballs............................313
539. Berry 'n' Smoked Turkey Twirls 314
540. Bone Crunching Meatballs 314
541. Butter Chicken Meatballs..........................315
542. Cabbage Bowl Nibbler Dip 315
543. Crab Stuffed Jalapenos 316
544. Cranberry Turkey Crostini........................316
545. Deli Sandwich Party Platter.....................317
546. Festive Holiday Sliders 317
547. Festive Turkey Meatballs 318
548. Flavorful Turkey Meatballs.......................318
549. Game Day Miniature Peppers...................319
550. Gooey Pizza Dip 320
551. Greek Party Pitas 320
552. Healthy House 320
553. Healthy Steamed Dumplings.....................321
554. Hearty Poppers...........................322
555. Honey Mustard Turkey Meatballs 322
556. Horseradish Meatballs...............................323
557. Hot Mexican Dip 323
558. Italian Pizza Bread 324
559. Italian Sausage Stuffed Mushrooms.........324
560. Layered Three Cheese Spread...................324
561. Leftover Turkey Turnovers 325
562. Lemon Marinated Antipasto 326
563. Makeover Hot Pizza Dip 326
564. Mandarin Turkey Pinwheels.....................327
565. Meatballs With Cranberry Sauce...............327
566. Meaty Salsa Dip..........................328
567. Mediterranean Pockets 328
568. Mexican Fiesta Dip....................................329
569. Microwave Texas Nachos 329
570. Mini Hot Browns 330
571. Mini Pizza Cups 330
572. Mini Sausage Bundles................................331
573. Mongolian Fondue.....................331
574. Party Cranberry Meatballs 332
575. Party Pinwheels 332

576. Pepperoni Pizza Bread 333
577. Pepperoni Pizza Pita..................................333
578. Phyllo Turkey Egg Rolls 334
579. Pistachio Turkey Meatballs In Orange Sauce 334
580. Polynesian Kabobs 335
581. Pomegranate Glazed Turkey Meatballs ...335
582. Pronto Mini Pizzas 336
583. Quesadilla...336
584. Quick Turkey Nachos Snack.....................337
585. Roasted Vegetable Turkey Pinwheels 337
586. Rustic Antipasto Tart 338
587. Saucy Asian Meatballs 338
588. Saucy Turkey Meatballs.............................339
589. Sausage Stuffed Red Potatoes 339
590. Silly Snake Sub 340
591. Southwest Turkey Spirals..........................340
592. Spinach Bacon Tartlets 341
593. Steamed Turkey Dumplings 341
594. Stromboli Ladder Loaf...............................342
595. Stuffed Turkey Spirals 343
596. Sun Dried Tomato Turkey Pinwheels 343
597. Sweet & Sour Turkey Meatballs................344
598. Tangy BBQ Meatballs 344
599. Tangy Turkey Meatballs............................345
600. Tender Turkey Meatballs 345
601. Thanksgiving Wontons 345
602. Turkey & Swiss Biscuit Sliders..................346
603. Turkey Bolognese Polenta Nests...............347
604. Turkey Cheese Ball 347
605. Turkey Crescents..348
606. Turkey Croquettes With Cranberry Salsa 348
607. Turkey Egg Rolls..349
608. Turkey Nachos 350
609. Turkey Quesadillas....................................350
610. Turkey Sandwiches With Red Pepper Hummus..351
611. Turkey Sliders With Chili Cheese Mayo ..351
612. Turkey Sliders With Sesame Slaw.............352
613. Turkey Sliders With Sweet Potato "Buns" 353
614. Turkey Taco Dip...353
615. Turkey Tea Sandwiches With Basil Mayonnaise 354
616. Turkey Wonton Cups.................................354
617. Turkey Cranberry Minis 355
618. Turkey Mushroom Egg Rolls....................355
619. Whole Wheat Pepperoni Pizzas................356

CHAPTER 5: TURKEY SIDE DISH RECIPES 357

620. After Thanksgiving Salad..........................357
621. After Thanksgiving Turkey Soup 357
622. After The Holidays Salad..........................358
623. Antipasto Tossed Salad 358
624. Artichoke Turkey Salami Salad 359
625. Autumn Acorn Squash...............................359
626. Autumn Pumpkin Chili..............................360
627. Avocado Turkey Salad 360
628. BLT Turkey Salad 360
629. Basic Turkey Soup 361
630. Beefy Vegetable Soup................................362
631. Big Batch Turkey Salad 362
632. Black Bean 'n' Pumpkin Chili....................363
633. Broccoli Turkey Salad................................363
634. Cabbage Parsley Slaw 364
635. California Burger Bowls............................364
636. Cannellini Comfort Soup...........................365
637. Cantaloupe Salami Salad 365
638. Cashew Turkey Pasta Salad 366
639. Chef's Spinach Salad..................................366
640. Chili With Potato Dumplings 367
641. Chinese Turkey Pasta Salad.......................367
642. Chunky Turkey Chili 368
643. Chutney Turkey Salad 368
644. Cincinnati Style Chili 369
645. Classic Turkey Noodle Soup.....................370
646. Club Sandwich Salad 370
647. Contest Winning Turkey Meatball Soup .371
648. Cranberry Turkey Salad.............................371
649. Cranberry Chutney Turkey Salad..............372
650. Cream Of Turkey And Wild Rice Soup ..372
651. Creamy Fruited Turkey Salad....................373
652. Creamy Turkey Noodle Soup 373
653. Creamy Turkey Soup.................................374
654. Creamy Turkey Vegetable Soup 374
655. Crispy Mashed Potato & Stuffing Patties 375
656. Crowd Pleasing Chicken Salad..................375
657. Crunchy Turkey Salad 376
658. Curried Turkey Salad 376
659. Curried Turkey And Rice Salad 377
660. Day After Thanksgiving Salad 377
661. Dressing For A Crowd...............................378
662. Dutch Potato Poultry Stuffing.................378

663. Easy Greek Pasta Salad 379
664. Easy Sausage Corn Chowder 379
665. Easy Turkey Noodle Soup........................380
666. Effortless Black Bean Chili.........................380
667. Fruit 'n' Spice Salad...................................381
668. Fruited Tarragon Turkey Salad 381
669. Fruited Turkey Salad..................................382
670. Garden Pasta Salad 382
671. Garden Fresh Chef Salad..........................382
672. Gizzard Soup 383
673. Greek Rice Salad 383
674. Grill Side Turkey Salad..............................384
675. Ham Salad 384
676. Ham And Turkey Pasta Salad 385
677. Ham, Turkey And Wild Rice Salad 385
678. Hamburger Soup..386
679. Harvest Turkey Soup.................................386
680. Healthy Italian Market Salad 387
681. Hearty Alfredo Potatoes 387
682. Hearty Brunch Potatoes............................388
683. Hearty Meatball Soup...............................388
684. Hearty Pasta Salad.....................................389
685. Hearty Sausage Chicken Chili 389
686. Homemade Kielbasa Bean Soup.............390
687. Hot Turkey Pecan Salad............................390
688. Hot Turkey Salad 391
689. Italian Sausage Kale Soup........................391
690. Italian Sausage Pizza Soup.......................392
691. Italian Sausage Tortellini Soup................392
692. Kielbasa Summer Salad 393
693. Lemony Turkey Rice Soup 394
694. Lentil Barley Soup.....................................394
695. Lentil Chili..395
696. Lentil Sausage Soup 395
697. Lentil Spinach Soup...................................396
698. Luncheon Spinach Salad..........................396
699. Makeover Pizza Pasta Salad.....................396
700. Makeover Sausage Pecan Stuffing............397
701. Makeover Twice Baked Potatoes 398
702. Mashed Potato Stuffing 398
703. Meatball Alphabet Soup...........................399
704. Mediterranean Tortellini Salad 399
705. Melon Turkey Salad 400
706. Mexican White Chili 400
707. Minute Minestrone 401
708. Mulligatawny Soup....................................401
709. Okra Pilaf..402
710. Parsley Tortellini Toss................................402
711. Pear Harvest Salad 403
712. Popover With Hot Turkey Salad 403
713. Potato Kale Sausage Soup 404
714. Quick Pantry Salad....................................404
715. Quick Pasta Sausage Soup 405
716. Quick Turkey Salad...................................406
717. Quick Turkey Bean Soup..........................406
718. Rainy Day Soup..407
719. Red Bean 'N' Sausage Soup 407
720. Refreshing Turkey Salad 408
721. Rosemary Split Pea Soup 408
722. Sausage & Cannellini Bean Soup.............409
723. Sausage Potato Salad 409
724. Sausage Tomato Soup...............................410
725. Sausage And Corn Bread Dressing 410
726. Sausage Pecan Turkey Stuffing................411
727. Savory Meatball Minestrone....................411
728. Shortcut Sausage Minestrone 412
729. Skinny Cobb Salad 413
730. Slow Cooker Turkey Chili 413
731. Slow Cooked Turkey White Bean Soup ..414
732. Smoked Turkey And Apple Salad 414
733. Southern Cornbread Dressing 415
734. Southwestern Turkey Dumpling Soup 415
735. Spice It Up Soup 416
736. Spicy Kielbasa Soup...................................416
737. Spicy Turkey Bean Soup 417
738. Spicy Turkey Chili......................................417
739. Submarine Sandwich Salad 418
740. Summer Spiral Salad 418
741. Summer Squash And Bell Pepper Saute With Bacon 419
742. Sweet And Savory Turkey Salad 419
743. Tangy Turkey Salad 419
744. Tarragon Turkey Salad 420
745. Tasty Reuben Soup 420
746. Tasty Turkey Soup 421
747. Texas Turkey Soup 421
748. Texican Chili..422
749. Thick Turkey Bean Chili 422
750. Thrive On Five Soup..................................423
751. Tomato Turkey Soup 423
752. Tropical Turkey Salad................................424
753. Turkey Almond Salad 424
754. Turkey Barley Soup....................................425
755. Turkey Barley Tomato Soup 426

#	Recipe	Page
756.	Turkey Bean Chili	426
757.	Turkey Bean Soup	427
758.	Turkey Cabbage Soup	427
759.	Turkey Cashew Salad	428
760.	Turkey Chili	428
761.	Turkey Chutney Salad	429
762.	Turkey Curry Salad	429
763.	Turkey Dumpling Soup	430
764.	Turkey Fried Rice	430
765.	Turkey Fruit Salad	431
766.	Turkey Ginger Noodle Soup	431
767.	Turkey Mandarin Salad	432
768.	Turkey Meatball Salad	432
769.	Turkey Meatball Soup	433
770.	Turkey Meatballs Soup	433
771.	Turkey Minestrone	434
772.	Turkey Noodle Soup	435
773.	Turkey Pasta Salad	435
774.	Turkey Pasta Soup	436
775.	Turkey Ramen Noodle Salad	436
776.	Turkey Ranch Salad	437
777.	Turkey Rice Salad	437
778.	Turkey Rice Soup	438
779.	Turkey Rice And Barley Soup	438
780.	Turkey Salad	439
781.	Turkey Salad Sundaes	439
782.	Turkey Salad For 50	440
783.	Turkey Salad For 60	440
784.	Turkey Salad With Grapes & Cashews	441
785.	Turkey Salad With Pear Dressing	441
786.	Turkey Salad With Raspberries	442
787.	Turkey Sausage Bean Soup	442
788.	Turkey Sausage Potato Salad	443
789.	Turkey Sausage And Lentil Soup	443
790.	Turkey Shrimp Salad	444
791.	Turkey Soup	445
792.	Turkey Soup With Slickers	445
793.	Turkey Vegetable Barley Soup	446
794.	Turkey Vegetable Pasta Salad	446
795.	Turkey White Chili	447
796.	Turkey Wild Rice Soup	447
797.	Turkey And Dumpling Soup	448
798.	Turkey And Fruit Salad	448
799.	Turkey And Ham Salad With Greens	449
800.	Turkey And Vegetable Barley Soup	449
801.	Turkey And Wild Rice Soup	450
802.	Turkey Berry Stuffing Balls	450
803.	Turkey Blue Cheese Pasta Salad	451
804.	Turkey Melon Pasta Salad	451
805.	Turkey White Bean Soup	452
806.	Two Bean Turkey Salad	452
807.	White Bean Bisque	453
808.	White Bean Sausage Soup	453
809.	White Bean Turkey Chili	454
810.	White Bean And Chicken Chili	455
811.	White Christmas Chili	455
812.	White Turkey Chili	456
813.	Wild Rice Stuffing	456
814.	Wild Rice Turkey Salad	457
815.	Wild Rice And Turkey Salad	457
816.	Williamsburg Inn Turkey Soup	458
817.	Wilted Green Salad	458
818.	Zesty Turkey Chili	458

CHAPTER 6: WHOLE TURKEY RECIPES 459

#	Recipe	Page
819.	Apple Stuffed Turkey	459
820.	Awesome Tangerine Glazed Turkey	460
821.	BBQ Turkey	460
822.	Best Greek Stuffed Turkey	461
823.	Brined Thanksgiving Turkey	462
824.	Brined Turkey	462
825.	Brined And Roasted Whole Turkey	463
826.	Brining And Cooking The Perfect Turkey With Delicious Gravy	464
827.	Cajun Deep Fried Turkey	465
828.	Carl's Turkey Stuffing	465
829.	Chef John's Boneless Whole Turkey	466
830.	Chef John's Roast Turkey And Gravy	467
831.	Classic Turkey And Rice Soup	468
832.	Cola Roast Turkey	468
833.	Deep Fried Turkey	469
834.	Dry Brine Turkey	469
835.	Easy Beginner's Turkey With Stuffing	470
836.	Easy Herb Roasted Turkey	471
837.	Easy Smoked Turkey	471
838.	English Honey Roasted Turkey	472
839.	Erick's Deep Fried Rosemary Turkey	473
840.	Evil Turkey	473
841.	Fruity Tutti Turkey Brine	474
842.	Garbage Can Turkey	474
843.	General Tso's Whole Turkey	475
844.	Greek Traditional Turkey With Chestnut And Pine Nut Stuffing	476

845. Grilled Turkey 477
846. Grilled Whole Turkey.......................477
847. Herb Glazed Roasted Turkey 478
848. Holiday Turkey With Honey Orange Glaze 478
849. Homestyle Turkey, The Michigander Way 479
850. Honey Brined Smoked Turkey 480
851. Honey Smoked Turkey 480
852. How To Cook A Turkey..........................481
853. Juicy Thanksgiving Turkey 481
854. Lauren's Apple Cider Roast Turkey 482
855. Lemon Herb Turkey................................483
856. Ma Lipo's Apricot Glazed Turkey With Roasted Onion And Shallot Gravy 483
857. Maple Basted Roast Turkey With Cranberry Pan Gravy 484
858. Maple Roast Turkey................................485
859. Maple Roast Turkey And Gravy..............486
860. McCormick® Savory Herb Rub Roasted Turkey...487
861. Megaturkey...488
862. Orange And Maple Glazed Turkey.........488
863. Perfect Turkey 489
864. Roast Peruvian Turkey 489
865. Roast Spatchcock Turkey 491
866. Roast Turkey With Tasty Chestnut Stuffing 491
867. Roast Turkey With Cranberry And Pomegranate Glaze 492
868. Roast Turkeys With Rich Pan Gravy.......493
869. Roasted Turkey, Navy Style 494
870. Rosemary Roasted Turkey......................495
871. Salvadorian Roasted Turkey....................495
872. Sherry's German Turkey 496
873. Simple Classic Roasted Turkey 496
874. Simple Deep Fried Turkey 497
875. Smoked Turkey 497
876. Sugar Free Citrus Turkey Brine 498
877. Super Easy Smoked Turkey.....................499
878. Thanksgiving Turkey Brine 499
879. The Attention Hungry Turkey Of Moistness..500
880. The Best Ugly Turkey..............................500
881. The Greatest Grilled Turkey 501
882. The World's Best Turkey 501
883. Thyme Roasted Turkey 502

884. Tiffany's Herb Roasted Turkey................502
885. Turducken 503
886. Turkey Mercedes.....................................504
887. Turkey And Stuffing................................504
888. Turkey In A Bag......................................505
889. Turkey In A Smoker................................505
890. Turkey With Cornbread Stuffing.............506
891. Upside Down Turkey..............................506
892. Very Moist And Flavorful Roast Turkey.507

CHAPTER 7: TURKEY BREAST RECIPES
....508

893. Aidan Special 508
894. Awesome Turkey Sandwich 508
895. Bacon Wrapped Turkey Breast Stuffed With Spinach And Feta...................................509
896. Baked Hawaiian Sandwiches 509
897. Bourbon And Molasses Glazed Turkey Breast 510
898. Cheater's Thanksgiving Turkey................510
899. Cranberry Stuffed Turkey Breasts 511
900. Croissant Club Sandwich 511
901. Deep Fried Turkey Breast 512
902. Easy Turkey Stuffing Roll Ups 512
903. Green Chile Posole (Low Fat) 513
904. Grilled Turkey Breast With Fresh Sage Leaves 513
905. Hatch Chile Turkey Panini 514
906. Heavenly Turkey Soup 514
907. Herbed Slow Cooker Turkey Breast 515
908. Inside Out Pizza......................................515
909. Instant Pot® Frozen Turkey Breast 516
910. Instant Pot® Thanksgiving Dinner 517
911. Instant Pot® Turkey Breast 517
912. Jamaican Turkey Sandwich......................518
913. Jeanne's Slow Cooker Spaghetti Sauce 519
914. Jill's Vegetable Chili 519
915. Karla's Nutty Turkey Cranwich 520
916. Kickin' Turkey Club Wrap......................520
917. Kids' Turkey And Cream Cheese Spread Bento Box 520
918. Low Carb Bacon Lettuce Turkey Wraps.521
919. Mama H's Fooled You Fancy Slow Cooker Turkey Breast..522
920. Maple Glazed Turkey Roast....................522
921. Marinated Turkey Breast.........................523
922. Mushroom Turkey Roulade 523

923. Oat And Herb Encrusted Turkey 524
924. Orange, Tea, Bourbon Brined Paprika Butter Turkey..525
925. Quick Turkey Peppers................................525
926. Roasted Turkey Breast With Herbs 526
927. Rotelle Pasta Salad 526
928. Slow Cooker Bacon Ranch Beer Can Turkey..527
929. Slow Cooker Boneless Turkey Breast......527
930. Slow Cooker Cranberry Turkey Breast....528
931. Slow Cooker Herbed Turkey Breast 528
932. Slow Cooker Italian Turkey......................529
933. Slow Cooker Mediterranean Roast Turkey Breast 529
934. Slow Cooker Thanksgiving Turkey 530
935. Slow Cooker Turkey Breast With Dressing 530
936. Slow Cooker Turkey Breast With Gravy.531
937. Slow Cooker Turkey And White Bean Chili 531
938. Soy, Garlic, And Chile Zoodles 532
939. Stuffed Turkey London Broil....................532
940. Sweet And Spicy Turkey Sandwich 533
941. Tender Breaded Turkey Cutlets.................533
942. Tex Mex Turkey Soup 534
943. Thanksgiving Won Tons............................534
944. The Hot Brown 535
945. Tunisian Slow Cooked Turkey Breast 536
946. Turkey Avocado Panini.............................536
947. Turkey Bacon Avocado Sandwich 537
948. Turkey Breast Roulade With Apple And Raisin Stuffing 537
949. Turkey Breast With Gravy........................538
950. Turkey Divan 539
951. Turkey Paupiettes With Apple Maple Stuffing 539
952. Turkey Sandwiches With Cranberry Sauce 540
953. Turkey Scallopini And Squash Ravioli With Cranberry Brown Butter 541
954. Turkey Taco Salad....................................541
955. Turkey A La King Deluxe 542
956. Turkey A La Matt.....................................543
957. Turkey A La Oscar 543
958. Turkey And Avocado Panini....................544
959. Turkey And Feta Grilled Sandwich..........544
960. Turkey And Stuffing Casserole 545

961. Wild Turkey Gumbo 545

CHAPTER 8: TURKEY LEG RECIPES ...546

962. African Turkey Stew.................................546
963. Colin's Turkey Casserole..........................546
964. Eva's Savory Turkey Legs.........................547
965. Fried Cabbage With Turkey 548
966. Grilled Turkey Legs 548
967. It's Way Better Than Thanksgiving Turkey Turkey..549
968. Meaty Potato Leek Soup..........................549
969. Old Man's Turkey Noodle Soup 550
970. Orangey Turkey Legs 551
971. Pammy's Slow Cooker Beans 551
972. Pressure Cooked Black Eyed Peas With Smoked Turkey Leg...552
973. Roasted Barbecued Turkey Legs 552
974. Roasted Potatoes And Smoked Turkey Legs 553
975. Roasted Turkey Legs 553
976. Slow Cooker Turkey Legs.........................554
977. Slow Cooker Turkey And Potatoes..........554
978. Slow Cooked Turkey Legs 555
979. Smoked Turkey Broth...............................555
980. Smoked Turkey Leg Salad 556
981. Smoked Turkey Split Pea Soup.................556
982. Smoked Turkey Wild Rice Soup...............557
983. Split Pea Smoked Turkey Soup.................557
984. Stuffed Turkey Legs..................................558
985. Super Soup 558
986. Super Easy Drumstick Casserole..............559
987. Tam's Black Eye Peas................................559
988. Tasty Collard Greens................................560
989. Turkey BBQ Sandwiches 560
990. Turkey Corn Chowder 561
991. Turkey Drumsticks Paprika......................561
992. Turkey Drumsticks Perfecto 562
993. Turkey Vegetable Soup 562
994. Tuscan Smoked Turkey Bean Soup 563

CHAPTER 9: TURKEY BRINE RECIPES 563

995. Apple Cider Turkey Brine.........................563
996. Grandma's Farmhouse Turkey Brine.......564
997. Incredible Turkey Brine 564
998. Make Your Turkey Melt In Your Mouth Turkey Brine 564

999. Salty And Sweet Cranberry Citrus Brine .565
1000. Terrific Turkey Brine..................................565
1001. Turkey Brine 566

INDEX 567

CONCLUSION..574

Chapter 1: Ground Turkey Recipes

***

1. 'Unstuffed' Cabbage With A Kick

Serving: 4 | Prep: 10mins | Cook: 40mins | Ready in:

Ingredients

- 1 pound ground turkey
- 1 tablespoon olive oil
- 1/2 tablespoon onion, diced
- 2 cloves garlic, minced
- 1 (14.5 ounce) can diced tomatoes
- 1 (8 ounce) can tomato sauce
- 1 tablespoon Italian seasoning
- 1 teaspoon dried basil
- 1 teaspoon red pepper flakes
- 1/2 teaspoon cayenne pepper
- salt and ground black pepper to taste
- 1 head cabbage, cut into 1-inch squares

Direction

- Set the large skillet over medium-high heat. Stir in ground turkey and cook for 5-7 minutes until crumbly and browned. Drain the ground turkey and discard any excess grease. Place the cooked turkey into the bowl.
- Put olive oil in a skillet and heat it over medium heat. Sauté the onion in the hot oil for 5 minutes until it is translucent. Add the garlic into onion and sauté for 1 minute until fragrant.
- Pour in tomato sauce and diced tomatoes. Season the mixture with red pepper flakes, black pepper, salt, Italian seasoning, cayenne pepper, and basil. Adjust the heat to medium-low. Simmer the mixture for 10 minutes until the tomatoes are softened.
- Mix in cabbage. Cook for 20-25 minutes until the cabbage is tender.
- Stir in ground turkey. Cook for 1-2 minutes to reheat turkey.

Nutrition Information

- Calories: 315 calories;
- Cholesterol: 84
- Protein: 28.2
- Total Fat: 12.6
- Sodium: 571
- Total Carbohydrate: 25.6

2. 30 Minute White Bean Chili

Serving: 4 | Prep: 15mins | Cook: 20mins | Ready in:

Ingredients

- 2 tablespoons olive oil
- 1 pound ground turkey breast
- 1 onion, diced
- 1 green bell pepper, diced
- 1 teaspoon minced garlic
- 1 (14.5 ounce) can diced tomatoes
- 2 stalks celery, diced
- 1 teaspoon ground cumin
- 1 teaspoon chili powder
- 1/2 teaspoon crushed bay leaf
- 1/2 teaspoon dried basil
- 1 cup water, or more to taste
- 1 (15 ounce) can navy beans, drained
- 1 (15 ounce) can lima beans, drained
- salt and ground black pepper to taste

Direction

- In a big pot, heat olive oil over medium heat. Add in garlic, green bell pepper, onion, and

turkey; cook and stir 5 minutes until onion is translucent and turkey is browned.
- Mix basil, bay leaf, chili powder, cumin, celery, and tomatoes into the pot. Add water, simmer 10-15 minutes with cover until chili reaches wanted level of thickness and celery is tender. Blend in lima beans and navy beans, cook 5-10 min till heated through. Season with pepper and salt.

Nutrition Information

- Calories: 446 calories;
- Sodium: 1106
- Total Carbohydrate: 48.7
- Cholesterol: 70
- Protein: 43.1
- Total Fat: 8.5

3. Actually Delicious Buffalo Turkey Burgers

Serving: 12 | Prep: 20mins | Cook: 5mins | Ready in:

Ingredients

- 2 pounds 99%-lean ground turkey
- 1 small onion, minced
- 1/2 cup panko bread crumbs
- 1/4 cup Buffalo wing sauce
- 1/4 cup chopped fresh parsley (optional)
- 1 egg
- 3 cloves garlic, minced
- 1/2 teaspoon celery seed
- 1/4 teaspoon ground black pepper
- 1 pinch cayenne pepper
- 1 pinch paprika
- 1 teaspoon salt
- 12 slices Monterey Jack cheese
- 12 hamburger buns, split
- 6 tablespoons ranch dressing, or to taste
- 6 tablespoons Buffalo wing sauce, or to taste

Direction

- Set an outdoor grill or George Foreman Grill® to medium-high heat for preheating.
- In a large bowl, mix a 1/4 cup of Buffalo wing sauce, celery seed, cayenne pepper, salt, paprika, black pepper, egg, ground turkey, panko, onion, garlic, and parsley. Form the mixture into 12 patties.
- Cook and grill the patties into the preheated grill for 3 minutes. Flip them up and cook for 2 more minutes until cooked through or when an inserted instant-read thermometer on its center reads at least 165°F or 74°C.
- Place a slice of Monterey Jack cheese on its top. Place each of the patties inside the bun.
- In a bowl, combine the ranch dressing and 6 tbsp. of Buffalo wing sauce. Spread the sauce onto each of the burgers.

Nutrition Information

- Calories: 389 calories;
- Sodium: 1067
- Total Carbohydrate: 28.4
- Cholesterol: 97
- Protein: 32.1
- Total Fat: 16.2

4. Actually Delicious Turkey Burgers

Serving: 12 | Prep: 15mins | Cook: 15mins | Ready in:

Ingredients

- 3 pounds ground turkey
- 1/4 cup seasoned bread crumbs
- 1/4 cup finely diced onion
- 2 egg whites, lightly beaten
- 1/4 cup chopped fresh parsley
- 1 clove garlic, peeled and minced
- 1 teaspoon salt
- 1/4 teaspoon ground black pepper

Direction

- Combine together in a big bowl with pepper, salt, garlic, parsley, egg whites, onion, seasoned bread crumbs and ground turkey. Shape the mixture into 12 patties.
- In a medium skillet, cook the patties on moderate heat while turning one time, until the internal temperature of patties reach 85°C or 180°F.

Nutrition Information

- Calories: 183 calories;
- Sodium: 354
- Total Carbohydrate: 2.3
- Cholesterol: 90
- Protein: 20.9
- Total Fat: 9.5

5. All White Meat Meatloaf

Serving: 6 | Prep: 20mins | Cook: 50mins | Ready in:

Ingredients

- 1/2 pound ground turkey
- 1/2 pound ground chicken breast
- 1/2 pound bulk pork sausage
- 1 egg, beaten
- 1 (4 ounce) packet crushed saltine crackers
- 1/2 cup sweet barbeque sauce
- 1 tablespoon prepared yellow mustard
- 1 teaspoon hickory-flavored liquid smoke
- 2 teaspoons dried parsley
- 1 teaspoon dried minced onion
- 1 teaspoon onion powder
- 1 teaspoon garlic salt
- 1 teaspoon seasoned salt
- Glaze:
- 1 tablespoon brown sugar
- 2 tablespoons sweet barbeque sauce
- 1 tablespoon prepared yellow mustard

Direction

- Preheat an oven to 175°C/350°F then grease a 9x9-in. baking pan.
- Mix together egg, sausage, chicken and turkey in a big bowl; mix in seasoned salt, garlic salt, onion powder, dried onion, parsley, liquid smoke, 1 tbsp. mustard, 1/2 cup barbeque sauce and saltine crackers and toss well. Press into prepped pan.
- In preheated oven, bake meatloaf for 25 minutes. To make a glaze, mix together 1 tbsp. mustard, the leftover 2 tbsp. barbeque sauce and brown sugar. Take meatloaf out of the oven; brush glaze. Put meatloaf back into oven; bake for about 25 minutes longer till not pink in middle anymore. An inserted instant-read thermometer in the middle should read at a minimum of 75°C/165°F.

Nutrition Information

- Calories: 369 calories;
- Total Fat: 16.6
- Sodium: 1439
- Total Carbohydrate: 29.3
- Cholesterol: 104
- Protein: 24.6

6. Allie's BIL's Thanksgiving Or Celebration Ground Turkey Meatloaf

Serving: 6 | Prep: 10mins | Cook: 1hours | Ready in:

Ingredients

- 3 pounds ground turkey, or more to taste
- 1 (16 ounce) can whole berry cranberry sauce, divided
- 1 (14 ounce) package herb-seasoned stuffing mix (such as Pepperidge Farm®)
- 4 eggs, beaten

Direction

- Set the oven to 175°C or 350°F to preheat.
- In a bowl, combine together eggs, stuffing mix, 2/3 of the cranberry sauce and ground turkey until well-mixed. Press into a loaf pan the turkey mixture, then scoop over top the leftover cranberry sauce.
- In the preheated oven, bake for an hour until it is not pink in the middle anymore. An instant-read thermometer should reach at least 75°C or 170°F after being inserted in the center.

Nutrition Information

- Calories: 746 calories;
- Sodium: 1102
- Total Carbohydrate: 78.1
- Cholesterol: 292
- Protein: 56.8
- Total Fat: 22.7

7. Amazing Ground Turkey Tomato Sauce

Serving: 4 | Prep: 15mins | Cook: 40mins | Ready in:

Ingredients

- 1/4 cup olive oil
- 1/2 white onion, chopped
- 1 tomato, chopped
- 6 basil leaves, chopped
- 4 cloves garlic, minced
- 1 (20 ounce) package ground turkey
- 1 teaspoon Italian seasoning
- 1/4 teaspoon oregano
- 2 (15 ounce) cans tomato sauce
- 1/2 (6 ounce) can tomato paste, or to taste
- salt and ground black pepper to taste

Direction

- In a big pot, heat olive oil over medium-high heat. Sauté garlic, basil, tomato and onion in the hot oil for about 5 minutes until the onion begins to soften.
- Break the ground turkey into small pieces then put it into the pot. Use oregano and Italian seasoning to season. Cook and stir mixture for 7 to 10 minutes until turkey is completely browned.
- Mix the tomato sauce into the turkey mixture then let it come to a boil. Turn the heat to low; simmer for 20 to 25 minutes until the sauce has slightly thickened.
- Mix tomato paste into the turkey mixture until it colors evenly. Use pepper and salt to season. Cook for another 1 to 2 minutes until the liquid is reheated.

Nutrition Information

- Calories: 413 calories;
- Total Fat: 24.8
- Sodium: 1352
- Total Carbohydrate: 19.4
- Cholesterol: 105
- Protein: 32.5

8. Amazing Turkey Jerky

Serving: 10 | Prep: 25mins | Cook: | Ready in:

Ingredients

- 1 1/2 pounds ground turkey
- 1/2 cup soy sauce
- 1 tablespoon honey
- 1 tablespoon Worcestershire sauce
- 1 tablespoon apple cider vinegar
- 1 tablespoon liquid smoke
- 1 tablespoon garlic powder
- 1 tablespoon coarsely ground black pepper
- 1 1/2 teaspoons ground ginger
- 1 teaspoon olive oil
- 1/2 cube beef bouillon
- wooden paint stir sticks

Direction

- Mix together beef bouillon, olive oil, ginger, pepper, garlic powder, liquid smoke, apple cider vinegar, honey, Worcestershire sauce, honey, soy sauce and ground turkey in a big bowl; stir well and cover. Marinate for 2-12 hours in the fridge.
- Tape 2 paint stir sticks on a flat work surface, 2-in. apart; use a big plastic wrap piece to cover. Put a golf ball-sized turkey mixture piece between sticks; use another plastic wrap piece to cover. Use a rolling pin to roll turkey mixture into a thin strips; put strip on a dehydrator tray. Repeat the process using the leftover turkey mixture.
- Dehydrate for 5-8 hours till thoroughly dried at 70°C or 160°F.

Nutrition Information

- Calories: 137 calories;
- Total Carbohydrate: 4.3
- Cholesterol: 50
- Protein: 14.6
- Total Fat: 7
- Sodium: 821

9. Amy's Delicious Turkey Burgers

Serving: 4 | Prep: 5mins | Cook: 10mins | Ready in:

Ingredients

- 1 pound ground turkey
- 1 tablespoon garlic powder
- 1 tablespoon red pepper flakes
- 1 teaspoon dried minced onion (optional)
- 1 egg
- 1/2 cup crushed cheese flavored crackers

Direction

- Prepare a grill by preheating over high heat.
- Combine the ground turkey, red pepper flakes, garlic powder, egg, minced onion, and crackers in a large bowl and mix them together using your hands. Divide the mixture and shape into four fat patties.
- Grill the patties and cook each side for 5 minutes, until the patties are well done.

Nutrition Information

- Calories: 239 calories;
- Sodium: 160
- Total Carbohydrate: 7.6
- Cholesterol: 131
- Protein: 25.5
- Total Fat: 12.2

10. Ang's Turkey Burritos

Serving: 8 | Prep: 20mins | Cook: 20mins | Ready in:

Ingredients

- 1 pound ground turkey
- 1 small onion, chopped
- 1 (15 ounce) can whole sweet corn, drained
- 1 (15 ounce) can black beans, drained and rinsed
- 1 (10 ounce) can diced tomatoes and green chile peppers, undrained
- 1/2 cup chopped red bell pepper, or to taste
- 2 teaspoons lime juice
- 3/4 teaspoon garlic powder
- 3/4 teaspoon chili powder
- 1/2 teaspoon ground cumin
- 8 (8 inch) whole wheat tortillas

Direction

- On moderately-high heat, heat one big skillet. In hot skillet, cook and mix onion and turkey for 5 to 7 minutes, till turkey browns and not anymore pink. Put in cumin, chili powder, garlic powder, lime juice, red bell pepper,

- tomatoes, black beans and corn. Lower the heat to moderately-low and simmer for 15 to 20 minutes till flavors meld.
- On microwavable plate, put the tortillas. In microwave, heat for 15 to 20 seconds, till warmed. Distribute turkey mixture on heated tortillas.

Nutrition Information

- Calories: 276 calories;
- Cholesterol: 42
- Protein: 19.7
- Total Fat: 5.4
- Sodium: 760
- Total Carbohydrate: 46

11. Asian Turkey Sliders

Serving: 8 | Prep: 20mins | Cook: 20mins | Ready in:

Ingredients

- cooking spray
- 1 pound lean ground turkey
- 1 1/2 cups panko bread crumbs, divided
- 1/2 cup thinly sliced green onions
- 1 egg, slightly beaten
- 3 tablespoons soy sauce
- 1 tablespoon brown sugar
- 2 1/2 teaspoons minced fresh ginger root
- 1 1/2 teaspoons minced garlic
- Sauce:
- 1/4 cup mayonnaise
- 1 teaspoon teriyaki sauce
- 1/4 teaspoon white sugar (optional)
- 4 (4 roll) packages Hawaiian bread rolls (such as King's®)

Direction

- Prepare the oven by preheating to 375°F (190°C). Use aluminum foil to cover a baking sheet then use cooking spray to grease.
- In a bowl, mix garlic, ginger, brown sugar, soy sauce, egg, green onions, 3/4 cup breadcrumbs, and turkey; combine well.
- Place the rest of the breadcrumbs in a shallow bowl. Turn turkey mixture to 16 1 1/2-inch balls using wet hands then place in breadcrumbs to coat. Place between your palms to flatten to form a patty and transfer to the baking sheet.
- Place in preheated oven and bake for 20-25 minutes until cooked well and not pink in the middle.
- In a bowl, mix teriyaki sauce and mayonnaise. Add sugar to season. Place turkey sliders on Hawaiian dinner rolls with a little mayo-teriyaki sauce to serve.

Nutrition Information

- Calories: 747 calories;
- Protein: 42.7
- Total Fat: 11
- Sodium: 969
- Total Carbohydrate: 101.4
- Cholesterol: 145

12. Awesome Sausage, Apple And Cranberry Stuffing

Serving: 10 | Prep: 15mins | Cook: 25mins | Ready in:

Ingredients

- 1 1/2 cups cubed whole wheat bread
- 3 3/4 cups cubed white bread
- 1 pound ground turkey sausage
- 1 cup chopped onion
- 3/4 cup chopped celery
- 2 1/2 teaspoons dried sage
- 1 1/2 teaspoons dried rosemary
- 1/2 teaspoon dried thyme
- 1 Golden Delicious apple, cored and chopped
- 3/4 cup dried cranberries
- 1/3 cup minced fresh parsley

- 1 cooked turkey liver, finely chopped
- 3/4 cup turkey stock
- 4 tablespoons unsalted butter, melted

Direction

- Preheat an oven to 175°C/350°F. Spread whole wheat and white bread cubes on a big baking sheet in 1 layer; in preheated oven, bake till evenly toasted for 5-7 minutes. Put toasted bread cubes in a big bowl.
- Cook onions and sausages in a big skillet till evenly browned, stirring and breaking up lumps, on medium heat. Add thyme, rosemary, sage and celery; cook to blend flavors for 2 minutes, stirring.
- Put sausage mixture on bread in bowl; stir in liver, parsley, dried cranberries and chopped apple. Drizzle melted butter and turkey stock over; lightly mix. Let cool stuffing completely; stuff into a turkey loosely.

Nutrition Information

- Calories: 235 calories;
- Sodium: 548
- Total Carbohydrate: 21.7
- Cholesterol: 80
- Protein: 12.5
- Total Fat: 11.6

13. Bab's Turkey Mushroom Lasagna Rolls

Serving: 8 | Prep: 20mins | Cook: 1hours | Ready in:

Ingredients

- cooking spray
- 8 uncooked lasagna noodles
- 2 tablespoons olive oil
- 1 pound ground turkey
- 1 (8 ounce) package sliced fresh mushrooms
- 2 tablespoons Italian seasoning
- 1/4 teaspoon salt
- 1/4 teaspoon ground black pepper
- 1 (10 ounce) package frozen chopped spinach, thawed and drained
- 2 cloves garlic, minced
- 1 (20 ounce) jar marinara sauce
- 1/2 cup shredded mozzarella cheese
- 1/2 cup ricotta cheese
- 1/4 cup grated Parmesan cheese
- 1 1/2 cups shredded mozzarella cheese

Direction

- Set oven to 350 0 F (175 0 C) to preheat.
- Use cooking spray to grease a large baking dish.
- Bring a large pot of lightly salted water to a boil. Place lasagna in the boiling water, cook while stirring occasionally for about 8 minutes until heated through but still firm to the bite. Drain and put aside pasta in a bowl of cold water.
- In a large skillet, heat olive oil over medium-high heat. Cook while stirring turkey, black pepper, salt, Italian seasoning and mushrooms until turkey is evenly browned.
- Mix spinach and garlic into turkey mixture until cooked through, about 1 more minute; take away from heat and let cool slightly.
- Spread over the bottom of the prepared baking dish with about 1/2 cup marinara sauce.
- Drain lasagna noodles.
- Mix 1/2 cup mozzarella cheese, ricotta cheese and parmesan cheese into the turkey mixture until well mixed.
- Spread down the center of each lasagna noodle with about 1/4 cup turkey and cheese mixture; at the end of the noodle, leave a space about 2 inches long.
- From the opposite end, roll the noodle up and put on the greased baking dish with seam sides down. Do the same steps with remaining rolls.
- Pour the rest of marinara sauce over lasagna rolls.
- Put in the prepared oven and bake for 30 to 40 minutes until sauce is bubbly. Use remaining 1

- 1/2 cups mozzarella cheese to sprinkle over the rolls and put back to oven.
- Keep baking until cheese is melted, for an additional 5 minutes.

Nutrition Information

- Calories: 364 calories;
- Sodium: 634
- Total Carbohydrate: 31.4
- Cholesterol: 64
- Protein: 25.8
- Total Fat: 15.7

14. Bacon Mushroom Turkey Burger

Serving: 4 | Prep: 15mins | Cook: 12mins | Ready in:

Ingredients

- 2 slices multigrain bread
- 1 pound ground turkey
- 6 white mushrooms, finely chopped
- 1 egg
- 2 green onions, finely chopped
- 3 slices cooked bacon, finely chopped, or more to taste
- 5 dashes hot sauce, or more to taste
- 1/2 teaspoon pureed garlic
- salt and ground black pepper to taste

Direction

- In a food processor, pulse bread and place the crumbs in a bowl. Add in ground turkey, egg, mushrooms, green onions, hot sauce, bacon, garlic, salt and pepper. Mix thoroughly and make four equal patties. Cook the patties in a pre-heated grill, 12-14 minutes or until not pink in the middle.

Nutrition Information

- Calories: 252 calories;
- Sodium: 314
- Total Carbohydrate: 7.4
- Cholesterol: 135
- Protein: 28.4
- Total Fat: 12.3

15. Baked Turkey Meatballs

Serving: 4 | Prep: 15mins | Cook: 15mins | Ready in:

Ingredients

- 1 pound ground turkey
- 1/2 cup Italian bread crumbs
- 1/4 cup thinly sliced baby spinach
- 1 egg
- 2 tablespoons onion powder
- 2 tablespoons garlic powder

Direction

- Set the oven to 375°F (190°C) and start preheating.
- In a bowl, mix garlic powder, onion powder, egg, spinach, bread crumbs and turkey. Roll mixture into palm-sized meatballs; arrange on a baking sheet, 2 inches apart.
- Bake in the prepared oven for 15-20 minutes until the center is no longer pink and it is browned on the outside. The inserted instant-read thermometer into the center should register at least 165°F (74°C)

Nutrition Information

- Calories: 267 calories;
- Total Carbohydrate: 16.1
- Cholesterol: 130
- Protein: 27.2
- Total Fat: 10.7
- Sodium: 350

16. Basil Turkey Burgers

Serving: 4 | Prep: 15mins | Cook: 15mins | Ready in:

Ingredients

- 1 pound ground turkey
- 1/2 onion, finely chopped
- 1/2 cup egg substitute
- 2 tablespoons minced fresh basil
- 1 teaspoon prepared horseradish
- 1 teaspoon light soy sauce
- 1/4 teaspoon ground black pepper
- 1 clove garlic, minced
- 4 whole wheat hamburger buns, split
- 4 leaves lettuce leaves
- 4 slices tomato

Direction

- Preheat the outdoor grill on high; grease the grate lightly.
- In a big mixing bowl, combine garlic, ground turkey, pepper, onion, soy sauce, egg substitute, horseradish, and basil; shape into four patties.
- Cook burgers for 6mins per side on the preheated grill until the juices are clear and the center is not pink. An inserted instant-read thermometer should register 74°C or 165°Fahrenheit. Serve turkey burgers with tomato and lettuce on buns.

Nutrition Information

- Calories: 326 calories;
- Sodium: 399
- Total Carbohydrate: 23.9
- Cholesterol: 84
- Protein: 31.2
- Total Fat: 12.3

17. Best Turkey Meatloaf

Serving: 8 | Prep: 15mins | Cook: 1hours | Ready in:

Ingredients

- Meatloaf:
- 1 1/2 pounds ground turkey
- 3/4 cup crushed buttery round crackers
- 1/2 cup milk
- 1 small onion, chopped
- 1 egg
- 1 1/2 teaspoons salt
- 2 cloves garlic, minced
- 1/4 teaspoon ground black pepper
- Topping:
- 1/2 cup ketchup
- 1/4 cup brown sugar
- 1 tablespoon Worcestershire sauce

Direction

- Set oven to 350°F (175°C) to preheat. Slightly put grease on a jelly-roll pan.
- In a bowl, mix together ground turkey, black pepper, garlic, salt, egg, onion, milk and buttery round cracker crumbs; form into a loaf and put on the prepared pan.
- In a separate bowl, combine Worcestershire sauce, brown sugar and ketchup; put aside.
- Bake the meatloaf for 30 minutes in prepared oven; take out of oven then drain out liquids. Put ketchup topping over the meatloaf. Put the loaf back to oven and keep baking for about 30 minutes more until no pink remains in the center. An instant-read thermometer should show at least 160°F (70°C) when inserted into the center.

Nutrition Information

- Calories: 296 calories;
- Total Fat: 13.2
- Sodium: 881
- Total Carbohydrate: 25.2
- Cholesterol: 85
- Protein: 19.7

18. Big Game Sunday Chili Dip

Serving: 8 | Prep: | Cook: 1hours5mins | Ready in:

Ingredients

- 1 (14 ounce) can black beans, drained
- 1 (8 ounce) jar salsa
- 1 pound ground turkey
- salt and ground black pepper to taste
- 1 (8 ounce) package shredded Mexican cheese blend

Direction

- In slow cooker set on low, mix salsa and black beans.
- In skillet, break ground turkey on medium heat; season with pepper and salt. Mix and cook turkey for 5-7 minutes till browned completely. Mix turkey into black bean mixture. Sprinkle the cheese on bean and turkey mixture.
- Cook mixture for 1 hour on high. Lower to low setting while serving to keep dip hot.

Nutrition Information

- Calories: 246 calories;
- Total Fat: 13.6
- Sodium: 630
- Total Carbohydrate: 10.9
- Cholesterol: 69
- Protein: 21

19. Breakfast Meatloaf

Serving: 16 | Prep: 30mins | Cook: 1hours | Ready in:

Ingredients

- 2 pounds ground turkey
- 2 cups textured vegetable protein
- 2 cups powdered milk
- 6 eggs, beaten
- 2 green bell peppers, chopped
- 1 small onion, chopped
- 4 stalks celery, chopped
- 1 (10 ounce) package frozen spinach, thawed and drained
- 1 teaspoon ground black pepper
- 1 teaspoon ground sage

Direction

- Preheat the oven to 175 ° C or 350 ° F. Slightly oil a baking dish, 8x11 inch in size.
- Combine eggs, powdered milk, tvp and ground turkey together in a big bowl till well incorporated. Mix in spinach, celery, onion and green peppers. Add sage and black pepper to season. Force mixture into prepped pan.
- In the prepped oven, bake for an hour, or till juices run clear and the middle is set. Rest for several minutes prior to cutting into 16 pieces.

Nutrition Information

- Calories: 252 calories;
- Protein: 28.8
- Total Fat: 11.5
- Sodium: 305
- Total Carbohydrate: 10
- Cholesterol: 130

20. Breakfast For Dinner Casserole

Serving: 6 | Prep: 15mins | Cook: 40mins | Ready in:

Ingredients

- 1 pound ground turkey breakfast sausage
- 1 (8 ounce) can refrigerated reduced-fat crescent roll dough

- 5 eggs, lightly beaten
- 1 cup shredded Cheddar cheese
- 1 cup shredded mozzarella cheese
- 2/3 cup milk
- 2/3 red bell pepper, chopped
- 1/2 cup chopped fresh spinach
- 1 scallion, chopped
- 1 tablespoon minced parsley
- salt and ground black pepper to taste

Direction

- Set the oven to 400°F (200°C) and start preheating. Grease a 9x13-inch baking dish lightly.
- Over medium-high heat, heat a large skillet. Cook while stirring turkey in hot skillet for 5-7 minutes until crumbly and browned; drain and get rid of grease.
- Unroll crescent roll dough; spread over the bottom of the greased baking dish evenly.
- Bake for 10 minutes in the prepared oven.
- In a bowl, mix eggs and sausage together. Add pepper, salt, parsley, scallion, spinach, red bell pepper, milk, mozzarella cheese and Cheddar cheese, stirring well after each addition. Top baked crescent rolls with egg mixture.
- Bake in the oven for 25-30 minutes until eggs are set.

Nutrition Information

- Calories: 461 calories;
- Protein: 32.4
- Total Fat: 27.6
- Sodium: 1270
- Total Carbohydrate: 19.7
- Cholesterol: 246

21. Brittany's Turkey Burgers

Serving: 8 | Prep: 15mins | Cook: 10mins | Ready in:

Ingredients

- 2 pounds ground turkey
- 1 green apple, chopped
- 1/4 cup chopped fresh mushrooms, or to taste
- 3 scallions, or more to taste, chopped
- 3 tablespoons barbeque sauce
- 2 tablespoons spicy mango chutney, or more to taste
- 2 tablespoons red pepper jelly
- 2 dashes Worcestershire sauce, or to taste
- 1 pinch seasoned salt, or to taste
- 1 pinch garlic powder, or to taste
- ground black pepper to taste

Direction

- Set grill to medium heat and start preheating; oil the grate lightly.
- In a large bowl, using hand, mix black pepper, garlic powder, seasoned salt, Worcestershire sauce, red pepper jelly, chutney, barbeque sauce, scallions, mushrooms, green apple and ground turkey; form into 8 patties.
- Cook turkey burgers on the prepared grill for about 4 minutes on each side until the center is no longer pink and juices run clear. The inserted instant-read thermometer into the center should register at least 165°F (74°C).

Nutrition Information

- Calories: 206 calories;
- Total Fat: 8.6
- Sodium: 163
- Total Carbohydrate: 10
- Cholesterol: 84
- Protein: 22.8

22. Buffalo Turkey Meatballs

Serving: 6 | Prep: 10mins | Cook: | Ready in:

Ingredients

- 1 pound ground buffalo meat

- 1 pound ground turkey
- 1/4 large sweet onion (such as Vidalia®), chopped
- 2 cloves garlic, chopped
- 2 teaspoons chopped fresh parsley
- 2 teaspoons sea salt
- 1 teaspoon Worcestershire sauce

Direction

- Preheat the oven to 225°F (110°C).
- In a bowl, combine Worcestershire sauce, sea salt, parsley, garlic, onion, turkey and buffalo then shape this mixture into big meatballs. It should be enough to create about twelve. In a glass casserole dish, put the meatballs inside.
- Put the dish into the preheated oven, baking for 1/2 hour. Turn the temperate up to 300°F (150°C) and proceed to bake for another 15 minutes until the meatballs are thoroughly cooked. When you insert an instant read thermometer in the middle, it should register a minimum of 165°F (74°C).

Nutrition Information

- Calories: 178 calories;
- Sodium: 666
- Total Carbohydrate: 1.1
- Cholesterol: 85
- Protein: 27.8
- Total Fat: 6.5

23. Buffalo Turkey Meatloaf

Serving: 4 | Prep: 20mins | Cook: 45mins | Ready in:

Ingredients

- Meatloaf:
- cooking spray
- 1 (20 ounce) package ground turkey
- 1 small onion, grated
- salt and ground black pepper to taste
- Buffalo Sauce:
- 1/4 cup butter
- 1/2 cup hot pepper sauce (such as Frank's RedHot®)
- 1 teaspoon garlic powder, or to taste
- 1 teaspoon onion powder, or to taste
- Blue Cheese Dressing:
- 1 cup sour cream
- 1/2 cup mayonnaise
- 1/2 cup blue cheese crumbles
- 1/2 teaspoon garlic powder, or to taste
- 1/2 teaspoon onion powder, or to taste
- 1 pinch black pepper, or to taste

Direction

- Set oven to 350°F (175°C) to preheat. Place aluminum foil into a 9x13-inch baking pan; grease slightly using cooking spray.
- In a large bowl, combine grated onion, ground turkey, black pepper and salt; mix well to combine. Move the turkey mixture into the prepared baking pan and form into a loaf.
- Bake the meatloaf for about 40 minutes in the prepared oven until lightly golden.
- In a small saucepan, melt butter on low heat. Stir in 1 teaspoon of onion powder, 1 teaspoon of garlic powder and hot pepper sauce. Evenly pour over the meatloaf.
- Put the meatloaf back to the oven and bake for about 5 minutes more until flavors are well absorbed. An instant-read thermometer should show at least 165°F (74°C) when inserted into the center.
- In a bowl, mix together blue cheese crumbs, mayonnaise and sour cream to create blue cheese dressing. Flavor with black pepper, 1/2 teaspoon of onion powder and 1/2 teaspoon of garlic powder. Serve along with the meatloaf.

Nutrition Information

- Calories: 707 calories;
- Sodium: 1363
- Total Carbohydrate: 7.4

- Cholesterol: 183
- Protein: 34.5
- Total Fat: 61.1

24. Buttermilk Turkey Meatloaf Muffins

Serving: 12 | Prep: 10mins | Cook: 25mins | Ready in:

Ingredients

- cooking spray
- 20 ounces 99% fat-free ground turkey
- 1 (6 ounce) package stuffing mix (such as Kraft® Stove Top®)
- 1 cup low-sodium chicken broth
- 2 tablespoons buttermilk
- 2 tablespoons Italian seasoning
- salt and ground black pepper to taste

Direction

- Heat up the oven to 190 degrees C or 375 degrees F. Use cooking spray to spray 12 muffin cups.
- In a bowl, combine pepper, salt, Italian seasoning, buttermilk, chicken broth, stuffing mix, and turkey, then divide between the muffin cups.
- Bake until cooked thoroughly, about 25 minutes. When you insert an instant-read thermometer in the center, it should read out at least 74 degrees C or 165 degrees F.

Nutrition Information

- Calories: 110 calories;
- Cholesterol: 24
- Protein: 13
- Total Fat: 1.3
- Sodium: 280
- Total Carbohydrate: 11.5

25. Butternut Squash And Turkey Chili

Serving: 12 | Prep: 20mins | Cook: 30mins | Ready in:

Ingredients

- 2 tablespoons olive oil
- 1 onion, chopped
- 2 cloves garlic, minced
- 1 pound ground turkey breast
- 1 pound butternut squash - peeled, seeded and cut into 1-inch dice
- 1/2 cup chicken broth
- 1 (4.5 ounce) can chopped green chilies
- 2 (14.5 ounce) cans petite diced tomatoes
- 1 (15 ounce) can kidney beans with liquid
- 1 (15.5 ounce) can white hominy, drained
- 1 (8 ounce) can tomato sauce
- 1 tablespoon chili powder
- 1 tablespoon ground cumin
- 1 teaspoon garlic salt

Direction

- Heat up a big pot with olive oil over medium heat and stir in garlic and onion, then cook while stirring for around 3 minutes. Add the turkey and stir until it is no longer pink and becomes crumbly.
- Add tomato sauce, hominy, kidney beans, tomatoes, green chilies, chicken broth, and butternut squash, then season this with garlic salt, cumin, and chili powder. Set to a simmer, then cut down the heat to a medium-low. Simmer while covered until the squash becomes tender, around 20 minutes.

Nutrition Information

- Calories: 164 calories;
- Protein: 13.3
- Total Fat: 3.3
- Sodium: 661
- Total Carbohydrate: 20.5

- Cholesterol: 23

26. California Turkey Burger

Serving: 4 | Prep: 15mins | Cook: | Ready in:

Ingredients

- 1 (16 ounce) package JENNIE-O® Ground Turkey
- 1/2 teaspoon kosher salt
- 1/4 teaspoon freshly ground pepper
- 4 slices Havarti cheese
- 1 cup arugula leaves
- 1 large tomato, sliced
- 1 avocado, sliced
- 4 small brioche or onion roll hamburger buns, toasted

Direction

- Heat the grill to 400°F.
- Mix pepper, salt, and ground turkey. Form the mixture into 4 patties.
- Follow the package directions on how to cook the patties. Make sure the meat is well-done, or when a meat thermometer reads 165°F.
- Serve it after topping the burger with arugula, avocado, tomato, and cheese.

Nutrition Information

- Calories: 524 calories;
- Protein: 37
- Total Fat: 29.3
- Sodium: 822
- Total Carbohydrate: 31.3
- Cholesterol: 117

27. Cameron's Ground Turkey Salsa Ranchera For Tacos And Burritos

Serving: 4 | Prep: 5mins | Cook: 30mins | Ready in:

Ingredients

- 1 teaspoon canola oil
- 1 1/4 pounds lean ground turkey
- 1 (7 ounce) can salsa ranchera (such as HERDEZ®)

Direction

- In multi-functional pressure cooker like Instant Pot(R), heat the oil on Sauté setting. Put in the ground turkey; cook and mix for 5 minutes till the majority are browned. Put in the salsa ranchera and mix to incorporate.
- Seal and latch the lid. Choose high pressure following manufacturer's directions; set timer for 15 minutes. Let pressure establish for 10 to 15 minutes.
- With quick-release method, let loose of pressure cautiously for 5 minutes following manufacturer's directions. Unlatch and take lid off.

Nutrition Information

- Calories: 234 calories;
- Sodium: 356
- Total Carbohydrate: 2.7
- Cholesterol: 105
- Protein: 28.7
- Total Fat: 12

28. Carrot, Tomato, And Spinach Quinoa Pilaf With Ground Turkey

Serving: 5 | Prep: 20mins | Cook: 40mins | Ready in:

Ingredients

- 2 teaspoons olive oil
- 1 cup quinoa
- 1/2 onion, chopped
- 2 cups water
- 2 tablespoons chicken-flavored vegetable bouillon
- 1 teaspoon ground black pepper
- 1 teaspoon ground thyme
- 1 carrot, chopped
- 1 tomato, chopped
- 1 cup baby spinach
- 2 tablespoons olive oil
- 1 pound ground turkey, or more to taste (optional)
- 1 (14.5 ounce) can black beans, rinsed and drained

Direction

- Heat 2 tsp. olive oil in saucepan on medium heat; mix and cook onion in hot oil for 5 minutes till translucent. Lower heat to medium low; mix quinoa with onion. Cook, constantly mixing, for 2 minutes till quinoa toasts lightly.
- Boil thyme, black pepper, bouillon granules and water in a saucepan. Cover saucepan; lower heat to low. Cook at simmer for 5 minutes till quinoa softens.
- Mix carrot into quinoa mixture; cover. Cook at simmer for 10 minutes till water is fully absorbed.
- Take off heat; mix baby spinach and tomato into quinoa mixture for 2 minutes till spinach wilts.
- Heat 2 tbsp. olive oil on medium high heat in big skillet; mix and cook turkey in hot skillet for 5-7 minutes till crumbly and browned. Drain; discard grease. Put heat on medium low. Mix black beans with turkey; mix and cook for 2-3 minutes till beans are hot. Add quinoa mixture; mix. Cook for 5 minutes till heated through.

Nutrition Information

- Calories: 422 calories;
- Total Fat: 16.6
- Sodium: 396
- Total Carbohydrate: 40.8
- Cholesterol: 67
- Protein: 28.6

29. Cheese Stuffed Turkey Meat Loaf

Serving: 5 | Prep: 10mins | Cook: 1hours | Ready in:

Ingredients

- nonstick cooking spray
- 1 pound ground turkey
- 1 egg
- 1/4 cup chopped fresh parsley
- 3/4 cup dry bread crumbs
- 1/2 teaspoon adobo seasoning
- 1 pinch salt
- 1 pinch pepper
- 1/2 cup shredded Cheddar cheese
- 1/4 cup shredded Cheddar cheese (optional)

Direction

- Set the oven to 350°F (175°C) and start preheating. Use nonstick cooking spray to spray a loaf pan.
- In a large bowl, combine pepper, salt, adobo, bread crumbs, parsley, egg and ground turkey. Combine well. Press 1/2 turkey mixture into bottom of sprayed loaf pan. Top half cup cheese in a mound down the pan's center; place the rest of meat on top to form a loaf.
- Bake meatloaf for about an hour in the prepared oven until cooked through and browned. If preferred, sprinkle with the optional 1/4 cup cheese in the last 5 minutes during baking time. Let cooked meatloaf stand for at least 5 minutes; slice.

Nutrition Information

- Calories: 293 calories;
- Sodium: 306
- Total Carbohydrate: 12.4
- Cholesterol: 125
- Protein: 26.3
- Total Fat: 15.2

30. Chef John's Turkey Burger

Serving: 4 | Prep: 15mins | Cook: 10mins | Ready in:

Ingredients

- 1 1/2 pounds ground turkey
- 1 1/2 tablespoons plain bread crumbs
- 1 1/2 tablespoons ground almonds
- 1 teaspoon chile paste
- 2 cloves garlic, crushed and minced
- 1 1/2 teaspoons finely grated fresh ginger
- 1 1/2 teaspoons salt
- 1 1/2 teaspoons garam masala
- 1 tablespoon lemon juice
- 2 tablespoons plain yogurt
- 2 tablespoons chopped fresh cilantro

Direction

- In a mixing bowl, combine ground turkey, almonds, breadcrumbs, garlic, ginger, chili paste, garam masala, yogurt, lemon juice and cilantro. Divide into four portions and shape each into a ball, chill for one hour. With damp hands, form a patty from every ball. Refrigerate while waiting for the grill to preheat. Over medium heat, on a pre-heated grill, cook the patties, 4-5 minutes each side. Or until the outside of the patty is cracked with the juices rising at the top.

Nutrition Information

- Calories: 301 calories;
- Total Fat: 16.3
- Sodium: 1026
- Total Carbohydrate: 5
- Cholesterol: 136
- Protein: 34.4

31. Chicken & Quinoa Stuffed Peppers

Serving: 4 | Prep: 20mins | Cook: 50mins | Ready in:

Ingredients

- 1 1/3 cups Swanson® Unsalted Chicken Stock
- 2/3 cup uncooked quinoa, rinsed
- 1 pound 98% fat-free ground chicken breast or 99% fat-free ground turkey breast
- 1 clove garlic, minced
- 1 medium onion, chopped
- 1 (10 ounce) package chopped frozen spinach, thawed and well drained
- 1 (10.5 ounce) can Campbell's® Healthy Request® Condensed Cream of Mushroom Soup
- 1/3 cup grated Parmesan cheese, divided
- 4 medium red bell peppers, cut in half lengthwise and seeded

Direction

- Set the oven to 350° F.
- In a 1-quart saucepan, heat the quinoa and stock to a boil over high heat. Lower the heat to low. Cook, covered, for 13 minutes or till the quinoa becomes tender.
- In a 12-inch nonstick frying pan, cook the onion, garlic, and chicken over medium-high heat while stirring often to separate meat till the chicken is cooked through. Mix in 3 tablespoons of cheese, quinoa, soup, and spinach.
- In an 11x8x2-inch baking dish, position the pepper halves. Fill the pepper halves with the chicken mixture.

- Bake for 30 minutes or until hot. Dust with the leftover cheese.
- Bake for 5 minutes or till cheese is melted.

Nutrition Information

- Calories: 393 calories;
- Total Carbohydrate: 38.2
- Cholesterol: 78
- Protein: 38.6
- Total Fat: 9.2
- Sodium: 547

32. Chili With Turkey And Beans

Serving: 15 | Prep: 30mins | Cook: 30mins | Ready in:

Ingredients

- 2 pounds ground turkey
- 1 cup chopped onion
- 1 cup chopped green bell pepper
- 4 (14.5 ounce) cans diced stewed tomatoes
- 1 (15.5 ounce) can chili beans, undrained
- 1 (16 ounce) can kidney beans, rinsed and drained
- 1 (15 ounce) can pinto beans, rinsed and drained
- 1 (15 ounce) can black beans, rinsed and drained
- 1 jalapeno pepper, seeded and chopped
- 4 cloves garlic, crushed
- 2 tablespoons chili powder
- 1 tablespoon molasses
- 2 teaspoons ground cumin
- 1 cube French onion bouillon
- 1 teaspoon dried oregano
- 1 teaspoon salt
- 1/4 teaspoon cayenne pepper

Direction

- Combine onion, green pepper, and turkey in a large soup pot or Dutch oven. Cook and stir for 10 minutes over medium heat until the turkey is no longer pink. Stirring often. Remove excess grease. Add jalapeno pepper, cumin, kidney beans, chili beans, black beans, pinto beans, bouillon cube, cayenne pepper, stewed tomatoes, chili powder, salt, garlic, oregano, and molasses into the turkey mixture.
- Boil the chili before reducing the heat to low. Cover the pot and let it simmer for 20 minutes until the flavors are well-blended and the vegetables are tender.

Nutrition Information

- Calories: 227 calories;
- Cholesterol: 45
- Protein: 19.3
- Total Fat: 5.6
- Sodium: 805
- Total Carbohydrate: 27.8

33. Chinese Firecrackers

Serving: 14 | Prep: 35mins | Cook: 20mins | Ready in:

Ingredients

- 1 teaspoon vegetable oil
- 1/2 pound ground turkey
- 1 cup shredded cabbage
- 1/2 cup shredded carrots
- 2 green onions, finely chopped
- 1 tablespoon chile paste
- 1 teaspoon cornstarch
- 1 tablespoon white wine
- 14 sheets phyllo pastry dough, halved into triangles
- 4 teaspoons vegetable oil
- 3/4 cup sweet and sour sauce for dipping

Direction

- Preheat oven to 190°C/375°F. Grease the baking sheet.
- In skillet, heat 1 teaspoon of vegetable oil on medium heat. Cook turkey in skillet till not pink; add green onions, carrots and cabbage. Cook for 5-7 minutes till veggies are slightly tender; mix chile paste through vegetable mixture.
- In small bowl, whisk cornstarch into white wine; add to mixture in skillet. Mix and cook till liquid in skillet is slightly thick; take off heat. Put aside; cool.
- On a flat surface, put 1 1/2 of phyllo dough sheet; brush a small amount vegetable oil on. Top with 2nd phyllo sheet. Put 2 tablespoons of turkey mixture on phyllo's short end. Form mixture to 4-inch log. Roll turkey mixture and phyllo. Twist log, 1-inch from every end to get firecracker shape; put on greased cookie sheet then repeat with leftover mixture and phyllo till all get used. Brush vegetable oil lightly on firecrackers.
- In preheated oven, bake for 18-22 minutes till phyllo dough is golden brown and crisp; serve with sweet and sour sauce.

Nutrition Information

- Calories: 120 calories;
- Cholesterol: 12
- Protein: 4.8
- Total Fat: 4.5
- Sodium: 164
- Total Carbohydrate: 15.2

34. Chipotle Fiesta Chili

Serving: 6 | Prep: 15mins | Cook: 10mins | Ready in:

Ingredients

- 1 pound lean ground turkey or chicken
- 1 onion, diced
- 1 clove garlic, minced
- 1 chipotle chile, canned in adobo sauce
- 2 teaspoons adobo sauce from chipotle peppers
- 2 teaspoons chili powder
- 1 (5.6 ounce) package Knorr® Fiesta Sides™ - Spanish Rice
- 1 (15 ounce) can low-sodium tomato sauce
- 1 (4 ounce) can diced green chiles
- Optional toppings:
- chopped fresh cilantro
- onion, chopped
- Shredded cheese

Direction

- In a medium saucepan, cook onion and ground turkey over medium heat; cook and mix till turkey is not pink anymore and cooked completely. Mix in chipotle peppers, chili powder garlic with adobo sauce; mix till turkey is covered and aromatic. Let excess fat from pan drain. To a bowl, put the mixture.
- In the same saucepan, prepare the Knorr(R) Fiesta Sides (TM) - Spanish Rice following packaging instructions. Once rice is cooked, put green chilies, tomatoes and ground turkey mixture; mix till heated through. Serve with shredded cheese, onion and/or chopped cilantro, if wished.

Nutrition Information

- Calories: 223 calories;
- Total Fat: 2.1
- Sodium: 301
- Total Carbohydrate: 15.6
- Cholesterol: 48
- Protein: 22.8

35. Chris's Incredible Italian Turkey Meatloaf

Serving: 6 | Prep: 20mins | Cook: 50mins | Ready in:

Ingredients

- 1 pound mild Italian turkey sausage, casings removed
- 1 pound ground turkey
- 2 eggs, beaten
- 1 1/2 cups rolled oats
- 1/2 cup chopped onion
- 1/2 cup milk
- 1 tablespoon Worcestershire sauce
- 1 teaspoon Italian-style seasoning
- 1/2 teaspoon garlic powder
- 1/2 teaspoon salt
- 2 cups spaghetti sauce
- 5 dashes hot pepper sauce
- 1 tablespoon Worcestershire sauce
- 1/2 teaspoon liquid smoke flavoring

Direction

- Preheat an oven to 175°C/350°F.
- Mix together milk, onion, oats, eggs, sausage and ground turkey in a big bowl; season with salt, garlic powder, Italian seasoning and 1 tbsp. Worcestershire sauce. Shape into a loaf; transfer into a 9x13-in. baking dish.
- Combine liquid smoke, 1 tbsp. Worcestershire sauce, hot sauce and spaghetti sauce in another small bowl; smooth over the whole meatloaf.
- In preheated oven, bake for 50-60 minutes.

Nutrition Information

- Calories: 434 calories;
- Total Fat: 19.9
- Sodium: 1327
- Total Carbohydrate: 28.8
- Cholesterol: 182
- Protein: 34.4

36. Christine's Meat Loaf

Serving: 8 | Prep: 15mins | Cook: 1hours | Ready in:

Ingredients

- 1 pound ground beef
- 1/2 pound ground turkey
- 1/2 pound bulk Italian sausage
- 1 (10.75 ounce) can vegetable beef soup (such as Campbell's®)
- 2 eggs, lightly beaten
- 1/2 cup plain bread crumbs
- 1/4 cup barbeque sauce
- 1/4 cup ketchup
- 1/4 teaspoon prepared yellow mustard
- 1 teaspoon minced garlic, or to taste
- 2 dashes Worcestershire sauce
- 2 dashes browning sauce (such as Kitchen Bouquet®)
- 2 pinches seasoned salt (such as Johnny's Seasoning Salt®)
- 2 pinches ground black pepper

Direction

- Set oven to 350°F (175°C) to preheat.
- In a mixing bowl, combine Italian sausage, ground turkey, ground beef, black pepper, seasoned salt, browning sauce, Worcestershire sauce, garlic, yellow mustard, ketchup, barbeque sauce, bread crumbs, eggs, and vegetable soup until well incorporated. Mold meat mixture into a loaf; arrange meatloaf in a 9x13-inch baking dish.
- Bake for 60 to 75 minutes in the preheated oven until browned outside and no longer pink inside. An instant-read meat thermometer inserted into the thickest part of the meatloaf should registers at least 160°F (70°C). Allow to stand for 10 minutes before cutting into slices about 1/2 inch thick.

Nutrition Information

- Calories: 298 calories;
- Sodium: 823
- Total Carbohydrate: 14
- Cholesterol: 114
- Protein: 23.2
- Total Fat: 16.3

37. Cilantro Turkey Burgers

Serving: 6 | Prep: 10mins | Cook: 10mins | Ready in:

Ingredients

- 1 1/4 pounds ground turkey
- 1/4 cup cilantro paste
- 1 lime, juiced (optional)
- 1 1/2 teaspoons reduced-sodium soy sauce
- 1 1/2 teaspoons garlic paste
- 1/2 teaspoon ground ginger
- 1/2 teaspoon ground black pepper

Direction

- In a bowl, combine pepper, ginger, garlic paste, soy sauce, lime juice, cilantro paste and turkey together; shape into 6 patties.
- Over moderately high heat, heat a skillet; let patties cook for 5 minutes on each side till juices run clear and not pink anymore in the middle.

Nutrition Information

- Calories: 158 calories;
- Total Fat: 7.1
- Sodium: 301
- Total Carbohydrate: 3.5
- Cholesterol: 70
- Protein: 18.9

38. Cocktail Turkey Meatballs

Serving: 8 | Prep: 20mins | Cook: 40mins | Ready in:

Ingredients

- Meatballs:
- 1 cup panko bread crumbs
- 1 egg, beaten
- 1/4 cup minced onion
- 1/4 cup minced water chestnuts
- 1/4 cup applesauce (such as Mott's® Natural Applesauce)
- 1/4 cup finely grated Parmesan cheese
- 1 tablespoon finely chopped fresh parsley
- 1/2 teaspoon salt
- 1/2 teaspoon dry mustard powder (such as Coleman's®)
- 1/2 teaspoon poultry seasoning
- 1 pound ground turkey
- Sauce:
- 1 cup apple jelly
- 1 cup applesauce (such as Mott's® Natural Applesauce)
- 1/2 cup cider vinegar
- 1/2 cup minced onion
- 1/4 cup ketchup
- 1/4 cup chili sauce (such as Heinz®)
- 2 tablespoons tomato paste
- 1 tablespoon brown sugar
- 1 tablespoon Dijon mustard
- 1 teaspoon dry mustard powder (such as Coleman's®)
- 1/2 teaspoon salt
- 1 tablespoon chopped fresh parsley, or more to taste

Direction

- Set the oven at 175° C (350° F) to preheat. Use aluminum foil to line a baking sheet.
- In a large bowl, mix together poultry seasoning, 1/2 teaspoon mustard powder, 1/2 teaspoon salt, 1 tablespoon parsley, Parmesan cheese, 1/4 cup applesauce, water chestnuts, 1/4 cup minced onion, egg, and bread crumbs. Put in the ground turkey and mix together gently until just combined.
- Next, roll the turkey mixture into 1 1/2-inch meatballs and arrange on the prepared baking sheet.
- Bake for around 20 minutes in the preheated oven until cooked through. Insert an instant-read thermometer into the center and it should state at least 74° C (165° F).

- In a saucepan, whisk together 1/2 teaspoon salt, 1 teaspoon dry mustard, Dijon mustard, brown sugar, tomato paste, chili sauce, ketchup, 1/2 cup minced onion, cider vinegar, 1 cup applesauce, and apple jelly; bring to a simmer and cook for about 10 minutes, stirring irregularly, until the flavors combine.
- Next, transfer the cooked meatballs to the simmering sauce, use a lid to cover the saucepan and continue to simmer for 10 minutes more, or until the flavors blend. Decorate with the remaining parsley.

Nutrition Information

- Calories: 303 calories;
- Cholesterol: 67
- Protein: 15.4
- Total Fat: 6.4
- Sodium: 716
- Total Carbohydrate: 50.6

39. Colorful Garlic Orzo

Serving: 6 | Prep: 15mins | Cook: 25mins | Ready in:

Ingredients

- 4 cups chicken broth
- 2 cups orzo pasta
- 1 1/2 pounds lean ground turkey
- 4 cloves garlic, minced, or more to taste
- 1/2 teaspoon red pepper flakes, or more to taste
- 4 cups fresh spinach leaves
- 4 cups frozen broccoli florets
- 1 pint cherry tomatoes
- 2/3 cup frozen peas
- 2/3 cup frozen carrots
- salt and ground black pepper to taste

Direction

- Boil the chicken broth. Let the orzo cook in the boiling broth for about 8-10 minutes, mixing from time to time, until completely cooked yet firm to chew. Take off from heat, but don't drain.
- Heat a big pan on medium-high heat. Cook and stir the turkey in the hot pan for about 10 minutes, until evenly brown and crumbly. Mix red pepper flakes and garlic into the turkey; cook for a minute. Then lower the heat to medium. Add broth, orzo, carrots, peas, tomatoes, broccoli and spinach to the turkey mixture and let it cook for 5-10 minutes, stirring frequently, until the tomatoes start to split and the spinach wilts. Sprinkle black pepper and salt to season.

Nutrition Information

- Calories: 484 calories;
- Total Fat: 10.5
- Sodium: 782
- Total Carbohydrate: 62.9
- Cholesterol: 87
- Protein: 37.3

40. Coriander, Barley, Leek Soup

Serving: 10 | Prep: 15mins | Cook: 1hours45mins | Ready in:

Ingredients

- 3 cups water
- 1 cup uncooked pearl barley
- 2 tablespoons olive oil
- 2 medium onions, chopped
- 1 bunch leeks, chopped
- 1 1/4 pounds ground turkey
- 2 1/2 quarts beef stock
- 1 1/2 cups Chinese rice wine
- 2 1/2 tablespoons ground coriander
- freshly ground black pepper to taste

Direction

- Boil 3 cups of water in a saucepan. Stir barley in. Lower heat and simmer for 30 minutes with lid on.
- In a stock pot, heat olive oil over medium-high heat. Sauté leeks and onions until soft. Mix turkey in and cook until heated through. Pour beef stock and stir cooked barley into the pot. On low heat, cook for 1 hour with lid on. Stir occasionally. Mix rice wine in and add coriander to season the soup. Cook for 10 more minutes. Pepper to season and serve.

Nutrition Information

- Calories: 319 calories;
- Protein: 16.7
- Total Fat: 9.2
- Sodium: 154
- Total Carbohydrate: 32.1
- Cholesterol: 45

41. Corn Noodle Casserole

Serving: 8 | Prep: 15mins | Cook: 25mins | Ready in:

Ingredients

- 1 (16 ounce) package uncooked egg noodles
- 1 pound ground turkey
- 1 (15 ounce) can canned or frozen corn
- 1 (10.75 ounce) can cream of mushroom soup
- salt and pepper to taste

Direction

- Turn oven to 350°F (175°C) to preheat. Lightly oil a medium casserole dish.
- Bring lightly salted water in a large pot to a boil. Cook noodles in boiling water until al dente, for 6 to 8 minutes; drain noodles.
- Cook turkey over medium heat in a skillet until evenly browned. Drain drippings.
- Combine soup, corn, turkey, and cooked noodles gently together in a mixing bowl. Season mixture with pepper and salt. Pour mixture into the greased baking dish.
- Bake in the preheated oven until bubbly, for 20 minutes.

Nutrition Information

- Calories: 352 calories;
- Protein: 19.6
- Total Fat: 9.9
- Sodium: 441
- Total Carbohydrate: 47.7
- Cholesterol: 83

42. Country Casserole

Serving: 6 | Prep: 20mins | Cook: 15mins | Ready in:

Ingredients

- 3/4 cup elbow macaroni
- 1 pound ground turkey
- 1 (15 ounce) can baked beans with pork
- 1/2 cup chopped green pepper
- 1 (10 ounce) can refrigerated biscuit dough
- 1 (5.5 ounce) can tomato-vegetable juice cocktail
- salt and pepper to taste
- 6 slices American cheese

Direction

- Turn oven to 375°F (190°C) to preheat. Bring lightly salted water in a small saucepan to a boil. Cook macaroni in boiling water until al dente for 8 minutes. Drain pasta; put to one side.
- In a large skillet, put green pepper and ground beef. Sauté over medium-high heat until browned. Drain drippings and return the skillet to heat. Mix in pepper, salt, vegetable juice, cooked macaroni, and beans. Cook

through; pour mixture into a 9-inch square casserole dish or baking dish. Split biscuits apart and slice into quarters. Arrange biscuits on a baking sheet.
- Bake casserole without covering and the biscuits for 15 minutes at the same time in the preheated oven until biscuits are cooked through. Take the casserole out of the oven just before the biscuits are done; place slices of cheese over top the casserole dish. Place back into the oven to melt.
- Take mixture in the casserole dish out onto serving plates and pat a couple of biscuit quarters into each serving to serve.

Nutrition Information

- Calories: 546 calories;
- Sodium: 1251
- Total Carbohydrate: 47.1
- Cholesterol: 109
- Protein: 35.9
- Total Fat: 24.3

43. Crazy Delicious Turkey Meatloaf

Serving: 8 | Prep: 10mins | Cook: 45mins | Ready in:

Ingredients

- cooking spray
- 1 (14 ounce) package frozen mixed red, yellow, and green bell pepper strips, thawed and drained
- 2 pounds 93% lean ground turkey
- 1 cup Italian-seasoned bread crumbs

Direction

- Set the oven to 400°F (200°C) and start preheating. Use aluminum foil to cover a baking sheet. Use nonstick cooking spray to spray foil.
- In a blender, puree peppers until smooth; transfer to a bowl. Add bread crumbs and turkey to bowl; mix. Form turkey mixture into a loaf pan; place on the prepared baking sheet.
- Bake in the prepared oven for 45-60 minutes until the center is no longer pink. The inserted instant-read thermometer into the center should register at least 160°F (70°C).

Nutrition Information

- Calories: 232 calories;
- Cholesterol: 84
- Protein: 25
- Total Fat: 9.4
- Sodium: 282
- Total Carbohydrate: 12.2

44. Cream Of Mushroom, Turkey, And Potato Soup

Serving: 6 | Prep: 15mins | Cook: 40mins | Ready in:

Ingredients

- 1 pound ground turkey
- 1 clove garlic
- 1/4 teaspoon dried thyme
- 1/4 teaspoon ground black pepper
- 5 medium potatoes, peeled and diced
- 1 (10.75 ounce) can condensed cream of mushroom soup
- 2 large onions, diced
- 1/2 cup water
- 2 quarts chicken stock, or as needed

Direction

- Heat a big pot on medium-high heat and add in the turkey, then cook, stirring, for 5 - 7 minutes until crumbled and brown. Add black pepper, thyme, garlic, water, onions, cream of mushroom soup, and potatoes. Then pour enough chicken stock in to cover potatoes.

Decrease the heat to medium-low and simmer for 20 minutes until the potatoes are soft.
- Use a slotted spoon to fill a blender half-full with the cooked potatoes and onions. Cover, holding the lid down using a potholder, and briefly pulse, then leave on to blend. Pour the puree back into the pot and repeat with the remaining potatoes and onions. Continue to simmer for another 15 - 20 minutes until the flavors blend.

Nutrition Information

- Calories: 326 calories;
- Total Fat: 9.7
- Sodium: 1292
- Total Carbohydrate: 40.7
- Cholesterol: 57
- Protein: 20.8

45. Crispy Ground Turkey Tostadas

Serving: 6 | Prep: 30mins | Cook: 29mins | Ready in:

Ingredients

- 1 red onion, halved and thinly sliced
- 1/4 cup Mexican crema
- 2 limes
- 1/4 teaspoon salt
- 2 tablespoons vegetable oil, divided
- 1 chayote - peeled, halved, seeded, and diced into 1/2-inch pieces
- 1 poblano pepper - seeds and white ribs removed, diced into 1/2-inch pieces
- 6 (6 inch) flour tortillas
- cooking spray
- 6 sprigs cilantro, minced, divided
- 1/2 teaspoon onion powder
- 1/4 teaspoon salt
- 1 1/4 pounds ground turkey
- 1/4 cup water
- 3 tablespoons taco seasoning mix
- 1 teaspoon chili powder
- 1 cup guacamole
- 1/2 cup shredded Cheddar cheese

Direction

- Preheat the oven to 375°F or 190°C.
- Prepare four small bowls and assign the following ingredients into their own individual bowl - red onion slices, crema and lime zest. Halve limes and squeeze juice into a fourth small bowl.
- In the crema bowl, add 1 teaspoon lime juice. Pour the remaining lime juice into the red onion bowl and stir in 1/4 teaspoon salt. At room temperature let mixture marinate for at least 20 minutes until pickled.
- Heat oil in a pan over medium heat. Toss in poblano pepper and chayote and sauté for about 10 minutes or until tender and golden. Stir constantly.
- On both sides of the tortillas to coat using cooking spray. Arrange tortillas on a big baking tray.
- Bake in the preheated oven for 8 to 10 minutes until lightly brown and crisped.
- In the poblano-chayote mixture, add in onion powder, 1/4 teaspoon salt, 1/2 of the cilantro and lime zest. Blend well then transfer mixture into a bowl.
- Pour 1 tablespoon oil that remains in the same pan and heat over medium temperature. Toss in ground turkey and cook for about 7 minutes or until browned. Stir occasionally. Add in the chili powder, taco seasoning and 1/4 cup water. Continue cooking for 4 minutes until water evaporates.
- Lay guacamole over each crisped tortilla then top with ground turkey, lime crema, pickled onions, remaining cilantro and the poblano-chayote mixture.

Nutrition Information

- Calories: 420 calories;
- Sodium: 815
- Total Carbohydrate: 26.3
- Cholesterol: 93

- Protein: 25.2
- Total Fat: 24.9

46. Cumin Turkey Burgers

Serving: 6 | Prep: 20mins | Cook: 10mins | Ready in:

Ingredients

- 1 egg
- 2 jalapeno peppers, seeded and minced
- 2 cloves garlic, minced
- 1/4 cup low-sodium soy sauce
- 1/4 cup Worcestershire sauce
- 2 teaspoons ground cumin
- 1 teaspoon mustard powder
- 1 teaspoon paprika
- 1/2 teaspoon chili powder
- 1/4 teaspoon kosher salt
- 1/4 cup dry bread crumbs
- 1 1/2 pounds ground turkey
- 6 hamburger buns, split and toasted

Direction

- In a big mixing bowl, combine garlic, jalapeno peppers, and egg until well blended. Thoroughly mix in turkey, soy sauce, bread crumbs, Worcestershire sauce, salt, cumin, chili powder, paprika, and mustard; shape into six patties.
- Preheat the outdoor grill on medium-high heat; grease the grate lightly.
- Cook turkey burgers in the preheated grill for 4mins on each side until the juices are clear and the center is not pink. An inserted instant-read thermometer in the middle should register at least 74°C or 165°Fahrenheit. Serve burgers on toasted buns.

Nutrition Information

- Calories: 344 calories;
- Sodium: 898
- Total Carbohydrate: 29.4
- Cholesterol: 115
- Protein: 28.8
- Total Fat: 12.3

47. Curried Fowl Balls

Serving: 16 | Prep: 20mins | Cook: 20mins | Ready in:

Ingredients

- 1 cup cooked rice
- 1/2 cup finely diced onion
- 1/2 cup mild curry powder
- 1/2 cup water
- 10 tortilla chips with a 'hint of lime', crushed, or as needed
- 1/4 cup vegetable oil
- 2 cloves garlic, minced
- 2 teaspoons salt
- 1 teaspoon dried tarragon
- 2 pounds ground turkey
- 2 teaspoons butter, or as needed

Direction

- In bowl, mix tarragon, salt, garlic, vegetable oil, tortilla chips, water, curry powder, onion and rice. Add turkey. Mix till combined thoroughly. Shape mixture to 1-in. balls.
- Preheat an oven to 60°C/140°F.
- Heat big nonstick skillet on medium heat; add butter. Place 12 balls in melted butter; press every ball using back of spatula to 1/2-in. thick patty. Cook, 2-3 minutes per side, till not pink in the middle anymore. Put cooked patties in oven-safe plate; keep warm in oven. Repeat with leftover balls, adding extra butter if needed.

Nutrition Information

- Calories: 159 calories;
- Sodium: 345

- Total Carbohydrate: 7.2
- Cholesterol: 43
- Protein: 12.2
- Total Fat: 9.3

- Total Carbohydrate: 9.9

48. Curried Turkey Meatballs

Serving: 4 | Prep: 15mins | Cook: 20mins |Ready in:

Ingredients

- 1 pound ground turkey
- 1 yellow onion, finely chopped
- 1/3 cup dry bread crumbs
- 1 egg, beaten
- 1 1/2 teaspoons Madras curry powder
- 1 teaspoon kosher salt
- 1/4 teaspoon ground cumin
- 1/4 teaspoon ground ginger
- 1 pinch ground cinnamon
- 2 tablespoons olive oil

Direction

- Preheat an oven to 175°C/350°F.
- Use your hands to mix cinnamon, ginger, cumin, salt, curry powder, egg, bread crumbs, onion and turkey in a bowl; shape to 20 balls.
- In a skillet, heat olive oil on medium high heat. In batches, cook meatballs in hot oil for 5 minutes till browned on all sides. Put browned meatballs in baking dish.
- In preheated oven, bake for 15 minutes till cooked through. An inserted instant-read thermometer in middle should register 70°C/160°F minimum.

Nutrition Information

- Calories: 294 calories;
- Cholesterol: 130
- Protein: 25.7
- Total Fat: 17.2
- Sodium: 629

49. Dana's Taco Salad

Serving: 4 | Prep: 25mins | Cook: 50mins |Ready in:

Ingredients

- 1/2 cup dry lentils
- 1 cup water
- 1/2 pound ground turkey
- 1 cup water
- 1 (1.25 ounce) package taco seasoning mix
- 1 head iceberg lettuce, chopped
- 1 avocado - peeled, pitted and diced
- 1 tomato, diced
- 1 (15 ounce) can pitted black olives, chopped
- 1 (15 ounce) can kidney beans, drained and rinsed
- 1/3 cup Catalina salad dressing

Direction

- In a pot, combine the water and lentils and let it boil. Reduce the heat and simmer. Allow it to cook for half an hour until tender.
- In a skillet, cook the turkey over medium heat for 8-12 minutes until it is no longer pinkish. Mix in cooked lentils, taco seasoning mix, and a cup of water. Let it boil. Adjust the heat to Low and let it simmer for about 5 minutes until the liquid is almost absorbed.
- In a large bowl, toss in olives, lentil and turkey mixture, tomatoes, avocado, kidney beans, Catalina dressing, and lettuce until well-combined.

Nutrition Information

- Calories: 584 calories;
- Sodium: 2057
- Total Carbohydrate: 55.6
- Cholesterol: 42
- Protein: 25.7

- Total Fat: 31.1

50. DannyZ's Turkey Pumpkin Chili

Serving: 6 | Prep: 15mins | Cook: 43mins | Ready in:

Ingredients

- 1 1/2 tablespoons extra-virgin olive oil
- 1 1/2 cups chopped yellow onion
- 1/2 cup chopped green bell pepper
- 1/2 cup chopped yellow bell pepper
- 1 jalapeno pepper, diced small
- 1 clove garlic, minced
- 1 pound ground turkey
- 2 (15 ounce) cans black beans
- 2 cups pumpkin puree
- 1 (14.5 ounce) can diced tomatoes
- 2 1/2 tablespoons chili powder
- 1 1/2 teaspoons ground chipotle chile pepper
- 1/2 teaspoon ground black pepper
- kosher salt to taste
- 1/2 cup fat-free sour cream
- 1/2 cup shredded low-fat Cheddar cheese
- 3 tablespoons chopped cilantro

Direction

- Heat olive oil over medium heat in a large pot; cook and stir for 3 to 4 minutes onion until slightly softened. Add jalapeno, green bell pepper, garlic, and yellow bell pepper; cook for 5 to 8 minutes until tender.
- Mix turkey into the pot and cook for about 5 minutes until evenly browned. Take away from the heat and drain off carefully the excess grease. Pour over the turkey mixture with tomatoes, pumpkin, and 1 can black beans. Drain the second can of beans and add to the pot.
- Ianthe pot, stir ground chipotle pepper, chili powder, salt, and black pepper. Simmer chili, stirring every 5 to 8 minutes, for about 30 minutes until flavors combine. Decorate on top each serving with sour cream, cilantro, and Cheddar cheese.

Nutrition Information

- Calories: 369 calories;
- Sodium: 888
- Total Carbohydrate: 40.1
- Cholesterol: 61
- Protein: 29.5
- Total Fat: 10.9

51. David's Favorite Football Dip

Serving: 8 | Prep: 10mins | Cook: 20mins | Ready in:

Ingredients

- 1 pound ground turkey
- 1 onion, chopped
- 1 green bell pepper, chopped
- 1 (28 ounce) can vegetarian baked beans
- 1 (16 ounce) can vegetarian refried beans
- 1 tablespoon coconut oil
- 1 cup salsa
- 1/2 cup taco seasoning mix
- 2 tablespoons ranch dressing
- 2 teaspoons soy sauce
- 2 teaspoons liquid smoke flavoring
- 1/2 cup shredded Cheddar cheese
- 1/2 cup shredded mozzarella cheese
- salt and ground black pepper to taste

Direction

- Heat big skillet on medium high heat; mix and cook ground turkey in hot skillet for 5-7 minutes till crumbly and browned. Add bell pepper and onion; cover skillet. Simmer for 5 more minutes till onion is softened. Put turkey mixture in bowl.
- In same skillet for turkey mixture, mix coconut oil, refried beans and baked beans; mix and cook on medium heat for 5-7 minutes till beans

are heated through. Mix liquid smoke, soy sauce, ranch dressing, taco seasoning and salsa into bean mixture. Sprinkle mozzarella cheese and cheddar cheese. Cover skillet. Cook for 3-5 minutes till cheese melts.
- Stir bean mixture into ground turkey mixture well. Season with pepper and salt.

Nutrition Information

- Calories: 367 calories;
- Total Carbohydrate: 40.8
- Cholesterol: 55
- Protein: 23.3
- Total Fat: 13.5
- Sodium: 1684

52. Delicious Spinach And Turkey Lasagna

Serving: 8 | Prep: 20mins | Cook: 35mins | Ready in:

Ingredients

- 9 whole-wheat lasagna noodles
- 1 teaspoon olive oil
- 1/2 cup chopped onion
- 1 pound ground turkey breast
- 3 cups tomato sauce
- 1/2 cup sliced fresh mushrooms
- 3 tablespoons Italian seasoning
- 1/4 teaspoon ground black pepper
- 1/4 teaspoon garlic powder
- 6 cups chopped fresh spinach
- 2 cups fat-free ricotta cheese
- 1/4 teaspoon ground nutmeg
- 2 cups shredded mozzarella cheese

Direction

- Heat oven to 190°C (375°F).
- Boil a big saucepan of slightly salted water. Put lasagna pasta in the saucepan for 8-10 minutes. Drain pasta, wash with cold water.
- Warm the olive oil on moderate heat in a pan. Add in onion; stir and cook until the onion is transparent and soft, 2 minutes. Put in ground turkey; stir to crumble large chunks of meat, 5-7 minutes. Put in mushrooms, tomato sauce, black pepper, garlic powder and Italian seasoning. Gently boil 2 minutes, sprinkle salt and pepper on to taste.
- Mix ricotta, nutmeg and spinach in a big bowl.
- To prepare: In a 9x 13-in. greased baking tray, place three pasta noodles, lengthwise in base. Layer with 1/3 of each, ricotta mixture, turkey mixture, and mozzarella. Make the layers again, finishing with the left mozzarella. Bake in the oven 25 minutes. Let it cool 5 minutes then serve.

Nutrition Information

- Calories: 326 calories;
- Total Fat: 6.3
- Sodium: 768
- Total Carbohydrate: 34.2
- Cholesterol: 69
- Protein: 33

53. Delicious Turkey Burgers

Serving: 8 | Prep: 20mins | Cook: 15mins | Ready in:

Ingredients

- 1/4 pound bacon
- 1 (20 ounce) package ground turkey
- 1/2 cup bread crumbs
- 1/2 cup shredded Cheddar cheese
- 1/3 cup finely chopped yellow onion
- 1 egg, beaten
- 1 jalapeno pepper, diced
- 2 cloves garlic, minced
- 1/4 teaspoon ground cumin
- salt and ground black pepper to taste

Direction

- Cook the bacon in a large skillet over medium-high heat for 10 minutes, flipping it occasionally until browned all over. Let it drain and cool on a paper towel-lined plate. Crumble the bacon once cooled.
- Combine garlic, pepper, salt, bread crumbs, bacon, egg, cumin, yellow onion, turkey, Cheddar cheese, and jalapeno pepper in a bowl. Form the mixture into eight 1/4-pound patties.
- Heat an outdoor grill over medium-high heat. Oil the grate lightly.
- Place the turkey burgers into the preheated grill and cook each side for 7-10 minutes until its juices run clear and its center is no longer pink. Check if an inserted instant-read thermometer on its center reads at least 165°F or 74°C.

Nutrition Information

- Calories: 198 calories;
- Total Fat: 10.6
- Sodium: 249
- Total Carbohydrate: 6.1
- Cholesterol: 88
- Protein: 19.3

54. Deluxe Egg Rolls

Serving: 20 | Prep: 45mins | Cook: 20mins | Ready in:

Ingredients

- 2 quarts oil for deep frying
- 1/2 pound ground turkey
- 2 tablespoons chopped fresh ginger root
- 3 cloves garlic, peeled and minced
- 2 teaspoons sesame oil
- 1 medium head bok choy, shredded
- 3/4 cup shredded carrots
- 2 green onions, finely chopped
- 1 teaspoon soy sauce
- 2 (12 ounce) packages wonton wrappers

Direction

- Heat oil in big heavy saucepan/deep-fryer to 190°C/375°F.
- In big deep skillet, put approximately 1/2 garlic, 1/2 ginger and ground turkey. Cook till evenly brown on medium high heat.
- In wok, heat sesame oil on medium high heat. Mix garlic and leftover ginger in. Mix soy sauce, green onions, carrots and bok choy in. Mix and cook till veggies are tender yet crisp; take off heat.
- Mix bok choy mixture and ground turkey in medium bowl.
- Use approximately 1 tablespoon bok choy and turkey mixture to fill double thickness of wonton wrappers. Fold wrappers on filling. To seal, moisten seam. Repeat with leftover filling and wrappers.
- Deep fry filled wontons in small batches for 3-5 minutes till golden brown and crisp.

Nutrition Information

- Calories: 206 calories;
- Sodium: 248
- Total Carbohydrate: 21.1
- Cholesterol: 12
- Protein: 6
- Total Fat: 10.8

55. Easiest Turkey Loaf

Serving: 6 | Prep: 10mins | Cook: 1hours | Ready in:

Ingredients

- 1 (14 ounce) package seasoned bread stuffing mix
- 1 2/3 cups very hot water
- 2 pounds ground turkey
- 2 eggs, beaten
- salt and ground black pepper to taste

Direction

- Preheat an oven to 190°C or 375°F. Oil a loaf pan, 5 3/4 x11 inches in size.
- Combine the hot water and stuffing mix in a bowl, and plump up bread crumbs by allowing the mixture to rest for 2 minutes. Combine ground turkey with black pepper, salt and beaten eggs in a separate bowl. Mix into stuffing till well incorporated. Scoop loaf mixture into the prepped pan.
- In the prepped oven, allow to bake for an hour till not pink anymore in the middle. An inserted instant-read thermometer into the middle should register a minimum of 70°C or 160°F. Allow to rest for 10 minutes prior to serving.

Nutrition Information

- Calories: 504 calories;
- Total Carbohydrate: 50.4
- Cholesterol: 182
- Protein: 35.8
- Total Fat: 16.4
- Sodium: 1217

56. Easy Easy Casserole

Serving: 5 | Prep: 15mins | Cook: 1hours | Ready in:

Ingredients

- 1 1/2 pounds ground turkey
- 4 potatoes, peeled and sliced
- 2 tablespoons butter
- salt and pepper to taste
- 1 (15 ounce) can cream-style corn
- 1 (10.75 ounce) can condensed tomato soup

Direction

- Set the oven to 350°F (175°C) and start preheating.
- Over medium-high heat, place the turkey in a large skillet; sauté until browned or for 5-10 minutes.
- In the bottom of a lightly greased 2-quart casserole dish, place potato slices, cover with butter and sprinkle with pepper and salt to season. Layer cream-style corn over the potatoes; place cooked turkey meat on top; pour tomato soup over top.
- Bake with a cover for an hour at 350°F (175°C).

Nutrition Information

- Calories: 486 calories;
- Total Carbohydrate: 55.3
- Cholesterol: 120
- Protein: 29.9
- Total Fat: 17.3
- Sodium: 784

57. Easy Gluten Free Turkey Burgers

Serving: 5 | Prep: 5mins | Cook: 14mins | Ready in:

Ingredients

- 1 pound ground turkey
- 1/2 white onion, finely chopped
- 1/4 cup almond flour
- 1 large egg
- 3 cloves garlic, minced
- 2 sprigs fresh basil, chopped
- 1 pinch garlic and herb seasoning blend (such as Mrs. Dash®), or to taste
- ground black pepper to taste

Direction

- Prepare the grill by preheating on medium heat and coat the grate lightly with oil.
- Combine the ground turkey, almond flour, onion, egg, basil, garlic, black pepper, and seasoning blend and mix them thoroughly

together in a bowl. Divide the mixture and form into 5 patties, about 1/3 cup of the mixture each.
- Grill the burgers and cook for 7 to 10 minutes per side until the center of the patties are no longer pink and the juices are running clear. Insert an instant-read thermometer into the center and it should read at least 165° F (74° C).

Nutrition Information

- Calories: 192 calories;
- Protein: 20.8
- Total Fat: 10.9
- Sodium: 66
- Total Carbohydrate: 3.2
- Cholesterol: 104

58. Easy Personal Turkey Pot Pies

Serving: 4 | Prep: 45mins | Cook: 30mins | Ready in:

Ingredients

- 2 teaspoons vegetable oil
- 1 1/2 pounds ground turkey
- 1 (16 ounce) package frozen mixed vegetables
- 2 (.87 ounce) packages turkey gravy mix
- 2 cups water
- 2 (9 ounce) packages pie crust mix (such as Jiffy®)
- 1/2 cup ice water, or as needed
- 4 disposable mini-loaf pans (5 5/8x2 inches)

Direction

- Set the oven to 425°F (220°C) and start preheating.
- Over medium heat, in a skillet, heat vegetable oil; cook ground turkey meat for about 10 minutes until crumbly and browned, as the meat cooks, break it apart. Drain excess fat if needed; transfer to a bowl. Pour enough water to cover the frozen vegetables (about 2 cups) in a saucepan and bring to a boil, then stir in the mixed vegetables; boil again over medium heat, cook for about 5 minutes until tender; drain. Transfer the mixed vegetables to the bowl with the turkey. In a small sauce pan, combine 2 cups of water with 2 packets of turkey gravy mix over medium heat. Lower the heat; simmer until the mixture comes to a boil. Simmer for about 2 minutes until thickened. Pour gravy into the bowl with vegetables and turkey; combine well.
- Stir 2 packages of pie crust mix with ice water, adding a tablespoon of water at a time, using a fork to stir until mixture forms a soft dough. Gather dough together; cut in half; cut each half into 4 pieces (8 pieces in total). Roll each piece out on a floured surface to about 6 inches square; fit 4 pie crusts into mini-loaf pans; retain the remaining 4 crusts. Scoop 1/4 vegetable and turkey mixture into each pan. Place the second crust on top of each pie; crimp 2 crusts together with a fork to seal. Cut excess dough away. Create 4 small slits with a knife into each top crust.
- Arrange the pies onto a baking sheet; bake in the prepared oven for 15-20 minutes until filling is hot and crusts turn golden brown. Let cool for about 10 minutes; serve.

Nutrition Information

- Calories: 1048 calories;
- Total Carbohydrate: 90.6
- Cholesterol: 127
- Protein: 47.4
- Total Fat: 56.2
- Sodium: 1531

59. Easy Slow Cooker Enchiladas

Serving: 6 | Prep: 15mins | Cook: 5hours15mins | Ready in:

Ingredients

- 1 pound ground turkey
- 1 cup chopped onion
- 3/4 cup chopped green bell pepper
- 2 cloves garlic, minced
- 1 (16 ounce) can kidney beans, rinsed and drained
- 1 (15 ounce) can black beans, rinsed and drained
- 1 (10 ounce) can diced tomatoes with green chile peppers
- 1/3 cup water
- 1 1/2 teaspoons chili powder
- 1/2 teaspoon ground cumin
- 1/4 teaspoon salt
- 1/4 teaspoon ground black pepper
- 2 cups shredded Cheddar cheese
- 2 cups shredded Monterey Jack cheese
- 6 (6 inch) corn tortillas

Direction

- Into big skillet, break up turkey on moderate heat. Into the turkey, mix garlic, bell pepper and onion. Cook and mix for 5 to 7 minutes till turkey is fully browned. Put in pepper, salt, cumin, chili powder, water, diced tomatoes, black beans and kidney beans; boil, lower heat to moderately-low, cover skillet, and let simmer for ten minutes.
- In bowl, stir together Monterey jack cheese and Cheddar cheese.
- Layer approximately 3/4 cup mixture of turkey, a tortilla, and half cup mixture of cheese in a 5-quart slow cooker base; redo piled till all ingredients are used, finishing with layer of cheese.
- Cook on Low until heated through, 5 to 7 hours.

Nutrition Information

- Calories: 614 calories;
- Total Fat: 31.1
- Sodium: 1216
- Total Carbohydrate: 41.5
- Cholesterol: 129
- Protein: 44.3

60. Easy Turkey Chili

Serving: 6 | Prep: 10mins | Cook: 45mins | Ready in:

Ingredients

- 1 teaspoon vegetable oil
- 1 pound ground turkey
- 1/2 onion, chopped
- 2 cups chicken broth
- 1 (28 ounce) can crushed tomatoes
- 1 (15 ounce) can black beans, rinsed and drained
- 1 (15 ounce) can kidney beans, rinsed and drained
- 1 (16 ounce) can refried beans
- 1 tablespoon minced garlic
- 2 1/2 tablespoons chili powder
- 1 teaspoon paprika
- 1 teaspoon dried oregano
- 1/2 teaspoon ground cumin
- salt and ground black pepper to taste
- 2 tablespoons shredded Cheddar cheese (optional)

Direction

- Pour vegetable oil into a big pot and heat it at a moderately high heat and stir in ground turkey. Start cooking and stirring until the turkey is crumbly and has no hint of pink left in it anymore. It is ready when the meat is equally brown everywhere. Drain off the surplus grease and get rid of it. Add onion, cooking and stirring for around 5 minutes until the onion becomes tender.
- Mix in black pepper, salt, cumin, oregano, paprika, chili powder, garlic, refried beans, kidney beans, black beans, tomatoes and chicken broth. Lead the mixture to boiling point. Adjust the setting to low heat then leave it simmering with a cover on for 1/2-hour. If

desired, top every bowl with a teaspoon of Cheddar cheese.

Nutrition Information

- Calories: 299 calories;
- Total Fat: 9.4
- Sodium: 655
- Total Carbohydrate: 31.2
- Cholesterol: 65
- Protein: 25.2

61. Easy Turkey Meatballs

Serving: 4 | Prep: 15mins | Cook: 20mins | Ready in:

Ingredients

- cooking spray
- 2 slices white bread, torn into pieces
- 2 1/2 tablespoons 1% milk
- 1/2 pound ground turkey
- 1/4 pound turkey Italian sausages, casings removed
- 2 1/2 tablespoons grated Parmesan cheese
- 1 1/2 tablespoons finely chopped fresh parsley
- 1 1/2 cloves garlic, finely chopped
- salt and ground black pepper to taste

Direction

- Set oven to 175 degrees C (350 degrees F) and start preheating. Line aluminum foil on a baking tray and grease with cooking spray.
- In a bowl, place bread pieces, cover with milk and let soak 1 minute. Squeeze to remove excess moisture from bread, put bread in a bowl; remove milk.
- In a bowl, combine pepper, salt, garlic, parsley, Parmesan cheese, turkey Italian sausage, and ground turkey. Add in soaked bread and kindly mix. Shape into 1 1/2 -inch balls; arrange on the prepared baking tray.
- Put into the preheated oven and bake 20-25 minutes till meatballs have been cooked through and inserting an instant-read thermometer into the center and it reads no less than 74° C (165° F)

Nutrition Information

- Calories: 183 calories;
- Total Carbohydrate: 7.4
- Cholesterol: 66
- Protein: 19.1
- Total Fat: 8.6
- Sodium: 406

62. Easy Turkey Taco Soup

Serving: 4 | Prep: 10mins | Cook: 30mins | Ready in:

Ingredients

- 1 pound ground turkey
- 1/2 cup chopped onion
- 1 (12 ounce) package frozen mixed vegetables (peas, carrots, green beans, corn)
- 2 (10 ounce) cans diced tomatoes with green chile peppers
- 1 (15 ounce) can ranch style chili beans
- 1 (15 ounce) can chicken broth
- 1 (1 ounce) package taco seasoning mix
- 1 (1 ounce) package ranch dressing mix

Direction

- Heat a big pot on medium-high heat and stir in onion and ground turkey. Cook, stirring, until the turkey crumbles, browns evenly, and is no longer pink. Drain and throw away excess grease. Add in ranch dressing mix, taco seasoning, chicken broth, ranch beans, tomatoes with green chiles, and mixed vegetables, then set to boil. Lower heat and simmer on low heat for 20 minutes.

Nutrition Information

- Calories: 390 calories;
- Total Carbohydrate: 43.8
- Cholesterol: 86
- Protein: 31.9
- Total Fat: 10.2
- Sodium: 2588

63. Egg, Cheese, And Turkey Breakfast Burritos

Serving: 10 | Prep: 15mins | Cook: 15mins | Ready in:

Ingredients

- 10 egg whites
- 6 eggs
- 2 teaspoons vegetable oil, or as needed, divided
- 1/2 (16 ounce) package frozen hash brown potatoes, thawed
- 1/2 pound ground turkey
- 1 cup chopped red onion
- 6 slices hickory ham (such as Farmland®), diced
- 1 1/2 cups shredded fat-free Cheddar cheese
- 10 low-carb, high-fiber tortillas, warmed

Direction

- In big bowl, whisk eggs and egg whites.
- Heat 1 teaspoon oil in big frying pan on medium high heat; mix and cook has browns for 5 minutes till crispy and browned. Put hash browns in big bowl.
- In same frying pan, heat 1 teaspoon oil on medium heat. Add ham, onion and turkey; mix and cook for 5 minutes till onion softens and turkey is crumbly. Add eggs; mix for 5-7 minutes till set and scrambled. Add cheese; melt for 3 minutes. Put mixture in bowl with hash browns; mix.
- Plate tortillas and add 3 tablespoons filling on each tortilla. Fold opposite tortilla edges to overlap filling. Roll 1 opposing edge around filling to make a burrito then repeat for leftover tortillas.

Nutrition Information

- Calories: 261 calories;
- Cholesterol: 140
- Protein: 25.5
- Total Fat: 12.6
- Sodium: 718
- Total Carbohydrate: 21.6

64. Eggless Organic Turkey Meatballs For Baby

Serving: 16 | Prep: 15mins | Cook: 45mins | Ready in:

Ingredients

- 1 medium sweet potato, peeled
- cooking spray
- 8 ounces ground turkey
- 1/4 cup infant oat cereal
- 1 1/2 ounces unsweetened applesauce

Direction

- Put sweet potato in a pot and cover with water. Bring to a boil; cook for 20-25 minutes until tender. Drain; allow to cool.
- Set the oven to 350°F (175°C) and start preheating. Use cooking spray to grease a baking pan.
- In a bowl, mash sweet potato. Add applesauce, oat cereal and turkey. Use hand to mix. Form mixture into 16-20 small balls; place them on the prepared baking pan.
- Bake into the prepared oven for about 20 minutes until the inserted thermometer into the center register at least 165°F (74°C). Take meatballs out of the oven; allow to cool. Break into pieces or serve whole.

Nutrition Information

- Calories: 38 calories;
- Protein: 3.1
- Sodium: 16
- Total Carbohydrate: 3.8
- Cholesterol: 10
- Total Fat: 1.2

- Total Carbohydrate: 24
- Cholesterol: 84
- Protein: 24.5
- Total Fat: 8.7

65. Elimination Meatballs With Zucchini

Serving: 4 | Prep: 15mins | Cook: 1hours | Ready in:

Ingredients

- 1 large sweet potato, peeled and diced
- 1/2 medium zucchini, shredded
- 1/2 medium yellow squash, shredded
- 1 pound ground turkey
- black pepper to taste

Direction

- Put sweet potatoes into a large pot; pour in salted water to cover; allow to boil. Turn the heat down to medium-low; simmer for around 20 minutes, till tender. Strain. Using a fork, mash the sweet potatoes properly in a large bowl; set aside and allow to cool slightly.
- Set the oven at 350°F (175°C) and start preheating.
- In the bowl of the sweet potatoes, combine yellow squash and zucchini. Include in black pepper and turkey. Roll into 1-in. balls and place on a 9x13-in. baking dish.
- Bake in the preheated oven for 35-40 minutes, till the meatballs are not pink in the center anymore.

Nutrition Information

- Calories: 269 calories;
- Sodium: 127

66. Enchilada Lasagna

Serving: 8 | Prep: 20mins | Cook: 1hours15mins | Ready in:

Ingredients

- 1 tablespoon vegetable oil
- 1 onion, chopped
- 3 cloves garlic, chopped
- 1 1/4 pounds ground turkey
- 1 (28 ounce) can enchilada sauce
- 1 (14.5 ounce) can diced tomatoes with lime juice and cilantro
- 1 (16 ounce) package small-curd cottage cheese
- 1 egg
- 1 tablespoon ground cumin
- 5 (6 inch) corn tortillas, halved
- 2 cups shredded Mexican cheese blend
- cooking spray
- 1 green onion, diced

Direction

- Put oil in a big pot and heat over medium heat setting. Sauté and stir garlic and onion for about 5 minutes or until the onion becomes translucent. Add in ground turkey and cook for 5 minutes or until meat is not pink. Drain excess oil.
- Mix diced tomatoes and enchilada sauce into the turkey mixture. Let it simmer for about 20 minutes until the flavors have fully blended. Remove the pot from heat.
- Preheat the oven at 375°F (190°C).
- In a small bowl, combine egg, cumin and cottage cheese.
- In an 8-inch pan, put 1/3 of turkey sauce evenly on bottom. Top the turkey sauce with 1/2 of corn tortillas. Put 1/2 of the cottage

cheese mixture evenly on top of the corn tortillas. Top with 1/3 of Mexican cheese. Do the whole layering process again finishing with the remaining turkey sauce and Mexican cheese at the very top.
- Cover the baking dish with greased aluminum foil.
- Put in heated oven and bake for about 30 minutes or until bubbling. Remove the foil cover and continue baking for about 15 minutes or until the cheese on top is brown. Let it cool down for 15 minutes then serve while still warm. Top with green onion.

Nutrition Information

- Calories: 428 calories;
- Total Carbohydrate: 22.1
- Cholesterol: 120
- Protein: 31
- Total Fat: 24.1
- Sodium: 930

67. Enoki Protein Egg Bakes

Serving: 12 | Prep: 25mins | Cook: 28mins | Ready in:

Ingredients

- 1 bunch enoki mushrooms, cut from stalk and separated
- 2 tablespoons garlic salt
- 2 tablespoons safflower oil
- 1/2 large shallot, chopped
- 2 cloves garlic, minced
- 1 pound extra-lean ground turkey breast
- 2 yellow bell peppers, finely chopped
- 12 eggs
- 2 tablespoons Italian seasoning
- salt and ground black pepper to taste

Direction

- Preheat the oven to 150 degrees C (300 degrees F).
- Toss the enoki mushrooms along with the garlic salt on a big plate.
- Heat the oil in a big wok or skillet. Put in the enoki mushrooms; cook and whisk for 2-3 minutes till firm and lightly browned on bottom. Bring back to the plate. Put the garlic and shallot into the skillet; cook and whisk for 1-2 minutes till becoming fragrant. Put to the mushrooms.
- Whisk the turkey into the skillet. Cook, whisk to crumble the clumps, for roughly 5 minutes till brown.
- Mix the turkey along with the mushroom mixture; cut finely. Whisk in the yellow bell peppers.
- Whip together the pepper, salt, Italian seasoning and eggs in a big bowl. Whisk in the turkey mixture and add into two a-third-cup muffin tins.
- Bake in preheated oven for roughly 20 minutes till the edges turn brown and a toothpick inserted in middle comes out clean.

Nutrition Information

- Calories: 140 calories;
- Sodium: 1008
- Total Carbohydrate: 1.8
- Cholesterol: 209
- Protein: 15.8
- Total Fat: 7.6

68. Fabulous Ground Turkey Meatloaf

Serving: 4 | Prep: 25mins | Cook: 1hours5mins | Ready in:

Ingredients

- 1 egg, beaten
- 1/4 cup vegetable juice (such as V-8®)

- 1/4 cup sour cream
- 2 tablespoons Worcestershire sauce
- 1 teaspoon dried sage
- 1 teaspoon dried parsley
- 1 teaspoon dried oregano
- 1 teaspoon salt
- 1/2 teaspoon ground black pepper
- 2 dashes hot pepper sauce (such as Tabasco®)
- 1/2 cup rolled oats
- 2 tablespoons butter
- 1/2 sweet onion, diced
- 1/2 green bell pepper, diced
- 2 stalks celery, diced
- 1 (16 ounce) can sliced mushrooms, drained
- 1 pound ground turkey
- 1 (8 ounce) can tomato sauce
- 1/2 cup chili sauce

Direction

- Set the oven to 350°F (175°C) to preheat.
- In a large bowl, beat together hot pepper sauce, black pepper, salt, oregano, parsley, sage, Worcestershire sauce, sour cream, vegetable juice and egg. Stir in oats and let soak.
- In a skillet, melt butter on medium heat; cook celery, bell pepper and onion for about 5 minutes while stirring until soft. Stir turkey, mushrooms and vegetable mixture into the oat mixture; form into a loaf and move into a broiling pan. In a bowl, combine chili sauce and tomato sauce; then pour over the turkey loaf.
- Bake for about 1 hour in the prepared oven until the center is no longer pink. An instant-read thermometer should reach at least 165°F (74°C) when inserted into the center.

Nutrition Information

- Calories: 405 calories;
- Total Fat: 19.9
- Sodium: 2083
- Total Carbohydrate: 30.2
- Cholesterol: 152
- Protein: 30.2

69. Fairuzah's Chili

Serving: 14 | Prep: 15mins | Cook: 2hours | Ready in:

Ingredients

- 1 1/2 pounds ground beef
- 1 1/2 pounds ground turkey
- 3/4 large white onion, diced
- 3 (15 ounce) cans kidney beans, drained
- 3 (15 ounce) cans baked beans with pork
- 1 (14.5 ounce) can stewed tomatoes
- 1 (12 ounce) can sliced mushrooms, drained
- 3 tablespoons chili powder
- 6 cloves garlic, minced
- 1 1/2 teaspoons garlic powder
- 1 teaspoon ground cinnamon
- salt and pepper to taste

Direction

- In a large pot, stir onion, ground turkey and ground beef. Keep stirring over medium heat until meat is well-cooked through, about 10 minutes.
- Combine in mushrooms, tomatoes, baked beans, and kidney beans. Flavor with pepper, salt, cinnamon, garlic powder, garlic, and chili powder. Lower the heat to low; simmer for at least 1 hour and stir on occasion. If you have time, keep simmering longer for better. After the first half-hour has gone, check the flavor and adjust seasonings to suit your taste.

Nutrition Information

- Calories: 427 calories;
- Total Fat: 19
- Sodium: 761
- Total Carbohydrate: 38.6
- Cholesterol: 86
- Protein: 27.4

70. Fajita Chili Con Carne

Serving: 4 | Prep: 10mins | Cook: 15mins | Ready in:

Ingredients

- 1 pound ground beef or ground turkey
- 1 medium onion, chopped
- 1 (5.4 ounce) package Knorr® Menu Flavors Rice Sides™ - Steak Fajitas
- 1 (14.5 ounce) can diced tomatoes, undrained
- 1 1/2 cups water
- 1 (16 ounce) can red kidney beans, rinsed and drained

Direction

- Cook onion and ground beef in a 4-quart stockpot until browned. You can drain it after cooking if you want.
- Mix the remaining ingredients and let it boil over high heat. Adjust the heat to low and let it simmer covered, stirring for some time, for about 7 minutes until the rice is tender.
- Garnish it with sour cream, sliced green onions, and/or shredded Cheddar cheese, if desired.

Nutrition Information

- Calories: 463 calories;
- Protein: 29.4
- Total Fat: 14.8
- Sodium: 957
- Total Carbohydrate: 51.3
- Cholesterol: 71

71. Family Favorite Slow Cooker Turkey Chili

Serving: 6 | Prep: 15mins | Cook: 4hours5mins | Ready in:

Ingredients

- 1 pound ground turkey
- 1 cup chopped onion
- 3/4 cup chopped green bell pepper
- 1 clove garlic, minced
- 2 (14.5 ounce) cans red kidney beans, undrained
- 1 (16 ounce) can diced tomatoes
- 1 (8 ounce) can tomato sauce
- 2 teaspoons chili powder
- 1/2 teaspoon dried basil
- 1/2 teaspoon salt
- 1/4 teaspoon ground black pepper

Direction

- Heat over medium-high heat a large skillet. Cook and stir garlic, bell pepper, onion, and turkey in the hot skillet until the turkey is browned fully, about 5 to 7 minutes; place to the crock of a slow cooker.
- Blend black pepper, salt, basil, chili powder, tomato sauce, diced tomatoes, and kidney beans into the turkey mixture.
- Cook on Low for 4 hours.

Nutrition Information

- Calories: 270 calories;
- Cholesterol: 56
- Protein: 24.1
- Total Fat: 6.5
- Sodium: 857
- Total Carbohydrate: 29.7

72. Famous Turkey Burgers

Serving: 4 | Prep: 10mins | Cook: 10mins | Ready in:

Ingredients

- 1 pound ground turkey
- 1/3 cup honey barbecue sauce, divided
- 1 green onion, chopped
- 1 teaspoon vegetable oil
- 1 teaspoon chili powder
- 1/2 teaspoon ground cumin
- 4 hamburger buns

Direction

- Prepare an outdoor grill by preheating on medium-high heat and coat the grate lightly with oil.
- Combine the turkey, green onion, 1/4 cup barbeque sauce, chili powder, oil, and cumin in a bowl and mix them together. Divide the mixture and form into 4 patties.
- Cook the patties on the grill for 4 to 5 minutes per side until they are cooked through. Insert an instant-read thermometer into the center and it should read 165° F (74° C). Put the patties on a bun and spread the remaining barbeque sauce over the burgers then serve.

Nutrition Information

- Calories: 332 calories;
- Total Fat: 11.8
- Sodium: 511
- Total Carbohydrate: 29.6
- Cholesterol: 84
- Protein: 26.7

73. Fantastic Black Bean Chili

Serving: 6 | Prep: 20mins | Cook: 1hours15mins | Ready in:

Ingredients

- 1 tablespoon vegetable oil
- 1 onion, diced
- 2 cloves garlic, minced
- 1 pound ground turkey
- 3 (15 ounce) cans black beans, undrained
- 1 (14.5 ounce) can crushed tomatoes
- 1 1/2 tablespoons chili powder
- 1 tablespoon dried oregano
- 1 tablespoon dried basil leaves
- 1 tablespoon red wine vinegar

Direction

- Heat a big heavy pot with oil over a medium heat and cook garlic and onion until the onion becomes translucent. Add the turkey and cook while stirring until browned. Stir in vinegar, basil, oregano, chili powder, tomatoes, and beans. Drop heat to low and simmer while covered for roughly 60 minutes or even more until the flavors blend well.

Nutrition Information

- Calories: 366 calories;
- Total Carbohydrate: 44.1
- Cholesterol: 56
- Protein: 29.6
- Total Fat: 9.2
- Sodium: 969

74. Fast Turkey Bolognese

Serving: 4 | Prep: 25mins | Cook: 1hours3mins | Ready in:

Ingredients

- 1/2 cup red lentils
- 1 cup water, or as needed
- cooking spray
- 3 carrots, minced
- 1 medium onion, minced
- salt and ground black pepper to taste

- 1 (16 ounce) package ground turkey
- 1/2 red bell pepper, chopped
- 2 cloves garlic, minced
- 1 (14.5 ounce) can diced tomatoes
- 1 (6 ounce) can tomato paste
- 1 (6 ounce) can tomato sauce
- 1 cup white wine
- 1 tablespoon Italian seasoning
- 3 dashes Worcestershire sauce
- 1/2 (16 ounce) package spaghetti

Direction

- In a saucepan, place lentils and pour in water to cover; bring to a simmer. Cook with a cover for about half an hour until lentils become tender, adding more water if needed.
- Use cooking spray to coat a large nonstick skillet; put over medium heat. Add a pinch of salt, onion and carrots. Cook while stirring often for 3-5 minutes until softened. Push vegetables to the sides of the pan. Cook turkey in the center of the pan, using a spoon to break it up for about 5 minutes until dry and browned. Mix turkey in with the vegetables.
- Stir garlic and red pepper to the skillet; cook for about 3 minutes until softened. Add tomato sauce, tomato paste and diced tomatoes; mix to combine. Stir in cooked lentils. Pour in wine; if needed, add water to thin sauce. Add Worcestershire sauce and Italian seasoning; sprinkle with pepper and salt.
- Boil a large pot of lightly salted water. Cook spaghetti while stirring occasionally in the boiling water for about 12 minutes until tender yet firm to the bite. Drain. Mix sauce and cooked pasta.

Nutrition Information

- Calories: 614 calories;
- Total Fat: 10.4
- Sodium: 834
- Total Carbohydrate: 79.3
- Cholesterol: 84
- Protein: 40.5

75. Fast And Friendly Meatballs

Serving: 6 | Prep: 10mins | Cook: 20mins | Ready in:

Ingredients

- 2 tablespoons olive oil
- 1 (20 ounce) package ground turkey
- 1 egg, beaten
- 1/3 cup Italian seasoned bread crumbs

Direction

- Heat an oven to 175°C or 350°F. Use olive oil to oil a baking dish, 9x13 inch in size and put in oven while it preheats.
- Use your hands to combine egg, bread crumbs and ground turkey in medium bowl. Shape meat with a scoop of ice cream if available, to meatballs size of golf ball. Put in hot baking dish, approximately an-inch away. Pat down to flatten the underside barely a little bit.
- Bake in prepped oven, about 15 minutes, then flip over, and keep baking for an additional of 5 minutes, or till outside is quite crispy. Serve along with sauce and pasta or anything you'd prefer.

Nutrition Information

- Calories: 218 calories;
- Sodium: 218
- Total Carbohydrate: 4.6
- Cholesterol: 106
- Protein: 18.5
- Total Fat: 13.5

76. Feta Cheese Turkey Burgers

Serving: 4 | Prep: | Cook: | Ready in:

Ingredients

- 1 pound ground turkey
- 1 cup crumbled feta cheese
- 1/2 cup kalamata olives, pitted and sliced
- 2 teaspoons dried oregano
- ground black pepper to taste

Direction

- Preheat the outdoor grill, lightly brush the grate with oil or spray with cooking spray. Prepare the patties, combine ground turkey, olives, feta cheese, oregano and pepper in a big bowl. Mix well and divide into equal patties. Grill the patties, 6 minutes per side or 10-12 minutes.

Nutrition Information

- Calories: 318 calories;
- Sodium: 800
- Total Carbohydrate: 3.6
- Cholesterol: 123
- Protein: 25.5
- Total Fat: 21.9

77. Feta And Turkey Stuffed Green Peppers

Serving: 6 | Prep: 15mins | Cook: 1hours10mins | Ready in:

Ingredients

- 6 green peppers, tops and seeds removed
- 3 tablespoons olive oil
- 1 pound ground turkey
- 1 white onion, chopped
- 1 1/2 teaspoons salt
- 1 1/2 teaspoons ground black pepper
- 1 (15.5 ounce) can sweet corn, drained
- 1 (14.5 ounce) can diced tomatoes, drained
- 1 1/2 teaspoons ground thyme
- 1 1/2 teaspoons dried rosemary
- 1 tablespoon crushed fennel seeds
- 1 cup water
- 1/3 cup white rice
- 1/4 cup sweet barbeque sauce
- 1 cup crumbled feta cheese

Direction

- Preheat oven to 175°C/350°F; put bell peppers, cavity side up, in casserole dish.
- Heat olive oil in skillet on medium heat; cook turkey in hot oil for 5 minutes till fully browned. Mix onion into turkey; season with pepper and salt. Mix and cook mixture for 3 minutes. Add fennel, rosemary, thyme, tomatoes and corn to turkey; mix. Put water on mixture then add rice; stir. Bring to a boil and cover; lower heat to low. Simmer for 15 minutes till rice is tender. Mix barbeque sauce through mixture; take off heat.
- Put enough turkey mixture in each bell pepper to fill 1/3 of the way full then divide 1/2 feta cheese into peppers to make a cheese layer over turkey mixture. Use leftover turkey mixture to fill peppers; put leftover feta cheese on top.
- In preheated oven, bake for 45 minutes till peppers are tender.

Nutrition Information

- Calories: 434 calories;
- Total Fat: 22.2
- Sodium: 1538
- Total Carbohydrate: 35.1
- Cholesterol: 93
- Protein: 24.9

78. Fiesta Chili

Serving: 4 | Prep: 15mins | Cook: 55mins | Ready in:

Ingredients

- 12 3/4 ounces ground turkey, broken into small portions
- 6 3/8 ounces bacon, chopped
- 1/4 cup chopped onion
- 1/4 cup chopped green bell pepper
- 1 medium jalapeno pepper, seeded and minced
- 1 (16 ounce) can kidney beans, rinsed and drained
- 1 (15 ounce) can black beans, rinsed and drained
- 1 (14.5 ounce) can stewed tomatoes, chopped
- 1/4 teaspoon chili powder
- 1/4 teaspoon ground cumin
- 1/4 teaspoon salt
- 1/8 teaspoon cayenne pepper

Direction

- Set the oven to 450°F (230°C) and start preheating.
- In a baking dish, mix jalapeno pepper, bell pepper, onion, bacon and turkey.
- Bake in the prepared oven while stirring occasionally for about 15 minutes until turkey is browned completely and bacon becomes crisp.
- In a large pot, stir cayenne pepper, salt, cumin, chili powder, tomatoes, black beans and kidney beans together; bring to a boil; lower the heat to medium-low.
- Stir turkey mixture into beans mixture. Cook chili while stirring occasionally at a simmer for about 40 minutes until beans become tender.

Nutrition Information

- Calories: 437 calories;
- Cholesterol: 82
- Protein: 36.8
- Total Fat: 13.9
- Sodium: 1413
- Total Carbohydrate: 43.1

79. Fiesta Stuffed Turkey Burgers

Serving: 4 | Prep: 15mins | Cook: 12mins | Ready in:

Ingredients

- 1 pound ground turkey
- 1 large clove garlic, minced
- 3 tablespoons minced onion
- 2 tablespoons minced red bell pepper
- 1 tablespoon minced green onion
- 2 teaspoons minced fresh cilantro
- 1 teaspoon cayenne pepper
- 1 teaspoon ground cumin
- salt and pepper to taste
- 2 slices pepperjack cheese, cut into quarters

Direction

- In a bowl, mix pepper, salt, cumin, cayenne pepper, cilantro, green onion, red bell pepper, onion, garlic and ground turkey. Divide mixture into 8 small patties. Place 2 of pepper jack cheese quarters onto each of 4 of the patties; place the other 4 patties on top so the center is filled with cheese. Press along edges of burgers to seal.
- Over medium-high heat, place a large skillet. In the skillet, cook the burgers for about 6 minutes on each side until the center is no longer pink and juices run clear.

Nutrition Information

- Calories: 233 calories;
- Sodium: 152
- Total Carbohydrate: 2.5
- Cholesterol: 99
- Protein: 25.9
- Total Fat: 13.3

80. Fiesta Turkey Tavern

Serving: 5 | Prep: 10mins | Cook: 40mins | Ready in:

Ingredients

- 2 tablespoons olive oil
- 1 1/4 pounds ground turkey
- 1 cup finely chopped white onion
- 1 clove garlic, minced
- 1/4 teaspoon ground black pepper
- 1 1/2 tablespoons prepared yellow mustard, divided
- 1/8 teaspoon cayenne pepper
- 1/8 teaspoon chili powder
- 1 cup water
- 1/4 cup finely chopped jalapeno
- 5 hamburger buns

Direction

- Over medium-low heat, heat olive oil; cook while stirring ground turkey with a back of a wooden spoon to break the meat into small crumbles as it cooks. When meat is about half browned, stir in black pepper, garlic and onion; cook while stirring until no longer pink and turkey is browned evenly and crumbly.
- Stir in a tablespoon of prepared mustard, water, chili powder, and cayenne pepper. Boil the mixture, lower the heat; simmer while stirring for about 20 minutes until water evaporates. Stir in the rest of mustard and chopped jalapeno; cook for about 5 more minutes until heated through. Scoop mixture onto hamburger buns.

Nutrition Information

- Calories: 356 calories;
- Sodium: 361
- Total Carbohydrate: 25.5
- Cholesterol: 84
- Protein: 26.8
- Total Fat: 16.4

81. Frank's Famous Spaghetti Sauce

Serving: 8 | Prep: 15mins | Cook: 30mins | Ready in:

Ingredients

- 1 tablespoon olive oil
- 1 onion, chopped
- 1 green bell pepper, chopped
- 3 cloves garlic, minced
- 4 fresh mushrooms, sliced
- 1 pound ground turkey
- 1 pinch dried basil
- 1 pinch dried oregano
- ground black pepper to taste
- 1 (14.5 ounce) can stewed tomatoes
- 2 (15 ounce) cans tomato sauce
- 1 (6 ounce) can tomato paste

Direction

- The first part of this dish is simply sautéing garlic, green bell pepper, and onions together in olive oil in a big skillet over medium heat until the bell pepper is tender and onions are translucent. Put in the ground black pepper, oregano, basil, ground turkey, and mushrooms; fry while stirring frequently until the turkey is cooked.
- To the same pan you used for the first part, add the can of stewed tomatoes with the liquid. Lower the heat once you've added this and allow it to simmer until the tomatoes turn soft and start to fall apart. Put in tomato sauce and stir; thicken it by adding tomato paste. Turn the heat down to very low and allow the sauce to simmer for 15 minutes. Serve this with your preferred pasta.

Nutrition Information

- Calories: 168 calories;
- Total Fat: 6.8
- Sodium: 885
- Total Carbohydrate: 15.6
- Cholesterol: 45

- Protein: 13.3

82. French Burgers

Serving: 4 | Prep: 20mins | Cook: 20mins | Ready in:

Ingredients

- 1/2 cup crumbled feta cheese
- 1/4 cup sliced green onion
- 1 teaspoon dried tarragon
- salt and ground black pepper to taste
- 1 1/2 pounds ground turkey
- 2 tablespoons olive oil
- 1 thin slice red onion
- 2 tablespoons flour
- 1/2 cup chicken broth
- 1/2 cup red wine
- 1/2 teaspoon chopped fresh parsley
- 1/2 teaspoon dried minced onion
- 1/2 teaspoon crushed bay leaf
- 1/4 teaspoon dried thyme
- salt and ground black pepper to taste

Direction

- Set the oven at 450°F (230°C) and start preheating.
- In a small bowl, combine tarragon, green onion and feta cheese; season with pepper and salt; set aside.
- Shape the ground turkey into 8 even-sized patties. Arrange four even portions of the cheese mixture on top of four of the patties. Place on top of the remaining patties on top of each. Seal by pinching the edges together.
- Bake the patties for 20-30 minutes in the preheated oven, turning once, till cooked through.
- Place a skillet on low heat; heat olive oil. Cook while stirring red onion into the hot oil till browned; take the onion away and discard. Mix in flour; cook till the mixture turns deep brown. Take the pan away from the heat; put in thyme, bay leaf, minced onion, parsley, red wine and chicken broth. Place the pan back to the heat; boil while stirring; season with pepper and salt. Spread the sauce over the prepared patties. Serve.

Nutrition Information

- Calories: 404 calories;
- Total Fat: 23.7
- Sodium: 308
- Total Carbohydrate: 5.7
- Cholesterol: 142
- Protein: 37.1

83. Fried Pot Stickers

Serving: 3 | Prep: 25mins | Cook: 3mins | Ready in:

Ingredients

- 1/4 pound ground turkey
- 1 egg, beaten, divided
- 1 teaspoon minced water chestnuts
- 1 teaspoon minced green onion
- 1/2 teaspoon light soy sauce
- 1/2 teaspoon minced fresh ginger
- 1/2 teaspoon freshly ground black pepper
- 1/4 teaspoon salt
- 1/4 teaspoon garlic powder
- 1/4 teaspoon red pepper flakes
- 12 wonton wrappers
- vegetable oil for frying

Direction

- In bowl, mix red pepper flakes, garlic powder, salt, black pepper, ginger, soy sauce, green onion, water chestnuts, 1 tablespoon beaten egg and turkey.
- Cut wonton wrappers to circles with a 3-in. biscuit cutter. In middle of every wonton wrapper, put 1 1/2 teaspoon turkey filling. Brush beaten egg on one side of every

wrapper. Fold wrapper on filling, pleating edges while sealing.
- In deep-fryer/big saucepan, heat oil to 190°C/375°F. 6 at a time, fry pot stickers for 3-6 minutes till browned. On paper towels, drain.

Nutrition Information

- Calories: 241 calories;
- Total Fat: 12.4
- Sodium: 472
- Total Carbohydrate: 19.5
- Cholesterol: 93
- Protein: 12.9

84. Gail's Turkey Lentil Stew

Serving: 10 | Prep: 15mins | Cook: 1hours11mins | Ready in:

Ingredients

- 2 teaspoons canola oil
- 1 1/4 pounds ground turkey
- 1 cup chopped onion
- 1 cup roughly chopped red bell pepper
- 6 cups water
- 1 (14.5 ounce) can diced tomatoes
- 1 (8 ounce) can tomato sauce
- 1 cup lentils
- 1 cup sliced carrots
- 3/4 cup pearl barley
- 6 cubes chicken bouillon
- 1 teaspoon salt
- 1 teaspoon Italian seasoning
- 1/2 teaspoon ground black pepper
- 1/8 teaspoon cayenne pepper

Direction

- Add oil to a frying pan, heat over moderate-high heat. Add red bell pepper, onion and turkey. Sauté for 6 to 8 minutes until the turkey is not pink any longer and pepper gets soft.
- In a big pot, mix cayenne pepper, black pepper, Italian seasoning, salt, bouillon, barley, carrots, lentils, tomato sauce, diced tomatoes and water together over moderate-high heat. Put in sautéed turkey mixture. Boil. Lower the heat and let simmer with a cover for about 60 minutes until the flavors combine together and the lentils get tender.

Nutrition Information

- Calories: 251 calories;
- Total Carbohydrate: 30.1
- Cholesterol: 42
- Protein: 19.3
- Total Fat: 6.2
- Sodium: 1053

85. Garlic And Ranch Turkey Burgers

Serving: 4 | Prep: 20mins | Cook: 10mins | Ready in:

Ingredients

- 1 pound ground turkey
- 1 (1 ounce) package ranch dressing mix
- 1 egg
- 3 cloves garlic, minced
- 1/4 cup Worcestershire sauce
- seasoned salt and pepper to taste

Direction

- Prepare an outdoor grill by preheating it on medium-high heat and coat the grate lightly with oil.
- Combine the turkey, egg, ranch mix, garlic, seasoned salt, Worcestershire sauce, and pepper, kneading them together in a bowl until they are well blended; form into 4 patties of equal proportions.

- Grill the patties on for about 5 minutes per side to be cooked well done. Insert an instant-read thermometer into the center and it should read 165° F (74° C).

Nutrition Information

- Calories: 219 calories;
- Sodium: 796
- Total Carbohydrate: 7.7
- Cholesterol: 130
- Protein: 24.2
- Total Fat: 9.8

86. Gary's Turkey Burritos

Serving: 6 | Prep: 5mins | Cook: 20mins | Ready in:

Ingredients

- 1 pound ground turkey
- 2 (7 ounce) cans hot tomato sauce
- 1 (15.25 ounce) can whole kernel corn, drained
- 1/2 small onion, diced
- 1 (16 ounce) can fat-free refried beans
- 1 (16 ounce) container fat free sour cream
- 3/4 cup shredded reduced-fat Cheddar cheese
- 6 (10 inch) flour tortillas

Direction

- Brown ground turkey in a large pan over medium high heat. Stir in onion, corn and the tomato sauce. Lower the heat to medium heat and simmer for 20 minutes until the liquids reduce, stirring occasionally.
- Heat beans in a separate medium pan over medium-low heat. Prepare cheese and sour cream for adding into the top of burritos. Heat the tortillas one by one over the stove burner, flipping a few times, about 1-2 minutes. Sprinkle with the beans, meat mixture, sour cream and cheese. Fold over and enjoy while they are still warm.

Nutrition Information

- Calories: 588 calories;
- Total Fat: 8.4
- Sodium: 1595
- Total Carbohydrate: 82.1
- Cholesterol: 76
- Protein: 34.5

87. Glazed Tofu Meatloaf

Serving: 12 | Prep: 15mins | Cook: 45mins | Ready in:

Ingredients

- 1 (14 ounce) package firm tofu, drained and mashed
- 2 pounds ground turkey
- 1/2 cup dry bread crumbs
- 1 (1 ounce) envelope dry onion soup mix
- 1/4 cup minced green bell pepper
- 2 eggs, beaten
- 1/4 cup brown sugar
- 1/4 cup soy sauce
- 1 teaspoon prepared yellow mustard

Direction

- Set the oven to 350°F (175°C) and start preheating. Grease a 9 inch square baking dish lightly.
- Mix eggs, green pepper, soup mix, bread crumbs, turkey and tofu in a bowl. Transfer mixture to the greased pan; mold into a loaf shape.
- Blend mustard, soy sauce and brown sugar over low heat in a saucepan.
- Bake the meatloaf in the prepared oven for half an hour. Drizzle with the sauce mixture; keep baking for 15 minutes or until the internal temperature reaches 180°F (80°C).

Nutrition Information

- Calories: 212 calories;
- Cholesterol: 91
- Protein: 20.6
- Total Fat: 10.3
- Sodium: 628
- Total Carbohydrate: 9.7

88. Gluten Free South Of The Border Spaghetti

Serving: 6 | Prep: | Cook: | Ready in:

Ingredients

- 1 (12 ounce) box Barilla® Gluten Free Spaghetti
- 2 cloves garlic, chopped
- 1 tablespoon extra virgin olive oil, divided
- 1 pound ground turkey
- 1 cup corn kernels
- 3 plum tomatoes, diced
- 1/2 small onion, diced
- 2 tablespoons chopped fresh parsley
- 1 Anaheim chile pepper, chopped
- 2 limes, juiced
- 1/2 cup sour cream
- 1/2 cup crumbled cotija cheese, divided
- Salt and black pepper to taste

Direction

- Boil a large pot of water.
- Meanwhile, place a large skillet on medium heat; sauté garlic in 1 tablespoon of olive oil for around 1 minute. Put in turkey; brown thorough till cooked through. Flavor with pepper and salt; set aside.
- To make salsa, in a small bowl, mix together lime juice, Anaheim pepper, parsley, onion, tomatoes and corn. Season to taste with salt; combine properly; set aside.
- Following the package instructions, cook pasta properly.
- Put 1 cup of the cooking water into the ground turkey; simmer the mixture. Put in sour cream; stir to mix.
- Strain the pasta; toss with sauce and the turkey.
- Take the skillet away from the heat; put in half of the salsa and half of the cheese. Stir to mix.
- Top with the remaining salsa and cheese before serving.

Nutrition Information

- Calories: 620 calories;
- Protein: 24.3
- Total Fat: 18.1
- Sodium: 239
- Total Carbohydrate: 91.1
- Cholesterol: 80

89. Gluten Free Casserole

Serving: 8 | Prep: 25mins | Cook: 45mins | Ready in:

Ingredients

- 8 cups water
- 2 cups green beans, chopped
- 1 teaspoon extra-virgin olive oil
- 1 small onion, chopped fine
- 1 1/2 pounds ground turkey
- salt and ground black pepper to taste
- 5 cloves garlic, minced
- 2 tablespoons chopped fresh basil
- 2 teaspoons chopped fresh thyme
- 1 cup frozen peas
- 1 cup mushrooms, chopped
- 2 zucchini, chopped
- 2 cups crushed tomatoes
- 1 cup shredded mozzarella cheese
- 2 tablespoons freshly grated Parmesan cheese

Direction

- Boil water in a big pot. Cook the green beans for about 3 minutes at a boil until it becomes soft, then drain.
- Set an oven to preheat to 175°C (350°F).
- In a big frying pan, heat the olive oil on medium-low heat. Cook and stir the onion for 3-5 minutes in hot oil until it becomes translucent.
- Crumble the ground turkey into the frying pan and turn up the heat to medium-high. Generously sprinkle pepper and salt on the turkey to season. Let it cook and stir for 7-10 minutes until the turkey turns brown completely. Lower the heat to medium. Stir in thyme, basil and garlic through the turkey mixture and let it cook for 3 minutes more, stirring from time to time.
- Using a slotted spoon, take out the turkey mixture from the frying pan and move to a 9x13-inch casserole dish. Set aside 2 tbsp of the pan drippings to be used later and get rid of the rest.
- In the frying pan, heat the reserved pan drippings on medium heat. Stir in zucchini, mushrooms, peas and green beans in the hot pan drippings, then sprinkle black pepper and salt to season. Cook and stir the vegetable mixture for around 5 minutes until it becomes hot, then add it to the casserole dish and mix to blend. Pour the crushed tomatoes on top of the vegetable and turkey mixture, then put a layer of mozzarella cheese on top. Sprinkle the Parmesan cheese on top of the mozzarella cheese.
- Let it bake in the preheated oven for about 20 minutes, until the vegetables become tender and the cheese melts. Allow the dish to rest for 10 minutes prior to serving.

Nutrition Information

- Calories: 217 calories;
- Total Fat: 9.9
- Sodium: 191
- Total Carbohydrate: 9.6
- Cholesterol: 73
- Protein: 23.6

90. Gluten Free Stuffing

Serving: 16 | Prep: 15mins | Cook: 1hours5mins | Ready in:

Ingredients

- 1 cup butter, softened, divided
- 1 1/2 loaves gluten-free bread
- 1 pound ground turkey
- 3 tablespoons sage
- 1 tablespoon celery salt
- 1 teaspoon ground black pepper
- 1 onion, diced
- 1 apple, diced
- 3 stalks celery, diced
- 1/2 (8 ounce) package mushrooms, diced
- 1 cup chicken broth
- 3/4 cup heavy whipping cream

Direction

- Set the oven to 175°C or 350°Fahrenheit. Grease a 9-in by 13-in baking dish lightly with butter.
- For both sides of each slice of bread, spread on butter then place on baking sheets.
- Bake for 5-10mins in the preheated oven until well toasted.
- On medium heat, cook and stir turkey in a big heated pan for 5-7mins until the turkey turns crumbly and brown; drain and get rid of the grease.
- In a big bowl, crumble the bread then stir in black pepper, sage, and celery salt.
- On medium heat, heat the remaining butter in a pot. Cook and stir mushrooms, onion, celery, and apple in hot butter for 5-10mins until tender.
- Into the bread mixture, mix onion mixture then gently stir in cream, chicken broth, and turkey until it is well incorporated. Spread the

mixture onto the buttered baking dish; use aluminum foil to cover.
- Bake for half an hour in the preheated oven; take off the foil cover then bake for another 20mins until brown on top.

Nutrition Information

- Calories: 405 calories;
- Total Fat: 28.1
- Sodium: 447
- Total Carbohydrate: 31.2
- Cholesterol: 67
- Protein: 7.9

91. Gluten Free Turkey Meatballs

Serving: 40 | Prep: 15mins | Cook: 30mins | Ready in:

Ingredients

- 3/4 pound ground turkey
- 1/2 pound chicken sausage, casings removed
- 2/3 cup gluten-free bread crumbs
- 3 tablespoons chopped fresh basil
- 3 tablespoons milk
- 2 teaspoons minced garlic
- 1/4 cup grated Parmesan cheese
- 1 teaspoon kosher salt
- 1/2 teaspoon ground black pepper
- 1 egg, lightly beaten

Direction

- Preheat an oven to 175°C/350°F. Line parchment paper on baking sheet.
- Mix black pepper, kosher salt, parmesan cheese, garlic, milk, basil, bread crumbs, chicken sausage and ground turkey in bowl; gently mix with fork. Drop mixture on prepped baking sheet with a spoon, 1 1/4-in. diameter per meatball.
- In preheated oven, bake for 30 minutes till lightly browned and cooked through. An inserted instant-read thermometer in middle should register 74°C/165°F minimum.

Nutrition Information

- Calories: 32 calories;
- Sodium: 114
- Total Carbohydrate: 1.3
- Cholesterol: 15
- Protein: 2.9
- Total Fat: 1.6

92. Goat Cheese And Spinach Turkey Burgers

Serving: 4 | Prep: 10mins | Cook: 15mins | Ready in:

Ingredients

- 1 1/2 pounds ground turkey breast
- 1 cup frozen chopped spinach, thawed and drained
- 2 tablespoons goat cheese, crumbled

Direction

- Preheat the oven broiler.
- Stir goat cheese, spinach, and ground turkey in a mid-sized bowl. Shape the mixture into 4 patties.
- Line them on a broiler pan and set pan in the middle of the prepared oven for 15 minutes, until done.

Nutrition Information

- Calories: 278 calories;
- Total Fat: 15.3
- Sodium: 207
- Total Carbohydrate: 1.7
- Cholesterol: 137
- Protein: 31.9

93. Grandma Gladys's Zucchini Soup

Serving: 6 | Prep: 25mins | Cook: 1hours10mins | Ready in:

Ingredients

- 10 ounces ground turkey
- 3 turkey Italian sausages, casings removed
- 1 cup chopped green bell pepper
- 2/3 cup chopped onion
- 4 stalks celery, thinly sliced
- 2 (28 ounce) cans stewed tomatoes
- 6 zucchini, cut into cubes
- 4 (10.75 ounce) cans low-sodium chicken broth
- 1 tablespoon Italian seasoning
- 1/2 teaspoon sea salt
- 1/2 teaspoon dried tarragon
- 1/2 teaspoon garlic powder
- ground black pepper to taste
- 1/4 cup grated Parmesan cheese, or to taste

Direction

- Mix and cook celery, onion, bell pepper, sausage and ground turkey in a big pot on medium high heat for 10-12 minutes till veggies are tender and meat isn't pink anymore.
- Mix black pepper, garlic powder, tarragon, sea salt, Italian seasoning, chicken broth, zucchini and tomatoes into the turkey mixture; boil. Lower the heat to low; simmer for 1 hour till flavors merge. Put soup into bowls; garnish using parmesan cheese.

Nutrition Information

- Calories: 277 calories;
- Sodium: 1283
- Total Carbohydrate: 25.4
- Cholesterol: 73
- Protein: 25.7
- Total Fat: 10

94. Grandma's Easy Turkey Taco Salad

Serving: 6 | Prep: 20mins | Cook: 10mins | Ready in:

Ingredients

- 1 pound ground turkey
- 1 (1.25 ounce) package taco seasoning mix
- 1 (15 ounce) can black beans, rinsed and drained
- 1 head iceberg lettuce, shredded
- 2 tomatoes, diced
- 1 (10 ounce) bag tortilla chips, coarsely crumbled
- 1 (8 fluid ounce) bottle thousand island dressing

Direction

- Heat the large skillet over medium-high heat. Add the ground turkey and let it cook and stir, until the turkey is browned evenly, crumbly and no longer pinkish. Follow the package directions on mixing the taco seasoning mix. Remove the mixture from heat.
- In a large bowl, mix the lettuce, tortilla chips, black beans, turkey, and tomatoes. Toss the mixture with the salad dressing. You can refrigerate it for an hour before serving or you can serve it immediately.

Nutrition Information

- Calories: 553 calories;
- Total Fat: 32.7
- Sodium: 1130
- Total Carbohydrate: 48.5
- Cholesterol: 69
- Protein: 19.8

95. Granny's Easy Turkey Pie

Serving: 6 | Prep: 10mins | Cook: 35mins | Ready in:

Ingredients

- 1 tablespoon vegetable oil
- 1 pound ground turkey
- 1 onion, chopped
- 1 pinch salt and ground black pepper to taste
- 1 pinch ground celery seed, or to taste
- 1 (10.75 ounce) can condensed cream of celery soup
- 1 cup milk
- 1 egg
- 1 (14.5 ounce) can peas and carrots, drained
- 1 cup shredded Cheddar cheese
- 1 (8 ounce) can refrigerated crescent rolls

Direction

- Set the oven to 350°F (175°C) and start preheating. Use cooking spray to coat a 9x12-inch baking dish.
- Over medium heat, in a skillet, heat vegetable oil; cook onion and ground turkey for about 10 minutes until the turkey is no longer pink. Season onion and turkey with ground celery seed, black pepper and salt; crumble the turkey as it cooks. Drain if needed. Mix carrots, peas, egg, milk and cream of celery soup together until combined thoroughly. Scoop the cooked turkey mixture into the prepared baking dish; top with the soup mixture. Place a layer of Cheddar cheese on top. Unroll crescent dough; top over cheese.
- Bake in the prepared oven for about 25 minutes until crescent dough turns golden brown and filling is bubbling.

Nutrition Information

- Calories: 464 calories;
- Total Fat: 26.4
- Sodium: 1044
- Total Carbohydrate: 29.8
- Cholesterol: 115
- Protein: 27.3

96. Greek Turkey Burgers

Serving: 8 | Prep: 15mins | Cook: 10mins | Ready in:

Ingredients

- 2 pounds ground turkey
- 1 1/2 cups fresh bread crumbs
- 1 1/2 cups chopped baby spinach
- 1/2 cup light Greek dressing
- 5 ounces feta cheese, cubed
- 1/4 large onion, finely chopped
- 1 egg
- salt and ground black pepper to taste

Direction

- Preheat outdoor grill to medium high heat; oil grate lightly.
- Mix black pepper, salt, egg, onion, feta cheese, Greek dressing, spinach, breadcrumbs and turkey in a bowl; shape to patties.
- On preheated grill, cook turkey burgers, 5-10 minutes per side, till juices are clear and not pink anymore in the center. An inserted instant-read thermometer in middle should read at least 74°C/165°F.

Nutrition Information

- Calories: 331 calories;
- Protein: 28.7
- Total Fat: 16.3
- Sodium: 583
- Total Carbohydrate: 17
- Cholesterol: 123

97. Grilled Turkey Burgers With Cranberry Horseradish Dressing

Serving: 8 | Prep: 25mins | Cook: 10mins | Ready in:

Ingredients

- 1 (14.5 ounce) can whole berry cranberry sauce
- 2 tablespoons prepared horseradish
- 3 tablespoons lemon juice, or to taste
- 1 pinch ground cumin
- salt and black pepper to taste
- 1 egg
- 1/2 cup minced celery
- 1/2 cup minced onion
- 1 1/2 pounds ground turkey
- 1 tablespoon chopped fresh thyme
- 1 tablespoon poultry seasoning
- 1 tablespoon chopped fresh parsley
- 1 cup dry bread crumbs
- 8 hamburger buns, split

Direction

- Prepare the outdoor grill and preheat it at medium-high heat. Oil the grate lightly. In a bowl, combine the cranberry sauce, cumin, horseradish, and lemon juice. Flavor them with salt and pepper; set aside.
- Use your hand to combine the onion, egg, and celery in a bowl until the egg is smooth. Stir in bread crumbs, thyme, parsley, poultry seasoning, and turkey until well-combined. Form the mixture into 8 patties.
- Place the patties onto the preheated grill and cook each side for 4 minutes until the juices run clear and the meat is no longer pink. Make sure that the inserted instant-read thermometer on its center reads at least 165°F (74°C). Assemble it into the hamburger buns and top with cranberry sauce. Serve.

Nutrition Information

- Calories: 395 calories;
- Total Fat: 10.1
- Sodium: 426
- Total Carbohydrate: 53
- Cholesterol: 86
- Protein: 23.4

98. Ground Turkey Burritos

Serving: 10 | Prep: 15mins | Cook: 16mins | Ready in:

Ingredients

- 1 (16 ounce) package ground turkey
- salt and ground black pepper to taste
- 1 (15 ounce) can black beans
- 1 (10 ounce) can diced tomatoes and green chiles (such as RO*TEL®)
- 1 tablespoon cooking oil, or as needed
- 10 (8 inch) flour tortillas (such as Mission®)
- 1 (16 ounce) package shredded Cheddar cheese

Direction

- Over medium heat, in a skillet, brown turkey for 5-7 minutes until no longer pink. Sprinkle with pepper and salt to season; drain and get rid of excess grease. Add diced tomatoes and black beans; cook for about 5 minutes until warm. Lower the heat to low.
- Set the oven to 300°F (150°C) and start preheating.
- Over low heat, in a skillet, warm cooking oil. Heat tortillas, one tortilla at a time, for about 1 minute each. Fill with turkey mixture; top with cheese. Arrange burritos on a baking sheet.
- Bake for about 5 minutes in the prepared oven until cheese melts.

Nutrition Information

- Calories: 462 calories;
- Total Fat: 23.3
- Sodium: 829
- Total Carbohydrate: 35.9
- Cholesterol: 81

- Protein: 27.2

99. Ground Turkey Burritos That Will Fool Your Kids

Serving: 12 | Prep: 20mins | Cook: 1hours | Ready in:

Ingredients

- water to cover
- 1 cup uncooked brown rice
- 1 head red cabbage
- 1/4 cup olive oil
- 1/2 red onion, chopped
- 1 stalk celery, finely chopped
- 1 clove garlic, minced
- 1 pound ground turkey
- sea salt to taste
- 1 (8 ounce) can crushed tomatoes
- 12 (10 inch) flour tortillas

Direction

- Boil brown rice and water in a saucepan. Lower heat to medium low then cover; simmer for 45-50 minutes till liquid is absorbed and rice is tender.
- Cut red cabbage stem off; gently peel off leaves, don't tear. Gently put individual leaves in a big pot of water; boil. Cook it for 5 minutes; lower heat. Simmer for 8-10 minutes till tender yet crunchy and red; drain.
- In a big skillet, heat olive oil on medium high heat. Sauté garlic, celery and onion for 5-7 minutes till soft. Mix turkey meat in; season with salt. Mix and cook for 5-7 minutes till crumbly and browned. Add cooked rice and crushed tomatoes; cook for 10-15 minutes till flavors combine, occasionally mixing.
- Put 1 cabbage leaf over each tortilla. Use turkey-rice mixture to fill. Fold the bottom end up; roll to a tight burrito.
- Heat a grill pan on medium heat. In batches, add burritos; cook, flipping if needed, for 5 minutes till outsides are crunchy.

Nutrition Information

- Calories: 401 calories;
- Total Fat: 13.4
- Sodium: 542
- Total Carbohydrate: 55.1
- Cholesterol: 28
- Protein: 15.9

100. Ground Turkey Enchilada Stew With Quinoa

Serving: 8 | Prep: 10mins | Cook: 4hours5mins | Ready in:

Ingredients

- 1 pound ground turkey
- 1 (19 ounce) can enchilada sauce
- 1 (15 ounce) can black beans, drained
- 1 1/2 cups uncooked quinoa
- 1 (10 ounce) can diced tomatoes and green chiles, undrained
- 1 cup water
- 1 cup frozen corn
- 1/2 cup salsa
- 1/2 cup chopped onion
- 1/2 cup chopped green bell pepper
- 1 tablespoon chili powder
- 1 teaspoon minced garlic
- 1 teaspoon ground cumin
- 2 cups shredded Mexican cheese blend
- 1/3 cup chopped fresh cilantro

Direction

- Heat a large frying pan over medium-high heat. In the hot skillet, cook and mix turkey for 5 – 7 minutes until crumbly and browned. Drain and remove the grease.
- In a slow cooker, blend cumin, garlic, chili powder, green bell pepper, onion, salsa, corn,

water, chiles, diced tomatoes, quinoa, black beans, enchilada sauce, and browned turkey.
- Cook on High for around 4 hours in the slow cooker until quinoa is softened and flavors are combined. Fold in cilantro and Cheddar cheese.

Nutrition Information

- Calories: 452 calories;
- Protein: 27.7
- Total Fat: 19.4
- Sodium: 943
- Total Carbohydrate: 43.6
- Cholesterol: 77

101. Ground Turkey Noodle Bake

Serving: 6 | Prep: 15mins | Cook: 35mins | Ready in:

Ingredients

- 3 cups wide egg noodles
- 1 pound ground turkey
- 1 onion, chopped
- 1 (15 ounce) can tomato sauce
- 1 teaspoon Italian seasoning
- 1/2 cup milk
- 4 ounces cream cheese
- 1 tablespoon minced fresh parsley
- 1 clove garlic, minced
- 1 1/4 cups shredded part-skim mozzarella cheese

Direction

- Set the oven at 375°F (190°C) and start preheating. Lightly coat an 8-in. square baking dish with a grease.
- Boil a large pot of lightly salted water. Cook egg noodles in boiling water while stirring occasionally for around 5 minutes, or till cooked through but still firm when bitten; drain.
- Place a large skillet over medium-high heat; stir in onion and turkey. Cook while stirring for around 10 minutes, or till the turkey mixture is not pink anymore, evenly browned and crumbly; drain. Mix in Italian seasoning and tomato sauce; boil. Turn the heat down to low; simmer with a cover for 10 minutes.
- In a small saucepan, mix garlic, parsley, cream cheese and milk together. Cook, stirring over medium heat for 5 minutes till the cream cheese melts.
- Toss the noodles with the cream cheese mixture; move to the prepared baking dish. Spread the turkey mixture on top; sprinkle mozzarella cheese over all.
- Bake in the preheated oven for 15-30 minutes, or till the cheese is melted.

Nutrition Information

- Calories: 346 calories;
- Protein: 26.7
- Total Fat: 17.4
- Sodium: 625
- Total Carbohydrate: 21.5
- Cholesterol: 109

102. Ground Turkey Taco Meat

Serving: 4 | Prep: 10mins | Cook: 16mins | Ready in:

Ingredients

- 1 1/2 tablespoons chili powder
- 2 teaspoons ground cumin
- 1 teaspoon ground paprika
- 1 teaspoon salt
- 1/2 teaspoon garlic powder
- 1/2 teaspoon onion powder
- 1/2 teaspoon dried oregano
- 1/4 teaspoon cayenne pepper

- 1 (12 ounce) package ground turkey
- 1/2 cup water
- 1 tablespoon cider vinegar
- 1 1/2 teaspoons brown sugar

Direction

- In a small bowl, combine cayenne, oregano, onion powder, garlic powder, salt, paprika, cumin and chili powder.
- In a large nonstick skillet over medium heat, cook turkey in 3-5 minutes until it is no longer pink, stir to break up clumps. Add water and chili powder mixture; stir well. Lower the heat; let it simmer for about 10 minutes with occasional stirs until almost all the liquid is absorbed.
- Add brown sugar and cider vinegar to the skillet and stir well. Let it simmer for 3-4 minutes until the flavors blend together. Serve in a serving bowl.

Nutrition Information

- Calories: 150 calories;
- Cholesterol: 63
- Protein: 17.6
- Total Fat: 7.2
- Sodium: 663
- Total Carbohydrate: 4.8

103. Ground Turkey Tacos

Serving: 4 | Prep: 10mins | Cook: | Ready in:

Ingredients

- Tacos:
- 1 tablespoon vegetable oil
- 1 pound lean (at least 93%) ground turkey
- 1 (1 ounce) package Old El Paso® taco seasoning mix
- 2/3 cup water
- 1 (4.6 ounce) package Old El Paso® taco shells
- Toppings:
- 2 medium avocados, pitted, peeled and sliced
- 1 cup sliced pineapple (fresh or canned)

Direction

- Heat up the oil in a 10-inch pan on medium-high heat. Cook the turkey until it is no longer pink, then drain.
- Stir in water and taco seasoning mix. Turn the heat down and simmer without a cover until it thickens, around 5-10 minutes.
- Spoon the filling into the taco shells. Add the toppings.

Nutrition Information

- Calories: 549 calories;
- Sodium: 872
- Total Carbohydrate: 39.1
- Cholesterol: 84
- Protein: 26.7
- Total Fat: 33.8

104. Ground Turkey Zucchini Boats

Serving: 6 | Prep: 10mins | Cook: 15mins | Ready in:

Ingredients

- 6 zucchini, ends trimmed
- salt and ground black pepper to taste
- 1 pound lean ground turkey
- 1 (16 ounce) bag fresh spinach
- 1 (14.5 ounce) can fire-roasted diced tomatoes
- 1 cup low-fat cottage cheese
- 1/2 cup shredded mozzarella cheese, or to taste
- 1 pinch red pepper flakes (optional)

Direction

- In a big skillet, put the zucchini with approximately half cup of water. Add pepper

- and salt to season, place on the cover, and let it steam for 10 minutes till soft. Allow to drain.
- In a skillet over medium heat, cook and mix the turkey until browned for approximately 8 minutes. Put in fire-roasted tomatoes and spinach. Let it simmer for about 4 minutes till spinach wilts. Mix in cottage cheese for about 3 minutes till heated through.
- Halve every zucchini lengthwise. Top with scoop of turkey mixture and jazz up with mozzarella cheese. For additional kick, put on several red pepper flakes.

Nutrition Information

- Calories: 225 calories;
- Sodium: 535
- Total Carbohydrate: 12.3
- Cholesterol: 65
- Protein: 26.6
- Total Fat: 8.5

105. Ground Turkey, Black Bean, And Kale Soup

Serving: 12 | Prep: 45mins | Cook: 30mins | Ready in:

Ingredients

- 2 pounds ground turkey
- 3 cups chopped red onion
- 2 cups diced celery
- 2 tablespoons minced garlic
- 1 tablespoon minced fresh ginger root
- 2 tablespoons water
- 8 cups vegetable broth
- 6 cups peeled and cubed butternut squash
- 6 cups roughly chopped kale
- 1 (15 ounce) can great Northern beans, drained and rinsed
- 1 (15 ounce) can black beans, drained and rinsed
- 1 (15 ounce) can butter beans, drained and rinsed
- 2 teaspoons dried basil
- 2 teaspoons dried thyme
- 1 teaspoon ground cumin
- salt and ground black pepper to taste

Direction

- In a big pot, combine ginger, garlic, water, celery, red onion, and turkey over medium-high heat. Sauté about 10 minutes until turkey is not pink anymore and vegetables are softened. Put in cumin, thyme, basil, butter beans, black beans, great Northern beans, kale, butternut squash, and broth; heat to a boil. Put cover and decrease to low heat. Allow to simmer for 15-20 minutes until vegetables are tender. Season with pepper and salt.

Nutrition Information

- Calories: 301 calories;
- Protein: 24.6
- Total Fat: 6.7
- Sodium: 659
- Total Carbohydrate: 38
- Cholesterol: 56

106. Guacamole Turkey Burger

Serving: 6 | Prep: 10mins | Cook: 15mins | Ready in:

Ingredients

- 8 Ball Park® Hamburger Buns
- 2 tablespoons extra virgin olive oil
- Burgers:
- 8 ground turkey breast patties
- 3 teaspoons garlic granules
- 1 teaspoon kosher salt
- 1 teaspoon ground black pepper
- 1 teaspoon ground cumin
- 1 teaspoon sweet paprika
- 1 tablespoon extra virgin olive oil

- Guacamole:
- 4 ripe avocados
- 1/4 cup finely chopped green onion
- 1/2 lemon, juiced
- 1/2 lime, juiced
- 1 teaspoon chili powder
- 2 tablespoons favorite Mexican salsa
- kosher salt to taste
- Trimmings: as desired, such as mayo, lettuce, tomato, onion and pickles

Direction

- For guacamole, halve the avocados lengthways. Get rid of the pit and take out the avocado flesh into a bowl using a spoon.
- Put in salt, salsa, chili powder and juices then use a fork to mash until nicely chunky.
- Use plastic to cover and put aside. If you want to make guacamole 1 hour in advance or so, press plastic wrap on the guacamole's surface to prevent air from reaching the avocado that makes it turn brown so you can keep it fresh in its bowl in the fridge.
- Mix together paprika, cumin, pepper, salt and garlic together in a bowl until blend thoroughly.
- Use olive oil to brush both sides of each patty and sprinkle on both sides with seasoning blend.
- Cook patties with a cover in a grill pan or skillet on moderately high heat until no pink left, about 5-6 minutes each side. If you are putting in cheese, do this for the final one minute of cooking process.
- Use melted butter to brush both sides of each bun and warm them in a separate skillet on moderately high heat just until toasty, about 15 seconds each side.
- Put on each bottom bun with patties then put guacamole and other preferred trimmings on top. Serve with some salsa alongside.

Nutrition Information

- Calories: 404 calories;
- Total Fat: 10

- Sodium: 740
- Total Carbohydrate: 36.2
- Cholesterol: 94
- Protein: 44.6

107. Hawaiian Stuffed Peppers

Serving: 6 | Prep: 30mins | Cook: 1hours20mins | Ready in:

Ingredients

- 1 tablespoon olive oil
- 1 tablespoon coconut oil
- 2 large onions, sliced
- 1 1/2 teaspoons Chinese five-spice powder
- 1 pound lean ground turkey
- 1 1/2 cups light coconut milk
- 1 cup water
- 1 cup jasmine rice
- 1 cup pineapple tidbits
- 6 large red bell peppers - halved, seeded, and stemmed
- 6 slices Monterey Jack cheese, halved
- 6 slices pepper jack cheese

Direction

- In a skillet set on low heat, add coconut and olive oil; stir and cook onions in the hot oil for approximately 1 hour until golden brown and tender. Take the caramelized onions from pan.
- Change the heat under skillet to medium-high. Dust Chinese five-spice powder on turkey. Stir and cook the turkey in hot skillet for approximately 10 minutes until crumbly and browned.
- Stir pineapple, caramelized onions, rice, water, and coconut milk in the ground turkey. Make it boil, lower heat, and simmer for approximately 25 minutes until rice becomes tender.
- Prepare the oven by preheating to 400°F (200°C). Prepare a 9x13-inch casserole dish that is greased.

- Place water in a pot and make it boil; add red bell pepper halves in the boiling water and cook for approximately 10 minutes until slightly tender. Strain.
- In prepared casserole dish, arrange the red bell pepper halves; scoop turkey mixture to every half. Put a slice of pepper jack cheese on each top of stuffed pepper.
- Place in preheated oven then bake for approximately 20 minutes until cheese is dissolved and bubbly.

Nutrition Information

- Calories: 580 calories;
- Cholesterol: 96
- Protein: 30
- Total Fat: 29.4
- Sodium: 297
- Total Carbohydrate: 48.7

108. Healthier World's Best Lasagna

Serving: 12 | Prep: 30mins | Cook: 2hours30mins | Ready in:

Ingredients

- 1 pound turkey sausage
- 3/4 pound lean ground turkey
- 1/2 cup minced onion
- 2 cloves garlic, crushed
- 1 (28 ounce) can crushed tomatoes
- 2 (6 ounce) cans tomato paste
- 2 (6.5 ounce) cans canned tomato sauce
- 1/2 cup water
- 1 1/2 teaspoons dried basil leaves
- 1/2 teaspoon fennel seeds
- 1 teaspoon Italian seasoning
- 1/4 teaspoon ground black pepper
- 2 tablespoons chopped fresh parsley
- 12 lasagna noodles
- 16 ounces ricotta cheese
- 3/4 pound low fat mozzarella cheese, sliced
- 3/4 cup grated Parmesan cheese

Direction

- Heat a big frying pan or Dutch oven on medium heat, then cook and stir the garlic, onion, ground turkey and turkey sausage for about 15 minutes until it turns well brown. Stir in water, tomato sauce, tomato paste and crushed tomatoes. Sprinkle 2 tbsp. of parsley, pepper, Italian seasoning, fennel seeds and basil to season. Let it simmer for about 1 1/2 hours without a cover, stirring from time to time.
- Set an oven to preheat to 190°C (375°F).
- Boil a big pot of lightly salted water. Cook the lasagna in the boiling water, stirring from time to time, for about 8 minutes until firm to the bite yet cooked through, then drain.
- In the bottom of a 9x13 baking dish, spread 1 1/2 cups of the turkey sauce and layout 6 noodles lengthwise on top of the sauce. Spread 1/2 of the ricotta on top of the noodles, then put 1/3 of the slices of mozzarella cheese on top. Spoon 1 1/2 cups of the turkey sauce on top of the mozzarella and sprinkle 1/4 cup Parmesan cheese on top. Redo the layers and put Parmesan cheese and leftover mozzarella on top. Use aluminum foil to cover, but make sure the foil doesn't touch the cheese to avoid it from sticking.
- Let it bake in the preheated oven for about 25 more minutes until the cheese melts and the sauce becomes hot. Take off the foil and let it bake for about 25 minutes until the cheese turns golden brown. Allow it to cool for 15 minutes prior to serving.

Nutrition Information

- Calories: 390 calories;
- Sodium: 1129
- Total Carbohydrate: 33.4
- Cholesterol: 81
- Protein: 33.1
- Total Fat: 15.4

109. Healthy Turkey Loaf

Serving: 5 | Prep: 15mins | Cook: 25mins | Ready in:

Ingredients

- 1/2 pound ground turkey
- 1 egg
- 1/4 cup salsa
- 1/8 cup chopped red bell pepper
- 1/8 cup chopped yellow bell pepper
- 1/4 cup chopped onion
- 1/4 cup dry bread crumbs
- lemon pepper to taste

Direction

- Set the oven to 350°F (175°C) and start preheating.
- Mix lemon pepper, bread crumbs, onion, yellow bell pepper, red bell pepper, salsa, egg and turkey in a large bowl. Use hands to well mix until blended. Roll into a small loaf; put on a baking sheet lined with foil.
- Bake for 25 minutes in the prepared oven.

Nutrition Information

- Calories: 112 calories;
- Total Carbohydrate: 6.1
- Cholesterol: 73
- Protein: 10.3
- Total Fat: 5.1
- Sodium: 174

110. Healthy Turkey Tex Mex Chili

Serving: 4 | Prep: 15mins | Cook: 1hours | Ready in:

Ingredients

- 1 1/2 cups dry black beans
- 2 tablespoons olive oil
- 1 pound ground turkey
- 1 large sweet onion, chopped
- 1 (28 ounce) can diced tomatoes
- 3 ears corn, kernels cut from cob
- 1 tablespoon maple syrup
- 1 tablespoon molasses
- 1 tablespoon Hungarian paprika
- 1 tablespoon chili powder
- 1 tablespoon garlic powder
- 1/2 teaspoon chipotle chile powder
- 1/4 teaspoon cayenne pepper
- sea salt to taste
- 1 (8 ounce) container plain yogurt (optional)
- 1 bunch green onions, diced (optional)

Direction

- Place black beans in a large pot, pour in water to cover; bring to a boil. Lower the heat to medium-low; cook at a simmer for 30-40 minutes until tender; drain. Place beans back to the pot.
- Over medium heat, in a large cast-iron skillet, heat olive oil. Cook while stirring turkey in hot oil for about 10 minutes until browned completely; add sweet onion and keep cooking while stirring for about 10 more minutes until onion becomes translucent. Add to black beans.
- Stir sea salt, cayenne pepper, chipotle chile powder, garlic powder, chili powder, Hungarian paprika, molasses, maple syrup, corn kernels and tomatoes into the black bean mixture; bring to a simmer; cook for 15-20 minutes until heated through. Place yogurt and green onions on top of servings of chili.

Nutrition Information

- Calories: 657 calories;
- Cholesterol: 87
- Protein: 45.2
- Total Fat: 18.3
- Sodium: 541

- Total Carbohydrate: 82.4

111. Healthy And Savory Turkey Meatballs

Serving: 6 | Prep: 20mins | Cook: 45mins | Ready in:

Ingredients

- cooking spray
- 1 pound lean ground turkey
- 1 pound artichoke- and spinach-flavored ground sausage
- 3/4 cup crushed buttery round crackers
- 2 eggs, beaten
- 1/2 cup soy milk
- 1/2 cup chopped onion
- 1 teaspoon Worcestershire sauce
- 1 teaspoon Italian seasoning
- 1 teaspoon garlic salt
- 1 cup ketchup
- 1/2 cup packed sucralose and brown sugar blend (such as Splenda® Brown Sugar)
- 1 tablespoon Worcestershire sauce
- 1/2 cup grated Parmesan cheese

Direction

- Set the oven to 400°F (200°C) and start preheating. Use cooking spray to spray 20 muffin cups.
- In a bowl, mix garlic salt, Italian seasoning, a teaspoon Worcestershire sauce, onion, soy milk, eggs, crackers, ground sausage and ground turkey. Fill turkey mixture 3/4 full in each muffin cup.
- In a bowl, mix a tablespoon Worcestershire sauce, brown sugar blend and ketchup together until smooth; scoop over each muffin cup; sprinkle with Parmesan cheese.
- Bake in the prepared oven for 45-50 minutes until meatballs are cooked through. The inserted instant-read thermometer into the center should register at least 165°F (74°C).

Nutrition Information

- Calories: 600 calories;
- Total Fat: 33.9
- Sodium: 1895
- Total Carbohydrate: 39
- Cholesterol: 167
- Protein: 33.1

112. Hearty Meatball Soup I

Serving: 6 | Prep: 30mins | Cook: 50mins | Ready in:

Ingredients

- 1 pound ground turkey
- 1 egg
- 1/4 cup chopped onion
- 1/2 teaspoon garlic salt
- 1/4 teaspoon ground black pepper
- 1 tablespoon vegetable oil
- 1 cube beef bouillon cube
- 1 1/2 cups water
- 1 (10.75 ounce) can condensed cream of mushroom soup
- 4 carrots, coarsely chopped
- 2 stalks celery, chopped
- 1 onion, chopped
- 1 (11 ounce) can whole kernel corn, drained

Direction

- Combine pepper, garlic salt, onion, egg, and ground turkey. Use a tablespoon measure to shape meatballs.
- In a frying pan, heat the oil over medium heat. Brown meatballs in the hot oil. On the paper towel, line the meatballs to drain.
- In a soup pot with boiling water, dissolve the bouillon cube. Mix in the undiluted mushroom soup. Add the corn, onion, celery, and carrots. Put meatballs into the soup, then let boil. Lower heat, then simmer for 25 - 30 minutes.

Nutrition Information

- Calories: 260 calories;
- Total Carbohydrate: 20
- Cholesterol: 91
- Protein: 17.3
- Total Fat: 13
- Sodium: 898

113. Herb & Garlic Turkey Burgers

Serving: 4 | Prep: 10mins | Cook: 20mins | Ready in:

Ingredients

- 1 pound ground turkey
- 1 (14.5 ounce) carton Campbell's® Creamy Herb & Garlic with Chicken Stock Soup
- 4 slices Swiss cheese
- 4 slices bacon, cut in half and cooked
- 4 Pepperidge Farm® Sesame Topped Hamburger Buns, split

Direction

- In a big bowl, combine 1/4 cup of soup and turkey together. Form the turkey mixture firmly into four burgers with the thickness of 1/2 inch.
- In a 10-in. skillet, heat 1 tbsp. of vegetable oil on moderately high heat. Put in burgers and cook until both sides are well-browned, about 10 minutes. Drain any fat.
- Put into the skillet with leftover soup and bring to a boil. Lower heat to low and cook with a cover until burgers are heated through. Put cheese on top of burgers and cook until cheese has melted.
- Put 1 tbsp. of soup and 2 bacon pieces on top of each burger, then serve burgers on buns together with leftover soup.

Nutrition Information

- Calories: 500 calories;
- Sodium: 926
- Total Carbohydrate: 33.3
- Cholesterol: 113
- Protein: 31.3
- Total Fat: 24.2

114. Hidden Veggie Meatloaf

Serving: 6 | Prep: 25mins | Cook: 1hours30mins | Ready in:

Ingredients

- 1 pound lean ground beef
- 2/3 pound ground turkey
- 1 egg
- 3/4 cup finely chopped celery
- 3/4 cup regular rolled oats
- 1/2 cup skim milk
- 1/2 cup ketchup
- 1/2 cup finely chopped onion
- 1/2 cup finely chopped green bell pepper
- 1 tablespoon dried parsley
- 1 teaspoon dry mustard powder
- 2/3 teaspoon salt
- 1/2 teaspoon minced garlic
- 1/2 teaspoon ground black pepper

Direction

- Set the oven to 325° F (165° C) to preheat.
- In a bowl, mix together black pepper, minced garlic, salt, dry mustard, parsley, green pepper, onion, ketchup, skim milk, rolled oats, celery, egg, ground turkey and ground beef, until completely combined; the mixture should be moist. Move the mixture to a 5x9-inch loaf pan.
- Bake for about 1 1/2 hours in the prepared oven until an instant-read meat thermometer reads at least 160° F (70° C) after inserted into the middle of the meatloaf. Due to ketchup, the meatloaf may still be pink inside.

Nutrition Information

- Calories: 310 calories;
- Sodium: 590
- Total Carbohydrate: 15.6
- Cholesterol: 118
- Protein: 28.4
- Total Fat: 14.8

115. Hill Country Turkey Chili With Beans

Serving: 8 | Prep: 10mins | Cook: 1hours35mins | Ready in:

Ingredients

- 3 tablespoons olive oil
- 1 pound ground turkey
- 3 cloves garlic, minced
- 1 (14 ounce) can beef broth
- 1 (28 ounce) can crushed tomatoes
- 1 onion, chopped
- 1 (15 ounce) can tomato paste
- 1 (10 ounce) can diced tomatoes and green chiles (such as RO*TEL®)
- 1 (15 ounce) can black beans, rinsed and drained

Direction

- Heat olive oil over medium heat in a large pot; cook and stir garlic and ground turkey in hot oil until completely browned, for 5 to 7 minutes.
- Transfer the beef broth over browned turkey mixture, heat to a boil, lower the heat to medium-low, and cook for 20 minutes.
- Mix green chiles, diced tomatoes, tomatoes paste, onion, and crushed tomatoes in the turkey mixture; heat to a boil, lower the heat to medium-low, and cook at a simmer until thickened, for approximately 1 hour.
- Blend black beans into the chili; cook until the beans are heated through, for extra 10 minutes.

Nutrition Information

- Calories: 273 calories;
- Sodium: 1089
- Total Carbohydrate: 30.3
- Cholesterol: 42
- Protein: 19.5
- Total Fat: 10.2

116. Homemade BBQ Meatballs

Serving: 30 | Prep: 45mins | Cook: 1hours | Ready in:

Ingredients

- 4 eggs, beaten
- 1/2 cup vodka
- 1/2 cup water
- 1 tablespoon Worcestershire sauce
- 2 tablespoons dried minced onion flakes
- 1 teaspoon garlic powder, or to taste
- 1/2 teaspoon salt, or to taste
- 1/2 teaspoon ground black pepper, or to taste
- 3 pounds ground beef
- 2 pounds ground turkey
- 1 (15 ounce) package Italian seasoned bread crumbs
- 2 (28 ounce) cans crushed tomatoes
- 2 (14.25 ounce) cans tomato puree
- 1 (18 ounce) bottle hickory smoke flavored barbeque sauce
- 1 (8 ounce) can crushed pineapple
- 1 cup brown sugar
- 1 (14 ounce) bottle ketchup
- 1/2 cup vodka
- 2 tablespoons dried minced onion flakes
- 1 teaspoon garlic powder, or to taste
- 1/2 teaspoon salt, or to taste

- 1/2 teaspoon ground black pepper, or to taste

Direction

- In a large bowl, combine Worcestershire sauce, half a cup of vodka and eggs. Put in garlic powder, 2 tablespoons onion flakes, pepper and salt to taste. Mix in bread crumbs, ground turkey and ground beef. Form into meatballs, and put aside.
- In a very large pot over medium heat, combine tomato puree, crushed tomatoes, pineapple, barbeque sauce, ketchup, brown sugar, and half a cup of vodka. Add garlic powder, onion flakes, pepper and salt for seasoning. Let it boil, lower the heat and let it simmer.
- Heat a large heavy skillet over medium heat. Cook meatballs until brown evenly on all sides. Carefully arrange into sauce, and simmer for at least one hour.

Nutrition Information

- Calories: 369 calories;
- Total Carbohydrate: 34.9
- Cholesterol: 87
- Protein: 17.3
- Total Fat: 16.3
- Sodium: 885

117. Homemade Dog Food

Serving: 5 | Prep: 5mins | Cook: 25mins | Ready in:

Ingredients

- 6 cups water
- 1 pound ground turkey
- 2 cups brown rice
- 1 teaspoon dried rosemary
- 1/2 (16 ounce) package frozen broccoli, carrots and cauliflower combination

Direction

- Put rosemary, rice, ground turkey ad water into a large Dutch oven. Stir until ground turkey is broken up and distributed evenly throughout the mixture; bring to a boil over high heat; lower heat to low and simmer for 20 minutes. Add frozen vegetables; cook for 5 more minutes. Take out of the heat; cool. Keep in the fridge until using.

Nutrition Information

118. Homemade Sausage

Serving: 4 | Prep: 10mins | Cook: 10mins | Ready in:

Ingredients

- 1 teaspoon salt
- 1 teaspoon crumbled dried sage
- 1/2 teaspoon ground black pepper
- 1/4 teaspoon ground nutmeg
- 1/8 teaspoon red pepper flakes
- 1 pinch ground ginger
- 1 pound ground turkey

Direction

- In a small bowl, stir ginger, red pepper flakes, nutmeg, black pepper, sage and salt. Put turkey in another bowl; mix in the spices thoroughly. Shape sausage into patties.
- Over medium heat, in a skillet, fry sausage patties for 3-5 minutes on each side until browned and the inside of meat is no longer pink.

Nutrition Information

- Calories: 170 calories;
- Protein: 22.5
- Total Fat: 8.7
- Sodium: 646
- Total Carbohydrate: 0.6

- Cholesterol: 84

119. Homemade Turkey Breakfast Sausage

Serving: 10 | Prep: 10mins | Cook: 10mins | Ready in:

Ingredients

- 2 teaspoons dried sage
- 2 teaspoons salt
- 1 teaspoon ground black pepper
- 1/2 teaspoon red pepper flakes
- 1/4 teaspoon dried marjoram
- 2 pounds ground turkey

Direction

- In a small bowl, combine marjoram, red pepper flakes, black pepper, salt and sage. Put turkey in a large bowl; use your hands to combine spice mixture into the turkey; shape into patties.
- Over medium-high heat, in a large skillet, cook patties for about 5 minutes on each side until the center is no longer pink and juices run clear. The inserted instant-read thermometer into the center should register at least 165°F (74°C).

Nutrition Information

- Calories: 135 calories;
- Sodium: 517
- Total Carbohydrate: 0.3
- Cholesterol: 67
- Protein: 18
- Total Fat: 6.9

120. Homemade Turkey Chorizo

Serving: 4 | Prep: 10mins | Cook: 10mins | Ready in:

Ingredients

- 1 pound ground turkey
- 1 tablespoon apple cider vinegar
- 2 teaspoons chili powder
- 2 teaspoons smoked paprika
- 2 teaspoons garlic powder
- 1 teaspoon kosher salt
- 1 teaspoon ground cumin
- 1 teaspoon ground coriander
- 1 teaspoon dried oregano
- 1/2 teaspoon ground black pepper
- 1/4 teaspoon red pepper flakes
- 1 tablespoon olive oil, or more to taste

Direction

- In a medium-size bowl, add the turkey, red pepper flakes, pepper, oregano, coriander, cumin, salt, garlic powder, paprika, chili powder, and vinegar. Mix thoroughly by hand. For best flavor, refrigerate for 8 hours to overnight.
- In a skillet, heat olive oil over medium heat. Cook chorizo while breaking apart the chorizo with a wooden spoon for 8 to 10 minutes, or until browned.

Nutrition Information

- Calories: 216 calories;
- Total Fat: 12.6
- Sodium: 560
- Total Carbohydrate: 3.4
- Cholesterol: 84
- Protein: 23.3

121. Idahoan Mexican Casserole

Serving: 6 | Prep: | Cook: | Ready in:

Ingredients

- 1 (4 ounce) package Idahoan® Bacon & Cheddar Chipotle Flavored Mashed Potatoes
- 1 tablespoon olive oil
- 1 medium onion, chopped
- 1 clove garlic, minced
- 2 teaspoons chili powder
- 1/2 teaspoon ground cumin
- 1 teaspoon salt
- 1/4 teaspoon black pepper
- 1 pound ground turkey (or ground beef)
- 1 (14.5 ounce) can diced tomatoes with chiles
- 1 (4 ounce) can chopped green chilies
- 1 cup corn, canned or frozen
- 1 (2.25 ounce) can sliced olives

Direction

- Prepare the oven by preheating to 350°F. Use cooking spray to coat a 9x9-inch baking dish. Ready mashed potatoes based on the directions of the package. Reserve.
- In a big sauté pan set on medium-high heat, add oil. Put the onions and cook for approximately 10 minutes until translucent.
- Place in the ground turkey then cook until browned.
- Mix in olives, corn (drained if using canned), green chiles, and tomatoes with the juice. Heat well.
- Transfer the meat mixture into prepared baking dish. Put a layer mashed potatoes on top.
- Bake in the preheated oven for 30 minutes. Allow it to stand for 10 minutes prior to serving.
- And grease, as it is, yet also yummy, served with hot sauce, salsa, or a dollop of sour cream.

Nutrition Information

- Calories: 210 calories;
- Protein: 17.1
- Total Fat: 10
- Sodium: 1194
- Total Carbohydrate: 15.2
- Cholesterol: 56

122. Italian Style Turkey Meatloaf

Serving: 6 | Prep: 10mins | Cook: 50mins | Ready in:

Ingredients

- cooking spray
- 1 pound ground turkey
- 1 egg
- 1/4 cup Italian seasoned bread crumbs
- 1 teaspoon Italian seasoning
- 1/2 clove garlic, minced
- 1/2 teaspoon ground black pepper, or to taste
- 1/4 teaspoon salt, or to taste
- 2 cups tomato sauce, divided

Direction

- Start preheating the oven to 200°C (400°F). Spray the cooking spray onto a baking dish.
- In a large bowl, combine salt, black pepper, garlic, Italian seasoning, breadcrumbs, egg and turkey; form the mixture into a loaf and place into the prepared baking dish.
- Bake it for 40 minutes in the preheated oven. Pour half of the tomato sauce over the loaf and keep baking for 10-15 minutes more, or until the meatloaf's middle is not pink anymore. If you insert an instant-read thermometer in the middle of the loaf, it should reach a minimum of 70°C (160°F). Let the meatloaf rest for 5-10 minutes before cutting to serve.
- Meanwhile, in a small saucepan, warm the remaining tomato sauce on medium-low heat;

serve the sliced meatloaf with the warmed tomato sauce.

Nutrition Information

- Calories: 163 calories;
- Total Fat: 7
- Sodium: 651
- Total Carbohydrate: 8.1
- Cholesterol: 87
- Protein: 17.8

123. Italian Turkey Meatloaf

Serving: 4 | Prep: 10mins | Cook: 1hours | Ready in:

Ingredients

- 1 pound ground turkey
- 1 cup Italian-style bread crumbs
- 2 eggs
- 1/4 cup finely chopped onion
- 1/4 cup grated Parmesan cheese
- 1/4 teaspoon ground black pepper
- 1 (14 ounce) jar marinara sauce, divided

Direction

- Set the oven to 350°F (175°C) to preheat.
- In a large bowl, mix together turkey, pepper, Parmesan cheese, onion, eggs and breadcrumbs. Stir in 1 cup of marinara sauce.
- Using wet hands, firmly pat and shape the turkey mixture into an 8x4-inch loaf pan. Pour the rest of the marinara sauce over the loaf.
- Bake for about 1 hour in the prepared oven until no pink remains in the center of the meatloaf. An instant-read thermometer should show at least 160°F (70°C) when inserted into the center. Allow to sit for 20 minutes before slicing.

Nutrition Information

- Calories: 420 calories;
- Total Fat: 16.5
- Sodium: 775
- Total Carbohydrate: 34.4
- Cholesterol: 183
- Protein: 33

124. Jan's Yummy Spaghetti

Serving: 8 | Prep: 20mins | Cook: 1hours10mins | Ready in:

Ingredients

- 1 pound Italian sausage links
- 1 pound ground turkey
- 1 onion, chopped
- 5 cloves garlic, minced
- 6 (8 ounce) cans tomato sauce
- 1 (15 ounce) can chopped tomatoes
- 2 (6 ounce) cans tomato paste
- 1 tablespoon white sugar
- 1 tablespoon dried oregano
- 1 tablespoon dried basil
- 1 tablespoon dried parsley
- 1 (16 ounce) package spaghetti

Direction

- Boil a pot of water; cook sausage in boiling water for about 5 minutes until cooked partially. Take sausage out of the water; slice.
- Over medium-high heat, heat a large skillet. In the hot skillet, cook while stirring garlic, onion and ground turkey for 5-7 minutes until crumbly and browned; drain and get rid of grease. Stir parsley, basil, oregano, sugar, tomato paste, chopped tomatoes, tomato sauce and sausage into ground turkey; bring to a boil; stir frequently. Lower the heat and simmer while stirring occasionally for about an hour until sausage is cooked fully and flavors have blended.
- Boil a large pot of lightly salted water. Cook spaghetti while stirring occasionally in the

boiling water for about 12 minutes until cooked through but firm to the bite. Drain; place spaghetti in a serving bowl; pour sauce on top. Toss to coat.

Nutrition Information

- Calories: 595 calories;
- Sodium: 1744
- Total Carbohydrate: 66.8
- Cholesterol: 85
- Protein: 31.7
- Total Fat: 23.6

125. Jay's Spicy Slow Cooker Turkey Chili

Serving: 8 | Prep: 20mins | Cook: 8hours | Ready in:

Ingredients

- 2 pounds ground turkey
- 1 (1.25 ounce) package taco seasoning mix
- 1 yellow onion, chopped
- 1 (14.5 ounce) can crushed tomatoes, drained
- 1 (15 ounce) can kidney beans, drained and rinsed
- 1 (10.75 ounce) can condensed tomato soup
- 1/2 (15 ounce) can black beans, drained and rinsed
- 1/4 cup chili powder
- 3 canned green chile peppers, sliced
- 1 tablespoon diced peppers from adobo sauce with chipotle peppers, or more to taste
- 2 teaspoons chile-garlic sauce (such as Sriracha®)
- 1 teaspoon ground black pepper
- 1 teaspoon salt
- 1 teaspoon dried basil
- 1 teaspoon paprika
- 1 teaspoon cayenne pepper

Direction

- Over medium-high heat, heat a big skillet. In hot skillet, cook and mix ground turkey for 5 to 7 minutes till crumbly and browned; let drain and throw the grease. Into the ground turkey, mix taco seasoning till equally coated.
- In a slow cooker, combine cayenne pepper, paprika, basil, salt, black pepper, chili-garlic sauce, chipotle peppers from adobo sauce, green chili peppers, chili powder, black beans, tomato soup, kidney beans, crushed tomatoes, onion and seasoned ground turkey.
- Allow to cook on Low for 8 to 9 hours or approximately 4 hours on High.

Nutrition Information

- Calories: 309 calories;
- Total Fat: 9.9
- Sodium: 1595
- Total Carbohydrate: 28.1
- Cholesterol: 84
- Protein: 28.9

126. Jesse's Spicy Veggie And Turkey Meatball Stew

Serving: 12 | Prep: 20mins | Cook: 1hours | Ready in:

Ingredients

- 2 pounds ground turkey
- 5 tablespoons vegetable oil, divided
- 2 large green bell peppers, cut into strips
- 1 large red bell pepper, cut into strips
- 1 large yellow bell pepper, cut into strips
- 2 large onions, cut into 1/2 inch chunks
- 2 cups sofrito sauce
- 1 (15 ounce) can tomato sauce
- 4 medium potatoes, cut into 1/2 inch chunks
- 4 carrots, sliced
- 2 cups broccoli
- 5 cups water
- 1 cup salsa
- 16 ounces low fat mozzarella cheese, shredded

Direction

- Roll the ground turkey into small meatballs. In a skillet, heat 1 tablespoon oil over medium heat; add meatballs and cook until browned evenly, or for 5 minutes. Drain and put aside.
- Heat the remaining oil over medium heat in a large pot; cook onions, yellow bell pepper, red bell pepper, and green bell pepper until softened. Mix in tomato sauce, and sofrito; keep cooking until thoroughly heated. Stir in broccoli, carrots, and potatoes. Add salsa, and water; bring to a boil. Put meatballs into the pot. Turn the heat to low, and simmer for about half an hour. Atop with mozzarella cheese before serving.

Nutrition Information

- Calories: 437 calories;
- Total Fat: 23.8
- Sodium: 827
- Total Carbohydrate: 27.6
- Cholesterol: 85
- Protein: 31.3

127. Jive Turkey Burgers

Serving: 8 | Prep: 15mins | Cook: 15mins | Ready in:

Ingredients

- 2 tablespoons olive oil
- 1 small onion, diced
- 1 large clove garlic, minced
- 1 pound ground turkey
- 1 pound turkey sausage, casings removed
- 1 egg
- 3 tablespoons chopped fresh flat-leaf (Italian) parsley
- salt and ground black pepper to taste (optional)

Direction

- Over medium heat, in a skillet, heat olive oil; cook while stirring garlic and onion for about 3 minutes until fragrant and soft; take out of the heat.
- In a large bowl, stir together pepper, salt, onion mixture, parsley, egg, turkey sausage and ground turkey. Measure 8 equal portions by an ice cream scoop; pat each into a burger shape gently.
- Over medium-low heat, in a large skillet, pan fry the burgers for about 4 minutes on each side until browned and the inside of the pink is no longer pink. The inserted instant-read meat thermometer into the burgers' center should register at least 160°F (70°C).

Nutrition Information

- Calories: 224 calories;
- Protein: 22.5
- Total Fat: 14.6
- Sodium: 538
- Total Carbohydrate: 1.2
- Cholesterol: 111

128. Joy's Lebanese Stuffed Zucchini

Serving: 6 | Prep: 25mins | Cook: 1hours15mins | Ready in:

Ingredients

- 6 zucchini, trimmed and halved lengthwise
- 2 teaspoons ground cinnamon
- 1 teaspoon minced garlic
- 1 teaspoon ground black pepper
- 2 (14 ounce) cans chicken broth
- 1 pound ground turkey
- 1 1/2 cups uncooked brown rice
- 1 tablespoon garlic powder

Direction

- Turn the oven to 450°F (230°C) to preheat.
- , scoop each zucchini half to remove the pulp and dispose. In a deep glass baking dish, put in the zucchini.
- Mix 1/2 teaspoon pepper, 1/2 teaspoon minced garlic, and 1 teaspoon cinnamon into each chicken broth can.
- Stuff the turkey mixture into each zucchini half. Top the bottom halves with the top halves to resemble whole zucchini. Pour into the baking dish and over the zucchini with the second seasoned chicken broth can. Put on aluminum foil to cover.
- Bake for 75 minutes in the preheated oven until the zucchini is tender and the rice is soft.

Nutrition Information

- Calories: 320 calories;
- Sodium: 683
- Total Carbohydrate: 42.8
- Cholesterol: 59
- Protein: 20.9
- Total Fat: 7.5

129. Kate's Turkey Meatballs

Serving: 15 | Prep: 30mins | Cook: 15mins | Ready in:

Ingredients

- 1 white onion, chopped
- 1 tablespoon minced garlic
- 2 pounds ground turkey
- 1 pound ground turkey breast
- 2 eggs
- 1 cup Italian-style bread crumbs (such as Progresso®)
- 1/4 cup skim milk
- 1 tablespoon ground black pepper
- 1 tablespoon dried oregano
- 1 tablespoon dried basil
- 1 tablespoon kosher salt
- 2 tablespoons olive oil, or as needed

Direction

- In a frying pan, mix together the garlic and onion on medium heat. Let it cook for 3-5 minutes until it becomes soft, then move to a big bowl.
- Add the salt, basil, oregano, black pepper, milk, bread crumbs, eggs, ground turkey breast and ground turkey to the bowl with the onions. Stir well and shape it into around 60 even-sized balls.
- In a big frying pan, heat the olive oil on medium heat. Fry the meatballs for around 10 minutes, until it has no visible pink color on the inside and turns brown on the outside. Add the cooked meatballs to the sauce.

Nutrition Information

- Calories: 184 calories;
- Protein: 21.6
- Sodium: 497
- Total Carbohydrate: 6.9
- Cholesterol: 88
- Total Fat: 7.7

130. Ke's Cajun (Dirty) Rice

Serving: 6 | Prep: 15mins | Cook: 1hours | Ready in:

Ingredients

- 1 1/2 cups water
- 2/3 cup uncooked brown rice
- 1/2 pound ground turkey
- 1/2 cup chopped green bell pepper
- 1/3 cup chopped onion
- 1/2 teaspoon minced garlic
- 1/2 teaspoon garlic powder
- 1/2 teaspoon dried celery flakes
- 1 teaspoon Cajun seasoning
- 1/4 teaspoon ground black pepper
- 1/3 cup water
- 1 pinch salt, or to taste

Direction

- Fill a saucepan with 1 1/2 cups of water and bring to a boil. Stir in brown rice, then reduce the heat. Simmer, covered, for 40 to 50 minutes, until the rice has absorbed the liquid and is tender. Set aside.
- Place a skillet over medium heat; cook and stir ground turkey for 2 to 3 minutes, until some of the fat gives up. Stir in minced garlic, onion, and green bell pepper. Cook and stir for 5 to 8 minutes more , until the vegetables are tender and the meat is not pink anymore and crumbly. If needed, drain off any excess grease. Stir in 1/3 cup of water, black pepper, Cajun seasoning, celery flakes, garlic powder, and cooked brown rice.
- Bring to a simmer and cook for 10 minutes, until the liquid is absorbed. If you'd like, add salt and extra black pepper to season.

Nutrition Information

- Calories: 141 calories;
- Cholesterol: 28
- Protein: 9.4
- Total Fat: 3.5
- Sodium: 107
- Total Carbohydrate: 18.1

131. Kelly's Enchiladas

Serving: 7 | Prep: 20mins | Cook: 40mins | Ready in:

Ingredients

- 1 pound lean ground turkey
- 2 large carrots, grated
- 2 tablespoons dried minced onion
- 1 diced fresh jalapeno pepper, or to taste
- 1 (1.25 ounce) package taco seasoning mix
- 1/2 teaspoon kosher salt
- 1/4 cup water
- hot garlic-pepper sauce (such as Tabasco® Garlic Pepper Sauce)
- 1 cup plain Greek yogurt
- 1 (10.75 ounce) can condensed cream of chicken soup
- 2 cups shredded queso quesadilla (Mexican melting cheese)
- 7 (6 inch) flour tortillas
- 1/2 (14.5 ounce) can red enchilada sauce

Direction

- Turn the oven to 350°F (175°) to preheat.
- Place a big frying pan on medium-high heat, and mix in kosher salt, 1/2 packet of taco seasoning, jalapeno pepper, onion, grated carrots, and ground turkey. Stir and cook until the turkey is not pink anymore, turning brown evenly, and crumbly. Mix in the leftover taco seasoning, a few dashes of hot sauce, and water. Simmer until the water evaporates.
- In a bowl, mix together queso quesadilla cheese, cream of chicken soup, and yogurt.
- On a work surface, put 1 tortilla, and then scoop some of the turkey mixture halfway between the middle and bottom edge of the tortilla. Put on the turkey with 2-3 tablespoons of the cheese mixture. Roll up the tortilla to the top edge to make a tight cylinder. Put in a 7x11-in. baking dish. Continue with the rest of the ingredients (You will not use all of the cheese sauce).
- Mix into the leftover cheese mixture with the enchilada sauce. Scoop on top of the tortillas. Put in the preheated oven and bake for 30-35 minutes until the cheese melts and the sauce is bubbling.

Nutrition Information

- Calories: 414 calories;
- Total Fat: 18.5
- Sodium: 1341
- Total Carbohydrate: 30.9
- Cholesterol: 84
- Protein: 29.1

132. Kelly's Hot Hash

Serving: 8 | Prep: 20mins | Cook: 35mins | Ready in:

Ingredients

- 1 pound ground turkey
- 2 tablespoons olive oil
- 1 leek, minced
- 1 red bell pepper, minced
- 1 carrot, peeled and minced
- 1 small zucchini, peeled and cut into small dice
- 4 crimini mushrooms, minced
- 1 pound baby kale, roughly chopped
- salt and ground black pepper to taste
- 1 dash Buffalo-style hot pepper sauce (such as Tabasco®)

Direction

- Heat a big skillet on medium heat; mix and cook turkey in hot skillet till crumbly and browned for 5-7 minutes. Drain grease; discard. Put browned turkey into a bowl.
- Heat olive oil on medium heat in the same skillet; mix and cook red bell pepper and leek for 5 minutes till leek is soft. Add carrot; cook for 5 minutes till carrot is soft. Mix crimini mushrooms and zucchini with leek mixture; mix and cook for 10 minutes till mushrooms are fully tender. Put kale over veggie mixture; mix into mixture while it wilts. Mix and cook for 5 minutes.
- Put browned turkey into skillet; mix with veggies. Season with pepper, salt and hot sauce; mix and cook for 2-3 minutes till turkey is reheated.

Nutrition Information

- Calories: 162 calories;
- Total Fat: 8.2
- Sodium: 93
- Total Carbohydrate: 9.8
- Cholesterol: 42
- Protein: 14.1

133. Kickin' Spicy Turkey Beer Chili

Serving: 8 | Prep: 30mins | Cook: 2hours15mins | Ready in:

Ingredients

- 1 tablespoon olive oil
- 1 pound ground turkey
- 1 teaspoon paprika
- salt and ground black pepper to taste
- 4 jalapeno peppers with seeds, chopped
- 1 large white onion, chopped
- 3 cloves garlic, minced
- 4 stalks celery, chopped
- 1 green bell pepper, chopped
- 3 chipotle peppers in adobo sauce, chopped
- 1 (28 ounce) can diced tomatoes with juice
- 1 (28 ounce) can tomato sauce
- 2 (16 ounce) cans spicy chili beans
- 1 (12 fluid ounce) can or bottle dark beer, such as porter
- 1/4 cup Worcestershire sauce
- 1 (1.25 ounce) package reduced-sodium chili seasoning (such as McCormick Chili Seasoning Mix 30% Less Sodium®)
- 1 dash liquid smoke flavoring, or to taste

Direction

- Heat olive oil in a big pot over medium heat, and let the turkey cook till not pink anymore; scatter black pepper, salt and paprika on turkey meat. Mix in chipotle peppers, green pepper, celery, garlic, onion and jalapeno peppers, then let cook for 15 minutes, mixing frequently, till onion is translucent and turkey meat is falling apart.
- Mix in liquid smoke flavoring, chili seasoning, Worcestershire sauce, dark beer, chili beans, tomato sauce and diced tomatoes. Lower the

heat and allow to simmer for a minimum of 2 hours, mixing from time to time.

Nutrition Information

- Calories: 298 calories;
- Total Fat: 7.4
- Sodium: 1422
- Total Carbohydrate: 38.4
- Cholesterol: 42
- Protein: 20.2

134. King Of The Hill Frito® Pie

Serving: 4 | Prep: 10mins | Cook: 10mins | Ready in:

Ingredients

- 1 pound lean ground turkey
- 2 (8 ounce) cans tomato sauce
- 1 (10 ounce) can petite diced tomatoes with green chiles
- 1 (6 fluid ounce) can tomato juice, or more to taste
- 1 (1.25 ounce) package mild chili seasoning mix
- 1 (16 ounce) package corn chips (such as Fritos®)
- 1/2 cup shredded Cheddar cheese, or to taste

Direction

- Heat a big frying pan on medium-high heat. Stir and cook the turkey in the hot frying pan for 5-7 minutes until turning brown and crumbly. Strain and dispose the grease.
- Mix chili seasoning mix, tomato juice, diced tomatoes, and tomato sauce into the turkey; simmer for another 5 minutes until the chili is hot.
- In a big bowl, put corn chips and put turkey chili on top. Sprinkle over the chili with Cheddar cheese.

Nutrition Information

- Calories: 871 calories;
- Total Fat: 46
- Sodium: 2663
- Total Carbohydrate: 85.6
- Cholesterol: 98
- Protein: 36.5

135. Kristin's Turkey Butternut Squash Casserole

Serving: 6 | Prep: 15mins | Cook: 35mins | Ready in:

Ingredients

- 1 tablespoon olive oil
- 1 pound lean ground turkey
- 2 cups cubed butternut squash
- 1 onion, chopped
- 1 cup 1% milk
- 1 cup shredded mozzarella cheese
- 1/4 cup butter, melted
- 2 eggs
- 1/2 teaspoon salt
- 1/4 teaspoon ground black pepper
- 1 cup crushed buttery round crackers (such as Ritz®)

Direction

- Start preheating the oven to 375°F (190°C). Lightly coat a 9-inch square baking dish with oil.
- In a skillet, heat olive oil over medium heat. Cook while stirring the ground turkey for 5-10 mins or until browned and crumbly. Put onion and butternut squash into the ground turkey; Cook while stirring for 5-10 mins until the squash is slightly tender. Drain the excess grease from pan.
- In a bowl, whisk together pepper, salt, eggs, butter, mozzarella cheese and milk. Mix into

the turkey mixture. Place the squash-turkey mixture into the prepared baking dish. Top with crackers.
- Bake in the prepared oven for 25-30 mins or until bubbling and cooked through.

Nutrition Information

- Calories: 509 calories;
- Protein: 26
- Total Fat: 31.2
- Sodium: 793
- Total Carbohydrate: 31.9
- Cholesterol: 152

136. Larb Gai Nikki Style

Serving: 4 | Prep: 20mins | Cook: 10mins | Ready in:

Ingredients

- Dressing:
- 2 lemons, juiced
- 1 lime, juiced
- 2 tablespoons fish sauce, or more to taste
- 1 tablespoon rice vinegar
- 1 teaspoon white sugar
- 1 teaspoon cayenne pepper
- 1 teaspoon lemon zest
- 1 pound ground turkey
- 1 clove garlic, minced
- 1 cup water to cover
- 1/2 red onion, thinly sliced
- 1 carrot, shredded
- 1/2 cup coarsely chopped chestnuts
- 3 Thai chile peppers, sliced
- 3 green onions, sliced
- 1/4 cup chopped fresh mint
- 1/3 cup chopped fresh Thai basil
- 2 tablespoons chopped fresh cilantro
- 3 tablespoons toasted rice powder
- 2 tablespoons Thai chile flakes

Direction

- In a bowl, mix lemon zest, cayenne, sugar, rice vinegar, fish sauce, lime juice and lemon juice till dressing is smooth in consistency.
- Spread ground turkey in a big skillet in a thin layer; add in garlic. Cover the turkey with enough water in the skillet; boil. Cook and stir turkey mixture, using fork to fluff meat apart, till turkey is crumbly and brown in color for 7 to 10 minutes. Drain liquid and transfer turkey into a big glass bowl.
- Combine cilantro, basil, mint, green onions, Thai chile peppers, chestnuts, carrot and red onion into turkey till combined well. Put in the refrigerator mixture till chilled for half an hour.
- Drizzle Thai chile flakes and rice powder on top of turkey mixture and combine well.

Nutrition Information

- Calories: 270 calories;
- Sodium: 630
- Total Carbohydrate: 22.3
- Cholesterol: 84
- Protein: 24.9
- Total Fat: 9.8

137. Laura's Quick Slow Cooker Turkey Chili

Serving: 8 | Prep: 15mins | Cook: 4hours | Ready in:

Ingredients

- 1 tablespoon vegetable oil
- 1 pound ground turkey
- 2 (10.75 ounce) cans low sodium tomato soup
- 2 (15 ounce) cans kidney beans, drained
- 1 (15 ounce) can black beans, drained
- 1/2 medium onion, chopped
- 2 tablespoons chili powder
- 1 teaspoon red pepper flakes
- 1/2 tablespoon garlic powder
- 1/2 tablespoon ground cumin

- 1 pinch ground black pepper
- 1 pinch ground allspice
- salt to taste

Direction

- In a skillet, heat oil on moderate heat. Put turkey into the skillet and cook until browned evenly, then drain.
- Use cooking spray to coat the inside of a slow cooker, then stir in onion, black beans, kidney beans, tomato soup and turkey. Season with salt, allspice, black pepper, cumin, garlic powder, red pepper flakes, and chili powder.
- Cover and cook on high for 4 hours or on low for about 8 hours.

Nutrition Information

- Calories: 276 calories;
- Cholesterol: 42
- Protein: 21.2
- Total Fat: 7.6
- Sodium: 547
- Total Carbohydrate: 32.8

138. Lazygirl's Ground Turkey Stroganoff

Serving: 4 | Prep: 15mins | Cook: 20mins | Ready in:

Ingredients

- 1 (8 ounce) package uncooked egg noodles
- 1 tablespoon vegetable oil
- 1 pound ground turkey
- 1 tablespoon minced onion
- 1 cube chicken bouillon, crumbled
- 1 (10.75 ounce) can condensed cream of mushroom soup
- 1/2 cup water
- 1 tablespoon paprika
- salt to taste

Direction

- Boil a pot of lightly salted water. Add the egg noodles into the pot. Cook the noodles for 6-8 minutes until al dente; drain.
- Put oil in a skillet and heat it over medium heat. Add the onion and turkey into the skillet and cook until the onion is tender and the turkey is browned evenly. Stir in bouillon.
- Mix the water and cream of mushroom soup into the skillet. Cook the mixture while stirring it until heated through. Season it with salt and paprika. Serve the mixture over the cooked egg noodles.

Nutrition Information

- Calories: 463 calories;
- Sodium: 852
- Total Carbohydrate: 41.8
- Cholesterol: 125
- Protein: 30.5
- Total Fat: 19.6

139. Lee's Taco Salad

Serving: 4 | Prep: 15mins | Cook: 15mins | Ready in:

Ingredients

- 1 tablespoon vegetable oil, or to taste
- 1 small white onion, diced
- 1 pound ground turkey
- 1 (1 ounce) package taco seasoning mix
- 1 head lettuce, chopped
- 1 (15 ounce) can corn, drained
- 1 (14 ounce) can black beans, drained
- 1 avocado - peeled, pitted, and diced
- 4 green onions, chopped (optional)
- 1/3 cup shredded Cheddar cheese
- 1/4 cup spicy ranch-style salad dressing

Direction

- Over medium heat, in a skillet, heat oil. Cook while stirring onion in hot oil for about 5 minutes until translucent. Break ground turkey into small chunks; add to skillet; cook while stirring for 2-3 minutes until starting to brown. Top turkey mixture with taco seasoning; keep cooking while stirring for 5-7 more minutes until turkey is browned through completely.
- Pile lettuce into the bottom of a large salad bowl; place turkey mixture, avocado, black beans, corn, green onions, Cheddar cheese and spicy ranch dressing on top.

Nutrition Information

- Calories: 619 calories;
- Total Carbohydrate: 52.8
- Cholesterol: 98
- Protein: 36.4
- Total Fat: 31.7
- Sodium: 1497

140. Light And Delicious Lasagna

Serving: 9 | Prep: 45mins | Cook: 1hours | Ready in:

Ingredients

- 2 1/3 tablespoons olive oil, divided
- 1 yellow onion, chopped
- 4 cloves garlic, chopped
- 1 pound ground turkey
- 3 cups fresh mushrooms, sliced
- 4 teaspoons dried basil
- 4 teaspoons dried oregano
- 1 teaspoon ground black pepper
- 2 (14.5 ounce) cans diced tomatoes
- 1 (6 ounce) can tomato paste
- 6 cups chopped fresh spinach, washed and dried
- 2 1/2 cups low-fat cottage cheese
- 4 egg whites
- 1/2 cup chopped fresh flat-leaf parsley
- 1/4 cup grated low-fat Parmesan cheese
- 8 no-boil lasagna noodles
- 3 cups zucchini, sliced
- 2 cups shredded low-fat mozzarella cheese

Direction

- Set oven temperature to 350 degrees F (174 degrees C) and leave aside for preheating. Use a teaspoon of olive oil to grease a baking tray measuring 9x13-inch.
- Add the remaining 2 tablespoons of olive oil into a large saucepan, heated to medium and cook onion and garlic for approximately 5 minutes, stirring until the onion turn translucent. Mix mushrooms, turkey, oregano, black pepper, and basil inside the saucepan, and stirring for 10-15 minutes, until turkey no longer appears rare and the mushrooms expelled their liquid. Mash the turkey meat into crumbles while cooking. Next, mix in diced tomatoes, spinach, and tomato paste into pan and stir. Continue stirring frequently for about 5 minutes and turn off the stove when the spinach leaves appear wilted.
- Combine in a bowl the egg whites, Parmesan cheese, cottage cheese, and parsley until mixed evenly. Leave to one side.
- Layer as follows; 4 lasagna noodles at the bottom of baking tray, overlapping as needed, and pour half of the turkey mix onto the noodles. Place half of the zucchini slices on the meat sauce, and add half of the cottage cheese mixture on top. Place another half of the mozzarella cheese above the cottage cheese. Continue layering in this arrangement, with four more noodles again as a base, and the remainder of the meat sauce, zucchini slices, cottage cheese mix, and mozzarella cheese.
- Bake in preheated oven for 45 minutes to an hour, until the cheese has melted and browned, and bubbles appear on the sauce.

Nutrition Information

- Calories: 351 calories;

- Sodium: 863
- Total Carbohydrate: 26.4
- Cholesterol: 56
- Protein: 34
- Total Fat: 12.6

141. Lighter Cretons

Serving: 10 | Prep: 15mins | Cook: 45mins | Ready in:

Ingredients

- 1 pound ground turkey
- 1 1/2 cups water, divided
- 1 cup chopped onion
- 1/8 teaspoon ground cloves
- 1/8 teaspoon sage
- 1/8 teaspoon ground cinnamon
- 1 (.25 ounce) package unflavored gelatin (such as Knox ®)

Direction

- Put together in a saucepan the cinnamon, sage, cloves, onion, 1 cup water and ground turkey. Make it boil, lower the heat and gently boil for 45 minutes, crushing the mixture regularly using a spatula while it's boiling; then get away from heat.
- Mix gelatin into left 1/2 cup water; add in the gelatin mixture into turkey mixture then mix. Then place it into a small container; let chill inside the refrigerator for 1 hour then serve.

Nutrition Information

- Calories: 76 calories;
- Total Carbohydrate: 1.5
- Cholesterol: 33
- Protein: 9.8
- Total Fat: 3.4
- Sodium: 29

142. Lighter Simple Lasagna Roll Ups

Serving: 4 | Prep: 40mins | Cook: 1hours | Ready in:

Ingredients

- 8 whole wheat lasagna noodles
- 1/2 pound ground turkey
- 6 cloves garlic, crushed
- 1 (10 ounce) package frozen chopped spinach, thawed and drained
- 1/2 cup chopped fresh chives
- 1/2 teaspoon dried oregano
- 1/2 teaspoon dried parsley
- 1/4 teaspoon dried basil
- 2 egg whites
- 1 (15 ounce) container reduced-fat ricotta cheese
- 2 tablespoons crumbled low-fat feta cheese
- 2 tablespoons grated Parmesan cheese
- 1/2 teaspoon ground black pepper
- 1 (28 ounce) jar low-fat tomato pasta sauce
- 1/2 cup shredded low-fat Cheddar cheese

Direction

- Set the oven at 190°C (375°F) to preheat.
- Boil a big pot of lightly salted water. Add lasagna noodles to the boiling water, cook while stirring occasionally for about 8 minutes, or until the pasta is cooked through. Drain.
- In a nonstick skillet, brown the ground turkey with garlic over medium heat for about 10 minutes, or until the turkey is not pink anymore. Break the turkey apart as it cooks. Mix the basil, parsley, oregano, chives and spinach into the ground turkey mixture. Cook until heated through, then take away from heat.
- In a bowl, lightly beat the egg whites and stir in the Parmesan, feta, and ricotta cheeses. Add black pepper to taste. Whisk the ground turkey mixture into the cheese mixture.

- On a sheet of waxed paper, line the cooked lasagna noodles flat. Equally divide the filling into eight portions and shape the fillings into balls. Arrange the balls on one end of the noodle and roll the pasta up around the filling. Repeat the process with the remaining filling and noodles.
- Spread a thin layer of pasta sauce onto the bottom of a 9x13 in. baking dish. Arrange the rolls into the baking dish, put the seam sides down. Add the remaining pasta sauce on the rolls and scatter with Cheddar cheese. Use aluminum foil to cover it.
- Bake for about 40 minutes in the preheated oven, until the cheese melts and the sauce is bubbling.

Nutrition Information

- Calories: 637 calories;
- Protein: 44.3
- Total Fat: 21.6
- Sodium: 1281
- Total Carbohydrate: 70.1
- Cholesterol: 87

143. Low Cholesterol Turkey Tacos

Serving: 6 | Prep: 20mins | Cook: 15mins | Ready in:

Ingredients

- 1 pound lean ground turkey
- 1 onion, diced
- 1/2 teaspoon chili powder
- 1/4 teaspoon garlic powder
- 1/4 teaspoon onion powder
- 1 cup Mexican salsa (such as Herdez®), drained
- 1 (4.5 ounce) can diced green chile peppers, drained
- 1 tablespoon chopped fresh cilantro, or to taste (optional)
- salt and ground black pepper to taste
- 12 taco shells
- 2 avocados, sliced, or to taste (optional)
- 1 cup shredded Monterey Jack cheese, or to taste (optional)
- 1 cup shredded lettuce, or to taste (optional)
- 1 cup diced tomatoes (optional)

Direction

- Over medium-high heat, heat a lightly oiled skillet. Sauté onion and turkey for about 8 minutes until browned. Drain; get rid of juice.
- Stir onion powder, garlic powder and chili powder into the turkey mixture until combined well. Mix in pepper, salt, cilantro, green chile peppers and salsa. Cook taco filling while stirring occasionally for 7-10 minutes until flavors meld.
- Fill taco filling into taco shells. Place tomatoes, avocado, lettuce and shredded Monterey Jack cheese on top.

Nutrition Information

- Calories: 468 calories;
- Total Fat: 27.7
- Sodium: 807
- Total Carbohydrate: 33.7
- Cholesterol: 73
- Protein: 24.8

144. Low Fat Turkey Burgers

Serving: 4 | Prep: | Cook: | Ready in:

Ingredients

- 1 pound ground turkey
- 2 cubes beef bouillon

Direction

- Set an outdoor grill to high heat to preheat and coat the grate slightly with oil.

- Mix well together bouillon and ground turkey in a big bowl, then shape the mixture into 4 patties.
- Grill patties on high heat until the internal temperature of patties reaches 70°C or 160°F, about 3 minutes each side.

Nutrition Information

- Calories: 172 calories;
- Total Fat: 9.4
- Sodium: 539
- Total Carbohydrate: 0.3
- Cholesterol: 90
- Protein: 20.1

145. Low Carb Turkey Quinoa Lasagna

Serving: 12 | Prep: 20mins | Cook: 1hours20mins | Ready in:

Ingredients

- 1/4 cup olive oil, divided
- 2 eggplants, peeled and sliced 1/8-inch thick
- 3 cloves garlic, minced
- 1 pound ground turkey
- 1 small yellow onion, chopped
- 1 cup quinoa
- salt and ground black pepper to taste
- 1 (24 ounce) jar spaghetti sauce (such as Hunt's®)
- 1 (16 ounce) package shredded mozzarella cheese
- 1 (16 ounce) package shredded Cheddar-Monterey Jack cheese blend
- 1 tablespoon Parmesan cheese (optional)

Direction

- Put 1 tbsp. of oil in a large skillet and heat it over medium-high. Working in a single layer at a time, fry slices of eggplant for 1 minute per side until soft and golden brown. Make sure to replenish oil between batches.
- Set the oven to 350°F (175°C) for preheating.
- Put 1 tbsp. of olive oil in a skillet and heat it over medium heat. Add the garlic. Cook and stir for 1 minute until fragrant. Add the onion and turkey. Cook and stir for 5 minutes until the turkey is already crumbled and not anymore pinkish. Mix in quinoa. Season the mixture with salt and pepper. Add the spaghetti sauce. Cook for 5-10 minutes until the sauce is bubbly.
- Spread the bottom of a 9x13-inches baking pan with a layer of sauce. Place an even layer of slices of eggplant and Cheddar-Monterey Jack cheese on top. Do the same layering for the remaining cheese, sauce, and eggplant. Make sure it ends with a sauce on top. Sprinkle the top with mozzarella cheese evenly. Use an aluminum foil to cover the pan.
- Let it bake inside the preheated oven for 45 minutes until the cheese is bubbly and melted. Remove the cover. Bake for 15 more minutes until the top is golden.

Nutrition Information

- Calories: 465 calories;
- Sodium: 755
- Total Carbohydrate: 25.3
- Cholesterol: 90
- Protein: 29.6
- Total Fat: 27.7

146. Low Carb, Low Fat Turkey Goulash

Serving: 6 | Prep: 15mins | Cook: 32mins | Ready in:

Ingredients

- 2 tablespoons olive oil
- 1 1/4 pounds ground turkey, or more to taste
- 2 yellow onions, diced

- 4 parsnips, diced
- 5 tablespoons paprika
- 1 clove garlic, chopped
- 1 teaspoon dried oregano
- salt to taste
- 3 cups chicken stock, or more as needed

Direction

- In a stockpot, heat the oil over medium heat. Put in turkey; cook for 5 to 7 minutes till browned and juices have cooked off. Put in onions; cook and mix for 5 minutes till transparent. Put in oregano, garlic, paprika and parsnips. Let it cook for 2 minutes, mixing often, till garlic is aromatic. Put in a pinch of salt and chicken stock. Simmer for 20 minutes to half an hour till thickened to a preferred consistency.

Nutrition Information

- Calories: 232 calories;
- Total Fat: 12.8
- Sodium: 427
- Total Carbohydrate: 11.1
- Cholesterol: 70
- Protein: 20.8

147. Low Fat Mexican Turkey Casserole

Serving: 10 | Prep: 20mins | Cook: 30mins | Ready in:

Ingredients

- 1 (16 ounce) package whole wheat rotini pasta
- 2 tablespoons olive oil
- 1 pound ground turkey
- 2 tablespoons chili powder
- 2 cloves garlic, minced
- 1 teaspoon ground cumin
- 1 teaspoon ground cayenne pepper
- 1 teaspoon dried oregano
- 1/2 teaspoon ground black pepper
- 1 (15 ounce) can yellow corn, drained
- 1 (10 ounce) can diced tomatoes and green chiles, undrained
- 1 green bell pepper, diced
- 1 onion, diced
- 1 celery stalk, diced
- 1 carrot, diced
- 1 (15 ounce) can tomato sauce
- 1 (8 ounce) package pepper Jack cheese, shredded

Direction

- Preheat oven to 175 degrees C (350 degrees F).
- Boil the big pot of the slightly-salted water; cook rotini at the boil for roughly 10 minutes or till softened but firm to bite; drain off.
- Heat the olive oil on medium-high heat in the big skillet. Put in the ground turkey and crumble using the wooden spoon. Put in the black pepper, oregano, cayenne pepper, cumin, garlic and chili powder; combine through. Cook and whisk for 5-7 minutes or till the turkey turns brown and crumbly. Put in the carrot, celery, onion, green bell pepper, chiles, diced tomatoes and corn; combine through.
- Put the lid on the skillet. Cook for roughly 8 minutes or till the veggies soften, whisk once in a while. Put in the tomato sauce; allow it to simmer for roughly 5 minutes or till thick. Move the turkey mixture into the 9x13-in. casserole plate and put in cooked pasta. Stir everything together. Add the pepper Jack cheese on top.
- Bake in preheated oven for roughly 10 minutes or till the cheese melts.

Nutrition Information

- Calories: 401 calories;
- Total Carbohydrate: 49.4
- Cholesterol: 58
- Protein: 22.8
- Total Fat: 14.8
- Sodium: 630

148. M's Sloppy Joe Sauce

Serving: 4 | Prep: 20mins | Cook: 15mins | Ready in:

Ingredients

- 1 tablespoon extra-virgin olive oil
- 1 large onion, diced
- 1 green bell pepper, diced
- 1 tablespoon minced garlic
- 1 pound ground turkey
- 1 cup canned pureed tomatoes
- 1/4 cup barbeque sauce (such as KC Masterpiece®)
- 2 tablespoons ketchup
- 2 tablespoons white vinegar
- 2 tablespoons Worcestershire sauce
- 1 tablespoon brown mustard
- 1 tablespoon chile-garlic sauce (such as Sriracha®)

Direction

- In a frying pan, heat olive oil over medium heat. In the hot oil, cook bell pepper and onion for 5 minutes until they start to get tender. Add ground turkey or garlic to the frying pan, stir and cook for 5-7 minutes until the turkey is brown and very crumbly.
- Mix chile-garlic sauce, mustard, Worcestershire sauce, vinegar, ketchup, barbeque sauce, and pureed tomatoes into the turkey mixture. Simmer for another 7-10 minutes until fully heated.

Nutrition Information

- Calories: 287 calories;
- Total Fat: 12.4
- Sodium: 865
- Total Carbohydrate: 21
- Cholesterol: 84
- Protein: 24.6

149. Maple Apple Turkey Sausage

Serving: 10 | Prep: 10mins | Cook: 6mins | Ready in:

Ingredients

- 1 pound lean ground turkey
- 1 small apple - peeled, cored, and finely chopped
- 1 tablespoon pure maple syrup, or more to taste
- 3/4 teaspoon salt
- 1/2 teaspoon dried sage
- 1/4 teaspoon garlic powder
- 1/4 teaspoon ground black pepper
- 1/4 teaspoon dried marjoram
- 1/8 teaspoon ground cinnamon
- 1 dash ground cloves
- 1 tablespoon olive oil

Direction

- Combine cloves, cinnamon, marjoram, black pepper, garlic powder, sage, salt, maple syrup, apple, and turkey in a bowl; stir to combine. Shape mixture into 10 small patties.
- Heat olive oil over medium heat in a skillet. Fry patties about 3 to 4 minutes on each side, until center is no longer pink and juices run clear. And instant-read thermometer pricked into the center should register at least 165°F (74°C).

Nutrition Information

- Calories: 92 calories;
- Cholesterol: 34
- Protein: 8.6
- Total Fat: 5.2
- Sodium: 206
- Total Carbohydrate: 3

150. Mexican Black Bean And Turkey Wraps

Serving: 4 | Prep: 10mins | Cook: 35mins | Ready in:

Ingredients

- 1 large onion, diced
- 1 pinch sea salt
- 1 pinch cayenne pepper
- 1 pound lean ground turkey
- 1 dash garlic powder
- 1 (15 ounce) can black beans, drained and rinsed
- 1 cup water
- 1 large green bell pepper, diced
- 1 (4 ounce) can chopped green chiles
- 6 tablespoons taco seasoning mix
- 1 cup cooked brown rice

Direction

- Heat a big skillet over medium-high heat and sauté onions with cayenne pepper and sea salt until they are softened, 7 minutes. Add in garlic powder and ground turkey, then cook while stirring for 5 minutes until the meat is no longer pink. Add taco seasoning, green chiles, green bell pepper, water, and black beans, mixing well. Bring heat down to low and allow to simmer, covered, for 10-15 minutes until the flavors combine.
- Stir in the cooked rice and simmer until heated through, around 3-5 minutes. Take off the heat and allow to sit for 10 minutes.

Nutrition Information

- Calories: 403 calories;
- Total Fat: 10.6
- Sodium: 1883
- Total Carbohydrate: 45.3
- Cholesterol: 90
- Protein: 30.6

151. Mexican Corn Bread Casserole With Turkey

Serving: 10 | Prep: 10mins | Cook: 20mins | Ready in:

Ingredients

- 2 pounds ground turkey
- 1 cup diced onion
- 2 cloves garlic, minced
- 1 1/2 cups salsa
- 2 teaspoons ground cumin
- 1/2 teaspoon salt
- 1/2 teaspoon ground black pepper
- 1/2 teaspoon chili powder, or to taste (optional)
- Corn Bread Base:
- 1 1/4 cups milk
- 1 cup polenta
- 1/2 cup butter, softened
- 1/2 cup corn flour
- 3 tablespoons egg whites
- 1 teaspoon baking soda
- 2 cups shredded Mexican-style Cheddar cheese blend, divided
- 2 cups salsa

Direction

- Bring a large skillet to medium-high heat. Cook while stirring garlic, onion, and turkey in the hot skillet, about 5 minutes, or until turkey is no longer pink inside. Stir in chili powder, black pepper, salt, cumin, and 1 1/2 cups salsa until well combined.
- Set oven to 425°F (220°C) to preheat.
- In a mixing bowl, stir baking soda, egg whites, corn flour, butter, polenta, and milk together. Transfer mixture to a 9x13-inch baking pan. Spread cooked ground turkey mixture over corn bread layer.
- Bake casserole for 10 minutes in the preheated oven. Scatter top with 1 1/2 cups shredded Mexican-style Cheddar cheese blend. Keep

baking for 5 minutes longer or until top is bubbly. Allow to cool for 10 minutes.
- Sprinkle the remaining 1/2 cup shredded Mexican-style cheese and 2 cups salsa over top of the casserole.

Nutrition Information

- Calories: 463 calories;
- Total Fat: 27
- Sodium: 1279
- Total Carbohydrate: 27.5
- Cholesterol: 121
- Protein: 29.8

152. Mexican Enchilada Casserole

Serving: 6 | Prep: 30mins | Cook: 30mins | Ready in:

Ingredients

- cooking spray
- 1 1/2 cups canned tomato sauce
- 1/3 cup chili powder (such as Gebhardt®)
- 1/2 cup water, or as needed
- 1 1/2 pounds ground turkey
- 1 1/2 cups chopped onion
- 2 (1 ounce) packages taco seasoning mix, divided
- 2/3 cup water
- 16 (5 inch) corn tortillas, cut in half
- 3 cups shredded sharp Cheddar cheese
- 3 cups shredded Monterey Jack cheese
- 1 1/2 (10 ounce) bags shredded iceberg lettuce
- 2 cups chopped fresh tomatoes

Direction

- Turn the oven to 425°F (220°C) to preheat. Spray cooking spray over a 3-qt. casserole dish.
- In a small saucepan, mix together 1/2 cup water or as you want, chili powder, and tomato sauce over medium heat. Simmer and whisk to form a pourable sauce. Take away from heat and put the enchilada sauce aside.
- In a big frying pan, stir and cook 1 envelope of taco seasoning mix, onion, and ground turkey over medium heat for 10 minutes, chopping turkey while cooking, until the meat is not pink anymore and crumbly. Mix in the leftover envelope of taco seasoning mix and 2/3 cup water and cook until the liquid of the turkey mixture evaporates, tossing frequently. Stir in the turkey mixture with 1 cup of enchilada sauce and take the frying pan away from heat.
- To layer the casserole, in the bottom of the prepared baking dish, spread 8 tortilla halves. If needed, overlap them to fit. In a bowl, combine Monterey Jack cheese and sharp Cheddar cheese and spread over the tortillas in an even layer of 1/4 of the cheese mixture. Put approximately 1/3 cup of the leftover sauce, 1/3 the chopped tomatoes, 1/3 the lettuce, and 1/3 the turkey mixture on top. Repeat layers twice more. Top the casserole with 8 tortilla halves and spread the leftover 1 1/4 cup shredded cheese mixture over.
- Put in the preheated oven and bake for 20-30 minutes until the cheese on top of the casserole turns brown and melts.

Nutrition Information

- Calories: 851 calories;
- Sodium: 1842
- Total Carbohydrate: 51.4
- Cholesterol: 193
- Protein: 57.3
- Total Fat: 47.8

153. Mexican Ground Turkey Dip

Serving: 18 | Prep: 20mins | Cook: 40mins | Ready in:

Ingredients

- 1 pound ground turkey
- 2 red bell peppers, chopped
- 1 large Spanish onion, chopped
- 1 jalapeno pepper, diced, or more to taste
- 2 cups salsa
- 1 cup sour cream
- 1 (1 ounce) packet taco seasoning
- 1 (1 pound) package processed cheese (such as Velveeta®), cubed
- 1 cup grated Cheddar cheese

Direction

- Preheat an oven to 175°C/350°F.
- Heat big skillet on medium high heat. Mix and cook turkey in hot skillet for 5-7 minutes till crumbly and browned. Add jalapeno pepper, onion and red bell peppers; sauté for 5 minutes till onion is just translucent.
- In big oven-safe casserole dish, mix taco seasoning, sour cream and salsa. Add processed cheese and turkey mixture; stir well. Put cheddar cheese on top.
- In preheated oven, bake for 30 minutes till top is bubbling.

Nutrition Information

- Calories: 194 calories;
- Cholesterol: 51
- Protein: 12.3
- Total Fat: 13.1
- Sodium: 667
- Total Carbohydrate: 7.1

154. Mexican Spaghetti Squash Stir Fry

Serving: 5 | Prep: 20mins | Cook: 30mins | Ready in:

Ingredients

- 1 spaghetti squash, halved and seeded
- 1 tablespoon olive oil
- 2 small green bell peppers, diced
- 1 onion, diced
- 2 cloves garlic, minced
- 1 pound lean ground turkey
- 1 (15 ounce) can black beans
- 1/4 cup sun-dried tomatoes
- 1 (6 ounce) can tomato sauce
- 1 cube chicken bouillon
- 1 tablespoon chili powder
- 1 tablespoon garlic powder
- 1 teaspoon seasoned salt
- 1/2 teaspoon ground cumin
- 1/2 teaspoon red pepper flakes (optional)

Direction

- Preheat an oven to 175°C/350°F.
- Put spaghetti squash halves on baking sheet, cut sides down.
- In preheated oven, bake for 20-30 minutes till a fork easily shreds it and flesh is tender. Use a fork to shred flesh carefully till it looks like spaghetti.
- In skillet, heat olive oil on medium heat; mix and cook garlic, onion and bell peppers in hot oil for 3-5 minutes till slightly tender. Put ground turkey in veggie mixture; mix and cook for 5-7 minutes till crumbly and browned. Drain; discard grease.
- Mix red pepper flakes, cumin, seasoned salt, garlic powder, chili powder, chicken bouillon, tomato sauce, sun-dried tomatoes and black beans into ground turkey mixture; cook for 10 minutes till flavors blend and heated through.
- Put spaghetti squash on each plate; put ground turkey mixture on top.

Nutrition Information

- Calories: 334 calories;
- Protein: 26.4
- Total Fat: 11.3
- Sodium: 1068
- Total Carbohydrate: 35.8

- Cholesterol: 67

155. Mexican Stuffed Shells

Serving: 8 | Prep: 10mins | Cook: 55mins | Ready in:

Ingredients

- 1 (12 ounce) box jumbo pasta shells
- 2 pounds ground turkey
- 1 (7 ounce) can chopped green chiles
- 3/4 cup water
- 1 (1.25 ounce) package taco seasoning
- 1 cup salsa
- 1 1/2 cups shredded Cheddar cheese

Direction

- Boil a big pot of slightly salted water. Cook the pasta shells in boiling water for 12 minutes, mixing from time to time, till soft but firm to the bite. Drain.
- Preheat the oven to 175 °C or 350 °F.
- In a big saucepan, mix taco seasoning, water, chopped green chilies and turkey; cook and mix for 8 to 10 minutes till turkey is cooked through and liquid is soaked up. Take away from heat.
- In the bottom of 9x13-inch baking pan, distribute the salsa.
- Fill some of turkey mixture into each pasta shell and set in baking dish over salsa. Scatter Cheddar cheese over top. Cover the pan using aluminum foil.
- In the prepped oven, bake for half an hour till cheese is bubbly and melted.

Nutrition Information

- Calories: 456 calories;
- Total Fat: 17.8
- Sodium: 1033
- Total Carbohydrate: 38
- Cholesterol: 111

- Protein: 35.1

156. Mexican Turkey Burgers

Serving: 6 | Prep: 20mins | Cook: 25mins | Ready in:

Ingredients

- 1 tablespoon olive oil
- 1 medium onion, finely chopped
- 1 medium green bell pepper, finely chopped
- 2 cloves garlic, minced
- 1 cup salsa
- 1 (15.25 ounce) can whole kernel corn, drained
- 1 pound ground turkey
- 1 (1.25 ounce) package taco seasoning mix
- 1/3 cup dry bread crumbs
- 6 (10 inch) flour tortillas
- 6 tablespoons sour cream
- 2 cups shredded lettuce

Direction

- Start preheating the oven to 450°F (230°C). Coat cooking spray over a medium baking dish.
- In a skillet, heat the olive oil over medium heat. Sauté garlic, green pepper and onion for 5 minutes. Discard from the heat, then slightly cool.
- Mix half of the corn and salsa in a small bowl. Mix 2 tablespoons of salsa mixture, taco seasoning and turkey with the onion mixture in a large bowl. Portion into six patties, then press all sides into breadcrumbs to coat lightly. Place the coated patties into prepared baking dish.
- In the prepared oven, bake patties for 10 minutes. Drain any liquid from the dish, turn the patties. Spread remaining salsa mixture over the patties. Bake 10 more minutes, until the internal temperature is 165°F (75°C).
- Microwave on high for 30 seconds to warm the tortillas. Cover cooked turkey patties by

warmed tortillas with lettuce and sour cream. Top with the remaining corn. Enjoy!

Nutrition Information

- Calories: 509 calories;
- Total Carbohydrate: 64.5
- Cholesterol: 62
- Protein: 25.2
- Total Fat: 17.5
- Sodium: 1445

157. Mexican Turkey Burgers With Pico De Gallo

Serving: 4 | Prep: 20mins | Cook: 10mins | Ready in:

Ingredients

- Pico de Gallo
- 3 medium tomatoes, chopped
- 1/3 cup chopped onion
- 2 cloves garlic, minced
- 1 serrano chile pepper, seeded and minced
- 1 lime, juiced
- 1/2 cup chopped fresh cilantro
- salt and pepper to taste
- Turkey Burgers
- 1 pound ground turkey
- 1 egg
- 1/2 onion, minced
- 2 cloves garlic, minced
- 1 teaspoon ground coriander
- 1/2 teaspoon celery salt
- 1 teaspoon chili powder
- 1/2 teaspoon cumin
- 1 tablespoon chopped fresh parsley

Direction

- Combine cilantro, lime juice, serrano chile pepper, 2 of the 4 cloves of minced garlic, 1/3 cup of chopped onion and tomatoes together in a bowl. Stir in pepper and salt to season to taste and put aside.
- In a bowl, add ground turkey, then put in chopped parsley, cumin, chili powder, celery salt, coriander, leftover 2 cloves minced garlic, 1/2 of the minced onion and egg. Work the mixture with your hands until entire of ingredients is blended evenly. Shape the mixture into four patties.
- Heat a big nonstick skillet on moderately high heat, then cook turkey burgers until juices run clear and not pink in the middle anymore, about 5 minutes each side. Lower heat as needed during the cooking process. Serve burgers together with Pico de Gallo salsa.

Nutrition Information

- Calories: 233 calories;
- Sodium: 576
- Total Carbohydrate: 10.4
- Cholesterol: 118
- Protein: 25.7
- Total Fat: 10.7

158. Mexican Turkey Corn Bread Casserole

Serving: 6 | Prep: 15mins | Cook: 50mins | Ready in:

Ingredients

- 1 tablespoon canola oil
- 1 pound ground turkey
- 1/4 cup fat-free chicken broth
- 1 tablespoon taco seasoning mix
- 2 ounces orzo pasta
- 1 (8 ounce) jar salsa, or to taste
- 1 (8.5 ounce) package dry corn muffin mix
- 1 (8.25 ounce) can cream-style corn
- 1 tablespoon milk
- 1 cup shredded Mexican cheese blend

Direction

- Preheat the oven to 175°C or 350°F.
- On medium-high heat, heat the oil in a big pot; add ground turkey. Cook and stir for 5-10mins, until crumbly and brown; drain the extra fat. Mix in taco seasoning mix and chicken broth; cook and stir for 3-5mins, until the liquid is thick and has reduced.
- Mix orzo with the turkey mixture, then let it simmer; cook for about 2mins, until slightly soft. Stir salsa into the turkey-orzo mixture. Move the mixture to a 2-qt. casserole dish.
- In a bowl, mix together the milk, creamed corn and muffin mix; spread on top of the turkey mixture.
- Bake for 35-40mins in the preheated oven, until an inserted skewer in the middle of the casserole comes out without residue. Spread Mexican cheese blend on top of the casserole. Bake for about 5mins, until the cheese melts.

Nutrition Information

- Calories: 466 calories;
- Sodium: 1123
- Total Carbohydrate: 46.2
- Cholesterol: 78
- Protein: 25.7
- Total Fat: 20.5

159. Mexican Turkey Dip

Serving: 16 | Prep: 5mins | Cook: 20mins | Ready in:

Ingredients

- 1 tablespoon olive oil
- 1 (16 ounce) package ground turkey
- 1/2 cup spicy salsa
- 1 (1.25 ounce) package dry taco seasoning mix
- 1 (16 ounce) can refried beans
- 1 (8 ounce) package tortilla chips
- 1/2 cup enchilada sauce
- 6 slices American cheese
- 1 (8 ounce) can sliced black olives (optional)

Direction

- Set an oven to 175°C (350°F) and start preheating.
- In a skillet, heat the olive oil on medium heat. Put in the ground turkey and cook it for 5 minutes until it is no longer pink. Combine in taco seasoning and salsa.
- In a 9x13-inch pan, place the American cheese, enchilada sauce, tortilla chips, refried beans, and turkey mixture in a layer in reverse order. Place with olives on top.
- In the prepared oven, bake for 15-20 minutes until heated thoroughly.

Nutrition Information

- Calories: 215 calories;
- Protein: 11
- Total Fat: 11.7
- Sodium: 675
- Total Carbohydrate: 17.3
- Cholesterol: 33

160. Mexican Style Spaghetti And Meatballs

Serving: 6 | Prep: 30mins | Cook: 45mins | Ready in:

Ingredients

- 1 pound ground turkey
- 1 1/2 teaspoons Mexican-style chili Powder
- 1 teaspoon guajillo chile powder
- 1/2 teaspoon salt
- 1/2 teaspoon ground black pepper
- 1 tablespoon grated Parmesan cheese
- 1 egg
- 1 tablespoon olive oil
- 1/2 onion, finely chopped
- 1 small jalapeno pepper, seeded and minced
- 1/2 Anaheim (New Mexico) chile pepper, seeded and minced
- 2 tostada shells, crushed into fine crumbs

- 1/4 cup bread crumbs
- 1 (16 ounce) package spaghetti
- 1 (14.5 ounce) can diced tomatoes
- 1/2 onion, diced
- 1 chipotle chile in adobo sauce, finely chopped
- 1 (24 ounce) jar spaghetti sauce
- 1 tablespoon taco seasoning mix

Direction

- Start preheating the oven at 175°C (350°F). On a baking sheet, lay a sheet of aluminum foil and lightly spray with cooking spray.
- In a big mixing bowl, add the ground turkey and top with the Parmesan cheese, black pepper, salt, guajillo chile powder, and Mexican chili powder. Put in Anaheim pepper, jalapeno pepper, chopped onion, olive oil, and the egg. Use your hands to mix all the ingredients together till evenly blended, then top with breadcrumbs and tostada crumbs. Mix again till the breadcrumbs are incorporated. Shape the mixture into one-inch balls and arrange on the prepared baking sheet.
- Bake the meatballs in the preheated oven for 40 minutes, or until their middles are not pink anymore and the color turns light brown. To ensure even cooking, flip the meatballs over after 20 minutes.
- Boil a big pot of lightly salted water to a rolling boil on high heat. Stir in the spaghetti once the water is boiling, then return to a boil. Do not cover the pot, cook while stirring occasionally for 12 minutes, or until the pasta is well cooked yet firm to the bite. Set a colander in the sink and strain the spaghetti well.
- After turning the meatballs, mix together taco seasoning, spaghetti sauce, chipotle chile, diced onion, and diced tomatoes in a big saucepan. Simmer the mixture on medium-high heat, then lower the heat to medium-low and simmer the mixture for 10-15 minutes until the onion becomes soft.
- Add the cooked meatballs to the sauce, cook and stir for 5 more minutes. Use a spoon to pour the meatballs and the sauce on the spaghetti, serve.

Nutrition Information

- Calories: 595 calories;
- Total Fat: 15.2
- Sodium: 1041
- Total Carbohydrate: 83.6
- Cholesterol: 94
- Protein: 28.2

161. Mexican Style Taco Salad

Serving: 6 | Prep: 25mins | Cook: 20mins | Ready in:

Ingredients

- 2 teaspoons olive oil
- 1 large onion, finely chopped
- 3 cloves garlic, minced
- 1 pound ground turkey
- 2 tablespoons chili powder
- 2 teaspoons ground cumin
- 1 teaspoon dried oregano
- 1 dash cayenne pepper
- 1 (19 ounce) can kidney beans, rinsed and drained
- 1 cup salsa
- 2 cups shredded iceberg lettuce
- 2 small carrots, julienned
- 2 red bell peppers, cut into thin strips

Direction

- Put olive oil in a skillet and heat it over medium heat. Mix in garlic and onion; cook and stir for about 5 minutes until the onion is translucent and softened. Add the turkey and then stir until it is crumbly and no longer pink. Season it with cayenne pepper, salsa, kidney beans, oregano, chili powder, and cumin. Let it cook over medium-high heat for about 5

minutes until the beans are heated through and the mixture is simmering.
- Split the lettuce, red bell peppers, and carrots into each of the 4 serving plates. Top each with the turkey mixture. Serve.

Nutrition Information

- Calories: 300 calories;
- Protein: 27.7
- Total Fat: 10.7
- Sodium: 553
- Total Carbohydrate: 25.7
- Cholesterol: 77

162. Miami Street Style Turkey Tacos

Serving: 8 | Prep: 20mins | Cook: 9mins | Ready in:

Ingredients

- 1 (16 ounce) package JENNIE-O® Lean Taco Seasoned Ground Turkey
- 3 cups shredded napa cabbage
- 1 mango, peeled and cut into thin strips
- 1/2 red bell pepper, cut into strips
- 1/4 cup chopped fresh cilantro leaves
- 1 tablespoon lime juice
- 1 tablespoon olive oil
- 1/4 teaspoon kosher salt
- 8 soft taco shells

Direction

- Cook turkey following package directions. Cook until well done, a meat thermometer should read 165 degrees F.
- In a medium bowl, mix salt, olive oil, lime juice, cilantro, red bell pepper, mango and cabbage.
- Spoon ground turkey mixture in the taco shells. Put slaw mixture on top.

Nutrition Information

- Calories: 191 calories;
- Total Fat: 9.5
- Sodium: 456
- Total Carbohydrate: 15.2
- Cholesterol: 40
- Protein: 11.2

163. Middle Eastern Rice With Black Beans And Chickpeas

Serving: 8 | Prep: 15mins | Cook: 45mins | Ready in:

Ingredients

- 1 tablespoon olive oil
- 1 clove garlic, minced
- 1 cup uncooked basmati rice
- 2 teaspoons ground cumin
- 2 teaspoons ground coriander
- 1 teaspoon ground turmeric
- 1 teaspoon ground cayenne pepper
- 1 quart chicken stock
- 1 1/2 pounds ground turkey
- 2 (15 ounce) cans garbanzo beans (chickpeas), drained and rinsed
- 2 (15 ounce) cans black beans, drained and rinsed
- 1 bunch chopped fresh cilantro (optional)
- 1 bunch chopped fresh parsley (optional)
- 1/4 cup pine nuts (optional)
- salt to taste
- ground black pepper to taste

Direction

- Heat olive oil on medium heat in the big sauce pan. Whisk in the garlic, and cook for 60 seconds. Whisk in the cayenne pepper, turmeric, coriander, cumin and rice. Cook while stirring for 5 minutes, then add the chicken stock. Boil. Lower the heat to low, covered, and let simmer for 20 minutes.

- Put turkey on medium heat in the skillet, and cook till becoming browned equally.
- Lightly mix the pine nuts, parsley, cilantro, black beans, garbanzo beans and cooked turkey to the cooked rice. Use the pepper and salt to season.

Nutrition Information

- Calories: 349 calories;
- Total Fat: 11.6
- Sodium: 267
- Total Carbohydrate: 37.7
- Cholesterol: 63
- Protein: 23.8

164. Middle Eastern Turkey Dogs

Serving: 4 | Prep: 5mins | Cook: 15mins | Ready in:

Ingredients

- 1 teaspoon ground cumin
- 1 teaspoon ground coriander seed
- 1 teaspoon ground ginger
- 1 teaspoon ground cinnamon
- 1 teaspoon fresh ground black pepper
- 1/4 teaspoon kosher salt
- 1 pound ground turkey

Direction

- Preheat the oven to 230°C or 450°F. With non-stick cooking spray, coat the baking sheet.
- Combine together salt, pepper, cinnamon, ginger, coriander and cumin in a small bowl. Break ground turkey up into crumbles in a big bowl; using your hands, gently work in seasoning mixture, dividing seasoning as equal as can be. Distribute into 8 even balls. Roll out every turkey ball on a flat area into a tube shape.

- With nonstick cooking spray, coat a big skillet, and place it on moderate heat. Put the turkey tubes into skillet; let cook, flipping often, till golden brown on every side. Turn onto a baking sheet.
- In prepped oven, let bake for 6 minutes.

Nutrition Information

- Calories: 177 calories;
- Total Fat: 9.6
- Sodium: 228
- Total Carbohydrate: 1.6
- Cholesterol: 90
- Protein: 20.1

165. Mild Mannered Chili

Serving: 10 | Prep: 15mins | Cook: 3hours5mins | Ready in:

Ingredients

- cooking spray
- 1 pound ground turkey
- 1 (28 ounce) can crushed tomatoes
- 1 (15 ounce) can black beans, rinsed and drained
- 1 (15 ounce) can kidney beans, rinsed and drained
- 1 (14.5 ounce) can diced tomatoes
- 1 (6 ounce) can tomato paste
- 3 tablespoons chili powder
- 2 teaspoons ground black pepper
- 1 teaspoon salt
- 1/2 teaspoon garlic powder

Direction

- Use cooking spray to coat the inside of a slow cooker lightly.
- Heat a big skillet on moderate high heat. Cook and stir ground turkey in the hot skillet for 5-7 minutes until crumbly and browned; drain

and get rid of grease. Put the ground turkey to the slow cooker.
- Stir into ground turkey the garlic powder, salt, black pepper, chili powder, tomato paste, diced tomatoes, kidney beans, black beans and crushed tomatoes.
- Cook on low setting for about 3 hours.

Nutrition Information

- Calories: 197 calories;
- Total Fat: 4.4
- Sodium: 838
- Total Carbohydrate: 25.4
- Cholesterol: 33
- Protein: 16.5

166. Moist Spicy Turkey Burgers

Serving: 4 | Prep: 15mins | Cook: 30mins | Ready in:

Ingredients

- 1 pound ground turkey
- 1/4 cup dry bread crumbs
- 1 onion, finely chopped
- 1 green onion, chopped
- 1 egg
- 2 cloves garlic, minced
- 2 tablespoons parsley paste
- 1 1/2 tablespoons Worcestershire sauce
- 1 tablespoon hot pepper sauce (such as Tabasco®)
- 1/2 teaspoon salt

Direction

- In a bowl, combine together salt, hot pepper sauce, Worcestershire sauce, parsley paste, garlic, egg, green onion, onion, bread crumbs and ground turkey. Use plastic wrap to cover the bowl and chill for a minimum of an hour.

- Set the oven to 175°C or 350°F to preheat. Grease a baking dish slightly.
- Shape the turkey mixture into four patties and place in a baking sheet.
- In the preheated oven, bake burgers for a half hour, until juices run clear and is not pink in the middle anymore. An instant-read thermometer should reach a minimum of 74°C or 165°F after being inserted in the center.

Nutrition Information

- Calories: 260 calories;
- Sodium: 707
- Total Carbohydrate: 14.3
- Cholesterol: 125
- Protein: 25.6
- Total Fat: 10.1

167. Moist Turkey Burgers

Serving: 12 | Prep: 15mins | Cook: 25mins | Ready in:

Ingredients

- 3 1/2 teaspoons olive oil
- 2 1/3 cups finely chopped onions
- 1 slice whole wheat bread, chopped into crumbs
- 4 teaspoons Worcestershire sauce
- 1 1/2 tablespoons Dijon mustard
- 4 cloves garlic, finely chopped
- 1 3/4 teaspoons poultry seasoning
- 1 teaspoon ground mustard
- 1 teaspoon ground black pepper
- 1 pinch salt
- 3 1/2 pounds lean ground turkey
- nonstick cooking spray

Direction

- On medium heat, heat olive oil in a small pan; add onions. Cook and stir for 15mins until light brown and tender; move to a big bowl.

- Mix the onion with salt, bread crumbs, pepper, Worcestershire sauce, ground mustard, Dijon mustard, poultry seasoning, and garlic; crumble the turkey then mix in thoroughly until well combined. Form the mixture into a dozen patties; use plastic wrap to cover. Place in the refrigerator for at least 20mins.
- Use a cooking spray to coat a non-stick pan; heat on medium heat.
- Cook patties in the hot pan for 4-5mins on each side until the juices are clear and the center is not pink. An inserted thermometer in the middle should register at least 74°C or 165°Fahrenheit.

Nutrition Information

- Calories: 233 calories;
- Cholesterol: 98
- Protein: 27.1
- Total Fat: 11.6
- Sodium: 153
- Total Carbohydrate: 5.3

168. Momma's Sloppy Joes

Serving: 6 | Prep: 15mins | Cook: 40mins | Ready in:

Ingredients

- 1 pound ground turkey
- 1 cup ketchup
- 2 tablespoons white sugar
- 2 tablespoons white vinegar
- 2 tablespoons yellow mustard

Direction

- In a large skillet over medium heat, place the turkey; cook until browned evenly, allow to drain.
- Mix the sugar, ketchup, mustard, and vinegar in a large saucepan over medium heat. Add in the turkey. Cook for around 30 minutes, stirring often.

Nutrition Information

- Calories: 170 calories;
- Sodium: 547
- Total Carbohydrate: 14.5
- Cholesterol: 56
- Protein: 15.9
- Total Fat: 6

169. Mozzarella Stuffed Pesto Turkey Meatballs

Serving: 12 | Prep: 35mins | Cook: 35mins | Ready in:

Ingredients

- 3 pounds ground turkey
- 1 cup finely chopped onion
- 4 garlic cloves, minced
- 1 egg
- 1 cup Italian-style bread crumbs
- 1/2 cup grated Parmigiano-Reggiano cheese
- 1/2 cup chopped fresh flat-leaf parsley
- 1/4 cup prepared pesto
- 1/4 cup milk
- 1 tablespoon salt
- 2 teaspoons fresh ground black pepper
- 1 pound fresh mozzarella, cut into small cubes
- 3 tablespoons extra-virgin olive oil
- 2 (24 ounce) jars marinara sauce

Direction

- Start preheating the oven at 375°F (190°C).
- Put black pepper, salt, milk, pesto, parsley, Parmigiano-Reggiano cheese, bread crumbs, egg, garlic, onion, and ground turkey in a bowl. Combine until evenly-blended, and then shape into 1 3/4-inch meatballs. Use your finger to create a hole in the meatball and put a cheese cube in the hole. Seal the meatball

around the cheese and arrange on a nonstick baking sheet. Sprinkle the olive oil over the meatballs.
- Bake in the prepared oven until the meatballs are not pink in the center anymore, in around 30 minutes. In a saucepan, heat the marinara sauce over low heat. Heat to a simmer and put the baked meatballs into the marinara sauce for approximately 2 minutes.

Nutrition Information

- Calories: 486 calories;
- Sodium: 1621
- Total Carbohydrate: 26
- Cholesterol: 130
- Protein: 38.3
- Total Fat: 25.3

170. Mum's Dairy Free Stroganoff

Serving: 6 | Prep: 5mins | Cook: 25mins | Ready in:

Ingredients

- 1 (16 ounce) package ground turkey
- 2 teaspoons garlic powder
- 2 teaspoons onion powder
- 1 (16 ounce) package egg noodles
- 1/8 cup Merlot wine
- 1/2 teaspoon salt
- 1/2 teaspoon ground black pepper
- 1/2 teaspoon Italian seasoning
- 2 drops liquid smoke flavoring, or to taste (optional)
- 1 (10 ounce) can golden mushroom soup (such as Campbell's®)

Direction

- Heat a big skillet on medium high heat; sauté the turkey in hot skillet for about 3 minutes till beginning to brown. Add onion powder and garlic powder; mix and cook for another 3-5 minutes till slightly pink and mostly browned.
- Put a big pot filled of lightly salted water on a rolling boil; mix in egg noodles. Bring back to a boil; cook pasta for approximately 6 minutes till tender but firm to bite, occasionally mixing, uncovered. Drain.
- Put Merlot into the skillet with turkey; simmer for about 5 minutes till reduced to your liking, occasionally mixing. Add liquid smoke, Italian seasoning, pepper and salt; thoroughly mix. Mix in mushroom gravy; simmer for a minimum of 5 minutes till stroganoff is thick.

Nutrition Information

- Calories: 442 calories;
- Cholesterol: 121
- Protein: 26.6
- Total Fat: 10.7
- Sodium: 588
- Total Carbohydrate: 58.5

171. Mushroom Blue Cheese Turkey Burgers

Serving: 4 | Prep: 15mins | Cook: 10mins | Ready in:

Ingredients

- 1 pound ground turkey
- 8 ounces fresh mushrooms, finely chopped
- 1 onion, finely chopped
- 2 tablespoons soy sauce
- 1/2 teaspoon kosher salt
- 1/4 teaspoon black pepper
- 1/4 cup crumbled blue cheese

Direction

- Preheat the grill for high heat.
- Combine the soy sauce, onion, mushrooms and ground turkey in a medium bowl. Add

kosher salt and pepper to taste. Shape into 4 burger patties.
- Grease grill grate lightly with oil. On the prepped grill, put the patties, allow to cook till well done, about 10 minutes each side. Put blue cheese on top on the final few minutes.

Nutrition Information

- Calories: 225 calories;
- Total Fat: 11.2
- Sodium: 877
- Total Carbohydrate: 5.3
- Cholesterol: 90
- Protein: 26.8

172. My Italian Turkey Meatballs

Serving: 4 | Prep: 30mins | Cook: 20mins | Ready in:

Ingredients

- 1 pound ground turkey
- 1/2 cup Italian-style bread crumbs
- 1/2 cup grated Parmesan cheese
- 1 egg
- 1/4 cup chopped fresh parsley
- 1/2 teaspoon kosher salt (optional)

Direction

- Set oven to 190° C (375° F) and start preheating.
- In a big bowl, combine salt, parsley, egg, Parmesan cheese, bread crumbs, and turkey. With wet hands, shape the mixture into 1 1/2 - inch-diameter balls, do not pack or handle too hard.
- Put into the preheated oven and bake 20 minutes until browned. Inserting an instant-read thermometer into the center and it should show no less than 70° C (160° F).

Nutrition Information

- Calories: 280 calories;
- Sodium: 573
- Total Carbohydrate: 10.4
- Cholesterol: 133
- Protein: 29.6
- Total Fat: 13.2

173. New York Turkey Meatball

Serving: 8 | Prep: 15mins | Cook: 25mins | Ready in:

Ingredients

- 1 (16 ounce) package JENNIE-O® Lean Italian Seasoned Ground Turkey
- 2 cloves garlic, minced
- 3 tablespoons chopped fresh basil leaves
- 1 tablespoon finely chopped fresh oregano
- 2 teaspoons grated lemon rind
- 1 large egg, lightly beaten
- 2 tablespoons dried bread crumbs
- 1 (24 ounce) jar tomato-basil pasta sauce, heated
- 1 (16 ounce) package spaghetti, cooked according to package instructions
- Grated Parmesan cheese (optional)

Direction

- Heat oven to 400 degrees F.
- In a big bowl, mix bread crumbs, egg, lemon rind, oregano, basil, garlic and turkey. Form into 1 1/2 in. balls. Put on a lightly sprayed oil baking sheet.
- Bake for 25 minutes. Cook turkey to well-done always, once meat thermometer reached 165°F. Allow meatballs to stand for 10 minutes.
- In a big bowl, toss together heated pasta sauce and meatballs. Serve over pasta, dredge in Parmesan cheese, if wanted.

Nutrition Information

- Calories: 375 calories;
- Total Fat: 8.6
- Sodium: 685
- Total Carbohydrate: 52.9
- Cholesterol: 66
- Protein: 19

174. Non Dairy Baked Penne Pasta

Serving: 12 | Prep: 30mins | Cook: 1hours5mins | Ready in:

Ingredients

- cooking spray (such as Pam®)
- 1 teaspoon extra-virgin olive oil
- 1 1/2 teaspoons salt, divided
- 1 (1 pound) package whole wheat penne pasta
- 1 pound lean ground turkey
- 1 large sweet onion, diced
- 1 red bell pepper, diced
- 3 cloves garlic, minced
- 2 teaspoons ground black pepper, divided
- 6 mild Italian sausages
- 2 (24 ounce) jars tomato and basil pasta sauce (such as Bertolli®), divided
- 1 (14.5 ounce) can petite diced tomatoes, undrained
- 1 (10 ounce) block mozzarella-style vegan cheese (such as Follow Your Heart®), shredded
- 2 (8 ounce) packages shredded mozzarella-style vegan cheese (such as Daiya®)
- 2 teaspoons garlic powder
- 1 1/2 teaspoons Italian seasoning

Direction

- Set the oven to 175°C or 350°F to preheat. Use cooking spray to coat 2 13"x9" baking dishes.
- Bring water together with 1/2 tsp. of salt and olive oil in a big pot to a boil, then put in whole wheat penne and cook for 7-10 minutes while stirring sometimes, until tender but still firm to the bite. Drain pasta.
- In a big skillet, cook and stir together 1 tsp. of black pepper, leftover salt, garlic, red bell pepper, onion and turkey over moderately low heat for 7-10 minutes, until turkey is crumbly and browned. Drain and get rid of grease.
- In a pot, add sausages and cold water to cover, then bring water to a boil. Lower heat to moderate and simmer for 20 minutes, until sausages are not pink in the middle anymore. An instant-read thermometer should reach 70°C or 160°F after being inserted in the center.
- Get rid of the sausage casings and chop sausage, then mix into the turkey mixture. Stir leftover black pepper, Italian seasoning, garlic powder, 1 package shredded mozzarella-style vegan cheese, shredded block of mozzarella-style vegan cheese, diced tomatoes, 1 1/2 jars of tomato-basil sauce and penne into the turkey-sausage mixture.
- In the bottoms of prepped baking dishes, spread leftover tomato-basil sauce. Split the turkey-sausage mixture among 2 baking dishes and put leftover shredded mozzarella-style cheese on top.
- In the preheated oven, bake for a half hour, until sauce bubbles and cheese has melted.

Nutrition Information

- Calories: 625 calories;
- Total Fat: 31.8
- Sodium: 2127
- Total Carbohydrate: 49.7
- Cholesterol: 50
- Protein: 30.8

175. One Pot Ground Turkey Black Bean Taco Soup

Serving: 12 | Prep: 20mins | Cook: 30mins | Ready in:

Ingredients

- 1 1/2 tablespoons olive oil
- 1 1/2 pounds ground turkey
- 1 red onion, chopped
- 4 cloves garlic, minced
- 2 teaspoons salt-free garlic and herb seasoning blend (such as Mrs. Dash®)
- 1 teaspoon Cajun seasoning
- 1 teaspoon garlic powder
- 1/2 teaspoon black pepper
- 1/8 teaspoon cayenne pepper, or to taste
- 1/8 teaspoon smoked paprika, or to taste
- 1 dash curry powder
- 1 dash ground cumin
- 1 (32 fluid ounce) container chicken stock
- 1 (16 ounce) jar chunky salsa
- 1 (15 ounce) can chili beans in sauce
- 1 (15 ounce) can black beans, rinsed and drained
- 1 (15 ounce) can white hominy, drained
- 1 (2.25 ounce) can sliced black olives, drained
- 2 tablespoons hot sauce (such as Taco Bell®)
- 1 (11 ounce) can condensed Cheddar cheese soup
- 1 (1 pound) package shredded Mexican cheese blend

Direction

- In a big stockpot, heat olive oil on moderately high heat. Put in cumin, curry powder, paprika, cayenne pepper, black pepper, garlic powder, Cajun seasoning, salt-free seasoning, garlic, onion and turkey, then cook and stir the mixture for 5-7 minutes, until turkey is not pink anymore.
- Lower heat to moderately low and put in hot sauce, olives, hominy, black beans, chili beans, salsa and chicken stock. Stir soup and bring it to a boil. Lower heat and simmer for 15-20 minutes, until flavors blend.
- Whisk into the stockpot with condensed Cheddar cheese soup, then take away from the heat when soup is smooth and melted, for 5 minutes. Put 1/4 cup of shredded Mexican cheese blend on top of each bowl.

Nutrition Information

- Calories: 376 calories;
- Cholesterol: 85
- Protein: 26.2
- Total Fat: 21.7
- Sodium: 1443
- Total Carbohydrate: 22.2

176. Paleo Turkey Sweet Potato Casserole With Eggplant And Tomato

Serving: 6 | Prep: 20mins | Cook: 1hours16mins | Ready in:

Ingredients

- cooking spray
- Casserole:
- 1 pound extra-lean ground turkey breast
- 1/4 cup chopped onion
- 1 tablespoon minced garlic
- 1 (15 ounce) can petite diced tomatoes, drained
- 1 (8 ounce) can tomato paste
- 1 sweet potato, peeled and cut into noodle shapes
- 1 eggplant, sliced into 1/2-inch pieces
- 1 teaspoon tarragon flakes, divided
- 1/2 teaspoon salt
- 1/2 teaspoon ground black pepper
- 1/4 teaspoon chili powder
- 1/4 teaspoon ground cumin
- 1/8 teaspoon oregano
- 1/8 teaspoon ground cardamom
- Sauce:
- 1 1/2 tablespoons extra-virgin olive oil

- 1 tablespoon almond flour
- 1 tablespoon coconut flour
- 1 cup unsweetened almond milk

Direction

- Preheat an oven to 175°C/350°F. Spray cooking spray on square 8-in pan.
- Heat big skillet on medium heat. Add garlic, onion and ground turkey; mix and cook for 5-10 minutes till turkey is browned. Mix tomato paste and diced tomatoes in. Add sweet potatoes; mix and cook for 5 minutes till slightly softened.
- Mix cardamom, oregano, cumin, chili powder, pepper, salt, 1/2 tsp. tarragon flakes and eggplant in bowl; toss till eggplant gets coated.
- On bottom of prepped pan, layer coated eggplant; put turkey mixture on top.
- In preheated oven, bake casserole for 15 minutes till sweet potatoes are browned lightly.
- Heat saucepan on high heat. Add coconut flour, almond flour and olive oil; mix and cook for 1 minute till thick. Lower heat to medium high; slowly whisk almond milk in till mixed. Cook, constantly whisking, for 10 minutes till sauce reduces by half.
- Take casserole from oven; use sauce to cover.
- In preheated oven, bake for 40-45 minutes till top of casserole is browned. Put leftover 1/2 tsp. tarragon on top. Use a sharp knife to cut to 6 pieces.

Nutrition Information

- Calories: 267 calories;
- Total Carbohydrate: 25.5
- Cholesterol: 56
- Protein: 19.4
- Total Fat: 10.6
- Sodium: 697

177. Paleo Turkey Cashew Chili

Serving: 6 | Prep: 20mins | Cook: 1hours15mins | Ready in:

Ingredients

- 3 tablespoons olive oil
- 1 white onion, chopped
- 2 teaspoons minced garlic
- 1 teaspoon sofrito
- 1 (20 ounce) package ground turkey
- 1 (28 ounce) can whole peeled tomatoes
- 1 cup water, plus more if desired
- 3/4 (6 ounce) can tomato paste, divided
- 1 cup chopped cashews
- 2 teaspoons chili powder, or more to taste
- 1 teaspoon ground cumin
- 1 teaspoon unsweetened cocoa powder
- 1 teaspoon sea salt, or to taste
- 1 teaspoon ground black pepper, or to taste

Direction

- In a heavy-bottomed saucepan covered by a lid, heat the olive oil on medium-high heat. In the heated oil, sauté the onion for 3 minutes until it is fragrant. Stir sofrito and garlic into the onion; then sauté for 3 more minutes until the garlic is fragrant. Press the mixture to the side of the saucepan.
- Break the turkey into pieces, then add into the space free of the onion mixture in the saucepan; cook and stir often for 5-7 minutes until crumbly and browned.
- Stir 3/4 of the tomato paste, water, and tomatoes into the turkey mixture until they are even in color; add cocoa powder, cumin, chili powder, and cashews. To incorporate the seasoning, stir the mixture, then cover the saucepan with the lid and turn down the heat to medium-low, cook at a simmer, stir often and add water to thin as wanted for an hour until the tomatoes break down. Flavor with pepper and salt.

Nutrition Information

- Calories: 385 calories;
- Total Fat: 25.2
- Sodium: 869
- Total Carbohydrate: 19.8
- Cholesterol: 70
- Protein: 24.8

178. Peachy Turkey Burger Over Greens With Endive, Bacon, Avocado, And Gorgonzola

Serving: 4 | Prep: 30mins | Cook: 20mins | Ready in:

Ingredients

- 1 tablespoon canola oil
- 1/2 red onion, chopped
- 1/2 jalapeno pepper, seeded and minced
- 2 cloves garlic, minced
- 1 pound ground turkey
- 1 tablespoon gluten-free teriyaki sauce (such as Kikkoman®)
- 1 tablespoon tamari (gluten-free soy sauce)
- 1 peach, halved, divided
- salt and ground black pepper to taste
- 1 head endive, chopped
- 1 (5 ounce) bag spring mix lettuce
- 1 firm ripe avocado, cubed
- 1/4 cup crumbled Gorgonzola cheese
- 4 bacon strips, cooked and chopped

Direction

- Sauté onions, garlic and jalapeno with canola oil on a skillet on medium heat. Cook for ten to twelve minutes until onions are soft and translucent. Set aside and let cool, fifteen minutes. Lightly oil grate and preheat grill to medium heat. In a bowl combine ground turkey with onion mixture, soy sauce and teriyaki sauce, mix well with a fork. Put chopped peaches into the mixture and gently mix. Add salt and pepper. Divide in four equal patties. On the preheated grill, cook turkey patties four minutes each side until juices are clear and nor pink in the middle. Temperature in the middle should be 165 degrees F (74 degrees C). In a big bowl, toss together endive and spring mix, top with Gorgonzola cheese, chopped avocado and minced bacon. You can add mustard vinaigrette to the salad if you prefer. Serve as a side to the awesome turkey burgers.

Nutrition Information

- Calories: 391 calories;
- Total Fat: 24.8
- Sodium: 798
- Total Carbohydrate: 14.1
- Cholesterol: 100
- Protein: 30.8

179. Perfect Healthy Meatloaf

Serving: 6 | Prep: 20mins | Cook: 50mins | Ready in:

Ingredients

- Meatloaf:
- 1 tablespoon olive oil, or as needed
- 1 onion, diced
- 1/2 red bell pepper, diced
- 1/2 green bell pepper, diced
- 1 clove garlic, minced, or to taste
- salt and ground black pepper to taste
- 1 pound ground turkey
- 1 pound lean ground beef
- 2 cups cooked quinoa, or more to taste
- 1/2 cup milk
- 2 eggs, beaten
- 2 tablespoons Worcestershire sauce
- 2 tablespoons sweet chili sauce
- 3/4 teaspoon ground ginger
- 1/4 cup bread crumbs, or as needed (optional)

- Glaze:
- 1/4 cup brown sugar
- 1/4 cup ketchup
- 1 tablespoon Worcestershire sauce

Direction

- Set the oven to 350°F (175°C) and start preheating. Use aluminum foil to line a baking sheet.
- Over medium-high heat, in a large skillet, heat olive oil. Sauté green bell pepper, red bell pepper and onion in hot oil for about 5 minutes until translucent and soft. Add garlic to vegetable mixture; sauté for about 1 more minute until fragrant. Season with black pepper and salt; take out of the heat to cool.
- In a bowl, mix ground ginger, sweet chili sauce, 2 tablespoons Worcestershire sauce, eggs, milk, quinoa, beef and turkey together until combined well. Add sautéed vegetable mixture; stir until incorporated completely. Add bread crumbs to meat mixture gradually until mixture holds together and becomes moist. Shape into 6 mini loves; transfer to the prepared baking sheet.
- In a bowl, beat together a tablespoon Worcestershire sauce, ketchup and brown sugar until sugar dissolves and glaze becomes smooth.
- Bake meat loaves for half an hour in the prepared oven. Spread each loaf with glaze and keep cooking for 10-15 minutes until the center of loaves are no longer pink. The inserted instant-read thermometer into the center should register at least 160°F (70°C).

Nutrition Information

- Calories: 484 calories;
- Total Fat: 20.8
- Sodium: 440
- Total Carbohydrate: 37.5
- Cholesterol: 172
- Protein: 36.6

180. Polynesian Meatballs

Serving: 6 | Prep: | Cook: |Ready in:

Ingredients

- 2 cups Minute® Brown Rice, uncooked
- 1 (20 ounce) can crushed pineapple, divided
- 1 (20 ounce) package ground turkey or chicken
- 3/4 cup green onions, thinly sliced, divided
- 1/2 cup teriyaki sauce, divided
- 1 egg, lightly beaten
- 1 teaspoon ground ginger
- 1/2 teaspoon ground nutmeg
- 2 tablespoons orange marmalade

Direction

- Preheat an oven to 175 °C or 350 °F. Prepare the rice following packaging instructions.
- For the meatballs, drain half cup of crushed pineapple. Set aside the rest of pineapple and juice for the sauce.
- In a big bowl, mix together nutmeg, ginger, egg, quarter cup teriyaki sauce, half cup green onions, half cup pineapple, cooked rice and ground chicken or turkey. Combine thoroughly.
- Spoon the mixture and gently roll into preferred size of meatball, suggested approximately the size of a golf ball; put the meatballs on baking sheet lined with aluminum foil with sides. Bake for 25 minutes to half an hour or till meatballs are done.
- While baking the meatballs, prepare sauce, in a medium saucepan, mix together orange marmalade, the leftover 1/4 cup teriyaki sauce and the rest of pineapple and juice; heat to boiling. Lower the heat and let it simmer for 3 to 4 minutes without a cover. Mix in the leftover quarter cup of green onions.
- Put sauce on top of cooked meatballs.

Nutrition Information

- Calories: 352 calories;
- Total Fat: 9.7
- Sodium: 1033
- Total Carbohydrate: 46.8
- Cholesterol: 102
- Protein: 21.5

181. Popa's Simple White Chili

Serving: 10 | Prep: 15mins | Cook: 1hours10mins | Ready in:

Ingredients

- 1 1/4 pounds ground turkey
- 1 tablespoon low-sodium chicken base (such as Better Than Bouillon®)
- 3 cups boiling water
- 3 (14.5 ounce) cans Great Northern beans, drained
- 1 (28 ounce) can green enchilada sauce
- 2 (4 ounce) cans diced green chiles, undrained
- 1 onion, chopped
- 1 tablespoon granulated garlic
- 1/4 teaspoon ground cumin
- 2 teaspoons dried Mexican oregano
- 1 bunch fresh cilantro, finely chopped
- 1 onion, diced

Direction

- Into a Dutch oven, crumble ground turkey over medium heat; cook and stir until browned, for 10 to 15 minutes. Drain and discard all the excess grease.
- In a bowl, combine the chicken base and boiling water, until the base is dissolved; transfer over cooked ground turkey. Put in oregano, cumin, granulated garlic, chopped onion, green chiles, enchilada sauce, and Great Northern beans; blend well. Simmer until reach the blended flavors, for about 1 hour. Scoop the chili into bowls.
- Mix diced onion and cilantro in a bowl; scatter over chili for enjoying.

Nutrition Information

- Calories: 287 calories;
- Total Fat: 6.5
- Sodium: 576
- Total Carbohydrate: 36
- Cholesterol: 43
- Protein: 22.5

182. Pumpkin Turkey Chili

Serving: 6 | Prep: 10mins | Cook: 20mins | Ready in:

Ingredients

- 1 tablespoon vegetable oil
- 1 cup chopped onion
- 1/2 cup chopped green bell pepper
- 1/2 cup chopped yellow bell pepper
- 1 clove garlic, minced
- 1 pound ground turkey
- 1 (14.5 ounce) can diced tomatoes
- 2 cups pumpkin puree
- 1 1/2 tablespoons chili powder
- 1/2 teaspoon ground black pepper
- 1 dash salt
- 1/2 cup shredded Cheddar cheese
- 1/2 cup sour cream

Direction

- Put oil in a large skillet and heat it over medium heat. Sauté green bell pepper, garlic, yellow bell pepper, and onion in oil until tender. Stir in turkey and cook the meat until browned all over; drain. Mix in pumpkin and tomatoes. Season the mixture with salt, pepper, and chili powder. Adjust the heat to low. Cover the skillet and simmer the mixture for 20 minutes. Serve the dish with sour cream and Cheddar cheese on top.

Nutrition Information

- Calories: 285 calories;
- Total Fat: 16.6
- Sodium: 321
- Total Carbohydrate: 14.9
- Cholesterol: 76
- Protein: 21.2

183. Quick Bean And Turkey Italian Meatballs

Serving: 12 | Prep: 20mins | Cook: 10mins | Ready in:

Ingredients

- 1 (15 ounce) can butter beans, rinsed and drained
- 1 1/4 pounds extra-lean ground turkey breast
- 1 egg white, beaten
- 1 teaspoon onion powder
- 1/2 teaspoon garlic powder
- 1/2 teaspoon salt
- 1/4 teaspoon black pepper
- 1/2 cup Italian bread crumbs
- 1 tablespoon olive oil

Direction

- In big mixing bowl, mash butter beans. Add pepper, salt, garlic powder, onion powder, egg white and ground turkey; mix till evenly combined. Evenly fold breadcrumbs into mixture.
- Shape mixture to 1-in. meatballs.
- In skillet, heat oil over medium heat.
- In hot oil, cook meatballs for 5-7 minutes till browned on all sides. Cover skillet. Cook for 5 more minutes till meatballs aren't pink anymore in the middle. An inserted instant-read thermometer in the middle should read minimum 74°C or 165°F.

Nutrition Information

- Calories: 126 calories;
- Total Fat: 5
- Sodium: 340
- Total Carbohydrate: 8.1
- Cholesterol: 35
- Protein: 12.1

184. Quinoa With Ground Turkey

Serving: 6 | Prep: 15mins | Cook: 35mins | Ready in:

Ingredients

- 1 1/2 cups water
- 1 cup quinoa
- 2 tablespoons olive oil
- 1/2 onion, chopped
- 1 red bell pepper, chopped
- 1 pinch Himalayan salt to taste
- 1 1/4 pounds ground turkey
- 1 pinch freshly ground black pepper to taste
- 4 cloves garlic, minced
- 1 teaspoon minced fresh sage
- 1 teaspoon minced fresh rosemary
- 1/2 cup grated Mizithra cheese

Direction

- Boil quinoa and water in saucepan. Lower heat to medium low and cover; simmer for 15-20 minutes till water is absorbed and quinoa is tender.
- Heat olive oil on medium heat in a skillet; mix and cook red bell pepper and onion in hot oil for 10 minutes till beginning to brown and tender. Season using salt.
- Season ground turkey with pepper and salt generously. Put into onion mixture; put temperature on medium high. Mix and cook turkey mixture for 5-7 minutes till crumbly and nearly brown; drain extra grease. Put heat on medium low. Put rosemary, sage and garlic

- in turkey mixture; mix and cook for 2-3 minutes till turkey is browned and fragrant.
- Stir quinoa into turkey mixture; cook for 2-3 minutes till quinoa heats through. Put Mizithra cheese in quinoa and turkey; take off heat. Season with pepper and salt.

Nutrition Information

- Calories: 330 calories;
- Total Carbohydrate: 32.6
- Cholesterol: 77
- Protein: 24.6
- Total Fat: 15.1
- Sodium: 303

185. Quinoa, Bean, And Ground Turkey Chili

Serving: 8 | Prep: 15mins | Cook: 51mins | Ready in:

Ingredients

- 1 tablespoon ghee
- 1 pound ground turkey
- 1 large onion, chopped
- 5 cloves garlic, minced
- 1/4 teaspoon ground black pepper
- 1 (15 ounce) can diced tomatoes
- 1 (6 ounce) can tomato paste
- 2 stalks celery, chopped
- 2 tablespoons chili powder, or more to taste
- 1 tablespoon Worcestershire sauce
- 1 tablespoon ground cumin
- 1 teaspoon dried oregano
- 1/8 teaspoon garlic powder
- 1/8 teaspoon onion powder
- Himalayan pink salt to taste
- 4 cups vegetable broth
- 1 (15 ounce) can black beans, drained and rinsed
- 1 (15 ounce) can kidney beans, drained and rinsed
- 1 cup tri-colored quinoa

Direction

- Heat ghee over medium heat in a Dutch oven. Put in garlic, onion, turkey, and black pepper. Sauté for about 6 minutes until turkey turns brown. Drain; discard drippings.
- Mix salt, onion powder, garlic powder, oregano, cumin, Worcestershire sauce, chili powder, celery, tomato paste, and tomatoes into the turkey mixture. Mix in kidney beans, black beans, and broth until combined. Add quinoa; bring to a boil. Turn heat to low; simmer for about 40 minutes until quinoa is tender.

Nutrition Information

- Calories: 335 calories;
- Sodium: 889
- Total Carbohydrate: 43.5
- Cholesterol: 46
- Protein: 22.9
- Total Fat: 8.4

186. Rachel's Turkey Loaf

Serving: 6 | Prep: 15mins | Cook: 1hours | Ready in:

Ingredients

- 1 pound ground turkey
- 2 eggs, lightly beaten
- 1/2 cup chopped fresh mushrooms (optional)
- 1 1/2 cups Italian seasoned bread crumbs
- 1 (1 ounce) envelope dry onion soup mix
- 2/3 cup ready-to-serve creamy tomato soup, divided
- 1/4 cup ketchup, divided
- 1/4 cup barbeque sauce, divided
- 2 tablespoons Worcestershire sauce, divided
- chili powder to taste

Direction

- Set the oven to 350°F (175°C) and start preheating.
- Mix a tablespoon Worcestershire sauce, 2 tablespoons barbeque sauce, 2 tablespoons ketchup, 1/3 cup creamy tomato soup, soup mix, bread crumbs, mushrooms, eggs and turkey in a bowl. Mold the mixture into a loaf shape; transfer to a baking dish. Top with chili powder.
- Mix the rest of each of Worcestershire sauce, barbeque sauce, ketchup and creamy tomato soup in another bowl. Put aside.
- Bake loaf in the prepared oven for 45 minutes. Pour sauce on top; keep baking 15 minutes until it reaches a minimum internal temperature of 165°F (74°C).

Nutrition Information

- Calories: 308 calories;
- Total Fat: 9.5
- Sodium: 1282
- Total Carbohydrate: 34
- Cholesterol: 118
- Protein: 22.2

187. Robert's Homemade Italian Sausage

Serving: 24 | Prep: 25mins | Cook: | Ready in:

Ingredients

- 1/4 cup dry red wine, chilled
- 1 tablespoon raw sugar
- 1/4 teaspoon sea salt
- 1 tablespoon garlic powder
- 1 teaspoon dried oregano
- 2 teaspoons black pepper
- 2 teaspoons paprika
- 1 1/2 teaspoons fennel seed
- 1/2 teaspoon anise seed
- 1/2 teaspoon dried parsley flakes
- 1/2 teaspoon red pepper flakes
- 1/2 teaspoon cayenne pepper
- 1/4 teaspoon dried minced onion
- 1/8 teaspoon coriander seed, coarsely cracked
- 1/8 teaspoon ground mace
- 2 pounds extra-lean ground turkey breast
- 1 pound lean ground pork

Direction

- In a big bowl, add the chilled red wine. Put in salt and sugar, whisk until dissolved. Put in the mace, coriander seed, minced onion, cayenne pepper, red pepper flakes, parsley flakes, anise seed, fennel seed, paprika, black pepper, oregano, and garlic powder. Put in the pork and turkey breast and use your hands to mix. Mix thoroughly to evenly distributed the seasonings in the meat mixture.
- Line plastic wrap onto 2 or 3 baking sheets. Roll the meat mixture into quarter-cup balls, flatten to half-an-inch thick and arrange in a single layer on the baking sheet. Use another layer of plastic to cover and freeze them till solid. Store the patties in a resealable plastic bag once they are solid.

Nutrition Information

- Calories: 102 calories;
- Sodium: 50
- Total Carbohydrate: 1.2
- Cholesterol: 40
- Protein: 11
- Total Fat: 5.6

188. Rosemary Turkey Meatloaf

Serving: 8 | Prep: 15mins | Cook: 1hours | Ready in:

Ingredients

- 1 1/2 pounds ground turkey
- 2 cups dry bread crumbs
- 1 onion, chopped
- 1 egg, beaten
- 1 cup milk
- 1/2 cup balsamic vinegar
- 1 clove garlic, minced
- 1 teaspoon salt
- 1 teaspoon pepper
- 1 1/2 tablespoons chopped fresh rosemary
- 1 cup canned tomato sauce
- 3/4 cup brown sugar
- 1 tablespoon Dijon mustard

Direction

- Prepare the oven by preheating to 350°F (175°C). Prepare a lightly greased loaf pan (9x5-inch).
- Combine milk, egg, onion, bread crumbs, and ground turkey in a large mixing bowl. Add rosemary, pepper, salt, and balsamic vinegar to taste. Transfer to the prepared pan and press. Mix mustard, brown sugar, and tomato sauce; put evenly over the top of the loaf.
- Place in the preheated oven and bake for 1 hour, or until juices run clear once poked with a knife.

Nutrition Information

- Calories: 362 calories;
- Sodium: 807
- Total Carbohydrate: 47.1
- Cholesterol: 93
- Protein: 20.9
- Total Fat: 9.8

189. S.O.B. (South Of The Border) Casserole

Serving: 4 | Prep: 15mins | Cook: 20mins | Ready in:

Ingredients

- 1/2 pound ground turkey
- 1/4 cup chopped onion
- 1 (16 ounce) can stewed tomatoes, undrained
- 1 (.75 ounce) packet brown gravy mix
- 1 teaspoon chili powder, or to taste
- 1/2 cup frozen corn kernels
- 1/2 cup uncooked elbow macaroni
- 1 cup shredded lettuce
- 3 tablespoons sour cream
- 2 cups corn tortilla chips

Direction

- Boil the lightly salted water in small saucepan. Put in macaroni. Cook for about 6 mins until it is almost tender. Drain. Put aside.
- In a large pan, crumble the turkey set over medium heat. Cook while stirring until it is brown evenly, then drain. Put onion into the browned turkey meat. Cook for about 5 mins until the onion is tender. Stir in chili powder, gravy mix and tomatoes until they are combined. Mix in macaroni and corn. Cover and lower the heat to low. Simmer, stirring occasionally, for 10 mins.
- Arrange on a bed of tortilla chips to serve. Top with sour cream and shredded lettuce.

Nutrition Information

- Calories: 297 calories;
- Cholesterol: 47
- Protein: 16.7
- Total Fat: 10.6
- Sodium: 606
- Total Carbohydrate: 34.4

190. Sarah's Incredible Turkey Chili

Serving: 6 | Prep: 5mins | Cook: 20mins | Ready in:

Ingredients

- 1 pound Italian seasoned ground turkey
- 3/4 cup diced onion
- 1 (14.5 ounce) can fire-roasted diced tomatoes, undrained
- 1 (5.6 ounce) package Knorr® Fiesta Sides™ - Spanish Rice
- 2 3/4 cups water
- 2 teaspoons chili powder
- 1 1/2 teaspoons ground cumin
- 1 teaspoon ground coriander

Direction

- In a heavy pot over medium heat, stir turkey frequently to break it up and until brown. Cook for 8 minutes, or until browned.
- Increase to medium-high heat and add the onions. Cook for 4 minutes until onions are caramelized and browned. Add fire roasted tomatoes and stir until combined. Add in coriander, cumin, chili powder, water, and Knorr Fiesta Sides – Spanish Rice. Stir thoroughly to combine. Bring to a boil, then reduce to low heat. Simmer with lid on for 8 minutes, or until flavors have blended.

Nutrition Information

- Calories: 239 calories;
- Cholesterol: 56
- Protein: 18.4
- Total Fat: 6.8
- Sodium: 240
- Total Carbohydrate: 13.4

191. Seasoned Turkey Burgers

Serving: 6 | Prep: 10mins | Cook: 20mins | Ready in:

Ingredients

- 1 1/2 pounds ground turkey
- 1 (1 ounce) package dry onion soup mix
- 1/2 teaspoon ground black pepper
- 1/2 teaspoon garlic powder
- 1 1/2 tablespoons soy sauce
- 1 egg, lightly beaten (optional)
- 6 hamburger buns, split

Direction

- Combine the turkey with the pepper, onion soup mix, garlic, soy sauce, garlic powder, and egg and mix them in a large bowl. Leave the mixture to refrigerate for 10 minutes then shape into 6 patties.
- Prepare the grill by preheating over medium-high heat.
- Coat the grate lightly with oil. Grill the patties and cook for 20 minutes or until well done, turning it over once. The inside of the patties should look whitish in color when they are already cooked through. Put the patties on buns and serve.

Nutrition Information

- Calories: 314 calories;
- Protein: 28.2
- Total Fat: 11.3
- Sodium: 920
- Total Carbohydrate: 24.8
- Cholesterol: 115

192. Seattle Style Turkey Lettuce Wraps

Serving: 4 | Prep: 20mins | Cook: | Ready in:

Ingredients

- 1 (16 ounce) package JENNIE-O® Lean Ground Turkey
- 2 cloves garlic, chopped
- 1 tablespoon fresh grated ginger
- 2 tablespoons HOUSE OF TSANG® ginger-flavored soy sauce
- 1 tablespoon brown sugar

- 1/4 cup chopped green onions
- 1 red bell pepper, chopped
- 1/2 cup chopped fresh mint leaves
- 1 head butter lettuce

Direction

- Cook turkey following packaging directions. Cook to well done all the time, a meat thermometer should register 165°F.
- Put in the red bell pepper, green onions, brown sugar, soy sauce, ginger and garlic. Let cook for 7 minutes or till garlic is tender.
- Mix in the mint leaves. Quickly transfer the meat to shallow dish and refrigerate for an hour.
- Take core off head of lettuce; part, rinse and dry the leaves.
- In lettuce cups, scoop refrigerated turkey mixture.

Nutrition Information

- Calories: 165 calories;
- Cholesterol: 46
- Protein: 28
- Total Fat: 1.7
- Sodium: 443
- Total Carbohydrate: 9.3

193. Shannon's Stuffed Delicata Squash

Serving: 8 | Prep: 20mins | Cook: 38mins | Ready in:

Ingredients

- 2 delicata squash, halved lengthwise and seeded
- 2 tablespoons olive oil
- 1/2 sweet red onion, chopped
- 2 stalks celery, diced
- 1 pound ground turkey
- 1 tablespoon crumbled cooked bacon
- 2 garlic cloves, minced
- 1 teaspoon ground turmeric
- 1 teaspoon ground cumin
- 1 teaspoon safflower (Mexican saffron)
- sea salt to taste
- 1 bunch rainbow chard, stemmed and chopped
- 1/4 cup vegetable broth, or as needed
- 1 (4 ounce) log crumbled goat cheese
- 2 tablespoons olive oil
- 1 teaspoon saffron
- 1/2 cup panko bread crumbs (optional)
- 2 tablespoons butter, melted (optional)

Direction

- Preheat oven at 350°F (175°C).
- In a shallow baking dish with half-inch water at the bottom, position squash cut side-down.
- Roast in the preheated oven for 20 to 30 minutes till tender-fork.
- In a 12-inch skillet, heat 2 tablespoons of oil over medium heat. Add celery and onion; cook and mix for about 5 minutes until onions turn translucent. Add sea salt, safflower, turmeric, garlic, cumin, bacon, and turkey; cook and stir for about 6 minutes until turkey is no longer pink. Add just enough broth and chard to make steam. Cook for about 4 minutes, till chard turns wilted and liquid vaporizes.
- Drain any liquid left from under the squash. Turn squash cut side-up. Coat evenly each squash half with goat cheese; fill the holes with turkey combination.
- In a bowl, gently mix butter and bread crumbs; scatter equally over the squash halves. Position oven rack about 6 inches away from the heat source and heat the oven's broiler beforehand.
- Move squash back to the oven and bake under the broiler for 3 -5 minutes. Keep an eye on until bread crumbs turn golden brown.

Nutrition Information

- Calories: 302 calories;

- Sodium: 318
- Total Carbohydrate: 19.1
- Cholesterol: 62
- Protein: 17.2
- Total Fat: 19.2

194. Shepherd's Pie III

Serving: 6 | Prep: | Cook: |Ready in:

Ingredients

- 4 potatoes, peeled and cubed
- 1/2 cup skim milk, heated
- 1 tablespoon olive oil
- 1/2 pound lean ground turkey
- 1/4 pound lean ground beef
- 1 onion, chopped
- 2 carrots, sliced
- 1 cup low fat, low sodium beef broth
- 1 tablespoon cornstarch
- 2 tablespoons water
- 2 tablespoons tomato paste
- 1 cup frozen green peas, thawed
- salt and pepper to taste
- 1/4 cup shredded Cheddar cheese

Direction

- Set the oven to 350°F (175°C) and start preheating.
- Put potatoes in a pot, pour in water to cover; bring to a boil. Boil until tender or for 20 minutes. Drain off water; mash potatoes with olive oil and hot milk until fluffy. Put aside.
- Brown ground beef and turkey in a nonstick skillet. Add onion; sauté for 5 minutes. Add carrot; sauté for 5 more minutes.
- Drain off excess fat. Add beef broth to meat mixture; bring to a boil.
- Beat together water and cornstarch in a small bowl. Add tomato paste and cornstarch mixture to meat mixture. Simmer while stirring frequently until thickened. Add pepper, salt and peas. Stir well; scoop mixture into a 2 quart casserole dish. Place potatoes on top; top with cheese.
- Bake for 35 minutes in the prepared oven or until potatoes turn brown.

Nutrition Information

- Calories: 314 calories;
- Cholesterol: 49
- Protein: 17.4
- Total Fat: 11.4
- Sodium: 195
- Total Carbohydrate: 35.7

195. Shepherd's Turkey Pie

Serving: 6 | Prep: 30mins | Cook: 1hours10mins |Ready in:

Ingredients

- 4 potatoes, cut into chunks
- 1/2 head cauliflower, separated into florets
- 2 cups chicken broth
- salt and ground black pepper to taste
- 1 tablespoon olive oil
- 1/2 onion, chopped
- 3 carrots, shredded
- 1 1/2 pounds ground turkey
- 1 1/2 cups frozen peas
- 2 tablespoons low-sodium Worcestershire sauce

Direction

- In a pot, add the cauliflower and potatoes, then add the chicken broth. Pour in water almost covering the vegetables; bring it to a boil. Turn to low heat, and simmer for 20 minutes until the cauliflower and potatoes are soft. Drain the cauliflower and potatoes yet save about half cup of the cooking liquid. Transfer the cooked potatoes into large bowl. Put the cauliflower and about 1/4 cup of the cooking liquid in a food processor or a blender

and process until well pureed. Scoop the cauliflower puree into the bowl with the potatoes, and smash together until the potatoes and cauliflower mixture is white and smooth. Sprinkle with black pepper and salt to season the mixture. Mix in a few more spoonfuls of the cooking liquid to make the toping softer.
- Set the oven to 200 °C (400 °F) to preheat. Coat a 9x12-inch baking dish with cooking spray.
- In a large skillet on medium heat, heat the olive oil and cook carrots and onions for 5 minutes until the onion is transparent; mix in the ground turkey, and cook until the meat in not pink anymore, crumbling it into small chunks as it cooks. Mix in Worcestershire sauce and peas, then cook for 10 minutes until the meat has begun to brown. Mix in a few spoonfuls of the cauliflower cooking liquid to keep it moist if the filling mixture starts to look dried out. In the coated baking dish, place the filling, then spread it into an even layer. Place the mashed potato and cauliflower mixture on top of the filling, and use a fork to spread, leaving little peaks and swirls in the topping.
- Bake the pie in the prepared oven for 25 minutes until the filling is bubbling. Turn on the oven's broiler and broil the pie 6 inches away from heat source for 10 minutes more, until the mashed topping turns brown.

Nutrition Information

- Calories: 366 calories;
- Total Carbohydrate: 38.4
- Cholesterol: 85
- Protein: 29.1
- Total Fat: 11.4
- Sodium: 506

196. Simple Scandinavian Turkey Chili

Serving: 4 | Prep: 15mins | Cook: 1hours10mins | Ready in:

Ingredients

- 1 1/4 pounds ground turkey, (93% lean)
- 1 large onion, chopped
- 3 stalks celery, chopped
- 1 (16 ounce) can chili beans in mild sauce (such as Bush's Best®)
- 1 (15 ounce) can tomato sauce
- 1 (14.5 ounce) can diced tomatoes
- 1 teaspoon chili powder
- 1/2 teaspoon cayenne pepper
- 1 bay leaf

Direction

- Over medium-high heat, heat a large pot. Cook while stirring onion, celery and turkey in hot skillet for about 7 minutes until turkey becomes crumbly and browned; drain and get rid of grease.
- Stir bay leaf, cayenne pepper, chili powder, diced tomatoes, tomato sauce and chili beans with turkey mixture; bring to a simmer, use a lid to cover the pot, lower the heat to medium-low; cook for an hour.

Nutrition Information

- Calories: 384 calories;
- Protein: 36.5
- Total Fat: 13.5
- Sodium: 1342
- Total Carbohydrate: 33.9
- Cholesterol: 113

197. Sloppy Joe With Ground Turkey

Serving: 6 | Prep: 15mins | Cook: 20mins | Ready in:

Ingredients

- 1 teaspoon extra-virgin olive oil
- 2 cloves garlic, minced
- 1 1/2 pounds ground turkey
- 1 tomato, chopped
- 1 small onion, chopped
- 3/4 green bell pepper, chopped
- 2 tablespoons chopped fresh parsley
- 1 pinch red pepper flakes
- salt and ground black pepper to taste
- 4 ounces tomato paste
- 1 lemon, juiced
- 6 hamburger buns, split and toasted
- 6 slices American cheese (optional)

Direction

- Over medium heat, in a pot, heat olive oil. Cook while stirring garlic in hot oil for about 2 minutes until fragrant. Break ground turkey into the pot. Use lid to cover the pot; cook meat for 2-3 minutes until the outside turns brown. Using a slivered wooden spoon, break meat up into very small pieces; keep cooking while stirring for 3-5 minutes until nearly browned completely.
- Stir red pepper flakes, parsley, green bell pepper, onion and tomato into turkey mixture; season with black pepper and salt; cook for 3-4 minutes until tomato is softened. Add lemon juice and tomato paste; stir to coat vegetables with tomato paste. Use lid to cover pot, lower the heat to low; cook for 7-10 minutes until vegetables become tender. Top with cheese and serve on toasted hamburgers buns.

Nutrition Information

- Calories: 435 calories;
- Total Fat: 20.6
- Sodium: 878
- Total Carbohydrate: 29.5
- Cholesterol: 110
- Protein: 33.8

198. Slow Cooker 3 Bean Chili

Serving: 10 | Prep: 10mins | Cook: 4hours10mins | Ready in:

Ingredients

- 1 (20 ounce) package 93%-lean ground turkey
- 1 (28 ounce) can diced fire-roasted tomatoes
- 1 (16 ounce) can tomato sauce
- 1 (15.5 ounce) can pinto beans, rinsed and drained
- 1 (15.5 ounce) can kidney beans, rinsed and drained
- 1 (15 ounce) can reduced-sodium black beans, rinsed and drained
- 1 small onion, chopped
- 1 (4.5 ounce) can chopped green chiles
- 2 tablespoons chili powder
- 1 tablespoon minced garlic
- 1 teaspoon oregano
- 1 pinch ground cumin

Direction

- In a big skillet, cook and mix turkey for 7 to 10 minutes till fully browned; put to a slow cooker.
- In the slow cooker, mix cumin, oregano, garlic, chili powder, green chilies, onion, black beans, kidney beans, pinto beans, tomato sauce and tomatoes with the turkey.
- Allow to cook on High for 4 hours or for 7 hours on Low.

Nutrition Information

- Calories: 238 calories;
- Total Carbohydrate: 29
- Cholesterol: 42

- Protein: 19.8
- Total Fat: 5.2
- Sodium: 878

199. Slow Cooker Pumpkin Turkey Chili

Serving: 6 | Prep: 15mins | Cook: 3hours10mins | Ready in:

Ingredients

- 1 tablespoon olive oil
- 1 pound ground turkey
- 1 onion, chopped
- 1 (28 ounce) can diced tomatoes
- 2 cups cubed fresh pumpkin
- 1 (15 ounce) can chili beans
- 1 (15 ounce) can seasoned black beans
- 3 tablespoons brown sugar
- 1 tablespoon pumpkin pie spice
- 1 tablespoon chili powder

Direction

- In a big soup pot, heat olive oil on moderate heat, then brown turkey for 10 minutes while stirring frequently until it is not pink anymore and crumbly. Drain and get rid of any excess fat.
- Put turkey to a slow cooker and stir in chili powder, pumpkin pie spice, brown sugar, black beans, chili beans, pumpkin, diced tomatoes and onions. Set the cooker to low setting, then cover and cook for a minimum of 3 hours until pumpkin has begun to break apart and is softened.

Nutrition Information

- Calories: 338 calories;
- Total Carbohydrate: 41.9
- Cholesterol: 56
- Protein: 25.1
- Total Fat: 9.1
- Sodium: 857

200. Slow Cooker Sauce With Meatballs

Serving: 6 | Prep: 30mins | Cook: 6hours | Ready in:

Ingredients

- Sauce:
- 2 tablespoons extra virgin olive oil
- 1 large onion, chopped
- 6 garlic cloves, minced
- 1 (28 ounce) can RED GOLD® Crushed Tomatoes
- 1 (28 ounce) can RED GOLD® Tomato Sauce
- 1 (6 ounce) can RED GOLD® Tomato Paste
- 1 tablespoon dried basil
- 1 teaspoon dried oregano
- Salt and black pepper to taste
- 1 teaspoon fennel seed
- 2 tablespoons sugar
- 1/2 cup water
- Mozzarella Meatballs:
- 2 pounds lean ground beef or ground turkey
- 1/2 cup quick cooking oats
- 1 teaspoon dried basil
- 1/4 teaspoon black pepper
- 2 cloves garlic, minced
- 2 eggs
- 8 ounces small fresh mozzarella balls
- 3 tablespoons extra-virgin olive oil

Direction

- Heat extra-virgin olive oil in a large skillet over medium heat. Place in garlic and onion. Cook until they become tender. Spray 5 qt. or bigger slow cooker. Throw in the garlic and onion together with the rest of the ingredients of the sauce. Mix well to combine. Leave it to cook on low for approximately 6 to 7 hours.

Pair it with the pasta of your choice when serving.
- If you want, meat can be added to the sauce. The following is a recipe for meatballs that should be added to the sauce at the start of cooking time.
- To prepare the mozzarella meatballs, combine eggs, garlic cloves, black pepper, basil, oats, and turkey in a large bowl. Form into 2-inch balls. You should be able to make 14 to 16 meatballs with this. In the center of each meat ball, add and press 1 small ball of mozzarella then seal it.
- In a large skillet over medium-high heat, heat oil. Place the meatballs on the skillet and allow them to cook to let them brown evenly on every side. Take a slow cooker and pour in half of the sauce, put in the meatballs, then add the rest of the sauce. Let cook as previously mentioned.

Nutrition Information

- Calories: 709 calories;
- Cholesterol: 197
- Protein: 43.7
- Total Fat: 39.9
- Sodium: 1187
- Total Carbohydrate: 42.5

201. Slow Cooker Turkey Chili With Kidney Beans

Serving: 10 | Prep: 20mins | Cook: 4hours5mins | Ready in:

Ingredients

- 1 1/4 pounds ground turkey
- 2 onions, chopped
- 2 Anaheim chile peppers, chopped
- 2 (16 ounce) cans kidney beans, rinsed and drained
- 1 (16 ounce) can Mexican-style hot tomato sauce
- 1/4 cup chili powder
- 1/4 cup cornmeal
- 2 tablespoons minced garlic
- 1 tablespoon dried onion flakes
- 1 tablespoon unsweetened cocoa powder
- 1 tablespoon ground cumin
- 1 teaspoon ground black pepper
- 1 teaspoon white sugar
- 1 teaspoon dried parsley
- 1 teaspoon dried Mexican oregano
- 1 teaspoon beef base
- 1/2 teaspoon red pepper flakes
- 1/2 teaspoon ground coriander
- 1/2 cup water, or as desired

Direction

- Heat a big skillet on moderate high heat. Cook and stir in the hot skillet the Anaheim chile peppers, onions and turkey for 5-7 minutes until crumbly and browned; drain and move the turkey mixture to a slow cooker.
- Combine coriander, red pepper flakes, beef base, oregano, parsley, sugar, ground black pepper, cumin, cocoa power, onion flakes, garlic, cornmeal, chili powder, Mexican-style tomato sauce and kidney beans into turkey mixture. Put in enough water to get the preferred consistency.
- Cook on high setting for about 4 hours or on low setting for about 8-10 hours.

Nutrition Information

- Calories: 222 calories;
- Cholesterol: 42
- Protein: 17.8
- Total Fat: 5.6
- Sodium: 475
- Total Carbohydrate: 27.1

202. Smothered Mexican Lasagna

Serving: 6 | Prep: 20mins | Cook: 25mins | Ready in:

Ingredients

- 1 1/2 pounds ground turkey
- 1 bunch green onions, chopped
- 1 (1.25 ounce) package taco seasoning mix
- 2 cups water
- 1 (14.5 ounce) can diced tomatoes, undrained
- 1 (4 ounce) can diced green chile peppers, undrained
- 1 (15 ounce) container ricotta cheese
- 2 eggs
- 8 (10 inch) flour tortillas
- 1 (8 ounce) container sour cream
- 1/4 cup salsa

Direction

- Preheat an oven to 200 degrees C (400 degrees F). Into a large, deep skillet, put ground turkey and then cook with medium high heat until browned evenly. Mix in green chiles with juice, diced tomatoes with juice, water, taco seasoning mix and green onions. Lower the heat to medium.
- Combine together eggs and ricotta in a medium bowl. Put two tortillas at the bottom of 9x13 inch pan. Scatter 1/4 of ricotta mixture over tortillas. Pour 1/4 of meat mixture atop cheese. Repeat layering until all are used up.
- Bake for about 20 minutes in preheated oven or until the sauce is bubbly. Combine salsa and sour cream together in a small bowl. Then serve in bowl alongside.

Nutrition Information

- Calories: 716 calories;
- Total Fat: 31.9
- Sodium: 1660
- Total Carbohydrate: 63.9
- Cholesterol: 190
- Protein: 40.5

203. Sophia's Spicy Sriracha Meatballs

Serving: 4 | Prep: 15mins | Cook: 40mins | Ready in:

Ingredients

- 1 red onion, diced
- 1 pound ground turkey
- 1 cup rolled oats
- 1/2 cup ricotta cheese
- 2 medium eggs
- 1/2 cup bread crumbs
- 1/4 cup pickled banana peppers, diced
- 1/4 cup grated Parmesan cheese
- 2 tablespoons medium chunky salsa
- 1 teaspoon sriracha sauce, or more to taste
- salt and ground black pepper to taste
- 1/2 tablespoon olive oil, or as needed
- 1 (16 ounce) jar spaghetti sauce, or to taste

Direction

- In a heavy-bottomed pan over medium heat, cook the onion for 5 minutes till onion begins to sweat. Turn heat to low and allow to brown and soften while you have other ingredients ready.
- In a big bowl, put the ground turkey. Put pepper, salt, sriracha sauce, salsa, Parmesan cheese, banana peppers, bread crumbs, eggs, ricotta cheese and oats. Mix till equally blended. Put the cooked onion last. Allow the meatball mixture to rest for 10 minutes to let texture thicken and the flavors to incorporate.
- Preheat an oven to 175 °C or 350 °F. Line aluminum foil on a jellyroll pan; on top, brush 1 layer of olive oil.
- Form ground turkey mixture into rounds and place on jellyroll pan.
- In the prepped oven, bake for 20 to 25 minutes till browned lightly.
- In a big saucepan, heat sauce over medium heat. Put the meatballs; mix till coated with

sauce. Allow to simmer for a minimum of 15 minutes till flavors intensify.

Nutrition Information

- Calories: 521 calories;
- Total Fat: 21.5
- Sodium: 916
- Total Carbohydrate: 44.3
- Cholesterol: 192
- Protein: 37.8

204. Southwest Stuffed Zucchini

Serving: 4 | Prep: 30mins | Cook: 45mins | Ready in:

Ingredients

- 2 large zucchini, halved and quartered
- 1 1/4 pounds lean ground turkey
- 1/2 small green bell pepper, finely chopped
- 1/4 onion, finely chopped
- 1 egg
- 1/4 cup bread crumbs
- 1 jalapeno pepper, seeded and minced
- 2 tablespoons chopped fresh cilantro
- 2 cloves garlic, minced
- 2 teaspoons steak seasoning (such as Montreal Steak Seasoning®)
- 2 teaspoons ground cumin
- 1 teaspoon dried thyme
- 1 cup salsa
- 1 cup shredded sharp Cheddar cheese

Direction

- Set an oven to preheat to 200°C (400°F).
- Use a spoon to scoop out the flesh from the zucchini, then create boats.
- In a big bowl, mix the thyme, cumin, steak seasoning, garlic, cilantro, jalapeno pepper, breadcrumbs, egg, onion, green bell pepper and turkey. Fill turkey mixture on the zucchini boats, then cover it with Cheddar cheese and salsa.
- Let it bake for about 45 minutes in the preheated oven, until the zucchini becomes very tender and the turkey has no visible pink color in the middle.

Nutrition Information

- Calories: 427 calories;
- Protein: 41.2
- Total Fat: 22.4
- Sodium: 1189
- Total Carbohydrate: 18.3
- Cholesterol: 181

205. Southwestern Macaroni And Cheese With Ground Turkey

Serving: 6 | Prep: 10mins | Cook: 20mins | Ready in:

Ingredients

- 2 (6 ounce) boxes Horizon® ClassicMac™ Macaroni & Mild Cheddar Cheese
- 4 tablespoons Horizon® organic butter
- 1/2 cup Horizon® organic milk
- 1 tablespoon olive oil
- 20 ounces extra-lean ground turkey breast
- 1/2 large red onion, diced small
- 1 red bell pepper, diced small
- 1 cup cooked black beans
- 1 tablespoon taco seasoning, or to taste
- 6 ounces Horizon® Organic Mexican finely shredded cheese
- 3 green onions, thinly sliced

Direction

- Prepare Horizon macaroni and cheese as directed on the package.
- Over medium-high heat, in a large skillet, heat olive oil. Add red bell pepper, red onion and

turkey. Sauté, breaking up turkey, until onions become translucent and turkey is cooked through.
- Stir in shredded cheese, prepared macaroni and cheese, taco seasoning and black beans. Keep cooking until cheese melts.
- Top with green onion slices and serve.

Nutrition Information

- Calories: 658 calories;
- Total Fat: 22.2
- Sodium: 895
- Total Carbohydrate: 66.5
- Cholesterol: 117
- Protein: 47.1

206. Southwestern Mini Turkey Meatballs

Serving: 24 | Prep: 15mins | Cook: 30mins | Ready in:

Ingredients

- 2 pounds ground turkey
- 1 cup finely crushed tortilla chips
- 1 egg
- 2 cups Dannon Oikos Plain Greek Nonfat Yogurt
- 1/2 cup chopped cilantro
- 1 cup prepared (jar) picante sauce or salsa, divided
- 1 cup frozen corn kernels, thawed
- 1 cup black beans
- 1 teaspoon cumin
- 1 teaspoon ground chipotle chili powder, divided

Direction

- Mix chipotle chili powder, cumin, salsa and yogurt in a bowl. In the fridge, put aside 1 1/2 cups.
- Mix black beans, corn, cilantro, leftover seasoned yogurt, egg, crushed chips and turkey in another bowl. Make tablespoon sized balls with small scoop spoon; put on lightly greased shallow baking sheet. In preheated 400°F oven, bake till lightly browned for 20-25 minutes.
- On shredded lettuce, serve meatballs with leftover sauce for a dip.

Nutrition Information

- Calories: 111 calories;
- Protein: 11.8
- Total Fat: 3.5
- Sodium: 103
- Total Carbohydrate: 8.7
- Cholesterol: 37

207. Spaghetti Casserole I

Serving: 8 | Prep: 30mins | Cook: 15mins | Ready in:

Ingredients

- 1 pound spaghetti
- 1 pound ground turkey
- 1 large onion, chopped
- 1 large green bell pepper, chopped
- 2 cloves garlic, minced
- 2 tomatoes, chopped
- 2 cups ketchup
- 1 cup shredded reduced-fat Cheddar cheese

Direction

- Turn oven to 350°F (175°C) to preheat.
- Bring lightly salted water in a large pot to a boil. Cook pasta in boiling water until al dente, for 8 to 10 minutes; drain off water and put to one side.
- Cook turkey over medium heat in a large skillet until browned. Transfer browned

turkey to a large mixing bowl; retaining all of the drippings in the skillet.
- Add bell pepper and onion to the skillet; sauté until tender. Stir in garlic; sauté to 2 minutes, then add tomatoes; stir to combine and turn off the heat.
- Pour vegetable mixture over turkey in the mixing bowl; mix in ketchup until well coated. Spread mixture into a 9x13-inch baking dish; top with spaghetti, then cheese.
- Bake for about half an hour in the preheated oven until thoroughly heated and cheese is melted; enjoy.

Nutrition Information

- Calories: 379 calories;
- Cholesterol: 40
- Protein: 25
- Total Fat: 3.8
- Sodium: 801
- Total Carbohydrate: 61.8

208. Spanish Rice Soup

Serving: 4 | Prep: 5mins | Cook: 40mins | Ready in:

Ingredients

- 1 pound ground turkey
- 1 onion, chopped
- 1 clove crushed garlic
- 1 (6.8 ounce) package Spanish-style rice mix
- 1 (14.5 ounce) can Mexican-style stewed tomatoes
- 2 (8 ounce) cans tomato sauce
- 4 1/2 cups water

Direction

- Brown garlic, onion and turkey. Add water, tomato sauce, stewed tomatoes and rice; bring to a boil. Lower the heat to low; simmer for 20 minutes. Serve hot.

Nutrition Information

- Calories: 389 calories;
- Sodium: 1808
- Total Carbohydrate: 49.5
- Cholesterol: 90
- Protein: 26.9
- Total Fat: 10.2

209. Spicy Bacon Cheeseburger Turkey Wraps

Serving: 7 | Prep: 5mins | Cook: 8mins | Ready in:

Ingredients

- 1 pound lean ground turkey
- 2 tablespoons Worcestershire sauce (such as French's®)
- 1 tablespoon Cajun seasoning, or to taste
- 1/4 cup bacon bits (such as Hormel®)
- 2 tablespoons diced jalapeno pepper
- 1 tablespoon minced garlic
- 7 light flatbreads (such as Flatout®)
- Condiments:
- 28 dill pickle slices
- 3 1/2 cups fresh spinach
- 7 slices pepper Jack cheese (such as Borden®)

Direction

- In a bowl, mix the turkey with the Cajun seasoning and the Worcestershire sauce.
- In a skillet, cook minced garlic, jalapeno pepper and bacon bits over medium-high heat for 4 mins or until the bacon bits begin to stick. Put in turkey mixture and cook while stirring for 4 mins or until it is no longer pink.
- In each flatbread, add 2 ounces of turkey mixture. In each wrap, put four slices of pickle, half a cup of spinach and one slice of the pepper Jack cheese.

Nutrition Information

- Calories: 273 calories;
- Total Fat: 13
- Sodium: 1080
- Total Carbohydrate: 20.1
- Cholesterol: 66
- Protein: 27.4

210. Spicy Breakfast Meatballs

Serving: 15 | Prep: 10mins | Cook: 20mins | Ready in:

Ingredients

- 1 (20 ounce) package bulk spicy Italian turkey sausage
- 1 (20 ounce) package spicy Italian ground turkey
- 3 eggs
- 4 ounces 2%-fat Cheddar cheese
- 1/4 onion, minced
- 1/4 teaspoon ground black pepper

Direction

- Set the oven at 350°F (175°C) and start preheating.
- In a large bowl, combine black pepper, onion, Cheddar cheese, eggs, ground turkey and sausage together; form into 1 1/2-in. balls. Arrange on your baking sheets.
- Bake in the preheated oven for 18-20 minutes, till the meatballs are not pink in the center anymore and the juices run clear. When done, an instant-read thermometer should read at least 165°F (74°C) when inserted into the center.

Nutrition Information

- Calories: 146 calories;
- Total Carbohydrate: 0.6
- Cholesterol: 95
- Protein: 17.7
- Total Fat: 8.2
- Sodium: 395

211. Spicy Chipotle Turkey Burgers

Serving: 4 | Prep: 25mins | Cook: 10mins | Ready in:

Ingredients

- 1 pound ground turkey
- 1/2 cup finely chopped onion
- 2 tablespoons chopped fresh cilantro
- 1 chipotle chile in adobo sauce, finely chopped
- 1 teaspoon garlic powder
- 1 teaspoon onion powder
- 1 teaspoon seasoned salt
- 1/4 teaspoon black pepper
- 4 slices mozzarella cheese
- 4 hamburger buns, split and toasted

Direction

- Lightly oil grate and preheat grill to medium heat. In a bowl, make the patties by combining ground turkey, cilantro, onion, garlic powder, chipotle chile peppers, onion powder, black pepper and seasoned salt, mix well and shape into four equal patties.
- Grill the turkey patties on the prepared grill, four minutes each side. Top patties with mozzarella on the last two minutes and let it melt. Serve on top of crisp toasted buns.

Nutrition Information

- Calories: 376 calories;
- Total Carbohydrate: 25.8
- Cholesterol: 102
- Protein: 33.3
- Total Fat: 15.3
- Sodium: 725

212. Spicy Turkey Burgers

Serving: 8 | Prep: 20mins | Cook: 20mins | Ready in:

Ingredients

- 2 pounds lean ground turkey
- 2 tablespoons minced garlic
- 1 teaspoon minced fresh ginger root
- 2 fresh green chile peppers, diced
- 1 medium red onion, diced
- 1/2 cup fresh cilantro, finely chopped
- 1 teaspoon salt
- 1/4 cup low sodium soy sauce
- 1 tablespoon freshly ground black pepper
- 3 tablespoons paprika
- 1 tablespoon ground dry mustard
- 1 tablespoon ground cumin
- 1 dash Worcestershire sauce

Direction

- Set the grill on high heat. Combine ground turkey, ginger, garlic, red onion, cilantro, chili peppers, soy sauce, salt, paprika, black pepper, cumin, mustard and the Worcestershire sauce in a big bowl. Mix well and divide into 8 patties. Brush the grill lightly with oil and cook the turkey burgers until well done. Five to ten minutes each side.

Nutrition Information

- Calories: 204 calories;
- Total Fat: 9.6
- Sodium: 626
- Total Carbohydrate: 6.4
- Cholesterol: 84
- Protein: 24.4

213. Spicy Turkey Four Bean Chili

Serving: 12 | Prep: 15mins | Cook: 1hours30mins | Ready in:

Ingredients

- 3 (15 ounce) cans diced tomatoes with green chile peppers
- 2 (15 ounce) cans chili beans in spicy sauce
- 1 (16 ounce) jar hot salsa
- 1 (15 ounce) can dark red kidney beans
- 1 (15 ounce) can light red kidney beans
- 1 (15 ounce) can seasoned black beans
- 2 small onions, chopped
- 6 cloves garlic, crushed
- 2 tablespoons chili powder
- 2 tablespoons red pepper flakes
- 2 tablespoons coarsely ground black pepper
- 2 tablespoons ground cumin
- 1 (1.25 ounce) package taco seasoning mix
- 1 teaspoon hot sauce
- 2 pounds ground turkey

Direction

- Blend hot sauce, taco seasoning mix, cumin, black pepper, red pepper flakes, chili powder, garlic, onions, black beans, dark and light red kidney beans, salsa, chili beans, green chiles, and diced tomatoes in a large soup pot. Heat to a boil, lower the heat to low, and close with the cover. Simmer until onions are transparent, and soup is heated, for approximately 20 minutes.
- Heat over medium-high a large skillet. Cook and stir ground turkey in the hot skillet until crumbled and browned, for about 10 minutes; drain and discard the grease. Blend the crumbled turkey into the chili.
- Cover pot and simmer chili until flavors are well-blended, for about 1 hour.

Nutrition Information

- Calories: 319 calories;

- Sodium: 1480
- Total Carbohydrate: 40.6
- Cholesterol: 56
- Protein: 26.4
- Total Fat: 8.8

214. Spicy Turkey Sloppy Joes

Serving: 12 | Prep: 20mins | Cook: 30mins | Ready in:

Ingredients

- 2 pounds ground turkey
- 2 onions, chopped
- 1/2 cup chopped green bell pepper
- 1/2 cup chopped red bell pepper
- 1 serrano chile pepper, minced
- 1 fresh chile pepper, minced
- 2 cloves garlic, minced
- 2 cups ketchup
- 1 cup barbeque sauce
- 1/4 cup cider vinegar
- 1/4 cup packed brown sugar
- 2 tablespoons prepared mustard
- 1 tablespoon Worcestershire sauce
- 1 teaspoon Italian seasoning
- 1 teaspoon onion powder
- 1/2 teaspoon ground black pepper
- hamburger buns, split

Direction

- Place a large skillet on medium heat; cook while stirring in garlic, fresh chile pepper, serrano chile pepper, red bell pepper, green bell pepper, onions and ground turkey for around 10 minutes, till the turkey is not pink anymore. Drain fat from the turkey mixture.
- Mix black pepper, onion powder, Italian seasoning, Worcestershire sauce, mustard, brown sugar, cider vinegar, barbeque sauce and ketchup together into the turkey mixture. Boil; turn the heat down to medium-low; simmer for around 20 minutes, till the vegetables becomes completely softened.
- Serve on split hamburger buns.

Nutrition Information

- Calories: 347 calories;
- Total Carbohydrate: 49.2
- Cholesterol: 56
- Protein: 20.1
- Total Fat: 8.3
- Sodium: 1009

215. Spicy And Thick Turkey Chili

Serving: 6 | Prep: 20mins | Cook: 1hours25mins | Ready in:

Ingredients

- 3 tablespoons extra-virgin olive oil
- 2 yellow onions, chopped
- 1 green bell pepper, seeded and minced
- 1 red bell pepper, seeded and minced
- 6 cloves garlic, minced
- 1 1/3 pounds ground turkey
- 2 tablespoons chili powder
- 2 tablespoons dried oregano
- 1 tablespoon paprika
- 1 tablespoon ground cumin
- 2 teaspoons seasoned salt
- 1 1/2 teaspoons red pepper flakes
- 1 teaspoon ground black pepper
- 1 teaspoon unsweetened cocoa powder
- 2 (14.5 ounce) cans diced tomatoes with green chile peppers, liquid drained and reserved
- 1 (15 ounce) can red chili beans, rinsed and drained
- 1 (15 ounce) can black beans, rinsed and drained
- 1 (6 ounce) can tomato paste
- 3/4 cup light beer (such as Miller Lite®)
- 1 tablespoon Worcestershire sauce
- 1/2 teaspoon hickory-flavored liquid smoke

- 1/2 cup low-sodium tomato juice
- 2 tablespoons hot pepper sauce (such as Tabasco®)

Direction

- Heat olive oil in a big pot on medium heat; mix and cook garlic, red and green bell peppers and onions in hot oil for 7-10 minutes till onions are translucent.
- Crumble ground turkey into small pieces; put into the pot. Cover pot; cook for about 5 minutes till turkey isn't pink anymore and cooked through, occasionally mixing.
- Season turkey with cocoa powder, ground black pepper, red pepper flakes, seasoned salt, cumin, paprika, oregano and chili powder; add tomato juices, liquid smoke, Worcestershire sauce, light beer, tomato paste, black beans, red chili beans and diced tomatoes with the green chile peppers. Cover pot loosely; cook at a simmer for approximately 1 hour till thick but still moist, occasionally mixing. Mix reserved liquid from the diced tomatoes with the green chilies into chili while simmering to keep it from being too dry.
- Mix hot pepper sauce through chili; lower the heat to low. Simmer for 10 minutes longer; slightly cool. Serve.

Nutrition Information

- Calories: 458 calories;
- Total Fat: 17.1
- Sodium: 1823
- Total Carbohydrate: 48.7
- Cholesterol: 75
- Protein: 32.7

216. Spinach And Feta Turkey Burgers

Serving: 8 | Prep: 20mins | Cook: 15mins | Ready in:

Ingredients

- 2 eggs, beaten
- 2 cloves garlic, minced
- 4 ounces feta cheese
- 1 (10 ounce) box frozen chopped spinach, thawed and squeezed dry
- 2 pounds ground turkey

Direction

- Lightly brush grate with oil and preheat grill to medium heat. While waiting for the grill to heat, make the patties by combining ground turkey, eggs, garlic, spinach and feta cheese in a bowl. Mix thoroughly and divide into 8 patties. Grill patties for 15 to 20 minutes, until center is not pink.

Nutrition Information

- Calories: 233 calories;
- Total Carbohydrate: 2.4
- Cholesterol: 143
- Protein: 27.4
- Total Fat: 13
- Sodium: 266

217. Spinach, Turkey, And Mushroom Lasagna

Serving: 12 | Prep: 30mins | Cook: 1hours | Ready in:

Ingredients

- 12 lasagna noodles
- 1 Vidalia onion, diced
- 2 cloves garlic, minced
- 1 pound ground turkey
- 1 (8 ounce) package sliced white mushrooms
- salt and ground black pepper to taste
- 2 (9 ounce) packages frozen spinach, thawed
- 2 cups whole milk ricotta cheese
- 1/4 cup heavy whipping cream

- zest of 2 lemons
- 1/2 teaspoon Italian seasoning
- 1/4 teaspoon ground nutmeg
- 1 (28 ounce) jar spaghetti sauce
- 2 cups grated Asiago cheese
- 2 cups shredded Cheddar cheese

Direction

- Boil a big pot with lightly salted water; cook lasagna noodles, occasionally mixing, in boiling water for 8 minutes till tender but firm to chew. Drain.
- Mix garlic and onion on medium high heat in big skillet; mix and cook for 5 minutes till onion is translucent. Add turkey; cook for 5-7 minutes till not pink. Add mushrooms; season with pepper and salt. Cook for 6 minutes till soft; take off heat. Cool.
- In clean dish towel, wrap thawed spinach; wring spinach to extract as much water as you can above bowl. Mix nutmeg, Italian seasoning, lemon zest, heavy cream, ricotta cheese and spinach in another bowl.
- Preheat an oven to 190°C/375°F.
- Use 3 tbsp. spaghetti sauce to coat bottom of 9x13-in. baking dish; layer with 4 cooked lasagna noodles, 1/2 spinach mixture, 1/2 turkey mixture, 1/3 Asiago cheese, 1/3 cheddar cheese then 3/4 cup spaghetti sauce over. Layer 4 extra noodles, leftover turkey and spinach mixtures, extra 1/3 Asiago cheese, 1/3 extra cheddar cheese then 3/4 cup extra spaghetti sauce. Put leftover 4 lasagna noodles, the spaghetti sauce, the Asiago cheese then cheddar cheese over; use aluminum foil to cover.
- In preheated oven, bake for 35 minutes then remove aluminum foil; put oven temperature on 220°C/425°F. Bake for 15 minutes till crust is golden.

Nutrition Information

- Calories: 453 calories;
- Protein: 28.1
- Total Fat: 24.1
- Sodium: 709
- Total Carbohydrate: 32.7
- Cholesterol: 93

218. Spooky Slow Cooker Turkey Lentil Chili

Serving: 12 | Prep: 15mins | Cook: 6hours5mins | Ready in:

Ingredients

- 2 1/2 pounds lean ground turkey
- 2 (14.5 ounce) cans Italian-style diced tomatoes
- 1 pound cooked lentils
- 1 (14.5 ounce) can pumpkin puree
- 1 (14.5 ounce) can pinto beans, rinsed and drained
- 1 (12 ounce) package frozen pearl onions
- 1 (8 ounce) can chopped green chile peppers
- 3 cloves garlic, minced
- 1 cup water
- 1/4 cup brown sugar
- 1/4 cup chili powder
- 2 tablespoons pumpkin pie spice
- 1 tablespoon onion powder
- salt and ground black pepper to taste

Direction

- In a nonstick skillet, cook the turkey over medium heat for 5 to 8 minutes till browned. Let drain.
- To a slow cooker, put the turkey. Put garlic, green chili peppers, pearl onions, pinto beans, pumpkin puree, lentils and tomatoes. Mix in pepper, salt, onion powder, pumpkin pie spice, chili powder, brown sugar and water.
- Put cover and allow to cook on Low for 6 to 10 hours till flavors incorporate.

Nutrition Information

- Calories: 262 calories;

- Total Fat: 1.7
- Sodium: 689
- Total Carbohydrate: 29.9
- Cholesterol: 68
- Protein: 31.7

- Sodium: 1229
- Total Carbohydrate: 32.9
- Cholesterol: 68
- Protein: 21.6
- Total Fat: 14.7

219. Strange But True Casserole

Serving: 6 | Prep: 25mins | Cook: 35mins | Ready in:

Ingredients

- 1 pound ground turkey
- 2 tablespoons minced garlic
- 2 tablespoons ground black pepper
- 1 green bell pepper, seeded and chopped
- 1 yellow onion, chopped
- 1 (10.75 ounce) can condensed cream of mushroom soup
- 2 (14.75 ounce) cans spaghetti with meat sauce
- 1 cup Italian-style seasoned bread crumbs

Direction

- Set an oven to 175°C (350°F) and start preheating.
- In a large skillet, brown the turkey for 10-15 minutes until it is not pink anymore; then drain the turkey. Put onion, bell pepper, pepper, and garlic into the browned turkey meat; stir them together and sauté for 5-7 minutes until the onion turns transparent.
- Mix in soup and allow to cook for 2 minutes, then mix in spaghetti and stir, combine until well mixed. Place the mixture into a 2-1/2 liter casserole dish, then put into the oven.
- In the prepared oven, bake for 35 minutes. Take out of the oven, then dust breadcrumbs over the top and bake for 10 more minutes.

Nutrition Information

- Calories: 350 calories;

220. Stroganoff Casserole

Serving: 8 | Prep: 10mins | Cook: 43mins | Ready in:

Ingredients

- 1/4 cup butter, divided
- 1 (8 ounce) package egg noodles (such as Inn Maid® Fine Egg Noodles)
- 2 (4 ounce) cans mushroom pieces and stems, drained
- 1 small onion, finely chopped
- 2 pounds ground turkey
- salt and ground black pepper to taste
- 2 (10.75 ounce) cans condensed cream of mushroom soup
- 1 (8 ounce) container sour cream
- 1 packet Swedish meatballs seasoning and sauce mixes (such as McCormick®)
- 2 meatball seasoning packets
- 1/4 cup milk, or more to taste

Direction

- Set the oven at 350°F (175°C) and start preheating. In a 9x13-in. casserole dish, place 2 tablespoons of butter.
- Insert the casserole dish into the preheating oven to melt butter. Take away from the oven, leaving the heat on; spread the melted butter around the dish to evenly coat the bottom.
- Fill lightly salted water into a large pot; bring to a rolling boil. Mix in egg noodles; turn back to boil. Cook while stirring occasionally the noodles, uncovered, around 6 minutes, or till tender yet firm to bite. Strain.
- Place a large skillet on medium heat; melt the remaining 2 tablespoons of butter. Include in onion and mushrooms; cook while stirring for

around 5 minutes, or till the onions turn soft. Include in ground turkey. Cook while breaking the meat up, 5-7 minutes, or till crumbled and browned. Season with pepper and salt. Include in meatball seasoning packets, sour cream and mushroom soup. Stir properly, including in milk, 3-5 minutes longer, or till the sauce is thickened to your desired consistency.
- Mix sauce and the egg noodles, place into the casserole dish. Use aluminum foil to cover.
- Bake for around 30 minutes in the preheated oven, or till the top is bubbling.

Nutrition Information

- Calories: 491 calories;
- Total Fat: 27
- Sodium: 1100
- Total Carbohydrate: 33.3
- Cholesterol: 136
- Protein: 30.2

221. Stuffed Orange Peppers

Serving: 6 | Prep: 15mins | Cook: 45mins | Ready in:

Ingredients

- 6 orange bell peppers, tops and seeds removed
- 1 pound ground turkey
- 1/3 cup chopped onion
- 1 (14.5 ounce) can diced tomatoes, or more to taste
- 1/2 cup white rice
- 1/2 cup water
- 1 teaspoon liquid smoke flavoring
- 1 cup shredded Gouda cheese

Direction

- Boil big pot of water. Cook orange bell peppers for about 5 minutes till slightly soft; drain.
- Heat a big skillet on medium high heat; mix and cook onion and turkey in the hot skillet for 5-7 minutes till crumbly and browned. Drain; discard grease.
- Preheat an oven to 175°C or 350°F.
- Mix liquid smoke, 1/2 cup water, rice and tomatoes into turkey mixture and cover skillet; simmer for approximately 15 minutes till rice is tender. Take skillet off the heat; mix gouda cheese into the turkey mixture.
- Use turkey mixture to stuff every orange bell pepper; put peppers in a baking dish, open side up. Use aluminum foil to cover dish.
- In the preheated oven, bake for 25-35 minutes till cheese melts and heated through.

Nutrition Information

- Calories: 295 calories;
- Sodium: 317
- Total Carbohydrate: 23.4
- Cholesterol: 79
- Protein: 22.9
- Total Fat: 12.3

222. Stuffed Peppers With Turkey And Vegetables

Serving: 4 | Prep: 20mins | Cook: 30mins | Ready in:

Ingredients

- 4 green bell peppers, tops removed, seeded
- 1 pound ground turkey
- 2 tablespoons olive oil
- 1/2 onion, chopped
- 1 cup sliced mushrooms
- 1 zucchini, chopped
- 1/2 red bell pepper, chopped
- 1/2 yellow bell pepper, chopped
- 1 cup fresh spinach
- 1 (14.5 ounce) can diced tomatoes, drained
- 1 tablespoon tomato paste
- Italian seasoning to taste

- garlic powder to taste
- salt and pepper to taste

Direction

- Preheat an oven to 175°C or 350°F.
- In aluminum foil, wrap green bell peppers, and put in baking dish. Allow to bake in prepped oven for 15 minutes. Take off heat.
- Let the turkey cook in a skillet over moderate heat till equally brown. Reserve. In skillet, heat the oil, and cook spinach, yellow bell pepper, red bell pepper, zucchini, mushrooms and onion till soft. Return turkey to the skillet. Mix in the tomatoes and tomato paste, and season with Italian seasoning, garlic powder, salt, and pepper. Stuff the green peppers with the skillet mixture.
- Put peppers back to oven, and keep cooking for 15 minutes.

Nutrition Information

- Calories: 280 calories;
- Sodium: 433
- Total Carbohydrate: 10.2
- Cholesterol: 84
- Protein: 25.4
- Total Fat: 15.6

223. Stuffed Red Peppers With Quinoa, Mushrooms, And Turkey

Serving: 8 | Prep: 30mins | Cook: 1hours30mins | Ready in:

Ingredients

- 2 cups water
- 1 cup uncooked quinoa
- 1 tablespoon olive oil
- 1 onion, diced
- 1 pound ground turkey
- salt and ground black pepper to taste
- 12 mushrooms, chopped, or more to taste
- 1 (24 ounce) jar tomato sauce, or more to taste
- 1 (6 ounce) can tomato paste
- 8 large red bell peppers - tops, seeds, and membranes removed
- 1 (8 ounce) package shredded Cheddar cheese, or to taste

Direction

- Boil quinoa and water in a saucepan. Lower heat to medium low and cover; simmer for 15-20 minutes till quinoa is tender.
- Heat olive oil on medium heat in a big skillet. Add onion; cook for 5 minutes till soft. Add turkey; season with pepper and salt. Mix and cook for 5-7 minutes till turkey isn't pink. Add mushrooms; cook for 5 minutes till soft.
- Preheat an oven to 175°C/350°F.
- Put cooked turkey mixture into big bowl. Add tomato paste, tomato sauce and cooked quinoa. Mix well; as needed, add extra tomato sauce till filling has a casserole-consistency.
- Put red bell peppers into baking dish; in each, put even filling amount.
- In preheated oven, bake for 45 minutes then remove from oven. Put cheddar cheese over each stuffed pepper. Bake for 10 minutes till cheese melts.

Nutrition Information

- Calories: 389 calories;
- Cholesterol: 71
- Protein: 25.8
- Total Fat: 17.4
- Sodium: 850
- Total Carbohydrate: 34.6

224. Stuffed Shells IV

Serving: 14 | Prep: 30mins | Cook: 45mins | Ready in:

Ingredients

- 1 (12 ounce) package jumbo pasta shells
- 8 ounces mushrooms, diced
- 3 cloves garlic, minced
- 1 onion, chopped
- 1 pound ground turkey
- salt and pepper to taste
- 1 (10 ounce) package frozen chopped spinach, thawed and drained
- 2 tablespoons chopped fresh parsley
- 2 cups cottage cheese
- 1 cup freshly grated Parmesan cheese
- 1 (32 ounce) jar spaghetti sauce
- 1 (8 ounce) package mozzarella cheese, shredded

Direction

- Preheat the oven to 175 °C or 350 °F.
- Boil a big pot of slightly salted water. Put in the pasta and cook until al dente, about 8 to 10 minutes; drain. Reserve in warm water.
- Sauté onions, garlic and mushrooms in a big heavy skillet. Put in the ground turkey and cook till equally brown. Add pepper and salt to season. Take away from heat, and mix in Parmesan cheese, cottage cheese, parsley and spinach.
- With the mixture, fill the cooked shells, and arrange in a 9x13 inch baking dish. Cover with spaghetti sauce, and scatter mozzarella cheese on top.
- Cover using foil, and in prepped oven, bake till heated through, about 30 to 45 minutes.

Nutrition Information

- Calories: 323 calories;
- Total Fat: 11.3
- Sodium: 622
- Total Carbohydrate: 30.9
- Cholesterol: 54
- Protein: 24.4

225. Swedish Turkey Meatballs

Serving: 6 | Prep: 20mins | Cook: 33mins | Ready in:

Ingredients

- Meatballs:
- 1 1/2 pounds ground turkey
- 3/4 cup bread crumbs
- 1 egg, beaten
- 2 tablespoons grated Parmesan cheese
- 2 cloves garlic, minced
- 2 teaspoons dried Italian seasoning
- Sauce:
- 2 cups beef broth
- 3 tablespoons all-purpose flour
- 2 tablespoons butter
- 1 cup heavy whipping cream
- 1 tablespoon Worcestershire sauce (optional)
- 1/4 teaspoon ground black pepper

Direction

- In a large bowl, using your hand to combine Italian seasoning, garlic, Parmesan cheese, egg, bread crumbs and ground turkey. Shape the mixture into 1 1/2-in. meatballs.
- Pour beef broth in a microwave-safe container; microwave on high for 2 minutes or till hot. Blend flour into beef broth till smooth.
- Place a large skillet on medium heat; melt butter. Put in meatballs, in batches if needed; cook for about 2 minutes per side or till browned on all sides. Turn the heat down to low. Add beef broth slowly over the meatballs. Mix in black pepper, Worcestershire sauce and heavy cream. Cook while stirring sometimes for 10 minutes or till the meatballs are cooked through.
- Bring a large pot of lightly salted water to boil. Cook egg noodles while stirring sometimes for 8-10 minutes, till tender yet firm to bite; strain. Serve sauce and meatballs over noodles.

Nutrition Information

- Calories: 435 calories;
- Total Carbohydrate: 15.2
- Cholesterol: 181
- Protein: 28.3
- Total Fat: 29.4
- Sodium: 533

226. Swedish Turkey Meatballs With Cream Of Mushroom Soup

Serving: 12 | Prep: 20mins | Cook: 1hours | Ready in:

Ingredients

- Meatballs:
- 2 teaspoons vegetable oil, or as needed
- 1/2 cup milk
- 2 eggs
- 1 1/2 pounds ground turkey, or more to taste
- 1 cup crushed chicken-flavored crackers (such as Nabisco® Chicken in a Biscuit)
- 1/2 onion, minced
- 1 teaspoon salt
- 1 teaspoon ground nutmeg
- 1 teaspoon ground black pepper
- Sauce:
- 2 (10.75 ounce) cans cream of mushroom soup
- 2 (10.75 ounce) cans condensed golden mushroom soup
- 1 (12 fluid ounce) can evaporated milk
- 1 (8 ounce) carton sour cream
- 1/2 pound baby portobello mushrooms, sliced
- 2 cloves garlic, minced
- 1 cup grated Parmesan cheese
- 1 (16 ounce) package egg noodles

Direction

- Set the oven to 350°F (175°C) and start preheating. Oil a 2-quart casserole dish and a baking sheet lightly.
- In a bowl, mix eggs and milk. Add black pepper, nutmeg, salt, onion, crackers and turkey. Combine well. Form into 1-inch balls; transfer to prepared baking sheet.
- Bake in the prepared oven for about 20 minutes until browned. Drain meatballs on paper towels; place on prepared casserole dish. Leave the oven on.
- In a large bowl, mix garlic, mushrooms, sour cream, evaporated milk, golden mushroom soup and cream of mushroom soup; stir until smooth. Top over meatballs in the casserole dish.
- Bake in the hot oven for about 40 minutes until bubbling.
- Boil a large pot of lightly salted water. In boiling water, cook egg noodles while stirring occasionally for about 8 minutes until tender but firm to the bite. Drain. Serve gravy and meatballs over hot noodles; top with Parmesan cheese; serve.

Nutrition Information

- Calories: 500 calories;
- Protein: 26.1
- Total Fat: 23.4
- Sodium: 1171
- Total Carbohydrate: 46.5
- Cholesterol: 130

227. Sweet Potato Chili

Serving: 8 | Prep: 30mins | Cook: 6hours | Ready in:

Ingredients

- 2 sweet potatoes, diced
- 2 (14.5 ounce) cans diced stewed tomatoes with chili seasonings
- 1 (8 ounce) can tomato sauce
- 3/4 cup diced sweet onion
- 1/2 cup chopped celery
- 1/2 cup water
- 1 tablespoon chili powder
- 1 teaspoon ground cumin

- 1/2 teaspoon ground cinnamon
- 1 pinch salt
- 1 pinch ground black pepper
- 1 pinch cayenne pepper
- 1 pinch garlic powder
- 1 pinch onion powder
- 1/2 pound ground turkey
- 1/2 pound ground beef
- 1 (12 ounce) can black beans, drained and rinsed
- 1 cup corn

Direction

- In a slow cooker, add onion powder, garlic powder, cayenne pepper, black pepper, salt, cinnamon, cumin, chili powder, water, celery, onion, tomato sauce, stewed tomatoes and sweet potatoes. Cook on high setting while stirring from time to time, about 5 hours.
- Heat a big skillet on moderate high heat and stir in ground beef as well as ground turkey. Cook and stir for 10-15 minutes until meat is crumbly, not pink anymore and browned evenly. Drain and get rid of any excess grease. Put corn, black beans, cooked ground beef and cooked ground turkey into the slow cooker; cook for about 1 to 2 hours longer until flavors combined. Serve warm.

Nutrition Information

- Calories: 250 calories;
- Total Fat: 7.4
- Sodium: 621
- Total Carbohydrate: 32.5
- Cholesterol: 38
- Protein: 16

228. Sweet Potato And Turkey Shepherd's Pie

Serving: 6 | Prep: 30mins | Cook: 1hours30mins | Ready in:

Ingredients

- 2 large sweet potatoes, peeled and cubed
- 1 large russet potato, peeled and cubed
- 2 large carrots, peeled and diced
- 1/4 cup egg substitute
- 1/3 cup light sour cream
- salt and ground black pepper to taste
- 1 tablespoon olive oil
- 1 pound ground turkey
- 1/2 cup chopped onion
- 1 stalk celery, chopped
- 1 clove garlic, minced
- 1 teaspoon crumbled dried thyme
- 3/4 teaspoon poultry seasoning
- 1/2 cup chicken stock
- 1/2 cup hot milk
- 1 tablespoon all-purpose flour
- 1 dash Worcestershire sauce
- 1 dash browning sauce
- 1 1/3 cups herb-seasoned stuffing mix
- 1 cup peas
- 3/4 cup corn
- 1/2 teaspoon crumbled dried thyme
- salt and ground black pepper to taste
- 1 teaspoon ground nutmeg

Direction

- Preheat an oven to 190 degrees C (375 degrees F). Coat a 2-quart, deep-dish casserole pan lightly with grease.
- Put carrot, sweet potato, and russet potato each in separate saucepans. Add plenty of water into each saucepan to cover the veggies. Transfer each saucepan onto medium heat and heat to boil. Cook each for about 5 to 7 minutes until they are tender enough to pierce with a fork. Drain off water. Reserve the carrots.
- In a large mixing bowl, put the drained russet potato and sweet potato and then mash lightly. Add sour cream and egg substitute. Use an electric hand mixer that is set to medium to blend the potato mixture for about 2 minutes until fluffy and smooth. Add pepper and salt to taste. Reserve.

- Over medium heat, heat oil in a large skillet and add turkey. Cook in hot oil for 4 to 5 minutes until browned. Add the poultry seasoning, onion, 1 teaspoon thyme, celery, and garlic. Cook until turkey is no longer pink and is cooked through. Raise the heat to medium-high. Add chicken stock into turkey mixture. Whisk flour and hot milk together until smooth. Once the chicken stock starts to boil, pour the flour mixture into the stock and mix until it becomes thick. Take out from the heat and mix in browning sauce and Worcestershire sauce.
- Transfer turkey mixture into the bottom of the casserole dish. Drizzle the stuffing mix atop turkey mixture. Spread corn, peas, and carrots over the stuffing mix. Season with pepper, salt, and thyme. Ladle the potato mixture atop veggies and spread to cover all the way to the edges of dish. Drizzle with nutmeg.
- Bake for about 35 minutes until the top is browned slightly. Let to rest for 30 minutes prior to serving.

Nutrition Information

- Calories: 452 calories;
- Total Carbohydrate: 65.7
- Cholesterol: 64
- Protein: 23.5
- Total Fat: 10.5
- Sodium: 566

229. Sweet Potato Turkey Meatloaf

Serving: 4 | Prep: 25mins | Cook: 1hours10mins | Ready in:

Ingredients

- 1 large sweet potato, peeled and cubed
- 1 pound ground turkey breast
- 1 large egg
- 1 small sweet onion, finely chopped
- 2 cloves garlic, minced
- 1/4 cup honey barbecue sauce
- 1/4 cup ketchup
- 2 tablespoons Dijon mustard
- 2 slices whole-wheat bread, torn into small crumbs
- 1 tablespoon freshly ground black pepper, or to taste
- 1 tablespoon salt, or to taste

Direction

- Set an oven to preheat to 175°C (350°F). Grease a 2-qt. baking dish lightly.
- Boil a pot of lightly salted water, then add the sweet potato and let it cook for about 10 minutes until it becomes soft. Drain the sweet potatoes and whip or mash it until it becomes smooth.
- In a big mixing bowl, mix the ground turkey together with whole-wheat breadcrumbs, Dijon mustard, ketchup, barbecue sauce, garlic, sweet onion and egg, then season using pepper and salt to taste. Add the sweet potatoes and mix until blended evenly. Add more breadcrumbs if the mixture appears too wet. Shape the turkey mixture into a loaf shape using your hands and put it in the prepped baking dish.
- Let it bake for an hour in the preheated oven. Cut the loaf, then serve.

Nutrition Information

- Calories: 336 calories;
- Sodium: 2478
- Total Carbohydrate: 43
- Cholesterol: 117
- Protein: 33.8
- Total Fat: 2.7

230. Sweet Turkey Chili From RED GOLD®

Serving: 8 | Prep: 10mins | Cook: 1hours | Ready in:

Ingredients

- 1 pound ground turkey
- 1 (14.5 ounce) can RED GOLD® Diced Tomatoes
- 1 (46 ounce) can RED GOLD® Fresh Squeezed Tomato Juice
- 1 onion, chopped
- 1 teaspoon dill weed
- 1/2 teaspoon dried oregano
- 1 teaspoon garlic powder
- 1 (15.5 ounce) can chili hot beans in chili gravy
- 1 (15.5 ounce) can kidney beans, rinsed and drained
- 1 (15 ounce) can pinto beans, rinsed and drained
- 1 (14.5 ounce) can red beans, rinsed and drained
- 1 (1.25 ounce) package chili seasoning mix
- 1 tablespoon chili powder
- 1/2 cup sugar
- Salt and black pepper to taste

Direction

- In a big soup kettle, brown turkey and crumble into small pieces. Add the rest of the ingredients and simmer for 1 hour. You can either add extra tomato juice if you want the consistency to be thicker, or thin it by adding extra water.
- Put shredded cheese on top and enjoy with a Red Gold smile.

Nutrition Information

- Calories: 361 calories;
- Sodium: 1617
- Total Carbohydrate: 57.6
- Cholesterol: 42
- Protein: 24.3
- Total Fat: 6

231. Sweet And Spicy Pumpkin Turkey Pasta

Serving: 4 | Prep: 25mins | Cook: 30mins | Ready in:

Ingredients

- cooking spray
- 1 medium onion, chopped
- 3 cloves garlic, minced
- 1 pound lean ground turkey
- 1 1/4 cups chicken broth
- 1 cup pumpkin puree
- 1/3 cup low-fat milk
- 2 chipotle peppers in adobo sauce
- 2 teaspoons white sugar
- 2 teaspoons dried sage
- 1 teaspoon ground black pepper
- 1 teaspoon ground cinnamon
- 1/2 teaspoon ground coriander
- 1/2 teaspoon pumpkin pie spice
- 1/4 teaspoon ground nutmeg
- 1 tablespoon salt
- 1 (8 ounce) package rotini pasta

Direction

- Use cooking spray to spray a deep skillet. Add onions; cook for about 3 minutes over medium heat until translucent. Add garlic; cook for about a minute until fragrant. Add ground turkey; cook for 8-10 minutes until no longer pink.
- Pour chicken broth into the skillet; bring to a boil. Add nutmeg, pumpkin pie spice, coriander, cinnamon, black pepper, sage, sugar, chipotle peppers, milk and pumpkin puree. Lower to a simmer; cook until pasta ready.
- Boil a large pot of water; add a tablespoon salt and rotini. Cook the rotini at a boil for about 8 minutes until tender but firm to the bite; drain.
- Stir cooked pasta into the skillet with the pumpkin-turkey sauce until coated evenly.

Nutrition Information

- Calories: 445 calories;
- Sodium: 2367
- Total Carbohydrate: 56
- Cholesterol: 86
- Protein: 32.2
- Total Fat: 10.4

232. Taco Stuffed Zucchini Boats

Serving: 4 | Prep: 20mins | Cook: 50mins | Ready in:

Ingredients

- 4 zucchinis, halved lengthwise and seeded
- 1 pound ground turkey
- 1 (1.25 ounce) package taco seasoning
- 3/4 cup water, or as needed
- 2 red sweet pepper, finely chopped
- 1 (10 ounce) can diced tomatoes and green chiles (such as RO*TEL® Mexican Lime & Cilantro)
- 1/2 white onion, finely chopped
- 1/4 cup chopped fresh cilantro
- 1 cup sour cream
- 1 (1 ounce) packet sour cream seasoning mix (such as Old El Paso® Zesty Sour Cream Seasoning Mix)
- 1 bunch green onions, diced
- 1/2 cup shredded Muenster cheese
- 1/2 cup shredded Cheddar cheese

Direction

- Start preheating the oven at 400°F (200°C). Oil the base of a 13x9-inch baking dish.
- Heat a large pot of water to a boil. In boiling water, cook zucchini halves to barely soften slightly about 1 minute. Bring zucchini halves out from the water and place into the oiled baking dish, cut sides up.
- On medium-high heat, heat a large skillet. In the hot skillet, cook and stir ground turkey about 5 to 7 minutes until crumbly and brown; drain, discard grease.
- Set skillet back to medium-high heat; pour water on turkey and flavor with taco seasoning. Cook about 5 minutes until the water thickens and covers the turkey. Include in cilantro, onion, diced tomatoes and green chiles, and red peppers; cook and stir for an extra 5 minutes until the peppers are tender.
- Blend sour cream seasoning mix and sour cream in a bowl.
- With a slotted spoon, scoop the turkey mixture in the hollows of each zucchini half and press firmly. Top the turkey mixture with 1/2 the sour cream mixture. Spread sour cream mixture with green onions, Muenster cheese, and Cheddar cheese, respectively.
- Bake in the prepared oven for about 30 minutes until the zucchini cooks fully and cheese melts. Pour the remaining sour cream mixture on top.

Nutrition Information

- Calories: 527 calories;
- Total Fat: 30.1
- Sodium: 1570
- Total Carbohydrate: 31.8
- Cholesterol: 137
- Protein: 35

233. Tarragon Turkey Soup

Serving: 8 | Prep: 25mins | Cook: 45mins | Ready in:

Ingredients

- 1 tablespoon olive oil
- 1 pound ground turkey
- 1/2 cup diced onion
- 1/4 cup diced green bell pepper
- 1 (48 fluid ounce) can chicken broth

- 2 tablespoons dried tarragon
- 3 carrots, peeled and thinly sliced
- 5 small red potatoes, diced with peel
- salt and pepper to taste
- 3/4 cup quick-cooking barley

Direction

- Heat olive oil in a big pot on medium high heat then add ground turkey; mix and cook for 3-4 minutes till turkey starts to brown and is crumbled. Mix green pepper and onion in; continue to cook for 3 minutes till onion is translucent and softens.
- Add chicken broth, red potatoes, carrots and tarragon; boil on high heat. Lower the heat to medium low; simmer for 20 minutes till potatoes soften, occasionally mixing. Season with pepper and salt to taste; mix barley in. Simmer continuously for 15 minutes till barley is tender.

Nutrition Information

- Calories: 271 calories;
- Cholesterol: 46
- Protein: 16.7
- Total Fat: 6.9
- Sodium: 912
- Total Carbohydrate: 36.4

234. Tastes Like Beef Turkey Burgers

Serving: 4 | Prep: 10mins | Cook: 8mins | Ready in:

Ingredients

- 1 pound ground turkey
- 1 (1 ounce) package dry onion soup mix
- 2 tablespoons steak sauce
- cooking spray
- 4 hamburger buns

Direction

- Combine together steak sauce, onion soup mix and ground turkey in a big bowl, then form into four patties.
- Heat in a big skillet on moderate heat and use cooking spray to coat slightly. Cook burgers for 4 minutes per side, then serve on hamburger buns.

Nutrition Information

- Calories: 315 calories;
- Total Carbohydrate: 27.2
- Cholesterol: 90
- Protein: 24
- Total Fat: 11.7
- Sodium: 1078

235. Tasty Ground Turkey Tacos

Serving: 6 | Prep: 20mins | Cook: 35mins | Ready in:

Ingredients

- 1 1/2 pounds ground turkey
- 1 (8 ounce) can tomato sauce
- 8 fluid ounces water
- 1 (4 ounce) can diced green chile peppers
- 1/2 onion, chopped
- 1 (1.25 ounce) package taco seasoning mix
- 1 clove garlic, minced
- 12 (6 inch) flour tortillas
- 1 cup shredded lettuce, or to taste
- 1/2 cup Cheddar cheese, or to taste
- 1/2 cup diced tomatoes, or to taste
- 1/4 cup chopped green onion, or to taste
- 1/4 cup chopped cilantro, or to taste
- 2 tablespoons sliced olives, or to taste

Direction

- Heat up a big skillet on medium-high heat beforehand; add the turkey. Cook while stirring until brown, around 5 minutes. Add garlic, taco seasoning, onion, green chile peppers, water, and tomato sauce, then simmer, occasionally stirring, until thick, roughly 30 minutes.
- Spoon the turkey mix onto the tortillas and top with sliced olives, cilantro, green onion, tomatoes, Cheddar cheese, and lettuce.

Nutrition Information

- Calories: 421 calories;
- Total Fat: 16.8
- Sodium: 1340
- Total Carbohydrate: 36.2
- Cholesterol: 96
- Protein: 30.8

236. Tasty Shepherd's Pie With Mashed Cauliflower And Ground Turkey

Serving: 4 | Prep: 15mins | Cook: 45mins | Ready in:

Ingredients

- 1 head cauliflower, cut into florets
- 1 tablespoon olive oil
- 2 cloves garlic, mashed
- 1/4 cup Parmesan cheese
- 1 tablespoon reduced-fat cream cheese
- 1/2 teaspoon sea salt
- 1/8 teaspoon freshly ground black pepper
- 1 pound ground turkey
- 1 1/2 cups hot water
- 1/2 cup whole wheat elbow macaroni
- 1/2 cup frozen peas
- 1 (1.25 ounce) envelope dry onion soup mix
- 1/2 teaspoon paprika

Direction

- Prepare the oven by preheating to 425°F (220°C).
- Insert a steamer into a saucepan and load with water to just below the bottom of the steamer. Make water boil. Put in the cauliflower; steam and cover for 10-12 minutes until tender.
- In a skillet over medium heat, put olive oil to heat; stir and cook garlic for about 2 minutes until tender.
- In a blender, process pepper, salt, cream cheese, Parmesan cheese, garlic and cauliflower until smooth.
- Preheat a large skillet over medium-high. Stir and cook ground turkey in hot skillet for 5-7 minutes until crumbly and browned; strain and get rid of grease. Add soup mix, peas, macaroni and water into turkey; gently boil for 5-10 minutes until pasta is softened but firm to chew.
- Place pasta mixture into a 9x13-inch baking dish. Scatter cauliflower mixture over pasta mixture. Dust paprika over the top.
- Place in the preheated oven and bake for about 20 minutes until lightly browned.

Nutrition Information

- Calories: 329 calories;
- Protein: 30.4
- Total Fat: 14.6
- Sodium: 1211
- Total Carbohydrate: 22.2
- Cholesterol: 90

237. Tasty Turkey Meatloaf With Sauce

Serving: 6 | Prep: 15mins | Cook: 1hours | Ready in:

Ingredients

- Meatloaf:
- 1 pound lean ground turkey
- 1 cup oats

- 1/2 onion, chopped
- 3 tablespoons pear applesauce
- 3 tablespoons chili powder
- 1 egg, beaten
- 1 teaspoon minced garlic
- 1 teaspoon Italian seasoning
- 1 teaspoon salt
- 1 teaspoon ground black pepper
- Sauce:
- 2 teaspoons olive oil
- 2 tablespoons chopped onion
- 1/4 cup brown sugar
- 1/2 cup barbeque sauce (such as Sweet Baby Ray's®)
- 1 teaspoon chili powder

Direction

- Set the oven to 350°F (175°C) and start preheating.
- In a bowl, mix black pepper, salt, Italian seasoning, garlic, egg, 3 tablespoons chili powder, pear applesauce, half chopped onion, oats and ground turkey together; press into an 8-inch square baking dish.
- Over medium heat, in a small saucepan, heat olive oil; cook while stirring 2 tablespoons onion for 5-10 minutes until browned lightly and softened. Stir a teaspoon of chili powder, barbeque sauce and brown sugar into onion; cook over low heat for about 5 minutes until sauce is warm.
- Bake meatloaf in the prepared oven, brushing top with sauce occasionally, for about 50 minutes until cooked through. The inserted instant-read thermometer into the center should register at least 165°F (74°C).

Nutrition Information

- Calories: 269 calories;
- Total Carbohydrate: 28.6
- Cholesterol: 83
- Protein: 18.5
- Total Fat: 9.7
- Sodium: 722

238. Tequila Meatballs

Serving: 8 | Prep: 15mins | Cook: 30mins | Ready in:

Ingredients

- Meatballs:
- 1 pound lean ground turkey
- 1/2 cup Parmesan cheese
- 1/2 cup cornmeal (such as PAN®)
- 2 tablespoons Worcestershire sauce
- 1 egg
- 1 jalapeno pepper, finely chopped
- Sauce:
- 2 (12 fluid ounce) cans or bottles Mexican beers
- 1 (12 ounce) bottle chili sauce
- 1/2 cup pickle relish
- 1/4 cup tequila

Direction

- Mix together jalapeno pepper, egg, Worcestershire sauce, cornmeal, Parmesan cheese and turkey in a bowl. Shape into meatballs.
- In a separate bowl, combine tequila, pickle relish, chili sauce and beer till sauce is mixed evenly. Move sauce to saucepan. Place in meatballs.
- Over medium-low heat, simmer meatballs in the sauce for about 30 minutes, till meatballs are thoroughly cooked.

Nutrition Information

- Calories: 228 calories;
- Cholesterol: 70
- Protein: 15.2
- Total Fat: 6.6
- Sodium: 341
- Total Carbohydrate: 17.5

239. Teriyaki Meatballs From Reynolds Wrap®

Serving: 4 | Prep: 15mins | Cook: 12mins | Ready in:

Ingredients

- Meatballs:
- 16 ounces lean ground turkey
- 1/2 cup panko bread crumbs
- 1/4 cup finely chopped green onion
- 1 large egg
- 1 teaspoon freshly grated ginger
- 1 garlic clove, pressed
- 2 teaspoons sesame oil
- Reynolds Wrap® Aluminum Foil
- Teriyaki Sauce:
- 1/4 cup light brown sugar, lightly packed
- 2 tablespoons hoisin sauce
- 1 tablespoon soy sauce
- 1/2 tablespoon sesame oil
- 1 medium garlic clove
- 1/2 teaspoon freshly grated ginger
- Optional Garnishes:
- Sesame seeds
- Chopped green onion

Direction

- Line Reynolds Wrap(R) Aluminum Foil on a 17x12-in. rimmed baking tray. Set oven to 400° F and start preheating.
- In a big bowl, combine sesame oil, garlic, ginger, egg, green onion, bread crumbs, and turkey. Mix, with a spoon or using your hands, until nicely mixed.
- Form into 1 1/4 - 1 1/2 -inch meatballs. Bake 10-12 minutes at 400° F until tender and the juices run clear, a thermometer inserted in the meat shows 170° F.
- At the same time, in a small sauce pan, put sauce ingredients and simmer, mixing often, about 3-5 minutes until lightly thickened.
- Remove warm meatballs to a mixing bowl then drizzle warm sauce over top; toss to combine.

Nutrition Information

- Calories: 303 calories;
- Total Carbohydrate: 28.1
- Cholesterol: 129
- Protein: 33.6
- Total Fat: 7.2
- Sodium: 495

240. Teriyaki Pineapple Turkey Burgers

Serving: 4 | Prep: | Cook: | Ready in:

Ingredients

- 1/4 cup Kikkoman Teriyaki Baste & Glaze, divided
- 1 (8 ounce) can pineapple slices, drained, reserve 1/4 cup juice
- 1 pound ground turkey or chicken
- 1 teaspoon grated fresh ginger
- 1/4 cup Kikkoman Panko Bread Crumbs
- 4 whole grain hamburger buns
- 4 slices Cheddar or Monterey Jack cheese

Direction

- Mix pineapple juice and Kikkoman Teriyaki Base & Glaze in a bowl. Set 2 tablespoons aside for burgers.
- Combine turkey, 2 tablespoons of the teriyaki mix, ginger, and Kikkoman Panko Bread Crumbs. Mold into 4 patties.
- Grill the patties while brushing with the remaining teriyaki mix until done as desired. Grill pineapple slices until golden brown.
- Serve burgers with pineapple and cheese, on buns.

Nutrition Information

- Calories: 486 calories;
- Protein: 34
- Total Fat: 20.2
- Sodium: 896
- Total Carbohydrate: 41.6
- Cholesterol: 113

241. Terrific Turkey Chili

Serving: 6 | Prep: 15mins | Cook: 55mins | Ready in:

Ingredients

- 3 tablespoons vegetable oil, divided
- 1 1/2 pounds ground turkey
- 1 (1 ounce) package taco seasoning mix
- 1 teaspoon ground coriander
- 1 teaspoon dried oregano
- 1 teaspoon chili pepper flakes
- 2 tablespoons tomato paste
- 1 (14.5 ounce) can beef broth
- 1 (7 ounce) can salsa
- 1 (14.5 ounce) can crushed tomatoes, or coarsely chopped tomatoes packed in puree
- 1 (7 ounce) can chopped green chile peppers
- 1 medium onion, finely chopped
- 1 green bell pepper, diced
- 3 medium zucchini, halved lengthwise and sliced
- 1 bunch green onions, chopped
- 1 cup sour cream
- 1 cup shredded Cheddar cheese

Direction

- Warm 1 tbsp. of oil on medium-high heat in a big saucepan; crush in turkey with a wooden spoon, stirring to shatter it more. Mix in coriander, oregano, chili flakes, tomato paste and taco seasoning mix until meat is coated evenly with the flavoring. Lower the heat if necessary and continue cooking until turkey is browned well.
- Add in beef broth and let simmer about 5 minutes to slightly lessen the liquid. Put green chilies, tomatoes and salsa; continue cooking at medium simmer for 10 minutes. Add water to your desired consistency.
- While cooking the chili, warm 1 tbsp. of oil in a big skillet on medium-high power. Add onion and green bell pepper. Stir until green bell pepper is slightly browned and onion is transparent, stirring every now and then for 5 minutes. Add to the chili mixture and continue to cook on very low simmer.
- In the same skillet, warm the remaining tbsp. of oil on medium-high. Cook the zucchini, stir every now and then for 5 minutes until slightly browned. Put the zucchini to the chili mixture and turn heat to low then cook for 15 minutes longer. Again, add water as needed to your desired consistency.
- Pour chili on serving bowls. Garnish with green onion, cheddar cheese and sour cream. Serve.

Nutrition Information

- Calories: 506 calories;
- Total Fat: 31.9
- Sodium: 1521
- Total Carbohydrate: 24.1
- Cholesterol: 125
- Protein: 34.7

242. Tex Mex Turkey Chili With Black Beans, Corn And Butternut Squash

Serving: 6 | Prep: 10mins | Cook: 20mins | Ready in:

Ingredients

- 1/4 cup Mazola® Corn Oil
- 1 pound ground turkey
- 1 cup diced onion
- 1 teaspoon minced garlic

- 2 tablespoons chili powder
- 1 tablespoon ground cumin
- 1 tablespoon chicken-flavored bouillon powder or tomato-flavored bouillon
- 1 (15 ounce) can black beans, rinsed and drained
- 1 (11 ounce) can Mexi-corn, drained
- 1 (12 ounce) package frozen diced butternut squash, thawed
- 1 (28 ounce) can crushed tomatoes or tomato sauce
- 1 cup water
- 1/3 cup ketchup
- Garnishes:
- Shredded Mexican cheese, fresh cilantro, lime wedges, avocado slice

Direction

- In a large 4 to 6-quart saucepan, heat oil over medium heat and put in turkey. Brown the turkey for 5 to 7 minutes while crumbling.
- Put in bouillon powder, cumin, chili powder, garlic, and onions; cook for 3 to 5 minutes or until onions are tender. Blend in ketchup, water, tomatoes, and vegetables. Heat to a boil; lower the heat to low and simmer, for 10 minutes. When serve, ladle into bowls and sprinkle on the top with desired toppings.
- Note: If using fresh butternut squash, microwave, for 1 to 2 minutes, before putting in the chili or allow extra cooking time to ensure tenderness.

Nutrition Information

- Calories: 411 calories;
- Protein: 25.1
- Total Fat: 17.2
- Sodium: 1039
- Total Carbohydrate: 46.8
- Cholesterol: 57

243. Texas Ground Turkey Burrito

Serving: 4 | Prep: 5mins | Cook: 11mins | Ready in:

Ingredients

- 1 tablespoon olive oil
- 1 pound lean ground turkey
- 1 pinch garlic powder, or to taste
- 1 pinch onion powder, or to taste
- salt and ground black pepper to taste
- 1 cup salsa
- 1 (8 ounce) can black beans, rinsed and drained
- 4 (8 inch) flour tortillas
- 1/4 cup shredded reduced-fat Cheddar cheese

Direction

- Over medium heat, heat olive oil in a big skillet. Put ground turkey and cook for about 5 minutes, until no longer pink. Use black pepper, salt, onion powder and garlic powder to season. Stir in black beans and salsa. Cook for about 5 minutes until heated through.
- Use moist paper towels to cover tortillas. For 30 seconds, microwave on high.
- In each tortillas, spoon turkey mixture in. Use cheddar cheese to sprinkle.

Nutrition Information

- Calories: 441 calories;
- Sodium: 995
- Total Carbohydrate: 41.2
- Cholesterol: 86
- Protein: 33.3
- Total Fat: 16.3

244. Thai Style Turkey Burgers

Serving: 4 | Prep: 15mins | Cook: 15mins | Ready in:

Ingredients

- 1 egg, beaten
- 2 tablespoons soy sauce
- 1/3 cup minced fresh cilantro
- 2 green onions, thinly sliced
- 1 1/2 tablespoons minced fresh ginger, or more to taste
- 2 cloves garlic, minced
- 1 pinch salt and ground black pepper to taste
- 1 pound lean ground turkey
- 1/3 cup bread crumbs

Direction

- In a bowl, whisk together soy sauce and egg. Put in pepper, salt, garlic, ginger, green onions and cilantro. Mix bread crumbs and turkey into the mixture. Mix well; shape into four patties.
- Over medium heat, heat a large non-stick skillet. In the hot skillet, put the patties. Cook, covered, for 15 mins until burgers are no longer pink in middle, flipping once. An instant-read thermometer should register at least 165°F (74°C) when inserted into middle.

Nutrition Information

- Calories: 235 calories;
- Total Fat: 11.2
- Sodium: 655
- Total Carbohydrate: 8.7
- Cholesterol: 130
- Protein: 24.9

245. Thanksgiving Flavored Turkey Burgers

Serving: 16 | Prep: 15mins | Cook: 40mins | Ready in:

Ingredients

- 1/4 cup butter
- 1 onion, finely chopped
- 1/2 cup finely chopped celery
- 3 pounds ground turkey breast
- 1 (6 ounce) package chicken-flavored dry bread stuffing mix
- 2 eggs
- 16 hamburger buns, split
- 1 (16 ounce) can cranberry sauce
- whipped cream cheese

Direction

- Preheat grill to medium indirect heat. Brush or spray the grate of grill with oil lightly. On medium-low heat, melt butter in a skillet and sauté celery and onion 5 minutes or until onion is translucent. In a big bowl, combine ground turkey and cooked onion and celery, stuffing mix and eggs; mix well. Divide mixture in 16 patties, making sure they are even in size because turkey patties do not change shape while cooking unlike hamburgers. Cook the patties on the prepared grill for 5 minutes each side, or until inner temperature says 165 degrees F (74 degrees C). Top each hamburger bun with cooked patties, spread whipped cream cheese and drizzle with cranberry sauce and serve.

Nutrition Information

- Calories: 373 calories;
- Total Fat: 9.8
- Sodium: 539
- Total Carbohydrate: 42.6
- Cholesterol: 94
- Protein: 27.3

246. Thanksgiving Style Turkey Meatloaf

Serving: 8 | Prep: 20mins | Cook: 55mins | Ready in:

Ingredients

- 2 pounds ground turkey
- 2 eggs, beaten slightly
- 1 onion, coarsely chopped
- 3/4 cup regular rolled oats
- 1/2 cup fresh green beans, chopped
- 1/2 cup fresh cranberries, chopped
- 1 teaspoon dried rosemary
- 1 teaspoon bay leaf, crumbled
- salt and ground black pepper to taste
- 1/4 pound thinly sliced pancetta
- 2 tablespoons butter
- 2 tablespoons all-purpose flour
- 1 clove garlic, minced
- 1 teaspoon ground cinnamon
- 1 teaspoon freshly grated nutmeg
- 1 cup milk
- 1/2 cup chicken broth
- 1 teaspoon salt
- 1/2 teaspoon ground black pepper

Direction

- Set oven to 375°F (190°C) to preheat. Put grease on a 9x9-inch square baking dish.
- In a large bowl, combine the ground turkey with bay leaf, rosemary, cranberries, green beans, rolled oats, onion and eggs. Thoroughly blend together the ingredients using your hands. Flavor to taste with pepper and salt. Put the ground turkey mixture into the bottom of the greased dish and spread. Put a layer of pancetta on top.
- Bake the meatloaf for 45 minutes to 1 hour in the prepared oven. When juices run translucent, and an internal thermometer reads 160°F (70°C) when inserted into the meatloaf, check for doneness.
- Meanwhile, in a pan, melt the butter on medium heat to make the gravy. Mix in the flour, stir and cook for 1 to 2 minutes until the mixture turns lightly brown and paste-like. Stir in the nutmeg, cinnamon and garlic. Slowly whisk in the chicken broth and milk, boiling the mixture. Reduce the heat to medium and keep cooking while whisking until it reaches the wanted thickness. Use salt and pepper to flavor to taste. Spoon the gravy over sliced meatloaf to serve.

Nutrition Information

- Calories: 308 calories;
- Protein: 28.6
- Total Fat: 16
- Sodium: 516
- Total Carbohydrate: 13
- Cholesterol: 146

247. The Best Turkey Chili

Serving: 14 | Prep: 15mins | Cook: 2hours15mins | Ready in:

Ingredients

- 2 pounds ground turkey
- 1 (28 ounce) can crushed tomatoes
- 1 (15 ounce) can tomato sauce
- 1 (15.5 ounce) can kidney beans, rinsed and drained
- 1 (15.5 ounce) can pinto beans, rinsed and drained
- 1 (15.5 ounce) can black beans, rinsed and drained
- 1/2 cup chopped onion
- 1 clove garlic, minced
- 1/4 cup red wine
- 2 tablespoons chili powder
- 1 teaspoon ground cumin
- 1 teaspoon dried parsley
- 1 teaspoon dried oregano
- 1/2 teaspoon black pepper
- 1/4 teaspoon crushed red pepper flakes (optional)
- 2 bay leaves

Direction

- Insert the ground turkey into a big pot. At moderate heat, cook the turkey, stirring from time to time, for around 5 minutes until it is crumbly and has no hint of pink left in it. Pour in the red wine, garlic, pinto beans, onion, black beans, kidney beans, tomato sauce and crushed tomatoes. Add bay leaves, black pepper, oregano, parsley, cumin, red pepper flakes and chilli powder to season. At a moderately high level of heat, lead it to a simmer. Adjust the heat to moderately low then leave it simmering with a cover on for 2 hours. During the process, stir from time to time. Before serving, extract the bay leaves out and throw them away.

Nutrition Information

- Calories: 214 calories;
- Total Carbohydrate: 22.2
- Cholesterol: 48
- Protein: 19.6
- Total Fat: 5.8
- Sodium: 562

248. Three Meat Meatloaf

Serving: 8 | Prep: 15mins | Cook: 1hours40mins | Ready in:

Ingredients

- 1 large onion, chopped
- 2 carrots, chopped
- 1 cup beef broth
- 2 eggs
- 1/2 cup bread crumbs
- 2 tablespoons minced fresh basil
- 1/2 teaspoon salt
- 1/2 teaspoon ground black pepper
- 1 pound ground turkey
- 3/4 pound ground beef
- 1/2 pound ground pork sausage
- 1/2 cup condensed tomato soup
- 1 tablespoon balsamic vinegar
- 1/2 teaspoon Dijon mustard

Direction

- Set oven to 350°F (175°C) to preheat. Grease a 9x5-inch loaf pan.
- Arrange carrots and onion in a saucepan, and add beef broth. Bring mixture to a boil over medium heat. Lower heat to a simmer; cook for about 8 minutes until vegetables are tender, stirring frequently. Set aside broth and vegetables.
- Whisk eggs together in a large mixing bowl; mix in black pepper, salt, basil, and bread crumbs. Let mixture rest for 5 minutes until crumbs are moistened; gently stir in pork sausage, beef, and turkey. Stir in the cooked onions, carrots, and beef broth. Transfer mixture to the prepared loaf pan. Combine Dijon mustard, balsamic vinegar, and tomato soup in a mixing bowl; distribute vinegar mixture over the meatloaf.
- Bake in the preheated oven for about 1 hour and 30 minutes until center of the meatloaf is no longer pink and a thermometer registers 160°F (70°C).

Nutrition Information

- Calories: 305 calories;
- Sodium: 728
- Total Carbohydrate: 11.2
- Cholesterol: 130
- Protein: 25.7
- Total Fat: 17.3

249. Tim's Turkey Tortilla Soup

Serving: 6 | Prep: 10mins | Cook: 45mins | Ready in:

Ingredients

- 1 pound ground turkey breast
- 2 (14 ounce) cans chicken broth
- 1 (20 ounce) jar picante sauce

- 1/4 cup chopped fresh cilantro
- 1 tablespoon lime juice
- 1 tablespoon olive oil
- 1/2 cup crushed tortilla chips, or to taste

Direction

- Over medium-high heat, heat a large skillet. Cook while stirring turkey in the hot skillet for 5-7 minutes until crumbly and browned; drain and get rid of grease. Place turkey in a 5-quart pot.
- Combine olive oil, lime juice, cilantro, picante sauce and broth into turkey; bring to a boil. Lower the heat; simmer with a cover for about 40 minutes until flavors blend. Transfer soup into serving bowls; place tortilla chips on top.

Nutrition Information

- Calories: 191 calories;
- Sodium: 1233
- Total Carbohydrate: 6.9
- Cholesterol: 52
- Protein: 20.8
- Total Fat: 8.2

250. Travis's Turkey Burgers With A Bite

Serving: 3 | Prep: 15mins | Cook: 10mins | Ready in:

Ingredients

- 1 pound ground turkey
- 1 (1.1 oz) package dry mesquite flavored seasoning mix
- 1 fresh jalapeno pepper, seeded and chopped

Direction

- Prepare an outdoor grill by preheating on high and coat the grate lightly with grease.
- Combine the ground turkey, jalapeno pepper, and dry mesquite flavored seasoning mix in a medium bowl. Form into 3 thin and flat patties.
- Grill the patties for 5 minutes on each side or to your preferred doneness.

Nutrition Information

- Calories: 228 calories;
- Total Carbohydrate: 0.6
- Cholesterol: 119
- Protein: 26.5
- Total Fat: 12.5
- Sodium: 448

251. Turffaloaf

Serving: 12 | Prep: 15mins | Cook: 1hours | Ready in:

Ingredients

- 1 pound ground turkey
- 1/2 pound ground buffalo
- 4 slices day-old bread, processed into crumbs
- 1 (1 ounce) package dry onion soup mix
- 1/2 cup grated Parmesan cheese
- 2 teaspoons Italian seasoning
- 1 egg, lightly beaten
- 1/2 cup creamy dill dip
- 1/2 cup blue cheese dressing
- 2 tablespoons Worcestershire sauce

Direction

- Preheat the oven to 375°F (190°C). Prepare a loaf pan around 5 by 9 inches by greasing it gently. Combine Worcestershire sauce, blue cheese dressing, dill dip, egg, Italian seasoning, Parmesan cheese, dry onion soup mix, breadcrumbs, buffalo and turkey together in a big bowl. Move the mixture into the prepped pan.
- Use aluminium foil to cover it up then put it into the preheated oven, baking for 45 minutes. Remove the foil and bake for another

15 minutes. Stop when the internal temperature reads 160°F (70°C). Before slicing it up, leave it standing for 10 minutes.

Nutrition Information

- Calories: 251 calories;
- Total Fat: 17.8
- Sodium: 541
- Total Carbohydrate: 8.3
- Cholesterol: 65
- Protein: 14

252. Turkey Bolognese Recipe

Serving: 4 | Prep: 20mins | Cook: 50mins | Ready in:

Ingredients

- 1 tablespoon olive oil
- 1 onion, diced
- 2 carrots, diced, or more to taste
- 2 stalks celery, diced
- 8 cloves garlic, diced
- 1 pound lean ground turkey
- 1 pinch salt to taste
- 1 pinch garlic powder, or to taste
- 1 pinch onion powder, or to taste
- 1 pinch dried oregano, or to taste
- 1 pinch red pepper flakes, or to taste
- 1 1/2 cups white wine
- 1 (28 ounce) can diced tomatoes
- 2 cups hot water, or more to taste
- 2 tablespoons ketchup, or more to taste

Direction

- Take a large pot and heat the olive oil with the heat setting on medium. To the same pot, add and cook the celery, carrots, and onion for about 10 minutes, stir until it starts to become brown. Add garlic to the pot and stir, letting it cook for 1 to 2 minutes until it becomes fragrant. Take the turkey and add it to the pot, seasoning the sauce with red pepper flakes, oregano, onion powder, garlic powder, and salt. Let it cook for 5 to 8 minutes, stir until the turkey begins to brown.
- To finish the sauce, take the white wine and pour it into the same pot. With a wooden spoon, make sure to scrape any browned bits that might have stuck to the bottom of the pot. Add ketchup, hot water, tomatoes, and stir well. Let it simmer for about half an hour just to let the flavors come together.

Nutrition Information

- Calories: 374 calories;
- Total Fat: 12.2
- Sodium: 547
- Total Carbohydrate: 22.8
- Cholesterol: 84
- Protein: 25.9

253. Turkey Bolognese Sauce

Serving: 8 | Prep: 10mins | Cook: 3hours20mins | Ready in:

Ingredients

- 2 pounds ground turkey
- 2 onions, minced
- 4 cloves garlic, minced
- 3/4 cup grated carrots
- 1 1/2 teaspoons dried basil
- 2 tablespoons minced jalapeno peppers
- 1 cup milk
- 1 1/2 cups white wine
- 2 (28 ounce) cans whole peeled tomatoes
- 1 tablespoon tomato paste
- 1 pound spaghetti
- 1/2 cup grated Parmesan cheese

Direction

- In a big saucepan over medium heat, cook jalapeno, basil, carrot, garlic, onion and turkey until turkey turns brown. Add milk, decrease heat to low, then simmer till lessened by one-third. Mix in wine and lessen again. Put in tomato paste and tomatoes then simmer for 3 more hours.
- Boil a large pot of lightly salted water. Put in pasta then cook for 8 - 10 minutes or until al dente; drain. Mix with tomato sauce and sprinkle with Parmesan. Serve.

Nutrition Information

- Calories: 510 calories;
- Total Fat: 12.6
- Sodium: 506
- Total Carbohydrate: 58
- Cholesterol: 96
- Protein: 32.4

254. Turkey Bolognese With Penne

Serving: 6 | Prep: 15mins | Cook: 35mins | Ready in:

Ingredients

- 2 tablespoons olive oil
- 1 pound ground turkey
- 3/4 cup chopped carrots
- 1/2 cup chopped onion
- 1/2 cup chopped celery
- 4 cloves garlic, minced
- 1 tablespoon ground thyme
- 1 pinch red pepper flakes
- 1/4 cup dry white wine
- 2 cups tomato sauce
- 1/2 cup tomato juice
- 2 tablespoons dried parsley
- 1 (8 ounce) package penne pasta
- 1/2 cup grated Parmesan cheese
- salt and ground black pepper to taste

Direction

- In a large skillet, heat the oil on high heat. Add ground turkey and cook for 5-7 minutes until browned thoroughly. Add red pepper flakes, thyme, garlic, celery, onion, and carrots. Stir and cook for 5-10 minutes until the vegetables become tender. If needed, drain off the grease and discard. Add white wine; stir and cook for 5 minutes until almost evaporated entirely. Add parsley, tomato juice, and tomato sauce. Turn down the heat and let it simmer for 20 minutes until the sauce achieves a thick consistency.
- Fill a large pot with lightly salted water and bring to a boil. Add penne, cook and stir from time to time for 11 minutes until firm to the bite but tender. Drain the penne and place it back into the pot. Add Parmesan cheese and sauce; combine thoroughly. Flavor with pepper and salt.

Nutrition Information

- Calories: 365 calories;
- Total Fat: 13.3
- Sodium: 678
- Total Carbohydrate: 37.5
- Cholesterol: 62
- Protein: 24.4

255. Turkey Burgers With Brie, Cranberries, And Fresh Rosemary

Serving: 6 | Prep: 20mins | Cook: 12mins | Ready in:

Ingredients

- 1 slice white bread, torn into small pieces
- 1 clove garlic, minced
- 3 tablespoons boiling water
- 1 pound ground turkey
- 1/2 medium red onion, chopped

- 1/4 cup dried cranberries, chopped
- 2 ounces Brie cheese, cubed
- 2 tablespoons tomato ketchup
- 2 sprigs fresh rosemary, chopped
- salt and pepper to taste

Direction

- Preheat oven's broiler; position the oven rack around 6 inches from the heat source.
- In a mixing bowl, combine boiling water, garlic and white bread; mash to combine using a fork. Put in pepper, salt, ketchup, rosemary, Brie, cranberries, red onion, and turkey; use your hands to mix well. Form into 6 patties.
- Cook under the preheated broiler for 6 minutes per side, until juices run clear and turkey is no longer pink in the center. Insert an instant-read thermometer into the center and it should show no less than 74 degrees C (165 degrees F).

Nutrition Information

- Calories: 178 calories;
- Sodium: 187
- Total Carbohydrate: 8.6
- Cholesterol: 65
- Protein: 17.5
- Total Fat: 8.5

256. Turkey Cheeseburger Meatloaf

Serving: 6 | Prep: 20mins | Cook: 55mins | Ready in:

Ingredients

- 1 teaspoon vegetable oil
- 7 slices turkey bacon, or more to taste
- 1 pound extra lean ground turkey
- 1 cup shredded Cheddar cheese
- 1 egg
- 1/2 small onion, diced
- 1 slice French bread, crumbled
- 2 tablespoons Worcestershire sauce, or more to taste
- 2 teaspoons garlic powder
- 1/4 teaspoon ground black pepper
- 1/4 cup ketchup
- 2 tablespoons prepared yellow mustard
- 1 1/2 tablespoons brown sugar

Direction

- Set the oven to 350°F (175°C) and start preheating.
- Over medium heat, in a large skillet, heat vegetable oil; cook turkey bacon for about 5 minutes on each side until crisp and browned. Drain bacon on paper towels; break to crumble once cool.
- Combine cooked bacon with black pepper, garlic powder, Worcestershire sauce, crumbled French bread, onion, egg, Cheddar cheese and ground turkey; transfer turkey meatloaf mixture into a 9x13-inch baking dish and shape into a loaf shape in the middle of the dish.
- In a bowl, combine brown sugar, yellow mustard and ketchup; stir so that brown sugar dissolves. Top turkey loaf with the mixture and spread.
- Bake the turkey loaf in the prepared oven for 45-60 minutes until the middle of the loaf is no longer pink, juices run clear and the inserted instant-read meat thermometer into the thickest part of the loaf reads at least 160°F (70°F).

Nutrition Information

- Calories: 253 calories;
- Total Carbohydrate: 11.3
- Cholesterol: 107
- Protein: 27.1
- Total Fat: 10.8
- Sodium: 549

257. Turkey Chorizo Burger

Serving: 4 | Prep: 10mins | Cook: 15mins |Ready in:

Ingredients

- 1 pound lean ground turkey
- 4 links Mexican chorizo sausage, casings removed
- 4 cloves garlic, minced
- 1/4 teaspoon onion powder
- 1/4 teaspoon chipotle chile flakes
- 1 pinch ground black pepper
- 2 tablespoons buttery spread
- 4 slices pepperjack cheese
- 4 hamburger buns
- 1/4 cup mayonnaise, divided
- 2 cups spring mix lettuce, divided
- 1 lime, juiced

Direction

- In a big bowl, mix together black pepper, chipotle flakes, onion powder, garlic, chorizo and ground turkey. Use your hands to mix until well-combined, then form into 4 patties packed loosely.
- Heat a big skillet or griddle on moderate heat until hot and coat with buttery spread. Arrange on griddle with patties and cook them for 3 minutes, until browned. Lower heat to moderately low and keep on cooking about 5 minutes. Turn patties and cook the other side for 6 minutes, until browned.
- Put a pepperjack cheese slice on top of each patty, then cook for 1 minute longer, until cheese has melted.
- In a toaster oven, toast hamburger buns, then spread over each half with 1 1/2 tsp. of mayonnaise. Put over bottom buns with cooked patties and put 1/2 cup of spring mix lettuce on top of each patty. Sprinkle over lettuce with lime juice and place top buns to cover.

Nutrition Information

- Calories: 766 calories;
- Cholesterol: 158
- Protein: 45
- Total Fat: 53.3
- Sodium: 1253
- Total Carbohydrate: 26.3

258. Turkey Garbanzo Bean And Kale Soup With Pasta

Serving: 8 | Prep: 10mins | Cook: 30mins |Ready in:

Ingredients

- 16 ounces whole-wheat pasta shells
- 1 tablespoon extra-virgin olive oil
- 1 pound ground turkey
- 1 cup chopped onion
- 3 cloves garlic, minced
- 2 tablespoons chopped fresh sage
- 2 tablespoons chopped fresh rosemary
- 3 (14 ounce) cans chicken broth
- 3/4 cup water
- 1 (15 ounce) can garbanzo beans, drained and rinsed
- 1/3 cup tomato paste
- 2 cups roughly chopped kale
- salt and pepper to taste

Direction

- Boil a big pot of salted water and stir in the pasta, then bring back to boiling. Boil while occasionally stirring for 12 - 15 minutes until the pasta is cooked but still firm to chew, then drain.
- In a big soup pot, heat olive oil and add in garlic, onion, and turkey, then cook on a medium heat until onion becomes soft and the meat is brown, 5 minutes. Stir in the rosemary and sage, then cook for 1 minute without allowing them to brown. Pour in the water and broth with the tomato paste and garbanzo beans, then set to boil. Add in the kale and

simmer for 5 minutes until the kale is soft. Season with pepper and salt.
- Place a serving cooked pasta on the bottom of a soup bowl and ladle over with the hot soup to serve.

Nutrition Information

- Calories: 374 calories;
- Cholesterol: 45
- Protein: 23.2
- Total Fat: 7.7
- Sodium: 940
- Total Carbohydrate: 56.8

259. Turkey Goulash With Penne

Serving: 6 | Prep: 15mins | Cook: 45mins | Ready in:

Ingredients

- 2 teaspoons extra-virgin olive oil, or to taste
- 1 sweet onion, cut into thin slivers
- 1 pound lean ground turkey
- 8 ounces sliced mushrooms
- salt and ground black pepper to taste
- 1 (26 ounce) jar spicy roasted red pepper tomato sauce
- 1 (14 ounce) can diced tomatoes
- 1 teaspoon bottled minced garlic
- 8 ounces multi-grain penne pasta

Direction

- Over medium heat, in a large skillet, heat olive oil. Cook while stirring sweet onion in hot oil for about 5 minutes until translucent. Add turkey to the skillet in small chunks; cook while stirring for 5-7 minutes until the turkey is no longer pink. Stir mushrooms into turkey mixture; cook while stirring for 3-5 minutes until softened. Season with pepper and salt.
- Pour diced tomatoes and tomato sauce over turkey mixture; add garlic; stir. Bring the mixture to a simmer; cook for about 20 minutes until tomato sauce is thickened.
- Boil a large pot of slightly salted water; add penne; cook while stirring occasionally for about 11 minutes until tender yet firm to the bite. Drain pasta; stir into turkey mixture; toss to coat.

Nutrition Information

- Calories: 358 calories;
- Total Carbohydrate: 38.4
- Cholesterol: 60
- Protein: 25.4
- Total Fat: 10.4
- Sodium: 523

260. Turkey Joes

Serving: 5 | Prep: 10mins | Cook: 20mins | Ready in:

Ingredients

- 2 tablespoons olive oil
- 1 yellow onion, diced
- 1 1/4 pounds ground turkey
- 1 cup ketchup
- 1 tablespoon red wine vinegar
- 1 tablespoon Worcestershire sauce
- 1 tablespoon Dijon mustard
- 1 tablespoon brown sugar
- 1 tablespoon chili powder

Direction

- Over medium heat, in a large skillet, heat oil; cook while stirring onion in hot oil for 5-7 minutes until translucent. Break ground turkey into small pieces; add to skillet; cook while stirring, breaking the turkey more into smaller pieces, for 7-10 minutes until browned completely.

- Stir chili powder, brown sugar, Dijon mustard, Worcestershire sauce, vinegar, and ketchup into the turkey; cook at a simmer for about 10 minutes until thick and hot.

Nutrition Information

- Calories: 302 calories;
- Sodium: 726
- Total Carbohydrate: 21.3
- Cholesterol: 84
- Protein: 24
- Total Fat: 14.4

261. Turkey Kofta Kabobs

Serving: 12 | Prep: 15mins | Cook: 25mins | Ready in:

Ingredients

- 1 pound ground turkey
- 1 small onion, minced
- 2 cloves garlic, minced
- 1/4 cup chopped fresh cilantro
- 1 egg
- 1/4 teaspoon chopped green chile pepper
- 1/4 teaspoon ground coriander
- 1/4 teaspoon ground paprika
- 1/4 teaspoon chili powder
- salt to taste

Direction

- Preheat the grill over medium heat and brush the grate lightly with oil.
- In a large bowl, mix together chile pepper, ground turkey, onion, cilantro, chili powder, garlic, egg, coriander, salt and paprika. Combine well.
- Divide the turkey mixture into twelve 1/4-cup parts, fold to form log-shaped ovals, and then transfer onto a baking sheet.
- Grill the ovals while turning often on top of indirect heat on the middle rack for about 25 to 30 minutes until pink color disappears in the middle. The temperature at the middle should be at least 74 degrees C (165 degrees F).

Nutrition Information

- Calories: 65 calories;
- Protein: 8.1
- Total Fat: 3.2
- Sodium: 41
- Total Carbohydrate: 0.9
- Cholesterol: 42

262. Turkey Lasagna With Butternut Squash, Zucchini, And Spinach

Serving: 8 | Prep: 30mins | Cook: 2hours | Ready in:

Ingredients

- 2 tablespoons vegetable oil
- 1 onion, diced
- 4 cloves garlic, chopped
- 1 (20 ounce) package ground turkey
- 1 (28 ounce) can crushed tomatoes
- 3 (6 ounce) cans tomato paste
- 1 1/2 cups water
- 1 1/2 teaspoons dried basil
- 1 teaspoon fennel seeds
- 1 teaspoon Italian seasoning
- 1/4 teaspoon ground black pepper
- 1/4 cup chopped fresh parsley
- 3 1/2 cups peeled and cubed butternut squash
- 1 (10 ounce) package fresh spinach
- 1 (15 ounce) container fat-free ricotta cheese
- 1 egg
- 2 tablespoons chopped fresh parsley
- 1/4 teaspoon ground black pepper
- 1 (6 ounce) package shredded part-skim mozzarella cheese, divided
- 9 no-boil lasagna noodles
- 2 zucchini, sliced lengthwise

Direction

- In a big frying pan heat vegetable oil on medium. Cook garlic and onion in pan until aromatic 5-7 minutes. Break the turkey in crumbs in pan; stir and cook until brown, 7-10 minutes. Add the crushed tomatoes, water, tomato paste, basil, fennel seeds, 1/4 tsp. black pepper, Italian seasoning, and 1/4 cup parsley to the mixture. Put on medium-low heat. Simmer, stir from time to time, until the sauce is consistency desired, 60-90 minutes.
- While the sauce is simmering, put squash in a microwavable bowl. Cover with some plastic wrap and cook on high until soft, 5 minutes. Set aside.
- Stir and cook the spinach in a big pan on medium heat until it wilts, 5 minutes. Set aside.
- Mix the ricotta cheese, 2 tbsp. parsley, egg, 1/4 tsp. black pepper and 2/3 of mozzarella cheese in a bowl. Set aside.
- Turn oven to 190°C (375°F).
- Put 1 1/2 cups of sauce in bottom of a 9 in. x 13 in. baking pan. Layer with 3 pasta noodles, 1 cup ricotta cheese mixture, 1/2 of squash, 1/2 of spinach, and 1/2 of slices of zucchini. Repeat the layers. Top with the last three pasta noodles. Pour remaining ricotta cheese on and top with the remaining sauce mixture. Cover with foil.
- Bake in the oven for half an hour. Remove the cover and drizzle remaining mozzarella on top. Put in the oven and bake without cover until golden brown on top, 30 minutes. Take out and let it set for 15 minutes before slicing and serving.

Nutrition Information

- Calories: 477 calories;
- Total Fat: 14.3
- Sodium: 907
- Total Carbohydrate: 56.9
- Cholesterol: 98
- Protein: 34.7

263. Turkey Lettuce Wraps With Shiitake Mushrooms

Serving: 4 | Prep: 40mins | Cook: 20mins | Ready in:

Ingredients

- 2 cups water
- 2 ounces mai fun (angel hair) rice noodles
- 1 teaspoon vegetable oil
- 4 shiitake mushrooms, sliced
- 2 teaspoons vegetable oil
- 1 (16 ounce) package ground turkey
- 6 green onions, chopped
- 1/4 cup chopped water chestnuts
- 4 teaspoons finely minced fresh ginger root
- 2 teaspoons minced garlic
- 3 tablespoons soy sauce
- 2 tablespoons brown sugar
- 1 tablespoon rice vinegar
- 1 teaspoon sesame oil
- 1 teaspoon finely grated orange zest
- 12 leaves green leaf lettuce
- Toppings
- 1/2 cup bean sprouts
- 1 carrot, grated
- 1/2 cup salted peanuts
- 1/2 cup chopped fresh cilantro
- 1/2 cup sweet chili sauce

Direction

- Boil 2 cups of water in a small saucepan. Turn heat off. Mix in rice noodles. Cover and let noodles soak for 5-7 minutes until soft. Rinse using cold water. Thoroughly drain.
- In a big skillet, heat 1 teaspoon oil on medium-high heat. Cook mushrooms in hot oil for about 2 minutes until soft and brown. Take mushrooms out of pan. Put aside.
- Heat leftover 2 teaspoons oil in the pan. Sauté turkey in oil for 5-7 minutes until it's not pink. Mix in green onions, garlic, ginger, and water chestnuts. Keep cooking for a minute. Mix in brown sugar, soy sauce, and reserved

mushrooms. Briefly simmer to merge flavors. Take pan off heat. Mix in orange zest, sesame oil, and rice vinegar.
- Put a little turkey filling on every lettuce leaf to make lettuce wraps. Place cooked noodles on top of each one. Add a sprinkle of cilantro, peanuts, carrots, and bean sprouts. Use sweet chili sauce as a dip.

Nutrition Information

- Calories: 481 calories;
- Total Fat: 22.4
- Sodium: 1284
- Total Carbohydrate: 43.5
- Cholesterol: 84
- Protein: 29.9

264. Turkey Loaf

Serving: 8 | Prep: 15mins | Cook: 1hours30mins | Ready in:

Ingredients

- 1 1/2 pounds ground turkey
- 1 egg, lightly beaten
- 1 onion, chopped
- 1 1/2 cups bread crumbs, or as needed
- 2 teaspoons salt
- ground black pepper to taste
- 1 tablespoon poultry seasoning

Direction

- Preheat the oven to 175°C or 350°F.
- Combine the bread crumbs, onion, egg and turkey in a medium bowl. To create a stiff mixture, adjust the amount of bread crumbs if necessary. Add pepper and salt to season. Turn the mixture onto a loaf pan, 9x5 inches in size, and scatter poultry seasoning on top.
- In the prepped oven, bake for 1 1/2 hour, or till meat is cooked completely and the inner temperature taken with a meat thermometer is at a minimum of 70°C or 170°F.

Nutrition Information

- Calories: 269 calories;
- Sodium: 805
- Total Carbohydrate: 16.3
- Cholesterol: 110
- Protein: 27
- Total Fat: 10.6

265. Turkey Meatballs

Serving: 4 | Prep: 15mins | Cook: 3hours | Ready in:

Ingredients

- 2 (1 ounce) envelopes dry onion soup mix
- water as needed
- 2 pounds ground turkey
- 1 (6.8 ounce) package beef flavored instant rice mix (e.g. Rice A Roni)
- 2 eggs, beaten

Direction

- Mix enough water to halfway fill slow cooker and onion soup mix in slow cooker. Put slow cooker to 175°C/350°F till soup boils.
- Meanwhile, make meatballs: Mix flavoring mix, rice and turkey in a big bowl. Add beaten egg; stir well. Shape mixture to 2-inch balls. Brown on medium high heat in a big skillet.
- When soup boils, put browned meatballs in slow cooker. Cook on medium setting for 3 hours or on low setting for 6 hours.

Nutrition Information

- Calories: 567 calories;
- Total Carbohydrate: 43.6
- Cholesterol: 272
- Protein: 48.4

- Total Fat: 22.2
- Sodium: 2213

266. Turkey Meatloaf And Gravy

Serving: 6 | Prep: 40mins | Cook: 1hours | Ready in:

Ingredients

- 1 tablespoon butter
- 2/3 cup minced white onion
- 3/4 cup minced green onions
- 1/2 cup minced carrots
- 1/2 cup minced celery
- 1/4 cup minced green bell pepper
- 1/4 cup minced red bell pepper
- 2 teaspoons minced garlic
- 1 teaspoon salt
- 1 teaspoon ground black pepper
- 1/2 teaspoon cayenne pepper
- 1/2 teaspoon ground nutmeg
- 1/2 teaspoon ground cumin
- 3 eggs
- 1/2 cup ketchup
- 1/2 cup half-and-half cream
- 1 1/2 pounds ground turkey
- 1/2 pound chicken sausage
- 3/4 cup fresh bread crumbs
- 2 tablespoons butter, divided
- 4 shallots, minced
- 1/4 cup minced red bell pepper
- 1/2 cup minced yellow bell pepper
- 1 sprig fresh thyme
- 1 bay leaves
- freshly ground black pepper to taste
- 1/2 cup half-and-half cream
- 2 tablespoons minced garlic
- 1 cup beef stock
- 1 cup chicken stock
- 2 roma tomatoes - peeled, seeded and chopped
- 1/2 cup ketchup
- salt and freshly ground black pepper to taste

Direction

- Prepare the oven by preheating to 350°F (175°C). Prepare a greased loaf pan (9x5-inch).
- In a large heavy skillet over medium heat, put butter to melt. Add garlic, red and green bell peppers, celery, carrots, green and white onions then sauté for about 10 minutes. Take away from the heat.
- Mix cumin, nutmeg, cayenne pepper, black pepper, and salt in a large bowl. Mix in half-and-half, ketchup, and eggs. Stir in the vegetable mixture from the skillet. Put in bread crumbs, chicken sausage, and ground turkey. Use your hands to stir well and form into a loaf. Transfer to a greased loaf pan (9x5-inch).
- Bake for 50-70 minutes in the preheated oven, or until nicely browned and cooked through. Allow it to rest for 10 minutes and serve with gravy.
- For the gravy: In a heavy skillet over medium heat, put 1 tablespoon butter to melt. Add yellow and red peppers, and shallots then sauté for about 10 minutes till tender. Add black pepper, bay leaf, and thyme to taste. Mix in chicken stock, beef stock, garlic and half-and-half. Raise the heat to high then boil for about 10 minutes, without cover, until liquid is reduced by 1/4. Mix in ketchup and tomatoes. Simmer for 20 minutes, uncovered. Mix in the rest tablespoon butter, and add pepper and salt to taste. Strain gravy, getting rid of the thyme and bay leaf before serving.

Nutrition Information

- Calories: 491 calories;
- Sodium: 1444
- Total Carbohydrate: 30.6
- Cholesterol: 236
- Protein: 33.6
- Total Fat: 26.5

267. Turkey Meatloaf With Kale And Tomatoes

Serving: 6 | Prep: 15mins | Cook: 55mins | Ready in:

Ingredients

- 1 pound lean ground turkey
- 1 1/2 sleeves buttery round crackers (such as Ritz®), crushed
- 1 1/2 cups thinly sliced kale
- 1 yellow onion, chopped
- 1/2 cup shredded Cheddar cheese
- 1/2 cup barbeque sauce
- 2 eggs
- 1/4 cup whole-grain mustard
- 4 cloves garlic, minced
- 2 tablespoons Worcestershire sauce
- 1 tablespoon cayenne pepper
- 1 tablespoon ground black pepper
- 1 teaspoon salt
- 6 cherry tomatoes, or as desired

Direction

- Preheat the oven to 190°C or 375°F.
- In a big bowl, combine salt, black pepper, cayenne pepper, Worcestershire sauce, garlic, mustard, eggs, barbeque sauce, Cheddar cheese, onion, kale, cracker crumbs and turkey together with your hands. Into a loaf pan, pat half of turkey mixture. Into the turkey mixture, insert tomatoes and put the rest of the turkey mixture on top.
- In the prepped oven, bake for 55 minutes to an hour till a knife pricked in the middle comes out clean. An inserted instant-read thermometer into the middle should register a minimum of 74°C or 165°F.

Nutrition Information

- Calories: 406 calories;
- Total Fat: 20.1
- Sodium: 1211
- Total Carbohydrate: 33.8
- Cholesterol: 130
- Protein: 23.6

268. Turkey Mushroom Stew

Serving: 10 | Prep: 15mins | Cook: 1hours | Ready in:

Ingredients

- 1 tablespoon vegetable oil
- 1 pound ground turkey
- garlic powder to taste
- Italian seasoning to taste
- ground black pepper to taste
- 2 (28 ounce) cans no-salt-added crushed tomatoes, with liquid
- 1 (28 ounce) can no-salt-added whole tomatoes, with liquid
- 1 (15 ounce) can kidney beans
- 1/2 cup hot pepper sauce
- 1 large green bell pepper, chopped
- 1 large onion, chopped
- 1 pound fresh mushrooms, chopped

Direction

- Add oil to a frying pan and heat over moderate heat, cook the turkey until browned evenly. Use pepper, Italian seasoning and garlic powder for seasoning. Drain and take turkey to a big pot.
- Stir in the hot sauce, kidney beans, whole tomatoes with liquid, and crushed tomatoes with liquid. Mix in the mushrooms, onion and the green bell pepper. Boil, lower to low heat and use pepper, Italian seasoning and garlic powder to season to taste. Keep cooking for 60 minutes or to get preferred thickness, stirring sporadically. Pour in some water and mix if the stew is too thick.

Nutrition Information

- Calories: 176 calories;
- Protein: 14.9

- Total Fat: 5.5
- Sodium: 439
- Total Carbohydrate: 19.9
- Cholesterol: 34

269. Turkey Mustard Burgers

Serving: 4 | Prep: 15mins | Cook: 10mins | Ready in:

Ingredients

- 1 pound ground turkey
- 1/4 cup minced red onion
- 1 tablespoon Dijon mustard
- 1 teaspoon coarse salt
- 1 tablespoon olive oil, or as needed
- 4 whole wheat hamburger buns
- 1 cup baby arugula
- 1 avocado - peeled, pitted, and sliced
- 4 slices green bell pepper
- 1/4 cup grated Parmesan cheese

Direction

- Combine the ground turkey, Dijon mustard, minced red onion, and coarse salt and mix them together in a bowl. Divide the mixture and form into 4 patties then leave for 30 minutes to refrigerate.
- Prepare an outdoor grill by preheating over medium-high heat and coat the grate lightly with oil.
- Brush the burgers with olive oil.
- Grill the patties on the grill for 4 to 5 minutes until the center is no longer pink and the juices are running clear. Insert an instant-read thermometer into the center of each patty and it should show at least 165° F (74° C).
- Place the patties on whole wheat buns and top with avocado, baby arugula, green bell pepper, and Parmesan cheese.

Nutrition Information

- Calories: 433 calories;
- Sodium: 1062
- Total Carbohydrate: 28.5
- Cholesterol: 88
- Protein: 29.3
- Total Fat: 23

270. Turkey Nacho Bake

Serving: 6 | Prep: 20mins | Cook: 25mins | Ready in:

Ingredients

- 1 pound ground turkey
- 2 cloves garlic, chopped
- freshly ground black pepper to taste
- 2 teaspoons crushed red pepper flakes
- 2 tablespoons chopped fresh chives
- 2 tablespoons hot sauce (optional)
- 1 (1 ounce) package dry taco seasoning mix
- 1 (14 ounce) can refried beans
- 1 (14.5 ounce) package tortilla chips
- 2 cups shredded Cheddar cheese
- 1 (4 ounce) can sliced black olives
- 1 ripe tomato, diced
- 1 bunch green onions, sliced

Direction

- Preheat an oven to 175°C/350°F.
- Start browning ground turkey in big skillet on medium heat. Mix 1 tablespoon of chives, 1 teaspoon of red pepper flakes, pepper and garlic in; mix 1 tablespoon of hot sauce in. Mix taco seasoning mix in following package instructions when turkey browns.
- Put beans in microwave safe bowl; heat till soft in microwave. Mix 1 tablespoon of hot sauce ant 1 tablespoon of chives in.
- Across the bottom of baking sheet, spread tortilla chips. Put beans mixture on chips; spread turkey mixture across top. Sprinkle the cheese then leftover 1 teaspoon of crushed red pepper flakes, green onions, tomatoes and olives on top.

- In preheated oven, bake for 15 minutes till cheese melts.

Nutrition Information

- Calories: 717 calories;
- Total Fat: 37.7
- Sodium: 1424
- Total Carbohydrate: 64.2
- Cholesterol: 105
- Protein: 32.8

271. Turkey Pasta Sauce

Serving: 14 | Prep: 10mins | Cook: 1hours12mins | Ready in:

Ingredients

- 2 tablespoons extra-virgin olive oil
- 1 large onion, diced
- salt and ground black pepper to taste
- 1 1/4 pounds ground turkey
- 1 tablespoon chopped garlic
- 1 1/2 teaspoons red pepper flakes
- 2 (28 ounce) cans crushed tomatoes
- 1 cup dry white wine
- 1 (6 ounce) can tomato paste
- 1 tablespoon dried oregano
- 1 tablespoon dried basil
- 2 tablespoons white sugar, or more to taste

Direction

- In a big pot, heat olive oil over medium heat and add the onion with a pinch of salt, then cook, stirring, for 5 minutes until soft. Add the turkey and cook while stirring for 5 minutes until brown. Stir in the garlic and cook for 2 minutes, then add red pepper flakes.
- Stir in the basil, oregano, tomato paste, white wine, and tomatoes. Let the sauce simmer, stirring sometimes, for about 1 hour until the raw flavor of wine cooks off. Stir in the sugar to reduce the acidity, then season with pepper and salt. Puree the sauce using an immersion blender to make the sauce less chunky.

Nutrition Information

- Calories: 152 calories;
- Total Carbohydrate: 14.5
- Cholesterol: 30
- Protein: 10.7
- Total Fat: 5.5
- Sodium: 279

272. Turkey Patties

Serving: 4 | Prep: 10mins | Cook: 10mins | Ready in:

Ingredients

- 1 pound ground turkey
- 1/4 cup fine dry bread crumbs
- 1 egg
- 2 tablespoons minced green onions
- 1 clove garlic, minced
- 1 teaspoon minced fresh ginger root
- 2 tablespoons soy sauce
- 1 tablespoon vegetable oil
- 2 tablespoons chopped fresh parsley

Direction

- Blend together soy sauce, ginger, garlic, green onion, egg, bread crumb and turkey in a big bowl. Form the mixture into four patties.
- In a wide skillet, heat oil on moderate heat. Cook burgers until cooked through, about 5 minutes per side. Use chopped parsley to decorate.

Nutrition Information

- Calories: 251 calories;
- Protein: 22.9
- Total Fat: 14.4

- Sodium: 626
- Total Carbohydrate: 6.2
- Cholesterol: 136

273. Turkey Patties With Cranberry Cream Sauce

Serving: 4 | Prep: 15mins | Cook: 30mins | Ready in:

Ingredients

- 1 pound ground turkey
- 2 eggs
- 1 cup bread crumbs
- 1 tablespoon minced garlic
- 1 teaspoon salt
- 1 teaspoon ground paprika
- 1/2 teaspoon dried sage
- 1/2 teaspoon ground black pepper
- 1/4 teaspoon cayenne pepper
- 1 cup bread crumbs
- 1/4 cup vegetable oil
- 1 (8 ounce) can whole cranberry sauce
- 1 cup heavy cream
- 1 tablespoon cornstarch
- 1 tablespoon cold water

Direction

- Set the oven to 375°F (190°C) and start preheating.
- In a bowl, mix cayenne pepper, black pepper, sage, paprika, salt, garlic, a cup of bread crumbs, eggs and turkey. Divide mixture into 4 patties. Coat each patty with 1/4 cup breadcrumbs.
- Over medium heat, in a cast iron skillet, heat the oil. In the heated oil, cook patties for 4-5 minutes on each side until browned. With patties in the skillet, get rid of about half the remaining oil in the skillet; add cranberry sauce to the skillet; use aluminum foil to cover.
- Put covered skillet in the prepared oven; cook the patties for about 15 minutes until the internal temperature reaches 165°F (75°C). Take the patties out of the skillet; use aluminum foil to wrap to keep warm.
- Return skillet on stove at medium heat. Stir heavy cream into the cranberry sauce. Beat together water and cornstarch; add to the skillet slowly; cook while stirring until sauce is thickened. Drizzle patties with sauce; serve.

Nutrition Information

- Calories: 839 calories;
- Cholesterol: 258
- Protein: 34.3
- Total Fat: 50
- Sodium: 1111
- Total Carbohydrate: 64.6

274. Turkey Picadillo

Serving: 4 | Prep: 10mins | Cook: 15mins | Ready in:

Ingredients

- 2 tablespoons olive oil
- 1 small potato, cubed
- 1 jalapeno pepper, seeded and chopped
- 1 small onion, chopped
- 1 clove garlic, chopped
- 1 (20 ounce) package ground turkey
- 1/2 teaspoon ground cumin, or to taste
- salt and pepper to taste

Direction

- In a big skillet, heat olive oil over moderate heat. Put potato, and fry for 10 minutes, then put garlic, onion and jalapeno. Cook and mix till potatoes turn browned. Crumble in ground turkey, and add pepper, salt and cumin to season. Cook and mix till turkey is cooked completely and potatoes are soft.

Nutrition Information

- Calories: 310 calories;
- Total Fat: 17.6
- Sodium: 85
- Total Carbohydrate: 9.4
- Cholesterol: 105
- Protein: 29.3

275. Turkey Picadillo II

Serving: 6 | Prep: 15mins | Cook: 25mins | Ready in:

Ingredients

- 1 tablespoon olive oil
- 1 pound ground turkey
- 1 1/2 teaspoons olive oil
- 1 large yellow onion, chopped
- 1 green bell pepper, chopped
- 4 cloves garlic, minced
- 2 bay leaves
- 1/2 cup white wine
- 1 (8 ounce) can tomato sauce
- 1/3 cup chopped green olives
- 1/3 cup raisins
- 1/2 cup canned black beans
- 1 tablespoon olive brine
- 1 tablespoon capers
- 2 teaspoons cayenne pepper, or to taste
- 2 teaspoons ground cumin

Direction

- In a big skillet over moderately high heat, heat a tablespoon of olive oil and mix in ground turkey. Cook and mix till turkey is not pink anymore, equally browned and crumbly. Take out the turkey; drain and get rid of any extra oil.
- In the skillet, heat 1 1/2 teaspoons of olive oil over moderate heat. Put in bay leaves, garlic, bell pepper and onions; cook and mix for 5 minutes till onion becomes translucent and has softened. Mix in cumin, cayenne, capers, olive brine, black beans, raisins, olives, tomato sauce, wine and cooked turkey. Allow to simmer for 15 minutes.

Nutrition Information

- Calories: 246 calories;
- Total Fat: 10.8
- Sodium: 590
- Total Carbohydrate: 17.9
- Cholesterol: 56
- Protein: 17.9

276. Turkey Pinwheel

Serving: 5 | Prep: 20mins | Cook: 1hours | Ready in:

Ingredients

- 1 1/4 pounds ground turkey
- 3/4 cup soft bread crumbs
- 1 egg
- 1 teaspoon salt
- 1/3 teaspoon ground black pepper
- 1 (10 ounce) package frozen chopped spinach, thawed and drained
- 3/4 cup shredded Italian cheese blend
- 1 teaspoon Italian seasoning
- 1/8 teaspoon garlic powder
- 1/4 teaspoon salt
- 3 tablespoons ketchup
- 1/4 cup shredded Italian cheese blend
- 1/2 teaspoon Italian seasoning, or to taste (optional)

Direction

- Set oven to 175°C (or 350°F) and start preheating. Line parchment paper on a baking sheet. Put a rack into a broiler pan.
- In a bowl, combine black pepper, 1 teaspoon of salt, egg, bread crumbs, and ground turkey, then pat the meat mixture out into a 10x14" rectangle on the lined baking sheet.

- Put a quarter teaspoon of salt, garlic powder, 1 teaspoon of Italian seasonings, three quarters cup of Italian cheese and spinach in a mixing bowl. Mix lightly; spread the spinach mixture on the meat surface, leaving 3/4" of the edges bare. Starting from the short end, hold one side of the paper and roll the edge over. Roll and release the paper as you go, until you form a firm roll. Press down the seam and place the seamed side of the roll down to the rack on the roasting pan.
- Bake in the prepared oven for about 50 minutes until the roll is cooked through and the juices run clear. Insert an instant-read thermometer into the middle of the roll and it should register 70°C (160°F).
- Take the roasting pan out of the oven, and spread ketchup over the roll; top with half a teaspoon of Italian seasoning and a quarter cup of Italian cheese blend. Put back into the oven, and bake for an additional 10 minutes until the cheese is melted.

Nutrition Information

- Calories: 306 calories;
- Total Carbohydrate: 9.5
- Cholesterol: 139
- Protein: 31.9
- Total Fat: 16.4
- Sodium: 1043

277. Turkey Portobello Pizza

Serving: 4 | Prep: 20mins | Cook: 25mins | Ready in:

Ingredients

- 4 large portobello mushroom caps, stems removed
- 1/4 cup extra-virgin olive oil
- 3 tablespoons extra-virgin olive oil
- 1 small red onion, diced
- 2 cloves garlic, minced
- 1 pound ground turkey
- salt to taste
- 2 roma (plum) tomatoes, diced
- 1 (8 ounce) jar basil pesto
- 6 ounces fresh mozzarella cheese, sliced
- 2 ounces grated Parmesan cheese

Direction

- Start preheating the oven to 350°F (175°C).
- Lightly grease a baking sheet.
- Coat both sides of the portobello mushrooms with about a quarter cup of olive oil. Place mushrooms on a baking sheet, the gill-side facing up.
- In a large skillet, heat 3 tablespoons of olive oil over high heat. In hot oil, cook while stirring garlic and onion for 3-5 mins until the onion starts to be translucent.
- Stir the turkey into the onion mixture. Lower the heat to medium-high; add salt to season. Keep cooking and stirring for 5-7 mins until the turkey is no longer pink.
- Then drain the turkey, saving about one tablespoon of grease in skillet.
- Stir pesto sauce and tomatoes into turkey; then simmer for 5-7 mins, stirring occasionally, until sauce has heated through.
- In middle of each mushroom cap, put 1 mozzarella cheese slice. Evenly sprinkle Parmesan cheese over.
- Evenly distribute turkey pesto sauce over mushroom caps.
- Bake for 10-15 mins in prepared oven until the cheese is melted.

Nutrition Information

- Calories: 871 calories;
- Cholesterol: 143
- Protein: 49.7
- Total Fat: 71.3
- Sodium: 1012
- Total Carbohydrate: 9.1

278. Turkey Ragu With Fontina And Parmesan

Serving: 8 | Prep: 10mins | Cook: 50mins | Ready in:

Ingredients

- 1 (16 ounce) package elbow macaroni
- 1 tablespoon olive oil
- 1 sweet onion (such as Vidalia®), diced
- 3 cloves garlic, minced
- 1 pound lean ground turkey
- 1 (14.5 ounce) can canned diced tomatoes with their juice
- 1 (14.5 ounce) can canned crushed tomatoes
- 2 tablespoons dried parsley
- 1 teaspoon dried oregano
- 2 teaspoons dried basil
- 1 teaspoon salt
- 1/4 teaspoon pepper
- 1 cup grated fontina cheese
- 1/2 cup grated Parmesan cheese
- 3 tablespoons grated Parmesan cheese

Direction

- Pour slightly salted water into a big pot and let come to rolling boil on high heat. When boiling, mix macaroni in, and bring back to boil. Let the pasta cook with no cover for 8 minutes, mixing from time to time, till pasta has cooked completely, yet remain firm to bite. Thoroughly strain in colander placed in sink.
- In big skillet, heat the olive oil on moderately-high heat. Cook and mix onions for 10 minutes, till partially brown and clear. Lower the heat to low and mix garlic in. Let cook for a minute, then put in ground turkey. Cook and mix till turkey is not anymore pink. Stir in pepper, salt, basil, oregano, parsley, crushed tomatoes and diced tomatoes. Simmer for 20 minutes with no cover. In skillet, mix pasta and tomato sauce. Toss fontina cheese, half cup Parmesan cheese and pasta till cheese melts. Sprinkle 3 tablespoons Parmesan cheese over pasta in big bowl and serve.

Nutrition Information

- Calories: 421 calories;
- Protein: 26
- Total Fat: 13.2
- Sodium: 687
- Total Carbohydrate: 49.8
- Cholesterol: 64

279. Turkey Reuben Burgers

Serving: 4 | Prep: 15mins | Cook: 30mins | Ready in:

Ingredients

- 1 1/3 pounds ground turkey
- 1 large clove garlic, finely chopped
- 1/4 cup thousand island salad dressing
- 1/2 cup Italian-style bread crumbs
- 1/2 teaspoon garlic salt, or to taste
- 1/4 cup Italian-style bread crumbs
- 2 tablespoons olive oil
- 4 slices mozzarella cheese
- 1 large onion, cut into rings
- 1 pinch ground black pepper
- 2 tablespoons butter, softened
- 8 slices whole-grain sandwich bread
- 1 (14.5 ounce) can sauerkraut, drained

Direction

- In a bowl, mix together 1/2 cup of Italian-style bread crumbs, thousand island dressing, garlic and ground turkey, avoid over-working the mixture. Shape into four patties and move to a plate. Sprinkle more 1/4 cup of bread crumbs and garlic salt over patties, then press crumbs into patties to adhere.
- In a big nonstick skillet, heat olive oil on moderately high heat. Cook in the hot oil with patties for 7-10 minutes each side, until turn

golden brown. Remove to a plate and put a mozzarella cheese slice on top of each patty.
- In the same skillet, cook and stir onion rings for 10 minutes, until soft and put in more oil if needed. Sprinkle ground black pepper over top.
- Heat a nonstick griddle to moderate heat. Coat both sides of bread slices slightly with butter and cook each side for 2 minutes, until browned.
- For burgers assembly, layer between bread slices with turkey and cheese patties, sauerkraut and cooked onions.

Nutrition Information

- Calories: 728 calories;
- Cholesterol: 150
- Protein: 47.9
- Total Fat: 38.2
- Sodium: 1746
- Total Carbohydrate: 50.1

280. Turkey Salisbury Steak

Serving: 8 | Prep: 15mins | Cook: 30mins | Ready in:

Ingredients

- 1 cup water
- 3 tablespoons dry onion soup mix
- 1 tablespoon Worcestershire sauce
- 1 teaspoon minced garlic
- 1/2 teaspoon ground black pepper
- 1 1/2 pounds ground turkey
- 1 cup Italian-seasoned bread crumbs
- 1 egg
- 1 (10.75 ounce) can condensed cream of mushroom soup
- 1 (10.75 ounce) can water
- 3 tablespoons brown gravy mix

Direction

- Set an oven to 200°C (400°F) to preheat.
- In a bowl, whisk together the black pepper, garlic, Worcestershire sauce, onion soup mix and 1 cup water. Strain the mixture and set aside the broth and solids. Pour the solids and 1/2 cup broth into a big bowl, then stir the egg, breadcrumbs and turkey into the broth-solids mixture, until blended thoroughly. Use a 1/2 cup measure to scoop 8 portions and shape each into an oval patty, then lay them out on a baking sheet.
- Let bake for around 20 minutes in the preheated oven, until the juices run clear and the pieces have no visible pink color in the middle. An instant-read thermometer inserted in the middle must read at least 74°C (165°F).
- In a saucepan, whisk together the gravy mix, 1 can water, mushroom soup and the leftover broth until it becomes smooth, then boil, stirring continuously. Take it away from the heat.
- Turn the patties and pour the gravy on top of each. Keep cooking for about 10 minutes more, until the gravy becomes a bit thick.

Nutrition Information

- Calories: 238 calories;
- Sodium: 856
- Total Carbohydrate: 16
- Cholesterol: 86
- Protein: 20.5
- Total Fat: 10.1

281. Turkey Salisbury Steak With Cranberry Orange Gravy

Serving: 6 | Prep: 15mins | Cook: 25mins | Ready in:

Ingredients

- Turkey Salisbury Steaks:
- 1 pound ground turkey
- 2/3 cup bread crumbs, or to taste

- 1 egg, beaten
- 1 1/2 teaspoons onion powder, or to taste
- 1 1/2 teaspoons garlic powder, or to taste
- 1 1/2 teaspoons ground black pepper, or to taste
- Cranberry-Orange Gravy
- 1 (12 ounce) package fresh cranberries
- 1 cup orange juice
- 3 tablespoons granular no-calorie sucralose sweetener (such as Splenda®)
- 1/4 cup water
- 1 tablespoon cornstarch

Direction

- In a big bowl, combine black pepper, garlic powder, onion powder, egg, bread crumbs and ground turkey together; put aside for 5 minutes.
- In a saucepan, mix sweetener, orange juice and cranberries together; boil. In a bowl, mix cornstarch and water together; pour into boiling cranberry mixture in a stream while mixing. Return the liquid to a boil and cook for 5 to 10 minutes till thickened to your preferred consistency.
- Over moderate heat, heat a big skillet. Form turkey mixture into 6 patties. In skillet, fry the patties for 7 minutes till fully browned on bottom. Turn patties over and keep cooking for 3 to 4 minutes longer till juices run clear and not pink anymore in the middle. An inserted instant-read thermometer into the middle should register a minimum of 74°C or 165°F.
- Put cranberry-orange gravy on top of patties; simmer and keep cooking for an additional of 3 to 4 minutes till sauce thickens more.

Nutrition Information

- Calories: 225 calories;
- Cholesterol: 87
- Protein: 18.3
- Total Fat: 7.3
- Sodium: 145
- Total Carbohydrate: 22.3

282. Turkey Sausage Patties

Serving: 4 | Prep: 10mins | Cook: 30mins | Ready in:

Ingredients

- 1 pound ground turkey
- 2 tablespoons steak seasoning (such as KC Masterpiece ® Steak Seasoning with Garlic), or to taste
- 3/4 cup corn flake crumbs, or as needed
- 1 tablespoon real maple syrup, or to taste
- 3 tablespoons canola oil

Direction

- Preheat the oven to 175°C or 350°Fahrenheit.
- In a bowl, stir maple syrup, corn flake crumbs, steak seasoning and ground turkey until well blended. On medium-high heat, heat canola oil in a pan. Scoop a quarter cup of turkey mixture then form into a patty then place on the hot pan. Repeat with the rest of the turkey mixture. Pan fry for 5-8 minutes on each side until both sides of the patties are brown. Drain patties on a cooling rack then arrange in one layer on a baking dish.
- Bake for 20-25 minutes in the preheated oven until an inserted instant-read thermometer in the middle of the patty registers at least 70°C (160°Fahrenheit) or the inside of the patties are not pink anymore.

Nutrition Information

- Calories: 343 calories;
- Protein: 23.6
- Total Fat: 19.2
- Sodium: 1568
- Total Carbohydrate: 20.3
- Cholesterol: 84

283. Turkey Shepherd's Pie

Serving: 6 | Prep: 15mins | Cook: 45mins | Ready in:

Ingredients

- 3 large potatoes, peeled
- 2 tablespoons butter, room temperature
- 1/4 cup warm milk
- 1 tablespoon olive oil
- 1 onion, chopped
- 1 pound ground turkey
- 1 large carrot, shredded
- 1 (4.5 ounce) can sliced mushrooms
- 1 tablespoon chopped fresh parsley
- 1/4 teaspoon dried thyme
- 1 clove garlic, minced
- 1 teaspoon chicken bouillon powder
- 1 tablespoon all-purpose flour
- salt to taste
- ground black pepper to taste

Direction

- Boil potatoes for 15-20 minutes until soft. As the potatoes cook, assemble other ingredients.
- Mash potatoes with milk and butter. Use pepper and salt to season to taste. Put aside.
- Start preheating the oven to 375°F (190°C).
- In a frying pan, heat olive oil over medium heat, mix in onion. Sauté the onion for 5 minutes until translucent and tender. Mix in the chicken bouillon, garlic, thyme, parsley, mushrooms, carrot, and ground turkey. Stir and cook until the meat is fully heated and crumbled. Add pepper and salt to taste. Mix in flour and cook for another 1 minute.
- Remove the meat mixture into a casserole dish or deep-dish pie pan. Spread over the meat with mashed potatoes, use a fork to swirl.
- Put in the preheated oven and bake for 30 minutes until the mashed potatoes have turned light brown on top.

Nutrition Information

- Calories: 339 calories;
- Total Fat: 12.9
- Sodium: 342
- Total Carbohydrate: 38
- Cholesterol: 71
- Protein: 18.3

284. Turkey Sloppy Joes

Serving: 8 | Prep: 15mins | Cook: 15mins | Ready in:

Ingredients

- 2 1/2 pounds ground turkey
- 1/2 cup chopped onion
- 1/2 cup chopped green bell pepper
- 1/2 cup chopped tomato
- 1 cup no-salt-added ketchup
- 7 tablespoons barbeque sauce
- 2 tablespoons prepared yellow mustard
- 1 tablespoon vinegar
- 1/2 teaspoon celery seed
- 1/2 teaspoon ground black pepper
- 1/2 teaspoon red pepper flakes, or to taste
- 8 hamburger bun, split and toasted

Direction

- Over medium heat, heat a nonstick skillet and then cook while stirring tomato, bell pepper, onion and turkey for about 5 minutes until the turkey is no longer pink and it is crumbly. Mix in red pepper flakes, black pepper, celery seed, vinegar, mustard, barbeque sauce and ketchup. Decrease the heat to low and let it simmer while stirring from time to time for 10 minutes. Serve the turkey mixture over the toasted hamburger buns.

Nutrition Information

- Calories: 393 calories;
- Cholesterol: 105
- Protein: 32.8
- Total Fat: 13.3

- Sodium: 525
- Total Carbohydrate: 36.4

285. Turkey Soft Tacos

Serving: 12 | Prep: 15mins | Cook: 23mins |Ready in:

Ingredients

- 1/4 cup chopped onions
- 1/2 jalapeno pepper, seeded and chopped
- 4 cloves garlic, minced
- 2 pounds ground turkey
- 3 tablespoons taco seasoning
- 1/4 cup green bell pepper, chopped
- 12 (6 inch) flour tortillas

Direction

- In a grill pan, put garlic, jalapeno, and onions on medium heat; stir and cook for 3 minutes until fragrant. Stir in green bell pepper, taco seasoning, and ground turkey. Stir and cook for 20-30 minutes until the turkey is cooked thoroughly. Distribute the turkey mixture among tortillas.

Nutrition Information

- Calories: 222 calories;
- Total Fat: 8.2
- Sodium: 411
- Total Carbohydrate: 18.8
- Cholesterol: 56
- Protein: 17.8

286. Turkey Spaghetti Zoodles

Serving: 5 | Prep: 15mins | Cook: 9mins |Ready in:

Ingredients

- 1 teaspoon extra-virgin olive oil
- 1 1/4 pounds ground turkey breast
- 1 cup diced green bell pepper
- 1 tablespoon minced garlic
- 2 teaspoons Italian seasoning
- 1/2 teaspoon ground black pepper
- 1/4 teaspoon salt
- 1/4 teaspoon red pepper flakes
- 3 cups marinara sauce
- 2 cups baby spinach leaves
- 4 zucchini, cut into noodle-shape strands

Direction

- Place a large skillet on medium heat and heat olive oil. Put in red pepper flakes, salt, ground black pepper, Italian seasoning, garlic, green pepper and turkey breast; cook while stirring for 4-5 minutes, till the turkey lightly turns brown.
- Mix into the turkey mixture with baby spinach and marinara sauce; cook while stirring for 3 minutes, till the marinara sauce is warm through.
- Using tongs, mix zucchini noodles into the sauce; cook while stirring for 2-3 minutes, till the zucchini slightly turns tender.

Nutrition Information

- Calories: 301 calories;
- Total Carbohydrate: 26.8
- Cholesterol: 85
- Protein: 34.3
- Total Fat: 6.1
- Sodium: 803

287. Turkey Spinach Crispy Baked Egg Rolls

Serving: 12 | Prep: 20mins | Cook: 18mins |Ready in:

Ingredients

- 1 pound lean ground turkey
- 1 onion, diced
- 1 teaspoon ground cumin
- 1 teaspoon garlic powder
- 1/2 teaspoon onion powder
- 1/4 teaspoon salt
- 1/4 teaspoon ground black pepper
- 2 1/2 cups fresh spinach
- 1 cup black beans, rinsed and drained
- 1/2 cup finely chopped red cabbage
- 1 tablespoon low-sodium soy sauce
- 1 tablespoon red chile paste
- 2 teaspoons garlic paste
- 12 egg roll wrappers
- 3/4 cup bean sprouts
- coconut oil cooking spray

Direction

- Preheat the oven to 210 degrees C (415 degrees F). Use parchment paper to line a baking sheet.
- In a nonstick skillet, combine turkey, onion powder, garlic powder, cumin, onion, pepper, and salt. Over medium heat, cook and stir for 3 minutes. Then add garlic paste, red chile paste, soy sauce, cabbage, black beans, and spinach. Cook for 3-5 minutes, until the turkey is no longer pink. Let drain the excess grease.
- Put egg roll wrappers on a flat surface, sweep the edges with water. In the center, place a few bean sprouts diagonally; use 3 tablespoons of the turkey mixture to cover. Fold the bottom corner over the filling and roll up halfway. Tightly fold in both sides. Wet the edges of the last flap, then roll up and seal the top corner. Arrange the flap-side down on the baking sheet. Next, repeat the process with the remaining filling and wrappers.
- Use coconut oil spray to spray the tops of egg rolls lightly.
- Bake for 12-15 minutes in the preheated oven, or until golden brown.

Nutrition Information

- Calories: 112 calories;
- Total Fat: 3.3
- Sodium: 283
- Total Carbohydrate: 10.7
- Cholesterol: 29
- Protein: 10.1

288. Turkey Taco Soup

Serving: 8 | Prep: 15mins | Cook: 50mins | Ready in:

Ingredients

- 2 tablespoons olive oil
- 1 1/4 pounds ground turkey
- 1 onion, chopped
- 2 carrots, cut into 1/4 inch rounds
- 2 stalks celery, chopped
- 1 1/2 cups frozen corn
- 5 cloves garlic, chopped
- 1 (1 ounce) package taco seasoning mix
- 1/4 teaspoon ground cumin
- 1/4 teaspoon chili powder
- 1/4 teaspoon dried oregano
- 1/2 bunch chopped fresh cilantro, divided
- 1 (28 ounce) can diced tomatoes with juice
- 1 (15 ounce) can kidney beans, rinsed and drained
- 1 green chile pepper, halved lengthwise
- 1/2 cup sliced black olives
- 3 1/2 cups chicken broth
- 1 cup water, or more as needed
- 1/4 cup lime juice
- salt and ground black pepper to taste

Direction

- Put olive oil in a large pot and heat it over medium-high heat. Mix in ground turkey. Cook and stir the turkey until it is no longer pink, and the meat is crumbly and browned all over. Place the cooked turkey in a bowl; put aside.
- Add the onion into the same skillet. Cook and stir the onion for 5 minutes until it is nearly

translucent. Add the celery and carrots. Cook and stir for 8 more minutes until tender.
- Mix in the 1/4 cup of cilantro, cumin, dried oregano, chili powder, garlic, corn, taco seasoning, and the cooked turkey. Cook and stir the mixture for 2 minutes until fragrant.
- Stir in kidney beans, olives, water, lime juice, chicken broth, green chili pepper, and tomatoes. Season the mixture with black pepper and salt. Boil the mixture before reducing the heat to low. Simmer the mixture for 20 minutes. Remove the chili halves. Before serving, garnish the mixture with the remaining cilantro.

Nutrition Information

- Calories: 273 calories;
- Total Fat: 10.6
- Sodium: 1074
- Total Carbohydrate: 26.9
- Cholesterol: 55
- Protein: 19.8

289. Turkey Vegetable Soup With Red Potatoes

Serving: 8 | Prep: 20mins | Cook: 48mins | Ready in:

Ingredients

- 1 1/2 pounds ground turkey
- 2 onions, chopped
- 1/2 tablespoon minced garlic
- 5 cups chicken broth
- 3 large red potatoes, chopped
- 8 carrots, sliced
- 1 (15.5 ounce) can corn, drained
- 6 stalks celery, sliced
- 1 cup frozen peas
- 1 cup frozen green beans
- 2 tablespoons tomato paste
- 1 tablespoon Worcestershire sauce
- 1 tablespoon soy sauce
- 1 1/2 teaspoons dried basil
- 2 bay leaves
- salt and ground black pepper to taste

Direction

- In a big stockpot, mix onions and turkey over medium-high heat; cook for about 6 minutes, until onions are translucent and turkey has no pink left. Drain and eliminate fat. Add garlic then cook while sometimes stirring for about 2 minutes until fragrant.
- In the stockpot with the turkey, put chicken broth and set to a boil. Add pepper, salt, bay leaves, basil, soy sauce, Worcestershire sauce, tomato paste, green beans, peas, celery, corn, carrots, and potatoes. Bring back to a boil, cover, decrease heat to low. Simmer for about 30 minutes until vegetables are softened.

Nutrition Information

- Calories: 356 calories;
- Protein: 24.6
- Total Fat: 7.8
- Sodium: 1217
- Total Carbohydrate: 50.1
- Cholesterol: 67

290. Turkey Veggie Meatloaf Cups

Serving: 10 | Prep: 20mins | Cook: 25mins | Ready in:

Ingredients

- 2 cups coarsely chopped zucchini
- 1 1/2 cups coarsely chopped onions
- 1 red bell pepper, coarsely chopped
- 1 pound extra lean ground turkey
- 1/2 cup uncooked couscous
- 1 egg
- 2 tablespoons Worcestershire sauce
- 1 tablespoon Dijon mustard

- 1/2 cup barbecue sauce, or as needed

Direction

- Set the oven to 400°F (200°C) for preheating. Use a cooking spray to coat the 20 muffin cups.
- In a food processor, pulse the red bell pepper, zucchini, and onions several times until the ingredients are finely chopped but not liquefied. In a bowl, mix the vegetables, couscous, Dijon mustard, ground turkey, egg, and Worcestershire sauce until well-combined. Pour the mixture into the prepared muffin cups, filling each for about 3/4 full. Drizzle 1 tsp. of barbecue sauce into each of the cups.
- Allow them to bake inside the preheated oven for 25 minutes until all the juices run clear and the inserted instant-read meat thermometer registers at least 160°F (70°C). Allow them to stand for 5 minutes. Serve.

Nutrition Information

- Calories: 119 calories;
- Sodium: 244
- Total Carbohydrate: 13.6
- Cholesterol: 47
- Protein: 13.2
- Total Fat: 1

291. Turkey Zucchini Meatballs

Serving: 12 | Prep: 20mins | Cook: 40mins | Ready in:

Ingredients

- 1 tablespoon vegetable oil
- 1 cup shredded zucchini
- 3/4 cup grated onion
- 3 cloves garlic, minced
- 2 slices multigrain bread, cut into 1-inch cubes
- 1/4 cup milk
- 1 pound 93% lean ground turkey
- 1 teaspoon dried oregano
- 1 teaspoon salt
- 1/2 teaspoon ground black pepper
- 1/4 teaspoon ground nutmeg
- 2 large eggs
- 2 tablespoons grated Parmesan cheese
- 1 tablespoon chopped fresh parsley
- 1/3 cup all-purpose flour
- 1 tablespoon olive oil

Direction

- Set oven to 175° C (350° F) and start preheating. Slightly oil a 9x13-in. baking pan.
- In a medium saucepan, heat vegetable oil on medium high heat. Sauté onion and zucchini about 8 minutes until softened. Put in garlic and cook 2 minutes. Take away from heat, allow to cool to room temperature.
- In a small bowl, place bread and milk; let soak 2 minutes till milk is absorbed. Take bread out and kindly squeeze to remove excess milk. Add bread to a food processor, pulse till mixture forms fine crumbs that look like wet sand.
- In a big bowl, combine ground turkey with nutmeg, pepper, salt, oregano, bread crumbs and the sautéed zucchini mixture. Add in parsley, Parmesan cheese, and eggs; combine thoroughly. With a big ice cream scoop, shape mixture into 12 big meatballs.
- In a shallow dish place 1/3 cup flour. In flour, dredge meatballs. Arrange 1-in. apart in prepared baking pan. Drizzle meatballs with olive oil.
- Put into the preheated oven and bake for 30-38 minutes till meatballs are no longer pink inside and slightly browned on top. Inserting an instant-read thermometer into the center and it shows no less than 71° C (160° F).

Nutrition Information

- Calories: 126 calories;
- Total Carbohydrate: 6.6
- Cholesterol: 60

- Total Fat: 6.6
- Protein: 10.3
- Sodium: 262

292. Turkey And Couscous Stuffed Peppers With Feta

Serving: 6 | Prep: 20mins | Cook: 30mins | Ready in:

Ingredients

- 2 tablespoons olive oil
- 1 pound ground turkey
- 3 tomatoes, chopped
- 1/2 yellow onion, chopped
- 3 cloves garlic, minced
- 1 (5.9 ounce) package roasted garlic and olive oil couscous with flavor packet
- 1 tablespoon ground cumin, or to taste
- salt and ground black pepper to taste
- 1 (6 ounce) can tomato sauce
- 5 tablespoons ketchup
- 1 teaspoon Worcestershire sauce, or to taste
- 1 teaspoon hot sauce, or to taste
- 2 green bell peppers - tops, seeds, and membranes removed
- 2 red bell peppers - tops, seeds, and membranes removed
- 2 yellow bell peppers - tops, seeds, and membranes removed
- salt and ground black pepper to taste
- 1 (6 ounce) container crumbled feta cheese, or to taste

Direction

- Set the oven to 350°F (175°C) and start preheating.
- Over medium heat, in a nonstick skillet, heat oil. Add turkey; sauté for 5-7 minutes until crumbly and browned. Add garlic, onion and tomatoes. Add cumin and couscous flavor packet; season with pepper and salt. Add couscous; stir and cover. Lower the heat; simmer for 5-10 minutes until couscous become tender.
- In a bowl, mix hot sauce, Worcestershire sauce, ketchup and tomato sauce. Season sauce with pepper and salt.
- Boil a large pot of lightly salted water. Add yellow bell peppers, red bell peppers and green bell peppers. Cook without a cover for 3-4 minutes until slightly tender. Drain in colander; rinse under cold water for several minutes to stop it from cooking. Drain; shake to dry. Sprinkle pepper and salt inside peppers.
- Put a small amount of feta cheese in the bottom of each bell pepper. Fill turkey-couscous mixture in each pepper halfway; add more feta; fill more couscous to the top. Place more feta on top to cover; scoop sauce on top. Put peppers in the oven-proof baking dish.
- Bake in the prepared oven for about 20 minutes until it is browned on tops.

Nutrition Information

- Calories: 381 calories;
- Cholesterol: 81
- Protein: 25.3
- Total Fat: 17.3
- Sodium: 1050
- Total Carbohydrate: 34.2

293. Turkey And Potato Pockets

Serving: 6 | Prep: 25mins | Cook: 1hours20mins | Ready in:

Ingredients

- 3 potatoes, cut into bite-sized pieces
- 1 pound ground turkey
- 1/2 onion, chopped
- 1/4 cup salsa
- 3 tablespoons Worcestershire sauce

- 3 tablespoons steak sauce (such as A1®)
- 2 tablespoons spicy mustard
- 1 pinch garlic powder, or to taste
- salt and ground black pepper to taste
- 1/4 bunch fresh cilantro, chopped
- 1 (17.5 ounce) package frozen puff pastry, thawed

Direction

- Set the oven to 400°F (200°C) and start preheating. Grease 2 baking sheets.
- Put potatoes into a large pot; pour salted water in to cover; bring to a boil. Lower the heat to medium-low; simmer for about 5 minutes until softened but not cooked fully. Drain.
- Over medium-high heat, in a skillet, cook while stirring turkey for about 5 minutes until no longer pink. Lower the heat to medium; stir in pepper, salt, garlic powder, mustard, steak sauce, Worcestershire sauce, salsa, onion and potatoes. Simmer for 5-10 minutes until sauce reduces and no longer soupy. Stir in cilantro.
- Put a puff pastry sheet on each baking sheet. Cut pastry into 3 equal portions following the fold lines. Cut each portion into 2 rectangles.
- Drop turkey-potato mixture by large spoonful on one side on each pastry rectangle. Fold pastry over filling; pinch ends to seal.
- Bake for about an hour in the prepared oven until pastry puffed up and golden brown.

Nutrition Information

- Calories: 670 calories;
- Sodium: 605
- Total Carbohydrate: 61.2
- Cholesterol: 56
- Protein: 23.9
- Total Fat: 37.3

294. Turkey And Quinoa Meatballs

Serving: 5 | Prep: 35mins | Cook: 20mins | Ready in:

Ingredients

- 1 tablespoon olive oil
- 1 1/2 cups chopped celery
- 1/2 large onion, chopped
- 2 tablespoons minced garlic
- 1 1/3 cups tomato ketchup
- 1/3 cup balsamic vinegar
- 1/3 cup low-sodium soy sauce
- 1 1/2 pounds ground turkey
- 1 1/2 cups cooked quinoa
- 2 eggs
- 1 tablespoon dried parsley
- 1 teaspoon dried sage
- 1/2 teaspoon ground black pepper
- 1/2 teaspoon salt

Direction

- Set an oven to preheat to 190°C (375°F).
- In a big frying pan, heat the oil on medium heat. Add garlic, onion and celery and let it cook for 5-7 minutes, stirring from time to time, until it becomes soft yet not brown. Take it out of the heat.
- In a small bowl, combine the soy sauce, balsamic vinegar and ketchup.
- In a big bowl, mix together the salt, black pepper, sage, parsley, eggs, quinoa and turkey. Add 1/3 cup of the ketchup mixture and celery mixture, then stir until well blended.
- On the bottom of the two 9-inch square baking dishes, spread 1/3 cup of the ketchup mixture. Using damp hands, shape the turkey mixture into meatballs. Pour the leftover 1/3 cup of the ketchup mixture on top of the meatballs.
- Let it bake for 15-20 minutes in the preheated oven, until the ketchup mixture becomes thick and the meatballs have no visible pink color in the middle.

Nutrition Information

- Calories: 419 calories;
- Protein: 34.7
- Total Fat: 16.4
- Sodium: 1657
- Total Carbohydrate: 35.8
- Cholesterol: 175

295. Turkey And Quinoa Meatloaf

Serving: 5 | Prep: 30mins | Cook: 50mins | Ready in:

Ingredients

- 1/4 cup quinoa
- 1/2 cup water
- 1 teaspoon olive oil
- 1 small onion, chopped
- 1 large clove garlic, chopped
- 1 (20 ounce) package ground turkey
- 1 tablespoon tomato paste
- 1 tablespoon hot pepper sauce
- 2 tablespoons Worcestershire sauce
- 1 egg
- 1 1/2 teaspoons salt
- 1 teaspoon ground black pepper
- 2 tablespoons brown sugar
- 2 teaspoons Worcestershire sauce
- 1 teaspoon water

Direction

- Boil water and quinoa in a saucepan on high heat. Lower heat to medium low and cover; simmer for 15-20 minutes till water is absorbed and quinoa is tender. Put aside; cool.
- Preheat oven to 175°C/350°F.
- Heat olive oil on medium heat in a skillet. Mix in onion; mix and cook for 5 minutes till onion is soft and translucent. Add garlic; cook for 1 minute. Take off heat; cool.
- Mix pepper, salt, egg, 2 tbsp. Worcestershire, hot sauce, tomato paste, onions, cooked quinoa and turkey till well combined in a big bowl; it'll be very moist. Form to loaf on foil-lined baking sheet. Mix 1 tsp. water, 2 tsp. Worcestershire and brown sugar in small bowl. Rub pasta on top of meatloaf.
- In preheated oven, bake for 50 minutes till not pink in center. An inserted instant-read thermometer in middle should read 70°C/160°F; cool for 10 minutes then slice and serve.

Nutrition Information

- Calories: 259 calories;
- Sodium: 968
- Total Carbohydrate: 15.2
- Cholesterol: 121
- Protein: 25.3
- Total Fat: 11

296. Turkey And Rice Meatballs (Albondigas)

Serving: 6 | Prep: 25mins | Cook: 2hours | Ready in:

Ingredients

- 1 pound ground turkey thigh meat
- 1 cup packed, cooked white long grain rice
- 3 cloves crushed garlic
- 1/4 cup chopped Italian flat leaf parsley
- 1 large egg
- 2 teaspoons kosher salt
- 1 teaspoon smoked paprika
- 1 teaspoon ground cumin
- 1/2 teaspoon freshly ground black pepper
- 1/4 teaspoon dried oregano
- 1/8 teaspoon cayenne pepper
- 1 tablespoon olive oil
- Sauce:
- 2 1/2 cups prepared tomato sauce
- 1 cup chicken broth, plus more as needed
- 1/3 cup creme fraiche

- 1 tablespoon sherry vinegar
- 1 teaspoon paprika
- 2 tablespoons chopped Italian flat leaf parsley
- salt and pepper to taste

Direction

- Turn on the oven to 450°F to preheat. Use foil to line a rimmed baking sheet; lightly oil the surface.
- In a bowl, use a fork to combine olive, cayenne, oregano, pepper, cumin, paprika, salt, egg, parsley, garlic, cooked rice and ground turkey. Divide mixture into small scoop (between 1/4 and 1/3 cup each); transfer onto the baking sheet lined with foil. Shape each scoop into round meatballs with your wet hands. Put into the oven to bake for about 15 minutes until they turn brown.
- In a saucepan, combine prepped tomato sauce and chicken broth. Stir in paprika, sherry vinegar and crème fraiche; whisk well. Put meatballs into the tomato sauce. Cook over medium high heat until it simmers. Lower the heat to low; let it simmer for 60-90 minutes to soften. Pour in a splash or 2 of water or broth if the sauce is too thick. Take it off the heat. Add pepper, salt and parsley; stir well.

Nutrition Information

- Calories: 258 calories;
- Total Fat: 14.3
- Sodium: 1423
- Total Carbohydrate: 15.1
- Cholesterol: 106
- Protein: 19.1

297. Turkey And Veggie Nachos

Serving: 8 | Prep: 10mins | Cook: 15mins | Ready in:

Ingredients

- 1/2 pound ground turkey breast
- 1 tablespoon olive oil
- 1/4 onion, minced
- 1 zucchini, chopped
- 1 yellow squash, chopped
- 1 pinch kosher salt
- 1/3 cup water
- 1/2 (1 ounce) packet taco seasoning mix
- 1/2 (15 ounce) can fat-free refried beans
- 1/2 (15.5 ounce) jar queso dip
- 1 (14.5 ounce) package baked tortilla chips
- 1 tomato, chopped

Direction

- Heat big skillet on medium high heat; mix and cook ground turkey in hot skillet for 5-7 minutes till crumbly and browned. Take off heat; drain. Throw grease.
- In 2nd skillet, heat olive oil on medium heat. Add onion in hot pan; mix and cook for 3-5 minutes till soft and translucent. Add salt, yellow squash and zucchini; cook for 3-5 minutes till soft. Add taco seasoning, water and cooked turkey; cook for 1-3 minutes till some water evaporates.
- Put refried beans in microwave-safe bowl; warm for 1-3 minutes in microwave. Put queso dip into microwave-safe bowl; warm for 1-3 minutes in microwave.
- Meanwhile, put tortilla chips on serving plate. Spread queso dip and warm refried beans over chips. Put turkey-veggie mixture on. Top using chopped tomato.

Nutrition Information

- Calories: 338 calories;
- Total Carbohydrate: 53.1
- Cholesterol: 30
- Total Fat: 8.1
- Protein: 16.1
- Sodium: 916

298. Turkey And Yam Spicy Tacos

Serving: 8 | Prep: 20mins | Cook: 25mins | Ready in:

Ingredients

- 1 yam, peeled and diced
- 1 tablespoon olive oil
- 3/4 pound ground turkey
- 1/2 cup chopped sweet onion
- 1 clove garlic, minced
- 4 jalapeno peppers, seeded and minced
- 1 tablespoon chili powder
- 1 teaspoon ground cumin
- 1/2 teaspoon Cajun seasoning
- 1/2 teaspoon salt
- 1/2 cup tomatillo salsa
- 1/2 cup chopped fresh cilantro
- 16 warm flour tortillas

Direction

- Cook diced yam in a microwave-safe bowl for 5-7 minutes till fork tender and cooked through, mixing once in the microwave
- Use olive oil to coat the bottom of a big skillet; put on medium heat. Mix and cook turkey for 5-7 minutes till evenly browned and crumbled. Mix jalapeno pepper, garlic and onion into the turkey; continue to cook for 7-10 minutes till onions start to caramelize. Season with salt, Cajun seasoning, cumin and chili powder. Put salsa on all; fold the sweet potatoes into the mixture. Cook mixture till extra moisture evaporates; use cilantro to garnish. Serve with warm tortillas.

Nutrition Information

- Calories: 602 calories;
- Total Fat: 16.4
- Sodium: 1182
- Total Carbohydrate: 91.1
- Cholesterol: 31
- Protein: 21.6

299. Turkey Zucchini Enchilada Meatballs

Serving: 2 | Prep: 15mins | Cook: 25mins | Ready in:

Ingredients

- 1 1/4 pounds lean ground turkey
- 1 egg
- 1/2 teaspoon cumin
- 1/2 teaspoon onion powder
- 1/2 teaspoon garlic powder
- 1 tablespoon extra-virgin olive oil
- 1 (8 ounce) can enchilada sauce
- 3 cups chopped zucchini
- 1 green bell pepper, quartered

Direction

- In a bowl, combine turkey with garlic powder, onion powder, cumin, and egg. Shape turkey mixture into meatballs, about 2 inches in size.
- Heat olive oil over medium heat in a large skillet. Put in meatballs for about 3 to 5 minutes until all sides are browned. Add green bell pepper and enchilada sauce, cook for 10 minutes. Put in zucchini; keep cooking for about 8 minutes longer until zucchini is tender.

Nutrition Information

- Calories: 587 calories;
- Sodium: 545
- Total Carbohydrate: 18
- Cholesterol: 303
- Protein: 61
- Total Fat: 31.3

300. Veggie Sneak In Meatballs

Serving: 4 | Prep: 20mins | Cook: 1hours | Ready in:

Ingredients

- 1 egg
- 1/2 cup grated carrot
- 1/2 cup grated zucchini
- 1 small onion, grated
- 1 teaspoon kosher salt
- 1 teaspoon dried basil
- 1 teaspoon dried oregano
- 1 pound ground turkey
- 1/2 cup grated Parmesan cheese
- 1/2 cup dry bread crumbs

Direction

- Preheat the oven to 175°C or 350°F. Grease baking sheet lightly.
- In a mixing bowl, whisk the egg, then mix in oregano, basil, salt, onion, zucchini and carrot. Put in Parmesan cheese and turkey; combine till equally incorporated. Shape the turkey mixture to make 16 meatballs, roll in bread crumbs, and put onto the prepped baking sheet.
- In the prepped oven, bake for an hour till turkey is not pink anymore on the inner side, and meatballs turn golden brown.

Nutrition Information

- Calories: 298 calories;
- Sodium: 825
- Total Carbohydrate: 14
- Cholesterol: 139
- Protein: 30.3
- Total Fat: 13.5

301. Vietnamese Kabocha Squash Soup

Serving: 8 | Prep: 30mins | Cook: 25mins | Ready in:

Ingredients

- 12 dried shiitake mushrooms
- 1 (10.5 ounce) package bean-thread noodles, or to taste
- 1 kabocha squash, quartered and seeded
- 1 pound ground turkey
- 1 1/2 teaspoons fish sauce, or more to taste
- 1 pinch ground white pepper
- 3 quarts water
- 1 quart chicken stock
- 1 pound shrimp
- 2 scallions, chopped
- 3 tablespoons chopped cilantro, or to taste
- cracked black pepper to taste

Direction

- Set the oven for preheating to 425°F (220°C).
- Slice 4 of the shiitakes into smaller cubes and 8 of them into halves. Submerge in hot water and soak for half an hour to rehydrate. Meanwhile, soak noodles in cold water for 15 minutes.
- Place the kabocha squash on a baking pan and add some water to the pan.
- Roast the squash inside the preheated oven for about 15 minutes until softened.
- Drain the noodles and cut into small pieces. Stir together diced shiitakes, noodles, turkey, white pepper and fish sauce well with a fork. Mixing the mixture well makes a delicious and chewy meatballs.
- Bring the chicken stock and water to a boil in a big stockpot. Form the turkey mixture into a quenelles or shape of an egg balls with 2, wet and hot spoons. Put the meatballs and cook for 10 to 30 seconds into the boiling broth until they floats.
- Peel the squash if preferred and cut into cubes measuring 1 1/2-inch per each. Put into the soup with shrimp and the halved shiitakes.

Cook for 5 minutes more until shrimp is opaque.
- Taste and add more fish sauce if preferred. Place cilantro, black pepper and scallions on top.

Nutrition Information

- Calories: 411 calories;
- Total Fat: 5.5
- Sodium: 561
- Total Carbohydrate: 69.7
- Cholesterol: 128
- Protein: 25.7

302. Waistline Friendly Turkey Chili

Serving: 8 | Prep: 20mins | Cook: 1hours15mins | Ready in:

Ingredients

- 1 pound ground turkey
- 1/2 cup diced onion
- 1 clove garlic, minced
- 1/2 cup diced green bell pepper
- 1/2 cup diced red bell pepper
- 1 (14.5 ounce) can diced tomatoes
- 1 cup medium salsa
- 1 cup chipotle barbeque sauce
- 1 (4 ounce) can chopped green chilies
- 1 cup corn kernels
- 1 (15 ounce) can black beans, rinsed and drained
- 1 tablespoon lime juice
- 1 teaspoon ground cumin
- 1 tablespoon crushed red pepper flakes
- 1 tablespoon chili powder
- 1 tablespoon dried cilantro
- 1/2 teaspoon salt
- 1 cup fat-free sour cream, for garnish (optional)

Direction

- Over medium-high heat, heat a large, non-stick pot and stir in red pepper, green pepper, garlic, onion, and the ground turkey. Stir and cook for 10 minutes until the turkey is not pink anymore, browned evenly, and crumbly. Pour in black beans, corn, green chiles, barbeque sauce, salsa, and tomatoes. Flavor with cilantro, chili powder, red pepper flakes, cumin, and lime juice. Bring to a simmer over medium-high heat, turn down the heat to medium-low, put on a cover and simmer for 1-3 hours until the flavors develop. Dollop sour cream onto each serving to serve.

Nutrition Information

- Calories: 212 calories;
- Total Carbohydrate: 27
- Cholesterol: 47
- Protein: 15.5
- Total Fat: 5.1
- Sodium: 1030

303. Weeknight Crack Slaw

Serving: 4 | Prep: 15mins | Cook: 10mins | Ready in:

Ingredients

- 1 tablespoon chipotle hot sauce (such as Cholula®)
- 1 tablespoon rice vinegar
- 1 tablespoon soy sauce
- 1 1/2 teaspoons minced ginger
- 1 teaspoon agave syrup
- 1 tablespoon olive oil
- 1 tablespoon sesame oil
- 1 pound ground turkey
- 1/2 teaspoon salt
- 1/2 tablespoon ground black pepper
- 1 (8 ounce) package coleslaw mix
- 1/2 red bell pepper, diced

- 2 green onions, chopped, or more to taste
- 2 cloves garlic, minced
- 1 tablespoon sesame seeds

Direction

- In a small bowl, combine agave syrup, chipotle hot sauce, soy sauce, rice vinegar, and ginger to create the sauce.
- Heat sesame oil and olive oil in a big skillet or wok placed over medium heat. Put in the ground turkey; let it cook for about 6 minutes and stir to break the clumps or until its juices run clear. Put pepper and salt to taste. Place the cooked turkey in a bowl and keep the juices in the wok.
- Mix green onions, coleslaw mix, garlic, and red bell pepper into the same wok; let it cook for 1-2 minutes over medium heat while stirring or until the coleslaw is a bit wilted. Add and mix in the sauce for about 1 minute or until blended. Put the cooked turkey back into the wok and mix it for 2-3 minutes or until the mixture is heated thoroughly.
- Top it off with sesame seeds prior to serving.

Nutrition Information

- Calories: 302 calories;
- Total Fat: 18
- Sodium: 682
- Total Carbohydrate: 12.5
- Cholesterol: 88
- Protein: 24.3

304. White Chili With Ground Turkey

Serving: 8 | Prep: 15mins | Cook: 30mins | Ready in:

Ingredients

- 1 onion, chopped
- 3 cloves garlic, minced
- 1 1/2 pounds ground turkey
- 2 (4 ounce) cans canned green chile peppers, chopped
- 1 tablespoon ground cumin
- 1 tablespoon dried oregano
- 1 teaspoon ground cinnamon
- ground cayenne pepper to taste
- ground white pepper to taste
- 3 (15 ounce) cans cannellini beans
- 5 cups chicken broth
- 2 cups shredded Monterey Jack cheese

Direction

- Mix ground turkey, garlic and onion in a big pot on medium heat. Sauté till turkey is browned well for 10 minutes. Add white pepper, cayenne pepper, cinnamon, oregano, cumin and chile peppers to taste. Sauté for 5 minutes more.
- Add chicken broth and 2 cans beans to pot. Puree 3rd can of beans in a food processor/blender. Add this to pot along with cheese. Mix well. Simmer, letting cheese melt, for 10 minutes.

Nutrition Information

- Calories: 396 calories;
- Total Fat: 17.3
- Sodium: 1366
- Total Carbohydrate: 26.7
- Cholesterol: 92
- Protein: 31.5

305. Yummy White Bean Chili

Serving: 8 | Prep: 15mins | Cook: 40mins | Ready in:

Ingredients

- 1 tablespoon olive oil
- 1 onion, chopped
- 3 stalks celery, diced

- 3 poblano peppers, seeded and chopped
- 2 cloves garlic, minced
- 1 1/4 teaspoons ground cumin
- 1/2 teaspoon ground coriander
- 1/2 teaspoon cayenne pepper, or to taste
- 1 1/2 pounds ground turkey
- 4 cups chicken broth
- 2 (15 ounce) cans cannellini beans, drained and rinsed
- 3/4 teaspoon dried oregano
- 1 (15.5 ounce) can hominy
- 1 teaspoon salt

Direction

- In a big skillet, heat olive oil on medium heat. Cook and stir in the hot oil the poblano peppers, celery and onion for 5-10 minutes, until soft. Add into the onion mixture the cayenne pepper, coriander, cumin and garlic, then cook and stir for a minute, until garlic is aromatic.
- Combine the turkey into the onion mixture, then cook and stir for 5-7 minutes, until turkey is not pink anymore and cooked through. Add into the turkey mixture the oregano, cannellini beans and chicken broth, then place a cover on skillet and cook about 15 minutes. Stir in salt and hominy, then keep on cooking for 15 more minutes, until heated through.

Nutrition Information

- Calories: 294 calories;
- Protein: 23.3
- Total Fat: 9.6
- Sodium: 1170
- Total Carbohydrate: 28.3
- Cholesterol: 65

306. Zesty Turkey Burgers

Serving: 4 | Prep: 10mins | Cook: 40mins | Ready in:

Ingredients

- 1 pound ground turkey
- 1 cup honey mustard and onion pretzels, crushed
- 1/4 cup finely chopped green bell pepper
- 1 egg, beaten
- salt and pepper to taste
- 4 slices Colby cheese

Direction

- Preheat the oven to 190°C or 375°Fahrenheit. Use olive oil to grease a baking dish lightly.
- Combine egg, ground turkey, green bell pepper, and crushed pretzels in a bowl; sprinkle pepper and salt to season then shape into four patties. Place the patties in the prepared baking dish.
- Bake patties for half an hour, flipping once, until the internal temperature reaches 74°C or 165°Fahrenheit. Place one cheese slice on top of each patty on the last few minutes of cooking.

Nutrition Information

- Calories: 403 calories;
- Sodium: 433
- Total Carbohydrate: 14.7
- Cholesterol: 157
- Protein: 32.4
- Total Fat: 24.2

307. Zucchini Boats With Ground Turkey

Serving: 8 | Prep: 35mins | Cook: 34mins | Ready in:

Ingredients

- 4 zucchini
- 1 pound ground turkey
- 1/2 cup chopped green bell pepper

- 1/2 cup chopped sweet red pepper
- 1 small onion, chopped
- 1/2 cup chopped fresh mushrooms
- 1/2 cup chopped fresh spinach leaves
- 1 cup shredded Cheddar cheese
- 1 (6 ounce) can tomato paste
- 1 pinch garlic powder, or to taste
- salt and ground black pepper to taste

Direction

- Trim zucchini ends; cut in 1/2 lengthwise. Spoon out and set pulp aside, leaving a half inch shell.
- Set the oven to 350°F (175°C) and start preheating. Grease a 9x13-inch baking dish.
- Over medium heat, in a skillet, mix spinach, mushrooms, onion, sweet red pepper, green bell pepper, turkey and reserved zucchini pulp. Cook for 8-10 minutes until the turkey is no longer pink. Drain. Take out of the heat; add pepper, salt, garlic powder, tomato paste and half cup Cheddar cheese; combine well. Scoop mixture into zucchini shells; put in the greased baking dish. Top with the rest of Cheddar cheese.
- Bake in the prepared oven for 25-30 minutes, uncovered, until zucchini becomes tender.

Nutrition Information

- Calories: 184 calories;
- Total Fat: 9.3
- Sodium: 320
- Total Carbohydrate: 9.6
- Cholesterol: 57
- Protein: 17.4

Chapter 2: Turkey Sausage Recipes

***

308. Acorn Squash With Sweet Spicy Sausage

Serving: 8 | Prep: 20mins | Cook: 1hours | Ready in:

Ingredients

- 2 acorn squash, halved and seeded
- 2 tablespoons olive oil
- 1 1/2 pounds spicy turkey sausage, casings removed
- 1 cup brown sugar

Direction

- Preheat oven to 350°F (175°C).
- In a baking dish with 1-in. of water, place the squash halves face-down. Bake for about 45 minutes until flesh is tender. Meanwhile, in a large skillet, heat the olive oil over medium heat. Cook the sausage in oil until brown. Break the sausage into small pieces as it cooks and set them aside.
- Discard the water once the squash halves are tender. Sprinkle a generous amount of brown sugar into the center of each squash half. Save 1/4 cup of brown sugar for later use. Fill the squash halves with the sausages. Top with reserved brown sugar. Place the squash back into the baking dish and bake for about 15 minutes or until sugar begins to melt.

Nutrition Information

- Calories: 343 calories;
- Sodium: 1013
- Total Carbohydrate: 45.2
- Cholesterol: 64
- Protein: 17.3
- Total Fat: 12.1

309. Apple Sausage Wagon Wheel

Serving: 6 | Prep: 15mins | Cook: 25mins | Ready in:

Ingredients

- 1/2 cup vegetable oil
- 1 egg, beaten
- 1/2 cup brown sugar
- 1 cup quick cooking oats
- 1 cup whole wheat flour
- 1 cup buttermilk
- 1 teaspoon baking powder
- 1/2 teaspoon salt
- 1/2 tablespoon baking soda
- 2 apples - peeled, cored and sliced
- 1/2 pound smoked turkey sausage links, chopped

Direction

- Preheat the oven to 400°F (200°C).
- Combine the quick cooking oats, baking powder, vegetable oil, baking soda, egg, whole wheat flour, salt, brown sugar and buttermilk together in a medium-sized bowl.
- In a cast iron skillet or a medium-sized baking dish, put in the sausage and apples. Pour the prepared batter mixture evenly on top of the sausage and apples.
- Put it in the preheated oven and let it bake for 20-25 minutes until it turns golden brown in color and is already crispy.

Nutrition Information

- Calories: 463 calories;
- Sodium: 923
- Total Carbohydrate: 50.2
- Cholesterol: 61
- Protein: 14.1
- Total Fat: 24.5

310. Bean And Sausage Soup

Serving: 8 | Prep: 10mins | Cook: 1hours15mins | Ready in:

Ingredients

- 12 ounces dry mixed beans
- 1 1/2 pounds Italian turkey sausage links
- 1 (29 ounce) can diced tomatoes
- 2 (14 ounce) cans chicken broth
- 1 cup white wine
- 1 red bell pepper, chopped
- 1 onion, chopped
- 2 stalks celery, chopped
- 2 large carrots, chopped
- 2 cups frozen green peas, thawed

Direction

- Select and wash beans. In a 4-quart pot, add the beans and pour in water to cover by 2 inches or more. Set to a boil for 2 - 3 minutes. Allow to stand while covered in the refrigerator overnight.
- Drain and wash beans. In a slow cooker, add beans with vegetables, white wine, broth, and canned tomatoes. Cook on low while covered for 7 to 8 hours.
- In a frying pan over medium heat, cook the sausage until done. Cut links into half an inch pieces. Pour meat into the slow cooker, then cook soup for another 30 - 60 minutes.

Nutrition Information

- Calories: 383 calories;
- Total Carbohydrate: 37.8
- Cholesterol: 67
- Protein: 29.2
- Total Fat: 9.6
- Sodium: 1560

311. Breaklava

Serving: 10 | Prep: 40mins | Cook: 40mins | Ready in:

Ingredients

- 1 (10 ounce) package frozen chopped spinach, thawed and drained
- 1 cup sour cream
- salt and ground black pepper to taste
- 6 eggs
- 1 1/2 cups shredded sharp Cheddar cheese
- 1 1/2 cups shredded Swiss cheese
- 1/2 (16 ounce) package phyllo dough, thawed
- 1 cup melted butter, divided
- 1 (14 ounce) package smoked turkey sausage, chopped
- 1/2 teaspoon dried parsley, or to taste

Direction

- Set the skillet over medium-high heat. Add spinach to the skillet and cook for 5 minutes until the liquid is evaporated. Make sure you didn't scorch the spinach. Mix in sour cream. Season it with salt and pepper.
- In a bowl, whisk the Swiss cheese, eggs, and Cheddar cheese. Season the mixture with salt and pepper.
- Set the oven to 350°F or 175°C for preheating.
- Unroll the phyllo dough. Cover the dough with a damp cloth. Set 2 sheets in a 9x13-inches baking pan. Use a basting brush to coat the top layer with butter. Do the same procedure twice to have a total of 6 layered phyllo dough sheets.
- Spread the dough with the spinach mixture. Place 6 more sheets dough on top, coating each second layer with butter.
- Spread the dough evenly with 1/2 of the sausage. Add half of the egg and cheese mixture. Follow the same steps in layering and coating 4 sheets of dough. Place the remaining sausage and egg and cheese mixture on top. Add the remaining dough, without spreading butter on the top.
- Use a sharp knife to slice the breaklava into even squares. Spread the top layer with butter and sprinkle them with parsley.
- Let them bake inside the preheated oven for 35-45 minutes until the egg mixture is set and the top layer is browned lightly. Cut it again along the pre-cut lines.

Nutrition Information

- Calories: 540 calories;
- Total Fat: 43.1
- Sodium: 818
- Total Carbohydrate: 15.4
- Cholesterol: 237
- Protein: 24.2

312. Butternut Squash And Spicy Sausage Soup

Serving: 8 | Prep: 15mins | Cook: 1hours3mins | Ready in:

Ingredients

- 2 cups water
- 1/2 cup long grain white rice
- 1 unpeeled butternut squash, halved and seeded
- 1 tablespoon olive oil
- 1 large yellow onion, chopped
- 1 1/4 pounds spicy turkey sausage, casings removed
- 1 cup frozen corn
- 2 (13.75 ounce) cans chicken broth
- salt to taste
- 1 tablespoon ground black pepper, or to taste
- salt, to taste
- 1/2 cup heavy cream (optional)

Direction

- Preheat an oven to 190°C/375°F. In a 9x13-in. baking dish, put 1 cup water.

- Put butternut squash, cut side down, into the prepped baking dish.
- In the preheated oven, bake for 45 minutes till squash is pierced easily with a fork.
- Meanwhile, boil leftover 1 cup of water and rice into a saucepan on medium high heat, uncovered. Lower the heat to low and cover; simmer for 20 minutes till rice is fluffy and water is absorbed. Take off from heat; use a fork to fluff.
- In a big soup pot, heat olive oil on medium high heat. Mix onion in; cook for 5 minutes till transparent and tender. Mix turkey sausage in; cook till evenly browned and crumbly. Drain any extra fat; mix corn and cooked rice in.
- Scoop cooked squash out; put in food processor bowl/blender. Discard squash peels. Put chicken broth into the food processor bowl/blender with the squash; blend for 1 minute till smooth.
- Mix squash mixture into the sausage mixture till blended well; season with salt to taste and pepper. Mix heavy cream in if desired; simmer the soup for 15 minutes on medium heat till heated through. Don't boil.

Nutrition Information

- Calories: 317 calories;
- Cholesterol: 76
- Protein: 17
- Total Fat: 14.9
- Sodium: 1076
- Total Carbohydrate: 31.6

313. Caroline And Brian's Stuffed Mushrooms

Serving: 5 | Prep: 30mins | Cook: 40mins | Ready in:

Ingredients

- 5 portobello mushrooms
- 1 turkey sausage link, without casing
- 3 cloves garlic, peeled and chopped
- 1 tablespoon crushed garlic
- 1/2 teaspoon ground cayenne pepper
- 1 teaspoon ground black pepper
- 1/2 cup seasoned bread crumbs
- 1/2 cup cream cheese, softened
- 2 tablespoons grated Parmesan cheese

Direction

- Remove portobello mushroom's stems. Put mushroom caps on medium baking sheet, bottoms up. Chop stems; put aside.
- On small baking sheet, put turkey sausage link. In preheated oven, cook for 15 minutes, uncovered, till interior isn't pink. Take off heat; chop.
- Mix seasoned breadcrumbs, black pepper, cayenne pepper, crushed garlic, chopped garlic, chopped sausage and chopped mushroom stems in a medium saucepan on medium heat. Mix and cook slowly for 5-7 minutes till breadcrumbs start to brown; take off heat. Cool for 10 minutes; put in medium bowl.
- Preheat an oven to 175°C/350°F.
- Mix Parmesan cheese and cream cheese in mushroom stem mixture. Use mixture to stuff mushroom caps.
- In preheated oven, bake stuffed mushrooms till stuffing is lightly browned for 20 minutes.

Nutrition Information

- Calories: 171 calories;
- Cholesterol: 27
- Protein: 7.3
- Total Fat: 9.6
- Sodium: 318
- Total Carbohydrate: 16.1

314. Cheesy Sausage Lasagna Soup

Serving: 6 | Prep: 20mins | Cook: 20mins | Ready in:

Ingredients

- 1 pound Italian turkey sausage, casings removed
- 2 cups chopped onions
- 2 cups sliced fresh mushrooms
- 4 cloves garlic, minced
- 4 cups chicken broth
- 1 (15 ounce) can tomato sauce
- 1 (14.5 ounce) can Italian-seasoned diced tomatoes
- 1 cup uncooked mafalda pasta
- 2 cups chopped fresh spinach
- 1 cup shredded mozzarella cheese
- 1/4 cup Parmesan cheese
- 4 teaspoons thinly sliced fresh basil

Direction

- In big pot, cook and mix sausage for 5 minutes, till browned. Mix in mushrooms, garlic and onions. Add in tomato sauce, diced tomatoes and chicken broth; boil soup.
- Mix into soup with pasta. Cook for 10 minutes, mixing from time to time, till nearly soft. Mix in mozzarella cheese, Parmesan cheese and spinach. Take off heat; mix basil in and rest for 2 minutes longer till pasta becomes tender.

Nutrition Information

- Calories: 281 calories;
- Cholesterol: 75
- Protein: 24.6
- Total Fat: 12.3
- Sodium: 2113
- Total Carbohydrate: 19.8

315. Chicken And Sausage With Bowties

Serving: 8 | Prep: 15mins | Cook: 45mins | Ready in:

Ingredients

- 1 (16 ounce) package uncooked farfalle pasta
- 2 skinless, boneless chicken breasts
- 1 pound hot Italian turkey sausage, casings removed
- 1 tablespoon olive oil
- 2 cloves garlic, sliced
- 1 (14.5 ounce) can crushed tomatoes
- 1/2 cup red wine
- 2 tablespoons chopped fresh basil
- 1 teaspoon dried rosemary

Direction

- Boil a big pot filled with water that's slightly salted, and add the pasta, cook until they become al dente, about 8-10 minutes.
- Wash the chicken breasts, then cut into large bite-size chunks, and also cut the sausages into the big size portions. Combine garlic and oil in a big deep skillet and cook over a medium-low heat long enough to infuse oil with flavor. Remove the garlic from the oil.
- In the same skillet with the infused oil, add the sausage and chicken, gently brown both of them until opaque. Add the wine and tomatoes, then let boil then simmer for 20 minutes. Season the sauce with pepper, salt, rosemary, and basil to your taste. Add the cooked drained pasta into the skillet, toss to serve.

Nutrition Information

- Calories: 382 calories;
- Sodium: 526
- Total Carbohydrate: 47.6
- Cholesterol: 51
- Protein: 24
- Total Fat: 9.1

316. Chicken With Sausage And Dried Fruit

Serving: 4 | Prep: 10mins | Cook: 9hours | Ready in:

Ingredients

- 4 skinless, boneless chicken breast halves
- 1 (6 inch) smoked turkey sausage link, sliced
- 1 green bell pepper, seeded and chopped
- 1 small onion, chopped
- 3 cloves garlic, minced
- 3/4 cup chopped dried apples
- 1/2 cup sweetened dried cranberries
- 1 tablespoon dried parsley
- 2 teaspoons dried chives
- 1 cup chicken stock
- 1 pinch salt and pepper to taste

Direction

- In the bottom of a slow cooker, put chicken breasts. If you use frozen chicken, you don't need to thaw them. Lay cranberries, apples, garlic, onion, green pepper, and sausage over the chicken. Sprinkle chives and parsley over. Drizzle everything with chicken stock, and use pepper and salt to season. Put the lid on and cook for 8-9 hours on Low.

Nutrition Information

- Calories: 297 calories;
- Total Fat: 7
- Sodium: 591
- Total Carbohydrate: 27.2
- Cholesterol: 93
- Protein: 31.8

317. Classic Smoked Sausage Mac And Cheese

Serving: 10 | Prep: 15mins | Cook: 1hours | Ready in:

Ingredients

- 1 pound cavatappi (corkscrew) pasta, uncooked
- 1 tablespoon butter
- 1 (14 ounce) package Butterball® Smoked Turkey Dinner Sausage, halved lengthwise, and cut into 1/4-inch-thick slices
- 1 cup chopped onions
- 3 cups prepared Alfredo sauce
- 3 cups half and half
- 3 cups cubed pasteurized prepared cheese product
- 2 cups shredded sharp Cheddar cheese
- 1/2 teaspoon ground black pepper
- Cooking spray
- 1 cup panko bread crumbs
- 1/4 cup butter, melted

Direction

- Turn oven to 375°F to preheat.
- Cook pasta as directed on package; rinse and drain off water. Put to one side.
- Melt 1 tablespoon butter over medium heat large saucepan. Cook onions and sausage in melted butter for 3 to 5 minutes, stirring, until onions are softened. Mix in half-and-half and Alfredo sauce. Bring to a boil, stirring continuously; lower heat. Simmer mixture for 1 minute.
- Take the saucepan away from the heat. Whisk in black pepper, and cheese until cheese is melted. Mix in sausage mixture and pasta.
- Transfer mixture to a lightly greased 13x9-inch baking dish. Scatter evenly with combined 1/4 cup melted butter and bread crumbs. Bake in the preheated oven until pasta mixture is bubbly and heated through and crumbs turn golden brown, about 20 to 25 minutes.

Nutrition Information

- Calories: 922 calories;
- Total Fat: 64.3
- Sodium: 2162
- Total Carbohydrate: 56.5
- Cholesterol: 167
- Protein: 36

318. Drunk Turkey Bites

Serving: 8 | Prep: 5mins | Cook: 20mins | Ready in:

Ingredients

- 1 tablespoon olive oil
- 2 (16 ounce) packages turkey kielbasa, cut into bite-size pieces
- 1/2 cup diced onion
- 1 cup lager-style beer
- 2 tablespoons brown sugar
- 1 tablespoon Dijon mustard, or to taste
- salt and ground black pepper to taste

Direction

- In a skillet, heat oil over medium heat. Cook and stir onion and kielbasa in hot oil for about 5 minutes, or until the onion starts to soften.
- In a bowl, whisk mustard, brown sugar, and beer gently; pour into the skillet.
- Next, bring the mixture to a boil and cook for about 15 minutes, or until the liquid reduces by half in volume. Season with pepper and salt.

Nutrition Information

- Calories: 227 calories;
- Protein: 16.3
- Total Fat: 11.7
- Sodium: 1050
- Total Carbohydrate: 9.8
- Cholesterol: 70

319. Healthier Baked Ziti

Serving: 10 | Prep: 20mins | Cook: 1hours | Ready in:

Ingredients

- 1 pound ziti pasta
- 1 bunch fresh spinach, or more to taste
- 3/4 cup reduced-fat sour cream
- 1 pound Italian turkey sausage
- 1 onion, chopped
- 2 carrots, chopped
- 3 cloves garlic, minced
- 2 (26 ounce) jars spaghetti sauce
- 1 head broccoli, cut into florets
- 6 ounces smoked fresh mozzarella cheese, diced
- 1/2 cup shredded mozzarella cheese

Direction

- Start preheating the oven at 350°F (175°C).
- Heat a large pot of lightly salted water to a boil. In the boiling water, cook ziti, stirring from time to time, for 8 minutes until well-cooked but set to the bite. Drain and place the pasta to a bowl and mix with sour cream and spinach.
- Heat over medium heat a large skillet; cook and stir garlic, carrots, onion and sausage for about 7 minutes until onion is transparent and sausage is not pink anymore. Add broccoli and spaghetti sauce to the sausage mixture and simmer for about 15 minutes until sauce mixture is heated thoroughly.
- Layer 1/2 of the ziti mixture on a 9x13-inch baking dish. Spread 1/2 of the fresh mozzarella cheese, 1/2 of the sauce mixture, the leftover ziti mixture, and fresh mozzarella cheese, respectively, into the baking dish. Scatter shredded mozzarella cheese over. Cover with aluminum foil.
- Bake in the prepared oven for about 20 minutes until cheeses are melted. Take off the aluminum foil and cook for an extra 10 minutes until the top turns lightly brown.

Nutrition Information

- Calories: 485 calories;
- Sodium: 1088
- Total Carbohydrate: 61
- Cholesterol: 61
- Protein: 24
- Total Fat: 16.2

320. Hot Italian Turkey Sausage Spread

Serving: 5 | Prep: 10mins | Cook: 11mins | Ready in:

Ingredients

- cooking spray
- 5 (10 inch) flour tortillas, cut into quarters
- 1 (14 ounce) package hot Italian turkey sausage, casings removed
- 1/2 red onion, chopped
- 5 slices American cheese

Direction

- Spray cooking spray on skillet; heat on medium heat. Fry tortilla quarters, 1 minute per side, till light brown and crisp. Take chips out of skillet.
- Put sausage in skillet on medium high heat. Mix and cook for 3 minutes then add onion. Mix and cook for 5 more minutes till turkey is crumbly and browned. Add American cheese; mix for 1 minute till completely melted. Put spread in serving dish then surround with chips using a spoon.

Nutrition Information

- Calories: 459 calories;
- Cholesterol: 87
- Protein: 27
- Total Fat: 22.3

- Sodium: 1525
- Total Carbohydrate: 37.4

321. Italian Hot Turkey Sausage And Black Eyed Peas

Serving: 6 | Prep: 20mins | Cook: 35mins | Ready in:

Ingredients

- 2 tablespoons extra-virgin olive oil
- 1 small yellow onion, chopped
- 2 stalks celery, thinly sliced
- 3 cloves garlic, minced
- 2 teaspoons dried oregano
- 6 hot Italian turkey sausage links, skinned and coarsely chopped
- 1 (14.5 ounce) can no-salt-added diced tomatoes
- 1 (15 ounce) can black-eyed peas, rinsed and drained
- 2 (14 ounce) cans canned low-sodium chicken broth
- 8 ounces whole wheat thin spaghetti, broken into 3-inch pieces
- 1/4 cup grated Parmesan cheese

Direction

- Set a big skillet with olive oil over medium heat; sauté the celery and onion in the hot oil for about 3 minutes until tender. Add the oregano and garlic, stir and allow to cook for additional 1 minute. Move the sautéed ingredients to the sides of the pan. Place the sausage meat in the center of the pan and let it cook for roughly 5 minutes until the pinkish color is no longer visible in the meat.
- Add the black-eyed peas, chicken broth and tomatoes. Cover the pan and lessen the heat to medium-low. Allow the mixture to simmer until the vegetables have softened and the meat is cooked completely for about 18 to 20 minutes, stir from time to time. Stir in the broken spaghetti and allow the mixture to

cook for 6 to 8 minutes until the pasta is soft. Transfer into a heated serving bowl using a ladle and top it off with Parmesan cheese.

Nutrition Information

- Calories: 428 calories;
- Protein: 30
- Total Fat: 17.1
- Sodium: 1238
- Total Carbohydrate: 39.8
- Cholesterol: 73

322. Italian Sausage And Bean Soup

Serving: 4 | Prep: 20mins | Cook: 25mins | Ready in:

Ingredients

- 1 pound Italian turkey sausage, casings removed
- 2 carrots, thinly sliced
- 1 large onion, chopped
- 1 cup thinly sliced mushrooms
- 1/3 cup chopped fresh parsley, divided
- 1 clove garlic, minced
- 3 cups water
- 1 (15 ounce) can garbanzo beans (chickpeas)
- 2 cubes beef bouillon
- 1/2 teaspoon dried sage
- salt and ground black pepper to taste

Direction

- Over medium heat, heat a pot. Cook and stir turkey sausage for 5-7 minutes until it is crumbly and brown in color.
- Mix into the sausage the mushrooms, onion, carrots, garlic and a quarter cup of parsley. Cook and stir for 7 to 10 minutes until onion softens.
- In the sausage mixture, pour in sage, beef bouillon cubes, garbanzo beans with liquid

and water. Let it boil. Put the cover on and adjust heat to low. Let it simmer for 10 minutes until carrots become tender. Skim and remove any collected fat. Drizzle with pepper and salt. Put remaining 4 teaspoons parsley on top.

Nutrition Information

- Calories: 306 calories;
- Total Fat: 12.4
- Sodium: 1613
- Total Carbohydrate: 23.7
- Cholesterol: 86
- Protein: 26.3

323. Italian Sausage And Tomato Soup

Serving: 6 | Prep: 20mins | Cook: 35mins | Ready in:

Ingredients

- 1 tablespoon olive oil
- 1 (16 ounce) package bulk turkey sausage
- 1 large onion, cut into chunks
- 4 cloves garlic, chopped
- 1 pinch Italian seasoning, or to taste
- salt and ground black pepper to taste
- 2 carrots, thinly sliced
- 1 (15 ounce) can cannellini beans, drained and rinsed
- 1 (14.5 ounce) can diced tomatoes
- 1 (14.5 ounce) can beef broth
- 1/2 (14.5 ounce) can chicken broth
- 1 (6.5 ounce) can tomato sauce
- 2 bay leaves
- 1 cup rigatoni pasta

Direction

- In a big pot, heat olive oil on medium heat. Stir and cook turkey sausage for 5 minutes till browned. Add garlic and onion. Stir and cook

for 5 more minutes till onion is tender. Season with black pepper, salt and Italian seasoning. Mix carrots in. Stir and cook for 5-7 minutes till carrots begin to soften.
- Put tomato sauce, chicken broth, beef broth, diced tomatoes and beans into turkey mixture. Mix bay leaves in. Simmer for 5 minutes till carrots are tender. Put rigatoni pasta. Stir and cook for 13 minutes till pasta cooks through yet is firm to chew.

Nutrition Information

- Calories: 291 calories;
- Sodium: 1422
- Total Carbohydrate: 27.6
- Cholesterol: 58
- Protein: 20.9
- Total Fat: 10.8

324. Jenny's Jambalaya

Serving: 6 | Prep: 25mins | Cook: 25mins | Ready in:

Ingredients

- 1 tablespoon olive oil
- 2 large onions, chopped
- 2 (14.5 ounce) cans stewed tomatoes, drained
- 2 boneless chicken breast halves, cooked and shredded
- 1 pound turkey sausage links, without casings, cooked and chopped
- 1/4 teaspoon garlic powder
- 1 tablespoon hot sauce
- salt and pepper to taste
- 1 1/2 cups uncooked long-grain rice
- 3 cups chicken broth
- 1 pound large shrimp, peeled and deveined

Direction

- On the electric skillet, choose medium-high setting, cook oil in the hot skillet. Place onion into oil and cook until soft. Mix in sausage, chicken, and tomatoes. Season with pepper, salt, hot sauce, and garlic powder. Add rice and stir, then fill in broth and add in shrimp.
- Cook at 150° C (300° F) in the covered electric skillet until rice is tender, or for about 20-25 minutes.

Nutrition Information

- Calories: 524 calories;
- Sodium: 1662
- Total Carbohydrate: 52.4
- Cholesterol: 206
- Protein: 44.9
- Total Fat: 14.6

325. Loaded Stuffed Jalapeno Poppers

Serving: 12 | Prep: 10mins | Cook: 30mins | Ready in:

Ingredients

- 12 jalapeno peppers, seeded
- 8 turkey sausage
- 2 cups finely shredded sharp Cheddar cheese
- 1 (8 ounce) package cream cheese, softened
- 1 cup shredded Parmesan cheese
- 1 (1 ounce) package dry ranch-flavored seasoning mix
- 1 teaspoon minced garlic, or more to taste
- 1 1/2 cups panko bread crumbs
- 2 tablespoons butter, melted

Direction

- Fill a big bowl with cold water and ice; put aside. Slice a thin piece from bottom of every pepper to keep peppers from rolling on sides while baking.
- Boil a big pot of water on medium high heat. Carefully drop every pepper in water; boil for

- 2 minutes. Take peppers from water; put in bowl with ice water.
- In skillet, cook turkey sausage on medium heat for 3 minutes till browned. Drain extra fat. Mix garlic, ranch-flavored seasoning, Parmesan cheese, cream cheese and Cheddar cheese in.
- Take peppers from water; drain. Use sausage mixture to fill each pepper, making a mound. Put filled peppers on a baking sheet. Put in freezer for 20 minutes till frozen.
- Preheat an oven to 175°C/350°F.
- Mix butter and breadcrumbs. Press into top of sausage filling.
- In the preheated oven, bake for 25-30 minutes till cheese begins to bubble and breadcrumbs are golden brown.

Nutrition Information

- Calories: 341 calories;
- Total Fat: 24.1
- Sodium: 1012
- Total Carbohydrate: 12.5
- Cholesterol: 98
- Protein: 21.9

326. Mushroom St. Thomas

Serving: 10 | Prep: 20mins | Cook: 40mins | Ready in:

Ingredients

- 2 pounds Italian turkey sausage links, casings removed
- 4 teaspoons fennel seed
- 1/2 pound sliced fresh mushrooms
- 2 (10 ounce) packages frozen chopped spinach, thawed and drained
- 1 cup butter, melted
- 1 cup grated Parmesan cheese
- 3/4 cup half-and-half cream
- 2 pounds shredded Monterey Jack cheese
- 2 teaspoons dry mustard powder
- 1/2 cup dry vermouth

Direction

- Preheat an oven to 190°C/375°F; grease 9x13-in. baking dish.
- Brown fennel seeds and turkey sausage for 10 minutes in big skillet on medium heat; drain excess grease off. Add spinach and mushrooms; cook for 10-15 minutes longer till juice from mushrooms and spinach evaporates and mixture is hot. Spread turkey mixture into prepped baking dish.
- Mix vermouth, mustard powder, Monterey Jack cheese, half-and-half cream, Parmesan cheese and butter till well combined in bowl; put over sausage mixture in baking dish.
- In preheated oven, bake for 20-30 minutes till bubbling and topping is brown; after 20 minutes, check it.

Nutrition Information

- Calories: 754 calories;
- Protein: 46
- Total Fat: 60.1
- Sodium: 1544
- Total Carbohydrate: 7.1
- Cholesterol: 212

327. Omelet Muffins With Sausage And Cheese

Serving: 24 | Prep: 20mins | Cook: 30mins | Ready in:

Ingredients

- 1 (6 inch) turkey sausage, diced
- 1 tablespoon light olive oil
- 1 (6 ounce) can mushroom stems and pieces, drained
- 1 cup diced red onion
- 1 cup diced red bell pepper
- 1/2 teaspoon salt, divided

- ground black pepper to taste
- 12 eggs
- 1 cup shredded Mexican cheese blend
- 1 cup chopped fresh spinach
- 1/2 cup milk
- 1/3 cup chopped fresh chives

Direction

- Let a skillet heat up over medium heat setting. Put in the sausage and let it cook for about 5 minutes until it turns brown in color. Place the cooked sausage in a bowl.
- In the same skillet used for the sausage, put in the oil and let it heat up over medium-high heat setting. Put in the onion, red bell pepper, mushrooms, pepper and 1/2 of the salt and let it cook for about 5 minutes until the vegetables have softened.
- Preheat your oven to 375°F (190°C). Use paper liners to line a 12-cup muffin tin.
- In a large bowl, mix the pepper, remaining salt and the eggs together. Put in the milk, shredded Mexican cheese blend, sautéed vegetables and sausage, spinach and chives.
- Use an ice cream scoop to put the prepared egg mixture into each of the cups in the muffin tin not more than 3/4 full.
- Put it in the preheated oven and let it bake for 20-25 minutes until it turns golden brown in color.

Nutrition Information

- Calories: 84 calories;
- Total Fat: 5.7
- Sodium: 219
- Total Carbohydrate: 2.1
- Cholesterol: 104
- Protein: 6.2

328. Pasta Primavera With Italian Turkey Sausage

Serving: 8 | Prep: 20mins | Cook: 30mins | Ready in:

Ingredients

- 1 (16 ounce) package uncooked farfalle pasta
- 1 pound hot Italian turkey sausage, cut into 1/2 inch slices
- 1/2 cup olive oil, divided
- 4 cloves garlic, diced
- 1/2 onion, diced
- 2 small zucchini, chopped
- 2 small yellow squash, chopped
- 6 roma (plum) tomatoes, chopped
- 1 green bell pepper, chopped
- 20 leaves fresh basil
- 2 teaspoons chicken bouillon granules
- 1/2 teaspoon red pepper flakes
- 1/2 cup grated Parmesan cheese

Direction

- Boil a big pot of lightly salted water. In pot, put farfalle and cook for 8 to 10 minutes, till al dente; drain.
- In a big skillet, put sausage over medium heat and cook till equally brown; reserve. Heat quarter cup oil in skillet. Mix in onion and garlic, and cook till soft. Put in basil, bell pepper, tomatoes, squash and zucchini. Melt bouillon in the mixture. Put red pepper to season. Mix in leftover oil. Keep cooking for 10 minutes.
- Into skillet, combine cheese, sausage and pasta. Keep cooking for 5 minutes, or till heated through.

Nutrition Information

- Calories: 477 calories;
- Total Fat: 21.8
- Sodium: 621
- Total Carbohydrate: 50.1
- Cholesterol: 38
- Protein: 20.5

329. Pasta With Roasted Butternut Squash And Sage

Serving: 4 | Prep: 10mins | Cook: 55mins | Ready in:

Ingredients

- 2 tablespoons olive oil
- 1 2/3 cups cubed butternut squash
- 1 large onion, chopped
- salt and pepper to taste
- 8 ounces uncooked penne pasta
- 1/2 pound turkey sausage
- 1/4 cup heavy cream
- 2 teaspoons dried sage
- 3 cloves garlic, minced
- 3 1/2 tablespoons balsamic vinegar

Direction

- Preheat an oven to 175°C/350°F. Use olive oil to coat a roasting pan. Put onion and squash in the pan; season with pepper and salt. Roast till squash is tender or for 30 minutes.
- Boil a big pot with lightly salted water. Put penne pasta in pot; cook till al dente for 8-10 minutes. Drain.
- Cook turkey sausage till evenly brown in a big skillet on medium heat; put cooked pasta, onion and squash into the skillet. Add cream gradually; season with sage. Keep cooking till heated through; stir in garlic. Put into a big bowl; toss with balsamic vinegar. Serve.

Nutrition Information

- Calories: 481 calories;
- Sodium: 484
- Total Carbohydrate: 57.2
- Cholesterol: 63
- Protein: 20.3
- Total Fat: 19.4

330. Penne With Peppers And Sausage

Serving: 6 | Prep: 20mins | Cook: 34mins | Ready in:

Ingredients

- 1 1/2 cups whole wheat penne pasta
- cooking spray
- 2 green bell peppers, cut into thin strips
- 1 onion, thinly sliced
- 1 cup fresh mushrooms, sliced
- 1 clove garlic, minced
- 1 (16 ounce) package spicy Italian turkey sausage, casings removed
- 1/4 teaspoon red pepper flakes
- 1/4 teaspoon salt
- 1/8 teaspoon ground black pepper
- 1/8 teaspoon dried oregano
- 1 (14.5 ounce) can diced tomatoes
- 1/4 cup grated Parmesan cheese
- 2 tablespoons grated Parmesan cheese

Direction

- Boil the lightly salted water in a large pot. Put in penne; cook for about 11 mins until tender but firm to bite, stirring occasionally. Drain.
- Coat cooking spray over a large nonstick frying pan; set over medium-high heat. Put in garlic, mushrooms, onion and green bell peppers. Cook for 7-8 mins until almost tender, stirring frequently.
- In a skillet, put turkey sausage over medium heat; cook while stirring for about 6 mins until crumbly and browned, breaking the sausage up using wooden spoon. Put in oregano, black pepper, salt and red pepper flakes; mix in tomatoes. Simmer for about 5 mins until heated through.
- In serving bowl, put penne. Add sausage mixture on top; add a sprinkle of Parmesan cheese over.

Nutrition Information

- Calories: 210 calories;
- Total Fat: 9.4
- Sodium: 901
- Total Carbohydrate: 14.4
- Cholesterol: 62
- Protein: 18.9

331. Potato, Sausage And Egg Breakfast Casserole

Serving: 4 | Prep: | Cook: | Ready in:

Ingredients

- PAM® Original No-Stick Cooking Spray
- 1 (16 ounce) container Egg Beaters® Original
- 1/2 cup fat free milk
- 1/4 teaspoon garlic salt
- 4 frozen Banquet® Brown 'N Serve™ Turkey Sausage links, sliced
- 2 cups refrigerated shredded hash brown potatoes
- 1/2 cup chopped red bell pepper
- 1/2 cup shredded sharp Cheddar cheese

Direction

- Set the oven to 350°F for preheating. Use cooking spray to coat the 8x8-inch glass baking dish; put aside.
- In a big bowl, mix garlic salt, milk, and Egg Beaters®. Stir in potatoes, sausage, cheese, and bell pepper until well-combined. Pour the mixture into the prepared dish.
- Let it bake inside the preheated oven for 45 minutes. To check, insert a knife and see if it comes out clean. Let it cool before serving.

Nutrition Information

332. Pressure Cooker Italian Chicken Soup

Serving: 8 | Prep: 25mins | Cook: 25mins | Ready in:

Ingredients

- 2 teaspoons olive oil
- 4 Italian turkey sausage links, casings removed
- 1 medium onion, diced
- 3 cloves garlic, minced
- 1/2 cup pearl barley
- 1 cup green lentils
- 1 bone-in chicken breast half, skin removed
- 1/2 cup chopped fresh parsley
- 3 cups chicken stock
- 1 (15 ounce) can chickpeas (garbanzo beans), drained
- 1 (16 ounce) bag fresh spinach leaves, chopped
- 1 cup mild salsa

Direction

- On medium heat, heat a teaspoon of olive oil in a pressure cooker; add sausage meat. Cook the sausage until brown, break to crumbles. Transfer the sausage to a plate and remove the oil. Heat another teaspoon of olive oil in the cooker. Sauté garlic and onion until the onion becomes transparent. Stir in barley for a minute. Place the sausage back in the pressure cooker. Put in chicken, parsley, and lentils. Pour in chicken stock until the chicken is totally covered. Secure the lid and the pressure regulator on the vent pipe. On high heat, let the cooker reach maximum pressure for 15 minutes. Turn heat to medium-high and cook for another 9 minutes. Adjust the heat accordingly so the pressure regulator keeps its slow and steady rocking movement.
- Let the pressure drop naturally or use the quick-release method following the pressure cooker's manual. Uncover, take out chicken, shred the chicken meat and place it back in the soup. Stir in salsa, spinach, and garbanzo beans until blended. Heat through and serve.

Nutrition Information

- Calories: 245 calories;
- Total Carbohydrate: 37.3
- Cholesterol: 16
- Protein: 17.4
- Total Fat: 3.3
- Sodium: 527

333. Red Rice And Sausage

Serving: 6 | Prep: 30mins | Cook: 2hours | Ready in:

Ingredients

- 2 cups long grain white rice
- 4 cups water
- 3 slices turkey bacon
- 1 onion, chopped
- 1 teaspoon minced garlic
- 1 green bell pepper, seeded and chopped
- 1 (16 ounce) package smoked turkey sausage, halved and sliced
- 1 (14.5 ounce) can stewed tomatoes, drained
- 1 (14 ounce) jar spaghetti sauce
- dried Italian seasoning to taste
- salt and pepper to taste

Direction

- Mix water and rice together in a saucepan, and heat to a boil. Cover the saucepan, turn heat down to low, and simmer until water has been absorbed and rice is tender, about 15 to 20 minutes. Put to one side.
- Set oven to 350°F (175°C) to preheat.
- Set a large skillet over medium heat. Cook bacon in heated skillet until all sides are browned. Put in green peppers, garlic, and onion; cook, stirring often, until tender. Stir in sausage, and cook until heated through; add tomatoes, and cook until heated through. Mix in spaghetti sauce and cooked rice. Season mixture with pepper, salt, and Italian seasoning. Pour mixture into a large casserole dish, and cover with aluminum foil or lid.
- Bake in the preheated oven for 60 minutes; uncover the skillet; keep cooking for 15 minutes longer.

Nutrition Information

- Calories: 467 calories;
- Sodium: 1258
- Total Carbohydrate: 68.3
- Cholesterol: 61
- Protein: 19.4
- Total Fat: 11.9

334. Rice Dressing

Serving: 15 | Prep: 15mins | Cook: 15mins | Ready in:

Ingredients

- 1 pound Italian turkey sausage links
- 2 cups chopped onion
- 4 cups cooked rice
- 2 cups diced celery
- 8 cups bean sprouts
- 1 pound fresh mushrooms, sliced
- 2 (8 ounce) cans water chestnuts, drained
- 2 teaspoons poultry seasoning
- 1 teaspoon sage

Direction

- Put the onion and sausage in a big, deep skillet. Sauté over medium high heat until the sausage is cooked well and the onions turned translucent.
- Stir in the rice, sprouts, celery, water chestnuts, mushrooms, sage and poultry seasoning. Cook until all the ingredients are warmed completely.
- Put the dressing in a cheese cloth. It should be big enough to hold enough stuffing to fit

inside the cavity of a turkey. Any leftover dressing can be placed in cheese cloth and put it alongside the turkey while it bakes so it can just absorb all the turkey drippings.

Nutrition Information

- Calories: 158 calories;
- Protein: 9.1
- Total Fat: 3.4
- Sodium: 270
- Total Carbohydrate: 23.7
- Cholesterol: 23

335. Sausage With Mango Salsa

Serving: 3 | Prep: 25mins | Cook: 25mins | Ready in:

Ingredients

- 1 fresh mango, peeled and chopped
- 1/2 fresh peach, peeled and chopped
- 1 lime, juiced
- 1 tablespoon chopped red onion
- 1 tablespoon chopped fresh cilantro
- 2 cups water
- 1 cup white rice
- 1 lime, juiced
- 1 tablespoon chopped fresh cilantro
- cooking spray
- 3 Italian turkey sausage links
- 1/2 cup orange juice
- 2 pinches garlic salt, or to taste

Direction

- Arrange peach and mango in a small mixing bowl. Add lime juice squeezed from a lime over mango mixture; stir in 1 tablespoon cilantro and onion until well combined.
- Bring water in a saucepan to a boil over high heat. Add 1 tablespoon cilantro, juice squeezed from 1 lime, and rice; mix well. Turn heat down to medium-low; simmer, covered, 15 to 20 minutes, or until liquid has been absorbed and rice is tender. Put rice to one side and keep it warm.
- Apply cooking spray to a large nonstick skillet and set over medium heat. Cook sausages for 5 to 10 minutes in the heated skillet, stirring, until browned. Take sausages out of the pan; slice into bite-sized portions.
- Bring orange juice to a simmer in the same skillet used for sausage. Place chopped sausage back into the skillet; simmer, covered, for about 5 minutes, until orange juice is reduced and syrupy and sausage is cooked through. Stir mango salsa into sausage until incorporated, about half a minute. Scatter with garlic salt; spoon mixture over rice to serve.

Nutrition Information

- Calories: 290 calories;
- Sodium: 231
- Total Carbohydrate: 65.7
- Cholesterol: 0
- Protein: 5.1
- Total Fat: 0.7

336. Sausage, Mushroom And Cranberry Tart

Serving: 8 | Prep: 30mins | Cook: 30mins | Ready in:

Ingredients

- 1/2 (14.1 ounce) package refrigerated pie crust
- 1 (9.6 ounce) package Jimmy Dean® Original Hearty Turkey Sausage Crumbles
- 3 tablespoons butter
- 1 1/2 cups sliced fresh button mushrooms
- 1 1/2 cups sliced fresh baby portobello mushrooms
- 2 eggs, lightly beaten
- 1 1/2 cups shredded Gruyere or Swiss cheese
- 3/4 cup dried cranberries, divided

- 1/2 cup whipping cream
- 3 tablespoons minced fresh parsley
- 2 green onions, thinly sliced

Direction

- Preheat the oven to 450°F. In a 9-inch fluted tart pan with detachable bottom, push the pie crust down its bottom and sides and cut off any excess crust hanging from the edges; put the crust trimmings aside. Use a fork to stab the bottom of the pie crust. Put it in the preheated oven and let it bake for 10-12 minutes until it turns golden brown in color. Let the baked crust cool down. Lower the temperature of the oven to 375°F.
- In a large skillet, put in the sausage and let it cook over medium heat setting for 4-5 minutes while stirring it often until the sausage is hot. Take the cooked sausage from the skillet and put it aside.
- Put the butter in the same skillet used for the sausage and let it melt. Put in the mushrooms and let it cook in melted butter for 3 minutes while stirring it from time to time until it has softened. Transfer the cooked mushrooms in a large bowl. Put in the parsley, eggs, cream, cheese, sausage and 1/2 cup of cranberries and mix everything thoroughly. Transfer the sausage mixture evenly in the baked tart shell.
- Place the reserved pie crust trimmings onto a clean surface that is covered with a little bit of flour then roll it out. Cut the rolled out pie trimmings using different shapes of cookie cutters and place it on top of the filling mixture.
- Put it in the preheated oven and let it bake for 25-30 minutes until a knife poked in the middle comes out clean. Garnish it with the remaining cranberries and onions on top. Slice it into 8 wedges and serve.

Nutrition Information

- Calories: 453 calories;
- Total Fat: 35.2
- Sodium: 375
- Total Carbohydrate: 22.2
- Cholesterol: 111
- Protein: 13.1

337. Sheet Pan Baked Seville Chicken, Sausage, And Vegetables

Serving: 4 | Prep: 15mins | Cook: 35mins | Ready in:

Ingredients

- cooking spray
- 2 1/2 teaspoons olive oil
- 2 teaspoons smoked paprika
- 1 teaspoon dried oregano
- 1 teaspoon kosher salt
- 4 skinless, boneless chicken thighs, patted dry
- 1 1/2 pounds potatoes, cut into 1-inch pieces
- 1 red onion, cut into 1-inch pieces
- 1/2 (14 ounce) package fully cooked smoked turkey sausage, cut into bite-sized pieces
- 1 small orange, zested and juiced

Direction

- Preheat an oven to 230°C or 450°F. With cooking spray, grease a big sheet pan, 11x17 inches in size.
- In a big bowl, mix salt, oregano, paprika and olive oil. Put in the onion, potatoes and chicken, and coat by tossing. Put in 1 layer on prepped pan.
- In the prepped oven, roast for 25 minutes.
- Take pan out of oven and mix vegetables slowly. Nestle sausage pieces between vegetables and chicken. Put the pan back into the hot oven and roast for 10 to 15 minutes longer till potatoes are soft and chicken is not pink anymore in the middle. A pricked instant-read thermometer into the middle of thigh should register a minimum of 74°C or 165°F.

- Take pan out of oven and scatter orange zest and juice on vegetables and chicken. Toss softly; serve.

Nutrition Information

- Calories: 411 calories;
- Sodium: 947
- Total Carbohydrate: 36
- Cholesterol: 90
- Protein: 28
- Total Fat: 17.6

338. Slow Cooker Kosher Autumn Mashup

Serving: 1 | Prep: 10mins | Cook: 5hours | Ready in:

Ingredients

- 1 acorn squash, halved and seeded
- 1 cup water
- 1 maple tea bag
- 4 ounces kosher turkey sausage, cut into bite-size pieces
- 1 tablespoon peanuts
- 1/4 teaspoon vanilla extract
- 1 tablespoon dried cranberries
- 1 1/2 teaspoons golden raisins
- 1 teaspoon light brown sugar

Direction

- In slow cooker, put tea bag, water and acorn squash.
- Cook in slow cooker set on high for 1 hour till tender. Remove squash flesh from skin; put flesh in slow cooker. Throw tea bag and skin.
- Mix vanilla, peanuts and sausage into squash mixture.
- Cook in slow cooker for 4 hours set on high; mix brown sugar, raisins and cranberries into squash mixture till combined well.

Nutrition Information

- Calories: 491 calories;
- Sodium: 1020
- Total Carbohydrate: 68.9
- Cholesterol: 84
- Protein: 27
- Total Fat: 15.9

339. Smoked Sausage Frittata

Serving: 6 | Prep: 15mins | Cook: 30mins | Ready in:

Ingredients

- 1 (14 ounce) package Butterball® Smoked Turkey Dinner Sausage, halved lengthwise, and cut into 1/4-inch-thick slices
- 1 cup diced green onions, white and green parts
- 1 1/2 tablespoons olive oil
- 10 large eggs, slightly beaten
- 3/4 cup shredded mozzarella cheese
- 1/3 cup freshly grated Parmesan cheese
- 16 torn fresh basil leaves
- 1/4 cup chopped sun-dried tomatoes
- 1/4 teaspoon ground black pepper
- Freshly grated Parmesan cheese (optional)
- Fresh basil leaves (optional)

Direction

- Preheat the oven to 350°F.
- In a heavy and oven-safe 10-inch skillet, put in the oil, onions and sausage and let it cook in hot oil over medium heat setting for 5 minutes while stirring it until it turns light golden brown in color.
- In a medium-sized bowl, mix all the rest of the ingredients together. Add the egg mixture into the sausage mixture and mix everything together. Let it cook over medium heat setting and use a rubber spatula to lift up the eggs 1 or 2 times so that the uncooked parts run under the cooked part. Allow the egg mixture

to cook for about 6 minutes just until it has started to set.
- Put the skillet inside the preheated oven and let it bake for 5-7 minutes until the top surface of the mixture turns golden brown in color and the egg mixture has firmed up when touched.
- Take the skillet out from the oven. Use a spatula to gently loosen up the edges of the baked frittata. Flip the skillet over to release the frittata onto the serving platter. Slice the baked frittata into 4 equal portions. You may top each sliced frittata with basil and Parmesan cheese if you want.

Nutrition Information

- Calories: 325 calories;
- Total Fat: 19.6
- Sodium: 361
- Total Carbohydrate: 3.8
- Cholesterol: 366
- Protein: 32.9

340. Smoked Turkey Sausage Tex Mex Style Pizza

Serving: 2 | Prep: | Cook: 7mins | Ready in:

Ingredients

- Cooking spray
- 2 slices Butterball® Turkey bacon
- 2 ounces Butterball® Smoked Turkey Dinner Sausage
- 1 Flatout® Light Original Flatbread
- 1/4 cup salsa
- 1/2 cup shredded Cheddar cheese*
- 10 thin slices fresh jalapeno pepper, seeds removed*
- 8 thin slices ripe pitted peeled avocado
- 1 tablespoon Ranch dressing

Direction

- Preheat the oven to 350°Fahrenheit. Use cooking spray to grease the cookie sheet; set aside.
- Prepare turkey bacon following the package instructions; cool and break into crumbles. Set it aside.
- Prepare turkey sausage following the package instructions. Thinly slice into ten portions; set aside.
- Arrange Flatout Flatbread on the greased cookie sheet and bake for 2 mins. Take it out of the oven. Slather salsa on the flatbread; add sausage, peppers, and cheese evenly on top. Bake in the oven for 4-5 mins until the cheese melts. Take it out of the oven; add slices of avocado and bacon on top. Pour in dressing. Serve.

Nutrition Information

- Calories: 441 calories;
- Total Carbohydrate: 20.1
- Cholesterol: 63
- Protein: 22.7
- Total Fat: 33.3
- Sodium: 588

341. Southwestern Breakfast Tacos

Serving: 2 | Prep: 10mins | Cook: 10mins | Ready in:

Ingredients

- cooking spray
- 2 eggs
- 1/2 cup turkey sausage
- 1/4 cup chopped onion
- 1 tablespoon chili powder
- 1 tablespoon ground cumin
- 1 tablespoon chopped jalapeno pepper
- 1 teaspoon garlic salt
- 1/4 cup habanero-flavored Cheddar cheese
- 2 (6 inch) corn tortillas

Direction

- Use cooking spray to coat a big skillet; heat on moderately-high heat. In a bowl, beat together the eggs. Put into skillet; cook and mix for 5 minutes till eggs are firm.
- On moderately-high heat, heat a big skillet. Put in the garlic salt, jalapeno, cumin, chili powder, onion and turkey sausage. Cook and mix for 5 to 7 minutes till sausage is crumbly and browned.
- Distribute sausage mixture, Cheddar cheese and scrambled eggs among the tortillas.

Nutrition Information

- Calories: 321 calories;
- Total Fat: 18.2
- Sodium: 1609
- Total Carbohydrate: 17.8
- Cholesterol: 246
- Protein: 23.8

342. Spicy Sausage And Peppers Over Rice

Serving: 2 | Prep: 20mins | Cook: 40mins | Ready in:

Ingredients

- 1 cup brown rice
- 2 cups water
- 2 turkey sausage links, cut into 1-inch pieces
- 1 tablespoon minced garlic, or to taste
- 3/4 red onion, diced
- 1 green bell pepper, sliced
- 3/4 cup vegetable or chicken broth
- 1 cup grape tomatoes
- 2 tablespoons diced pimento
- crushed red pepper flakes to taste
- Cajun seasoning to taste
- black pepper to taste

Direction

- Put brown rice and water in a small saucepan. Simmer on medium-high heat. Turn heat to medium-low, put on the lid and let it simmer for 40 minutes until the rice is tender.
- On medium-high heat, preheat a pan. Place in the turkey sausage and cook until the inside is not pink and the outside is brown. Take out the cooked sausage and mix in the onion and garlic in the same pan. Cook for a couple of minutes until the onion is transparent and soft. Put in the green pepper, cook and stir for 2 minutes.
- Add pimiento, tomatoes and 1/2 of the vegetable stock. Sprinkle pepper, Cajun seasoning, and red pepper flakes to season. Cook until the stock nearly evaporates completely. Mix in sausage with the leftover vegetable broth, let it simmer until hot all the way through. Place the sausage mixture on top of the brown rice, serve.

Nutrition Information

- Calories: 412 calories;
- Sodium: 275
- Total Carbohydrate: 87.1
- Cholesterol: 0
- Protein: 9.6
- Total Fat: 3.3

343. Spicy Turkey Sweet Potato Gumbo

Serving: 6 | Prep: 30mins | Cook: 1hours15mins | Ready in:

Ingredients

- 2 teaspoons vegetable oil
- 1 pound skinless, boneless turkey thigh meat, trimmed and cut into 1-inch pieces
- 1 pound hot Italian-style turkey sausage links, casings removed
- 1 cup chopped onion

- 1 cup chopped celery
- 1 cup chopped green bell pepper
- 4 garlic cloves, minced
- 1/2 cup all-purpose flour
- 2 cups peeled cubed sweet potato
- 1 teaspoon dried thyme
- 1 teaspoon dried oregano
- 2 (14.5 ounce) cans chicken broth
- 1 (14.5 ounce) can diced tomatoes
- 1 bay leaf
- 1/2 teaspoon hot pepper sauce

Direction

- In a big pot place over medium heat, heat vegetable oil, add turkey thigh pieces and cook for about 10 minutes until evenly browned on all sides and the meat is not pink inside anymore, remember to stir while cooking. Remove turkey from pot and set aside. Place sausage in the same spot and break into small chunks using a spatula. Cook sausage, stirring, for about 10 minutes until crumbly and brown in color.
- Stir into the pot green pepper, celery and onion. Cook for another 5 minutes, stirring well, until onions are translucent. Mix in garlic and cook for about 1 minute until fragrant; then stir in the flour. Cook for another 5 to 8 minutes until flour creates a cover on sausage and vegetable starts to become brown, remember to stir the mixture while cooking.
- Mix in bay leaf, tomatoes, chicken broth, oregano, thyme and sweet potato, bring gumbo to a boil. Lower the heat to medium low and simmer for about 15 minutes until mixture thickens and sweet potatoes are softened, remember to stir often while simmering. Stir in hot sauce and cooked turkey and continue to simmer until meat is heated through. Throw away bay leaf. Serve.

Nutrition Information

- Calories: 380 calories;
- Cholesterol: 150
- Protein: 39.9

- Total Fat: 12.5
- Sodium: 1427
- Total Carbohydrate: 24.9

344. Stoplight Sausage Pasta

Serving: 6 | Prep: 10mins | Cook: 50mins | Ready in:

Ingredients

- 1 pound turkey Italian sausage, casings removed
- 1 (16 ounce) package sliced fresh mushrooms
- 1 green bell pepper, chopped
- 1 red bell pepper, chopped
- 1 yellow bell pepper, chopped
- 1/2 large onion, chopped
- 2 tablespoons minced garlic
- 1/2 cup dry white wine
- 1 (14.5 ounce) can beef broth
- 1 tablespoon Italian seasoning
- 1 teaspoon red pepper flakes (optional)
- 16 ounces whole wheat rigatoni
- 1/2 cup freshly grated Parmesan cheese

Direction

- Heat a large skillet on medium-high heat. In the heated skillet, stir and cook the turkey sausage for 5-7 minutes until crumbly and browned; drain and throw away grease. Put in garlic, onion, yellow, red and green bell peppers, and mushrooms; stir and cook for 5-10 minutes until the mushrooms become tender and their liquid is evaporated.
- Add white wine to the sausage mixture; cook for 5 minutes until the wine is reduced. Put in Italian seasoning and beef broth; allow to simmer for 15 minutes until the liquid reduces by half. Add the red pepper flakes into the sausage mixture and stir; allow to simmer for 5 more minutes.
- Boil a large pot of lightly salted water. In the boiling water, cook the rigatoni, stirring from

time to time, for 13 minutes until al dente. Drain rigatoni and place into a serving bowl.
- Pour the sausage mixture onto the pasta and put Parmesan cheese on top.

Nutrition Information

- Calories: 503 calories;
- Total Fat: 12.2
- Sodium: 970
- Total Carbohydrate: 66.2
- Cholesterol: 63
- Protein: 30.2

345. Sunchoke And Sausage Soup

Serving: 10 | Prep: 45mins | Cook: 1hours15mins | Ready in:

Ingredients

- 4 slices turkey bacon, diced
- 1 (16 ounce) package turkey sausage, casings discarded, coarsely chopped
- 1 pound Jerusalem artichokes, peeled, halved, and cut into 1/2-inch slices
- 6 small white potatoes, peeled and halved
- 3 stalks celery, diced
- 1/2 large onion, diced
- 1 leek, white and light green parts only, chopped
- 3 cups chopped fresh spinach
- 2 cloves garlic, minced
- 1 quart chicken stock
- 1/2 cup chopped fresh parsley
- 2 tablespoons chopped fresh basil
- 2 tablespoons chopped fresh oregano
- 1 pinch cayenne pepper
- 1 pinch ground paprika
- salt and pepper to taste
- 1/4 cup all-purpose flour
- 1 cup water

Direction

- In a large saucepan, put the turkey sausage, turkey bacon, potatoes, artichokes, celery, garlic, onion, spinach, and leek. Pour in the chicken stock, and add basil, parsley, oregano, pepper, cayenne pepper, salt, and paprika to taste. Cover, and let it simmer over medium-high heat. Lower to medium-low heat, and simmer for 45 minutes.
- Mix flour into the water until no lumps remain. Stir the mixture into the simmering soup, and continue simmering while covering for 30 minutes until thickened, stirring occasionally.

Nutrition Information

- Calories: 218 calories;
- Total Fat: 5.8
- Sodium: 723
- Total Carbohydrate: 30
- Cholesterol: 38
- Protein: 12.9

346. Ten Bean Soup II

Serving: 8 | Prep: | Cook: |Ready in:

Ingredients

- 1 (16 ounce) package dry mixed beans
- 1 (15 ounce) can tomato sauce
- 1 (14.5 ounce) can diced tomatoes with green chile peppers
- 3 stalks celery, diced
- 4 carrots, diced
- 16 ounces smoked turkey sausage, diced
- salt to taste
- ground black pepper to taste
- 1/4 teaspoon poultry seasoning
- 1/2 teaspoon onion powder
- 2 1/2 teaspoons minced garlic

Direction

- Steep the bean mix in the water overnight.
- Add the sausage, carrots, celery, chilies and tomatoes, tomato sauce, drained steeped beans in the slow cooker. Pour in enough water to cover all of the ingredients and use garlic, onion powder, chicken seasoning, pepper, salt to season the soup to taste. Let simmer over low heat till the beans soften or for 8 - 10 hours.

Nutrition Information

- Calories: 301 calories;
- Protein: 21.3
- Total Fat: 2.5
- Sodium: 1102
- Total Carbohydrate: 47.1
- Cholesterol: 20

347. Toscano Soup

Serving: 4 | Prep: | Cook: | Ready in:

Ingredients

- 1 (4 ounce) package Idahoan® Roasted Garlic Flavored Mashed Potatoes, dry
- 3 slices bacon, cooked and crumbled
- 3 Italian turkey sausage links
- 1/2 onion, diced
- 3 cloves garlic, minced
- 5 cups chicken stock
- 5 cups 2% milk
- 2 cups green Swiss chard or kale, chopped
- Pinch of crushed red pepper, or to taste
- Sea salt and freshly ground black pepper to taste

Direction

- On medium heat, cook bacon in a big Dutch oven; place on a paper towel to drain.
- Crumble the bacon and set it aside.
- Take off the turkey Italian sausage links from its casing; put it in a Dutch oven with diced onion.
- Sauté until the sausage is cooked and the onion is soft; put in garlic. Stir often for 45secs.
- Pour in milk and chicken stock; add the potatoes.
- Put in kale or Swiss chard. Sprinkle fresh cracked black pepper, sea salt, and crushed red pepper to taste.
- On medium-low heat, cook for 15mins until hot.
- Transfer into soup bowls then add crumbled bacon on top.

Nutrition Information

- Calories: 323 calories;
- Protein: 25.8
- Total Fat: 16
- Sodium: 1780
- Total Carbohydrate: 19.8
- Cholesterol: 80

348. Turkey Sausage Barley Soup

Serving: 6 | Prep: 15mins | Cook: 1hours30mins | Ready in:

Ingredients

- 1 tablespoon olive oil
- 1 large onion, diced
- 3/4 pound bulk turkey sausage
- 1 clove garlic, crushed
- 1 (32 fluid ounce) container chicken stock
- 6 ounces frozen chopped spinach
- 2 teaspoons kosher salt
- ground black pepper to taste
- 1/3 cup barley

Direction

- Over medium heat, heat olive oil in a large pot. Cook and stir onion in hot oil about 5 minutes, until soft. Add garlic and turkey sausage; a use a wooden spoon to crumble the sausage into small pieces; cook and stir for about 5 minutes, until browned. Pour the chicken stock over the sausage mixture. After that, put spinach into the broth, stir; simmer and season with black pepper and kosher salt. Boil the soup, reduce the heat to medium-low, and simmer for about 20 minutes.
- Next, stir barley into the soup and keep cooking until softened, for about 60 minutes.

Nutrition Information

- Calories: 175 calories;
- Cholesterol: 43
- Protein: 13.6
- Total Fat: 8.8
- Sodium: 1587
- Total Carbohydrate: 12

349. Turkey Sausage Breakfast

Serving: 6 | Prep: 15mins | Cook: 1mins | Ready in:

Ingredients

- 1 pound ground turkey sausage
- 4 eggs, lightly beaten
- 4 green onions, finely chopped
- 1 (16 ounce) package frozen hash brown potatoes
- 1/2 cup milk
- 1 1/2 cups shredded Cheddar cheese

Direction

- In a large and deep skillet placed over medium-high heat setting, put in the turkey sausage and let it cook until it turns evenly browned on all sides. Drain off any excess oil then crumble and put it aside.
- Preheat the oven to 350°F (175°C).
- Combine the cheddar cheese, hash browns, eggs, cooked sausage, green onions and milk together in a large bowl. Transfer it into a 9x13-inch baking pan.
- Put it in the preheated oven and let it bake for 60 minutes.

Nutrition Information

- Calories: 408 calories;
- Protein: 30.1
- Total Fat: 30.1
- Sodium: 765
- Total Carbohydrate: 15.5
- Cholesterol: 217

350. Turkey Sausage Noodles

Serving: 4 | Prep: 10mins | Cook: 10mins | Ready in:

Ingredients

- 2 tablespoons olive oil
- 1/2 pound turkey sausage, cut into pieces
- 1 large onion, chopped
- 3 (3 ounce) packages chicken flavored ramen noodles
- 3 tablespoons all-purpose flour
- 2 cups water
- 1 cup frozen green peas
- 1/4 cup sour cream

Direction

- Warm oil in a big skillet on medium heat. Sauté onion and sausage for 10 minutes. Meanwhile, boil a big pot with water.
- Whisk water, flour and 2 ramen noodles seasoning packets till smooth in a small bowl. Add peas and this sauce into skillet.
- Boil mixture; cover. Cook till heated through for 5 minutes.

- Put noodles into a big pot with boiling water. Cook for 3 minutes then drain.
- Take sausage mixture off heat. Mix sour cream in; don't boil. Stir noodles in then serve.

Nutrition Information

- Calories: 439 calories;
- Protein: 25.6
- Total Fat: 12.4
- Sodium: 772
- Total Carbohydrate: 55.4
- Cholesterol: 43

351. Turkey Sausage Pie

Serving: 4 | Prep: 20mins | Cook: 15mins | Ready in:

Ingredients

- 2 (10 ounce) cans refrigerated pizza dough
- 1 tablespoon olive oil
- 1 pound turkey sausage links, without casings
- 1 onion, diced
- 1 green bell pepper, diced
- 1 (8 ounce) can tomato sauce

Direction

- Set the oven to 190°C or 375°F to preheat. Coat one 10-inch quiche dish or pie pan lightly with oil.
- In the greased pan, put 1 sheet of pizza dough. Trim the edges of dough to fit the pan, if needed. In the preheated oven, bake dough about 7 minutes, then take out and put aside.
- While baking dough in the oven, heat oil in a big skillet over moderately high heat. Crumble sausage into the skillet and sauté about 2 minutes. Put in green peppers and onions, then sauté until onion is browned slightly and sausage is cooked through, about 5-7 more minutes. Put in tomato sauce and stir well.
- Put sausage mixture into the baked crust and place another sheet of pizza dough on top to cover. Trim the edges as needed and seal gently 2 crusts together. Cut steam vents in top.
- Bake at 190°C or 375°F until turning golden brown, about 15 minutes.

Nutrition Information

- Calories: 617 calories;
- Total Fat: 19.8
- Sodium: 2238
- Total Carbohydrate: 73.9
- Cholesterol: 86
- Protein: 34.8

352. Turkey Sausage Sauce

Serving: 6 | Prep: 5mins | Cook: 45mins | Ready in:

Ingredients

- 1 pound turkey sausage, casings removed
- 1 cup tomato-vegetable juice cocktail (such as V8®)
- 1 (14.5 ounce) can diced tomatoes, undrained
- 1/2 teaspoon onion powder
- 1 teaspoon dried oregano
- salt and ground black pepper to taste
- 1 tablespoon cornstarch
- 1/4 cup water

Direction

- Set a large skillet over medium high heat and mix in turkey sausage. Cook sausage, stirring, until no longer pink, evenly browned, and crumbly. Drain and pour off any excess drippings. Stir in black pepper, salt, oregano, onion powder, diced tomatoes, and tomato-vegetable juice cocktail. Turn heat down to medium-low, and simmer for half an hour.

- Stir water and cornstarch together. Gradually mix cornstarch mixture into the sauce. Simmer for about 5 minutes or until sauce is thickened.

Nutrition Information

- Calories: 150 calories;
- Total Fat: 7.7
- Sodium: 827
- Total Carbohydrate: 5.9
- Cholesterol: 57
- Protein: 15

353. Turkey Sausage And Egg Pie

Serving: 4 | Prep: 20mins | Cook: 40mins | Ready in:

Ingredients

- 1 pound spicy turkey sausage, casings removed
- 1 small onion, chopped
- 1/2 green bell pepper, chopped
- 1/2 cup sliced mushrooms
- 1 clove garlic, minced
- 2 eggs
- 1 cup milk
- 1/2 cup biscuit baking mix
- 1 cup shredded Cheddar cheese

Direction

- Preheat the oven to 400°F (200°C). Coat a 9-inch pie plate with oil.
- Put the green bell pepper, turkey sausage, garlic, onion and mushrooms in a large skillet and let it cook over medium heat setting for about 8 minutes while stirring it until the turkey sausage is not anymore pink inside. Transfer the cooked turkey mixture into the greased pie plate and distribute it in the pie plate.
- In a bowl, whisk the milk and eggs together then add in the biscuit mix and mix well. Pour the egg mixture on top of the turkey mixture. Top it off with Cheddar cheese.
- Put it in the preheated oven and let it bake for about 30 minutes until the pie filling is bubbly and thick in consistency, and the cheese topping has turned brown in color.

Nutrition Information

- Calories: 440 calories;
- Total Fat: 26.7
- Sodium: 1366
- Total Carbohydrate: 15.5
- Cholesterol: 213
- Protein: 35

354. Turkey Spinach Sweet Potato Breakfast Casserole

Serving: 6 | Prep: 15mins | Cook: 50mins | Ready in:

Ingredients

- cooking spray
- 1 tablespoon vegetable oil, or to taste
- 1 pound turkey sausage
- 2 cups fresh spinach
- 12 egg whites
- 1/4 cup almond milk
- 3/4 teaspoon dried sage
- 1/4 teaspoon dried thyme
- 1/4 teaspoon dried oregano
- 1/4 teaspoon red pepper flakes
- 1/4 teaspoon dried basil
- 1 pinch ground nutmeg
- salt and ground black pepper to taste
- 2 cups peeled and grated sweet potatoes
- 1 tablespoon grated Parmesan cheese

Direction

- Set the oven to 350°F (175°C) and start preheating. Coat a baking dish with cooking spray.
- In a skillet over medium heat, heat oil; stir in spinach and turkey sausage. Cook for about 5 minutes until spinach is wilted and sausage is browned, remember to stir while cooking.
- In a large bowl, mix together almond milk and egg whites; stir properly. Add pepper, salt, nutmeg, basil, red pepper flakes, oregano, thyme and sage.
- Arrange an even layer of grated sweet potatoes on the bottom of the baking dish. Add spinach and turkey on top. Add the egg mixture into the casserole. Dust Parmesan cheese on top.
- Bake in the preheated oven for about 45 minutes until the top of golden brown in color and bubble appears. Cut into 6 pieces.

Nutrition Information

- Calories: 225 calories;
- Total Fat: 10.4
- Sodium: 815
- Total Carbohydrate: 10.5
- Cholesterol: 58
- Protein: 22.8

355. Turkey Spinach Sweet Potato Casserole

Serving: 6 | Prep: 10mins | Cook: 50mins | Ready in:

Ingredients

- cooking spray
- 2 cups peeled and shredded sweet potatoes
- 1 (16 ounce) package lean breakfast turkey sausage links
- 2 cups fresh spinach
- 12 large egg whites
- 1/4 cup almond milk
- 3/4 teaspoon dried sage
- 1/4 teaspoon red pepper flakes
- 1/4 teaspoon ground thyme
- 1/4 teaspoon dried oregano
- 1/4 teaspoon dried basil
- 1 pinch ground nutmeg
- salt and ground black pepper to taste
- 1 tablespoon grated Parmesan cheese

Direction

- Set the oven to 350°F (175°C) and start preheating. Coat a baking dish with cooking spray.
- Arrange sweet potatoes evenly on the bottom of the prepared dish.
- Place a big saucepan over medium heat and start heating. Add spinach and turkey sausage and cook for about 5 minutes until turkey turns brown and spinach is wilted, stirring. Remove from heat and add on top of potatoes.
- In a big bowl, crack egg whites; add pepper, salt, nutmeg, basil, oregano, thyme, red pepper flakes, sage and almond milk. Stir properly. Add egg mixture to the top of casserole; add Parmesan cheese on top.
- Bake for about 45 minutes in preheated oven until set. Cut into 6 pieces and serve.

Nutrition Information

- Calories: 200 calories;
- Cholesterol: 58
- Protein: 22.7
- Total Fat: 8.1
- Sodium: 813
- Total Carbohydrate: 9.5

356. Turkey Lentil Chili

Serving: 12 | Prep: 35mins | Cook: 35mins | Ready in:

Ingredients

- 2 cups dry lentils

- 2 quarts vegetable broth
- 2 tablespoons extra-virgin olive oil
- 4 cloves garlic, minced
- 1 large onion, chopped
- 2 stalks celery, chopped
- 1 pound turkey sausage
- 2 tomatoes, peeled, seeded, and chopped
- 1 teaspoon ground turmeric
- 1 teaspoon ground cumin
- 1/2 teaspoon dried thyme leaves
- 1 pinch crushed red pepper flakes
- sea salt to taste
- 1 (8 ounce) container plain lowfat yogurt
- 1/4 cup chopped fresh parsley for garnish

Direction

- In a big pot on high heat, heat vegetable broth and lentils to a boil. Decrease to medium heat and cook at a simmer, about 10 minutes.
- At the same time, in a big skillet, heat olive oil on medium-high heat. Mix in sausage, celery, onion and garlic; stir and cook 10 minutes till sausage is no longer pink and is crumbly. Mix in red pepper flakes, thyme, cumin, turmeric and tomatoes; cook for 5 minutes longer.
- Mix sausage mixture into simmering lentils. Keep simmering for 20-30 minutes till lentils are tender. Season with salt to taste. Put a sprinkle of chopped parsley and a dollop of yogurt atop each serving; serve.

Nutrition Information

- Calories: 240 calories;
- Sodium: 670
- Total Carbohydrate: 26.8
- Cholesterol: 30
- Protein: 17.5
- Total Fat: 7.2

357. Uptown Red Beans And Rice

Serving: 5 | Prep: 5mins | Cook: 30mins | Ready in:

Ingredients

- 2 tablespoons vegetable oil
- 1 pound smoked turkey sausage, sliced
- 1 (8 ounce) package ZATARAIN'S® Red Beans and Rice Mix
- 3 1/4 cups water
- Chopped green onions (optional)

Direction

- In a medium saucepan, warm the oil over medium-high heat. Cook sausage until all sides are browned.
- Add water and rice mix and bring it to boil. Adjust the heat to low and simmer it for 20-25 minutes, covered, until the rice is tender. Be sure to stir it occasionally during cooking time.
- Remove it from heat before stirring in green onions. Allow it to cool for 5 minutes before serving.

Nutrition Information

- Calories: 348 calories;
- Sodium: 1704
- Total Carbohydrate: 31.9
- Cholesterol: 68
- Protein: 23.3
- Total Fat: 14.5

358. Yam Sausage Spread

Serving: 16 | Prep: 1hours | Cook: 20mins | Ready in:

Ingredients

- 1/2 cup whole wheat flour
- 1 cup heavy cream
- 3 eggs, beaten

- 4 medium beets, peeled and julienned
- 1/4 cup fresh chives, chopped
- 1 turkey sausage link, without casing, chopped
- 4 tablespoons ground allspice
- 2 tablespoons baking soda
- 1 tablespoon yam extract

Direction

- Mix heavy cream and flour in medium bowl. Let mixture stand for 1 hour till thick.
- Mix turkey sausage, chives, beets and eggs into heavy cream and flour. Mix yam extract, baking soda and allspice in.
- Put mixture in a medium saucepan; boil. Frequently mixing, cook for 20 minutes till liquid evaporates.

Nutrition Information

- Calories: 90 calories;
- Total Carbohydrate: 6.3
- Cholesterol: 55
- Protein: 2.4
- Total Fat: 6.7
- Sodium: 477

Chapter 3: Turkey Dinner Recipes

***

359. Apple Almond Stuffed Turkey

Serving: 12 servings (12 cups stuffing). | Prep: 40mins | Cook: 05hours00mins | Ready in:

Ingredients

- 1 loaf (1 pound) sliced bread
- 3 medium onions, chopped
- 3 medium tart apples, chopped
- 1-1/2 cups diced fully cooked ham
- 1 cup sliced celery
- 1 tablespoon dried savory
- 2 teaspoons grated lemon zest
- 1-1/2 teaspoon grated orange zest
- 1 teaspoon salt
- 1/2 teaspoon pepper
- 1/2 teaspoon fennel seed, crushed
- 1/2 cup butter
- 1-1/2 cups slivered almonds, toasted
- 1/2 cup dried currants
- 1 cup turkey or chicken broth
- 1/2 cup apple juice
- 1 turkey (14 to 16 pounds)

Direction

- Cut bread into 1/2 inches cubes. Arrange on unoiled baking sheets, in single layer. Bake for 30 to 40 mins at 225°, until dried partially, tossing occasionally.
- In the meantime, sauté next ten ingredients in butter in a skillet for 15 mins or until apples and onions become tender.
- Place into a large bowl. Put in juice, broth, currants, almonds and bread cubes; toss well.
- Stuff turkey just before baking. Skewer the openings and tie together drumsticks. Arrange on rack in the roasting pan.
- Bake at 325°, uncovered, until thermometer registers 165° for the stuffing and 180° for the turkey, about 4-1/2 to 5 hours. If needed, lightly wrap in foil and baste once turkey starts to brown.

Nutrition Information

- Calories: 778 calories
- Fiber: 5g fiber)
- Total Carbohydrate: 36g carbohydrate (13g sugars
- Cholesterol: 230mg cholesterol
- Protein: 87g protein.

- Total Fat: 30g fat (10g saturated fat)
- Sodium: 973mg sodium

360. Apricot Stuffed Turkey Breast

Serving: 8 servings. | Prep: 10mins | Cook: 60mins | Ready in:

Ingredients

- 1 boneless skinless turkey breast half (2-1/2 pounds)
- 1-1/2 cups soft bread crumbs
- 1/2 cup finely chopped dried apricots
- 1/4 cup chopped pecans, toasted
- 3 tablespoons water or unsweetened apple juice, divided
- 1 tablespoon canola oil
- 1/4 teaspoon garlic salt
- 1/4 teaspoon dried rosemary, crushed
- 1 tablespoon Dijon mustard

Direction

- Cut a crosswise slits into the thickest part of turkey to make a pocket, about 5x4-inch; put to one side.
- Combine rosemary, salt, garlic, oil, 2 tablespoons water, pecans, apricot, and bread crumbs in a small bowl. Fill mixture into the pocket of turkey. Use soaked wooden or metal skewers to secure opening.
- Set up the grill for indirect heat. Cover and grill turkey for 50 minutes over medium indirect heat. Stir together the remaining water and mustard; brush all over the turkey. Grill until a thermometer registers 170°, for 10 to 25 minutes more. Allow the turkey to rest for 10 minutes before slicing.

Nutrition Information

- Calories: 268 calories
- Sodium: 313mg sodium
- Fiber: 2g fiber)
- Total Carbohydrate: 20g carbohydrate (0 sugars
- Cholesterol: 81mg cholesterol
- Protein: 33g protein. Diabetic Exchanges: 4 lean meat
- Total Fat: 6g fat (0 saturated fat)

361. Arkansas Travelers

Serving: 5 servings. | Prep: 15mins | Cook: 0mins | Ready in:

Ingredients

- 1 pound turkey breast
- 1 block (5 ounces) Swiss cheese
- 1 avocado, peeled and pitted
- 1 large tomato
- 10 bacon strips, cooked and crumbled
- 1/3 to 1/2 cup ranch salad dressing
- 10 slices whole wheat bread, toasted

Direction

- Cut the tomato, avocado, cheese and turkey into a quarter inch cubes; add to a big bowl. Put in dressing and bacon. Scoop half a cup of the mixture between two toast slices.

Nutrition Information

- Calories: 464 calories
- Protein: 30g protein.
- Total Fat: 27g fat (8g saturated fat)
- Sodium: 1378mg sodium
- Fiber: 5g fiber)
- Total Carbohydrate: 30g carbohydrate (4g sugars
- Cholesterol: 66mg cholesterol

362. Baked Deli Focaccia Sandwich

Serving: 8 servings. | Prep: 10mins | Cook: 20mins | Ready in:

Ingredients

- 1 loaf (12 ounces) focaccia bread
- 1/4 cup prepared pesto
- 1/4 pound sliced deli ham
- 1/4 pound sliced deli smoked turkey
- 1/4 pound sliced deli pastrami
- 5 slices process American cheese
- 1/3 cup thinly sliced onion
- 1 small tomato, sliced
- 1/4 teaspoon Italian seasoning

Direction

- Halve the focaccia horizontally and spread cut sides with pesto. Layer ham, pastrami, turkey, onion, tomato and cheese on the bread bottom. Use Italian seasoning to sprinkle over top and replace top. Use foil to wrap the sandwich, then arrange on a baking sheet.
- Bake at 350 degrees until heated through, about 20 to 25 minutes. Allow to stand about 10 minutes then slice into wedges.

Nutrition Information

- Calories: 240 calories
- Protein: 15g protein.
- Total Fat: 9g fat (3g saturated fat)
- Sodium: 817mg sodium
- Fiber: 1g fiber)
- Total Carbohydrate: 26g carbohydrate (3g sugars
- Cholesterol: 30mg cholesterol

363. Barbecue Turkey Wings

Serving: 6 servings. | Prep: 15mins | Cook: 50mins | Ready in:

Ingredients

- 3 pounds turkey wings
- 1-1/4 cups barbecue sauce
- 2 green onions, sliced
- 1 teaspoon paprika
- 1/2 teaspoon garlic powder
- 1/2 teaspoon salt
- 1/2 teaspoon pepper
- 1/4 teaspoon soy sauce

Direction

- Slice the turkey wings into sections; remove the wingtips. Mix the remaining ingredients in a large resealable plastic bag; put in the wing sections. Seal closed and turn the bag to coat; then put in the fridge overnight.
- Set an oven to 350 degrees. Drain the marinade from the wings and discard. In a 15x10x1-inch baking pan, arrange the wings. Without the cover, bake until the turkey becomes tender and a thermometer registers 180 degrees, 50-60 minutes.

Nutrition Information

- Calories: 293 calories
- Sodium: 702mg sodium
- Fiber: 1g fiber)
- Total Carbohydrate: 8g carbohydrate (6g sugars
- Cholesterol: 89mg cholesterol
- Protein: 31g protein.
- Total Fat: 15g fat (4g saturated fat)

364. Barley Wraps

Serving: 1 dozen. | Prep: 20mins | Cook: 60mins | Ready in:

Ingredients

- 1-1/2 cups water
- 1/2 cup medium pearl barley
- 1/4 teaspoon salt
- 3/4 pound ground turkey
- 1 cup chunky salsa
- 1 cup fresh or frozen corn
- 1 can (4 ounces) chopped green chilies, drained
- 1 can (2-1/4 ounces) sliced ripe olives, drained
- 1 teaspoon ground cumin
- 1/2 teaspoon dried oregano
- 1/2 teaspoon garlic powder
- 3 cups shredded cheddar cheese
- 12 flour tortillas (6 to 7 inches), warmed

Direction

- Mix salt, barley and water in a saucepan, boil. Lower the heat; simmer with a cover till tender, 45 minutes. Cook turkey in a skillet till not pink anymore, drain. Pour in seasonings, olives, chilies, corn, salsa and the barley; simmer with a cover for 15 minutes. Mix in cheese. Using a spoon, place into tortillas; roll up.

Nutrition Information

- Calories: 303 calories
- Protein: 15g protein.
- Total Fat: 16g fat (7g saturated fat)
- Sodium: 653mg sodium
- Fiber: 3g fiber)
- Total Carbohydrate: 25g carbohydrate (2g sugars
- Cholesterol: 49mg cholesterol

365. Big Sandwich

Serving: 8 servings. | Prep: 20mins | Cook: 15mins | Ready in:

Ingredients

- 1 unsliced round loaf of bread (8 inches)
- 2 tablespoons horseradish
- 1/2 pound thinly sliced cooked roast beef
- 2 tablespoons prepared mustard
- 1/2 pound thinly sliced fully cooked ham or turkey
- 4 slices Swiss cheese
- 2 tablespoons mayonnaise
- 1 small tomato, thinly sliced
- 6 bacon strips, cooked
- 4 slices American cheese
- 1 small onion, thinly sliced
- 1/4 cup butter, melted
- 1 tablespoon sesame seeds
- 1/2 teaspoon onion salt

Direction

- Cut the bread into 5 even layers horizontally. Use horseradish to spread on the bottom layer, then put roast beef on top. Top beef with the next bread slice, then spread with mustard and put turkey or ham and Swiss cheese on top. Put in the next bread slice, then spread with mayonnaise and put tomato and bacon on top. Put in the next bread slice, then put American cheese and onion on top. Put the leftover bread on top to cover. Mix together onion salt, sesame seeds and butter, then brush on top and sides of loaf. Put on a baking sheet and use heavy-duty foil to tent loosely. Bake at 400 degrees until heated through, about 15 to 20 minutes. Cut into 8 wedges carefully.

Nutrition Information

- Calories: 408 calories
- Cholesterol: 66mg cholesterol
- Protein: 22g protein.

- Total Fat: 21g fat (10g saturated fat)
- Sodium: 1162mg sodium
- Fiber: 2g fiber)
- Total Carbohydrate: 32g carbohydrate (4g sugars

366. Breaded Turkey Breasts

Serving: 4 | Prep: 15mins | Cook: 30mins | Ready in:

Ingredients

- 1 cup dry bread crumbs
- 1/4 cup grated Parmesan cheese
- 2 teaspoons Italian-style seasoning
- 1 cup milk
- 1 pound skinless, boneless turkey breast meat - cut into strips
- 1/4 cup olive oil

Direction

- Mix the Italian seasoning, bread crumbs, and Parmesan cheese in a shallow bowl. In a separate shallow bowl, pour the milk. Slowly dip the turkey in the milk, and then in the crumb mixture.
- Put olive oil in a large skillet and heat it over medium heat. Cook the turkey for 8-10 minutes or until the juices run clear and the turkey is golden brown.

Nutrition Information

- Calories: 428 calories;
- Sodium: 362
- Total Carbohydrate: 22.8
- Cholesterol: 89
- Protein: 34.5
- Total Fat: 21.4

367. Butter & Herb Turkey

Serving: 12 servings (3 cups gravy). | Prep: 10mins | Cook: 05hours00mins | Ready in:

Ingredients

- 1 bone-in turkey breast (6 to 7 pounds)
- 2 tablespoons butter, softened
- 1/2 teaspoon dried rosemary, crushed
- 1/2 teaspoon dried thyme
- 1/4 teaspoon garlic powder
- 1/4 teaspoon pepper
- 1 can (14-1/2 ounces) chicken broth
- 3 tablespoons cornstarch
- 2 tablespoons cold water

Direction

- Rub butter over the turkey. Mix pepper, garlic powder, thyme, and rosemary; scatter on the turkey. Arrange in a 6-quart slow cooker. Pour broth on the top. Put a cover and cook on low until tender, for 5-6 hours.
- Transfer the turkey onto a serving platter; then keep it warm. Remove the fat from cooking juices; then place into a small saucepan. Boil. Mix water and cornstarch until smooth. Mix into the pan gradually. Boil; stir and cook until thicken, for 2 minutes. Serve along with the turkey.

Nutrition Information

- Calories: 339 calories
- Sodium: 266mg sodium
- Fiber: 0 fiber)
- Total Carbohydrate: 2g carbohydrate (0 sugars
- Cholesterol: 128mg cholesterol
- Protein: 48g protein.
- Total Fat: 14g fat (5g saturated fat)

368. Cashew Turkey Salad Sandwiches

Serving: 4 servings. | Prep: 15mins | Cook: 0mins | Ready in:

Ingredients

- 1/4 cup reduced-fat mayonnaise
- 2 tablespoons reduced-fat plain yogurt
- 1 green onion, chopped
- 1/4 teaspoon salt
- 1/4 teaspoon pepper
- 1-1/2 cups cubed cooked turkey breast
- 1/4 cup thinly sliced celery
- 2 tablespoons chopped dried apricots
- 2 tablespoons chopped unsalted cashews
- 8 slices pumpernickel bread
- 4 lettuce leaves

Direction

- Combine the first 5 ingredients in a bowl. Mix in cashews, apricots, celery and turkey.
- With lettuce, line 1/2 of the bread slices. Put turkey mixture and leftover bread on top.

Nutrition Information

- Calories: 298 calories
- Protein: 22g protein. Diabetic Exchanges: 2 starch
- Total Fat: 9g fat (2g saturated fat)
- Sodium: 664mg sodium
- Fiber: 4g fiber)
- Total Carbohydrate: 32g carbohydrate (4g sugars
- Cholesterol: 51mg cholesterol

369. Cassoulet For Today

Serving: 6 servings. | Prep: 45mins | Cook: 50mins | Ready in:

Ingredients

- 6 boneless skinless chicken thighs (about 1-1/2 pounds)
- 1/4 teaspoon salt
- 1/4 teaspoon coarsely ground pepper
- 3 teaspoons olive oil, divided
- 1 large onion, chopped
- 1 garlic clove, minced
- 1/2 cup white wine or chicken broth
- 1 can (14-1/2 ounces) diced tomatoes, drained
- 1 bay leaf
- 1 teaspoon minced fresh rosemary or 1/4 teaspoon dried rosemary, crushed
- 1 teaspoon minced fresh thyme or 1/4 teaspoon dried thyme
- 2 cans (15 ounces each) cannellini beans, rinsed and drained
- 1/4 pound smoked turkey kielbasa, chopped
- 3 bacon strips, cooked and crumbled
- TOPPING:
- 1/2 cup soft whole wheat bread crumbs
- 1/4 cup minced fresh parsley
- 1 garlic clove, minced

Direction

- Start preheating oven to 325 degrees. Season chicken with pepper and salt. Put 2 teaspoons of oil in a broiler-safe Dutch oven and heat on medium; add chicken and brown on both sides. Remove chicken. Put the remaining oil in the Dutch oven and on medium heat sauté onion until tender and crisp. Mix in garlic and cook for 1 more minute. Stir in wine and heat to boiling, stir to remove brown bits from pan. Mix in chicken, herbs, and tomatoes and bring back to a boil. Place in oven. Cover and bake for 30 minutes. Mix in kielbasa and beans and put back in oven. Cover; bake 20-25 minutes until chicken is tender. Take it out of the oven and turn on broiler. Remove and discard the bay leaf; mix in bacon. Mix bread crumbs with garlic and parsley, then sprinkle on top. Put in oven making sure the surface of the dish is 4-5 inches from the heat. Broil 2-3 minutes until bread crumbs are golden brown.

Nutrition Information

- Calories: 394 calories
- Total Fat: 14g fat (4g saturated fat)
- Sodium: 736mg sodium
- Fiber: 8g fiber)
- Total Carbohydrate: 29g carbohydrate (4g sugars
- Cholesterol: 91mg cholesterol
- Protein: 33g protein. Diabetic Exchanges: 4 lean meat

370. Champagne Basted Turkey

Serving: 16 servings (1-2/3 cups gravy). | Prep: 20mins | Cook: 03hours00mins | Ready in:

Ingredients

- 1/4 cup butter, softened
- 1 teaspoon salt
- 1 teaspoon celery salt
- 3/4 teaspoon pepper
- 1 turkey (14 to 16 pounds)
- Fresh sage and parsley sprigs, optional
- 2 medium onions, chopped
- 1-1/2 cups minced fresh parsley
- 1/2 teaspoon dried marjoram
- 1/2 teaspoon dried thyme
- 2 cups champagne or other sparkling wine
- 1 cup condensed beef consomme, undiluted
- 1 tablespoon butter
- 1 tablespoon all-purpose flour

Direction

- Set an oven to 325 degrees and start preheating. Combine the first 4 ingredients. On a rack set in a roasting pan, arrange the turkey with breast side up; then pat it dry. Rub the inside and outside of the turkey with the butter mixture. Fill the cavity with parsley sprigs and sage if desired. Tuck the wings underneath the turkey; tie the drumsticks together.
- Roast with no cover for half an hour. Toss onions together with thyme, marjoram, and parsley; add into the roasting pan. Pour in consommé and champagne.
- Roast with no cover, basting with pan juices from time to time, for 2 1/2-3 hours until a thermometer registers 170-175 degrees when inserted into the thickest part of the thigh. If the turkey browns too fast, lightly cover it in foil. Take the turkey out of the oven; tent with foil. Before carving, allow to stand for 20 minutes.
- In the meantime, filter pan juices into a bowl. Melt the butter in a small saucepan. Add in flour and stir until smooth; add the filtered juices gradually. Boil; stir and cook for 1-2 minutes until thicken. Serve along with turkey.

Nutrition Information

- Calories: 518 calories
- Protein: 64g protein.
- Total Fat: 25g fat (9g saturated fat)
- Sodium: 522mg sodium
- Fiber: 1g fiber)
- Total Carbohydrate: 3g carbohydrate (1g sugars
- Cholesterol: 224mg cholesterol

371. Chili Stuffed Poblano Peppers

Serving: 4 servings. | Prep: 20mins | Cook: 10mins | Ready in:

Ingredients

- 1 pound lean ground turkey
- 1 can (15 ounces) chili without beans
- 1/4 teaspoon salt

- 1-1/2 cups shredded Mexican cheese blend, divided
- 1 medium tomato, finely chopped
- 4 green onions, chopped
- 4 large poblano peppers
- 1 tablespoon olive oil

Direction

- Preheat broiler. Cook turkey in a big skillet on moderate heat for 5 to 7 minutes while crumbling meat, until it is not pink anymore, then drain. Put in salt and chili then heat through. Stir in green onions, tomato and 1/2 cup of cheese.
- In the meantime, halve peppers lengthways and remove seeds. Arrange peppers on a 15-inch x10-inch x1-inch baking pan lined with foil, cut-side facing down, then brush oil over peppers. Broil 4 inches away from heat source for 5 minutes, until skins blister.
- Turn peppers using tongs. Stuff peppers with turkey mixture and sprinkle leftover cheese over top. Broil for 1 to 2 minutes more, until cheese melts.

Nutrition Information

- Calories: 496 calories
- Protein: 40g protein.
- Total Fat: 30g fat (11g saturated fat)
- Sodium: 913mg sodium
- Fiber: 4g fiber)
- Total Carbohydrate: 17g carbohydrate (5g sugars
- Cholesterol: 134mg cholesterol

372. Citrus Herb Turkey

Serving: 12 servings. | Prep: 40mins | Cook: 02hours30mins | Ready in:

Ingredients

- 1 package (1 ounce) fresh rosemary, divided
- 1 package (1 ounce) fresh thyme, divided
- 3/4 cup softened unsalted butter, divided
- 1 turkey (12 to 14 pounds)
- 2 teaspoons seasoned salt
- 1/2 teaspoon garlic powder
- 1/2 teaspoon pepper
- 1 medium apple, chopped
- 1 medium orange, chopped
- 1 small red onion, chopped
- 1 small sweet orange pepper, chopped

Direction

- Set the oven to 400° and start preheating. Use 3 pieces of heavy-duty foil to line a roasting pan (3 pieces should be long enough to be able to cover the turkey). Mince 1/2 the rosemary and thyme from each package (about 1/4 cup in total). Beat minced herbs and half cup of butter until blended in a small bowl. Use fingers to loosen skin carefully from the turkey breast; rub butter mixture under the skin. Use toothpicks to secure skin to the breast's underside. Combine pepper, garlic powder and seasoned salt; sprinkle inside turkey cavity and over turkey.
- Cube the remaining butter. Mix remaining herb sprigs, orange pepper, onion, orange, apple and butter in a large bowl; spoon to fill inside cavity. Tucks wings under turkey, tie together drumsticks. Put turkey with its breast side up in the prepared pan.
- Cover turkey with edges of foil. Cover and roast for 1 hour. Open foil carefully and fold foil down. Lower the oven setting to 325°. Roast without a cover for 1-1/2 to 2 more hours or until the inserted thermometer in the thigh's thickest part reads 170°-175°. Use foil to cover loosely to prevent the turkey from browning too fast.
- Take turkey out of the oven; use foil to tent it. Allow to stand for 20 minutes, then carve. Remove fruit mixture from cavity. If preferred, skim fat and thicken pan drippings for gravy. Serve with turkey.

Nutrition Information

- Calories: 434 calories
- Protein: 49g protein.
- Total Fat: 24g fat (10g saturated fat)
- Sodium: 286mg sodium
- Fiber: 1g fiber)
- Total Carbohydrate: 3g carbohydrate (2g sugars
- Cholesterol: 184mg cholesterol

373. Classic Stuffed Turkey

Serving: 12 servings (10 cups stuffing). | Prep: 20mins | Cook: 03hours45mins | Ready in:

Ingredients

- 2 large onions, chopped
- 2 celery ribs, chopped
- 1/2 pound fresh mushrooms, sliced
- 1/2 cup butter
- 1 can (14-1/2 ounces) chicken broth
- 1/3 cup minced fresh parsley
- 2 teaspoons rubbed sage
- 1 teaspoon salt
- 1 teaspoon poultry seasoning
- 1/2 teaspoon pepper
- 12 cups unseasoned stuffing cubes
- Warm water
- 1 turkey (14 to 16 pounds)
- Melted butter

Direction

- Sauté mushrooms, celery and onions in butter till tender in a big skillet. Add seasonings and broth; stir well. Put bread cubes into a big bowl. Add the mushroom mixture; toss till coated. Mix in enough warm water to get desired moistness.
- Loosely stuff turkey then bake. Put any leftover stuffing into a greased baking dish and cover; refrigerate till baking time. Skewer turkey openings; use kitchen string to tie drumsticks together. Put onto a rack in a roasting pan, breast side up; brush with melted butter.
- Bake without cover for 3 3/4-4 1/2 hours at 325° till a thermometer reads 165° for the stuffing and 180° for the turkey, occasionally basting using pan drippings (if turkey browns very quickly, loosely cover with foil). Bake extra stuffing for 30-40 minutes, covered. Uncover; bake till lightly browned for 10 minutes. Use foil to cover turkey; stand for 20 minutes prior to carving and removing stuffing. Thicken pan drippings for the gravy, if desired.

Nutrition Information

- Calories: 571 calories
- Total Carbohydrate: 42g carbohydrate (5g sugars
- Cholesterol: 153mg cholesterol
- Protein: 44g protein.
- Total Fat: 26g fat (11g saturated fat)
- Sodium: 961mg sodium
- Fiber: 4g fiber)

374. Cranberry Turkey Loaf

Serving: 4 servings. | Prep: 10mins | Cook: 55mins | Ready in:

Ingredients

- 1/2 cup herb-seasoned stuffing mix, crushed
- 1 egg, lightly beaten
- 3/4 cup whole-berry cranberry sauce, divided
- 1/4 teaspoon salt
- 1/8 teaspoon pepper
- 1 pound ground turkey

Direction

- Mix the pepper, salt, egg, stuffing mix and 1/4 cup of cranberry sauce together in a big bowl.

- Crumble the turkey on this mixture and stir thoroughly.
- Press the mixture into an 8x4-inch ungreased loaf pan and leave it uncovered. Bake the turkey at 350°F for around 55-65 minutes. It is ready when a thermometer says at 165°F.
- In a microwave, heat the leftover cranberry sauce on high for a minute or until thoroughly heated. Slice the turkey loaf up and serve together with sauce.

Nutrition Information

- Calories: 349 calories
- Protein: 21g protein.
- Total Fat: 18g fat (6g saturated fat)
- Sodium: 419mg sodium
- Fiber: 1g fiber)
- Total Carbohydrate: 26g carbohydrate (14g sugars
- Cholesterol: 130mg cholesterol

375. Creamy Turkey Tetrazzini

Serving: 8-10 servings. | Prep: 25mins | Cook: 50mins | Ready in:

Ingredients

- 1 package (1 pound) linguine
- 6 tablespoons butter
- 6 tablespoons all-purpose flour
- 1/2 teaspoon salt
- 1/4 teaspoon pepper
- 1/8 teaspoon cayenne pepper
- 3 cups chicken broth
- 1 cup heavy whipping cream
- 4 cups cubed cooked turkey
- 1 cup sliced fresh mushrooms
- 1 jar (4 ounces) diced pimientos, drained
- 1/4 cup chopped fresh parsley
- 4 to 5 drops hot pepper sauce
- 1/3 cup grated Parmesan cheese

Direction

- Cook pasta following the package instructions. Melt butter in large saucepan over medium heat. Stir in cayenne, pepper, salt and flour until they become smooth. Pour in broth gradually. Boil; cook while stirring until thickened, about 2 mins. Discard from heat; then stir in the cream.
- Drain the linguine. Put in 2 cups of the sauce; coat by tossing. Place into an oiled 13x9 inches baking dish. Create a well in middle of the pasta, creating a space about 6x4 inches.
- For remaining sauce: Put in pepper sauce, parsley, pimientos, mushrooms and turkey; then mix well. Transfer to middle of the dish. Sprinkle cheese over.
- Bake, covered, for half an hour at 350°. Uncover and bake until heated through and bubbly, about 20 to 30 mins more.

Nutrition Information

- Calories: 0
- Protein: 22 g protein.
- Total Fat: 20 g fat (11 g saturated fat)
- Sodium: 568 mg sodium
- Fiber: 1 g fiber
- Total Carbohydrate: 19 g carbohydrate
- Cholesterol: 96 mg cholesterol

376. Creole Stuffed Turkey

Serving: 6-8 servings. | Prep: 20mins | Cook: 03hours30mins | Ready in:

Ingredients

- 4 cups cubed corn bread
- 2 cups cubed crustless day-old whole wheat bread
- 1 cup chopped fully cooked ham
- 3/4 cup Johnsonville® Fully Cooked Polish Kielbasa Sausage Rope

- 1/2 cup chopped sweet red pepper
- 1/2 cup chopped green pepper
- 1/4 cup chopped celery
- 3 tablespoons finely diced onion
- 2-1/2 teaspoons Creole seasoning
- 1/2 cup egg substitute
- 1 to 1-1/2 cups chicken broth
- 1 turkey (8 to 10 pounds)

Direction

- Mix the first 10 ingredients in a large bowl; add sufficient broth to moisten. Stuff the turkey lightly just before baking. Skewer the turkey openings; then tie together the drumsticks. Arrange on a rack set in a roasting pan, with the breast side up.
- Bake with no cover at 325 degrees, basting with the pan drippings from time to time, until a thermometer registers 165 degrees for stuffing and 180 degrees for turkey, for 3 1/2-4 hours. If the turkey browns too fast, cover them lightly in foil. Before taking the stuffing out and carving the turkey, cover it and allow to stand for 20 minutes.

Nutrition Information

- Calories:
- Protein:
- Total Fat:
- Sodium:
- Fiber:
- Total Carbohydrate:
- Cholesterol:

377. Deli Club Sandwich

Serving: 2 servings. | Prep: 15mins | Cook: 0mins | Ready in:

Ingredients

- 2 tablespoons Dijon mustard
- Dash dried basil
- Dash dill weed
- 2 sandwich buns, split or 4 slices sourdough bread
- 4 slices smoked turkey
- 10 slices pepperoni
- 4 to 6 slices tomato
- 4 slices Swiss cheese

Direction

- Mix together dill, basil and mustard, then spread the mixture over buns or 2 bread pieces. Put in layer of turkey, pepperoni, tomato and cheese, then use bun tops or leftover bread to cover.

Nutrition Information

- Calories: 510 calories
- Protein: 32g protein.
- Total Fat: 25g fat (14g saturated fat)
- Sodium: 1311mg sodium
- Fiber: 2g fiber)
- Total Carbohydrate: 39g carbohydrate (7g sugars
- Cholesterol: 73mg cholesterol

378. Effortless Alfredo Pizza

Serving: 6 slices. | Prep: 10mins | Cook: 10mins | Ready in:

Ingredients

- 1 package (10 ounces) frozen chopped spinach, thawed and squeezed dry
- 1 cup shredded cooked turkey breast
- 2 teaspoons lemon juice
- 1/4 teaspoon salt
- 1/4 teaspoon pepper
- 1 prebaked 12-inch pizza crust
- 1 garlic clove, peeled and halved
- 1/2 cup reduced-fat Alfredo sauce

- 3/4 cup shredded fontina cheese
- 1/2 teaspoon crushed red pepper flakes

Direction

- Prepare the oven by preheating to 450 degrees. Combine the first five ingredients in a large bowl until mixed.
- Put the crust on a 12-inch ungreased pizza pan; rub with cut sides of garlic. Get rid of the garlic. Pour Alfredo sauce over the crust and spread. Put pepper flakes, cheese, and spinach mixture on top. Bake for 8 to 12 minutes or until the crust turns light brown.

Nutrition Information

- Calories: 302 calories
- Total Fat: 10g fat (4g saturated fat)
- Sodium: 756mg sodium
- Fiber: 1g fiber)
- Total Carbohydrate: 33g carbohydrate (1g sugars
- Cholesterol: 45mg cholesterol
- Protein: 20g protein. Diabetic Exchanges: 2 starch

379. Fiesta Fry Pan Dinner

Serving: 6 servings. | Prep: 30mins | Cook: 0mins | Ready in:

Ingredients

- 1 pound ground turkey or beef
- 1/2 cup chopped onion
- 1 envelope taco seasoning
- 1-1/2 cups water
- 1-1/2 cups sliced zucchini
- 1 can (14-1/2 ounces) stewed tomatoes, undrained
- 1 cup frozen corn
- 1-1/2 cups uncooked instant rice
- 1 cup shredded cheddar cheese

Direction

- Cook the onion and turkey in a skillet until the meat is not pink anymore; if needed, drain. Stir in corn, tomatoes, zucchini, water, and taco seasoning; boil. Put in rice. Turn down the heat; put on a cover and bring to a simmer until the liquid is absorbed and rice becomes tender, 5 minutes. Dust with cheese; put on a cover and allow to stand until the cheese melts.

Nutrition Information

- Calories: 377 calories
- Sodium: 651mg sodium
- Fiber: 2g fiber)
- Total Carbohydrate: 38g carbohydrate (7g sugars
- Cholesterol: 71mg cholesterol
- Protein: 20g protein. Diabetic Exchanges: 3 lean meat
- Total Fat: 17g fat (8g saturated fat)

380. Garlic Rosemary Turkey

Serving: 10 servings. | Prep: 10mins | Cook: 03hours00mins | Ready in:

Ingredients

- 1 turkey (10 to 12 pounds)
- 6 to 8 garlic cloves, peeled
- 2 large lemons, halved
- 2 tablespoons olive oil
- 2 teaspoons dried rosemary, crushed
- 1 teaspoon rubbed sage

Direction

- Set an oven to 325 degrees and start preheating. Make 6-8 small slits in the turkey skin; place the garlic under the skin. Squeeze 2 lemon halves inside the turkey; then squeeze

the remaining halves on the outside of the turkey. Insert lemons in cavity.
- Tuck the wings under the turkey; tie together drumsticks. Arrange, breast side up, on a rack set in a shallow roasting pan. Brush oil over; dust with sage and rosemary. Roast for an hour.
- Use foil to cover the turkey; roast until a thermometer registers 170-175 degrees when inserted into the thickest part of the thigh, for 2-2 1/2 more hours. Baste with the pan drippings from time to time.
- Take the turkey out of the oven. Before carving, allow to stand for 20 minutes. Thicken the pan drippings and remove the fat for gravy if desired. Serve along with the turkey.

Nutrition Information

- Calories: 414 calories
- Sodium: 159mg sodium
- Fiber: 0 fiber)
- Total Carbohydrate: 2g carbohydrate (0 sugars
- Cholesterol: 171mg cholesterol
- Protein: 66g protein.
- Total Fat: 14g fat (4g saturated fat)

381. Garlic Ginger Turkey Tenderloins

Serving: 4 servings. | Prep: 5mins | Cook: 25mins | Ready in:

Ingredients

- 3 tablespoons brown sugar, divided
- 2 tablespoons plus 2 teaspoons reduced-sodium soy sauce, divided
- 2 tablespoons minced fresh gingerroot
- 6 garlic cloves, minced
- 1/2 teaspoon pepper
- 1 package (20 ounces) turkey breast tenderloins
- 1 tablespoon cornstarch
- 1 cup reduced-sodium chicken broth

Direction

- Start preheating the oven at 375°. In a small saucepan, blend pepper, garlic, ginger, 2 tablespoons of soy sauce, and 2 tablespoons of brown sugar.
- Put the turkey in a 13x9-inch baking dish greased with cooking spray; trickle with 1/2 the soy sauce mixture. Bake, without covering, for 25 to 30 minutes, or until a thermometer shows 165°.
- In the meantime, include soy sauce, brown sugar left, and cornstarch to the remaining mixture in saucepan; combine until smooth. Pour in broth. Heat to a boil; cook and stir about 1 to 2 minutes, or until thickened. Slice turkey into pieces; enjoy with sauce.

Nutrition Information

- Calories: 212 calories
- Total Carbohydrate: 14g carbohydrate (10g sugars
- Cholesterol: 69mg cholesterol
- Protein: 35g protein. Diabetic Exchanges: 4 lean meat
- Total Fat: 2g fat (1g saturated fat)
- Sodium: 639mg sodium
- Fiber: 0 fiber)

382. Golden Roasted Turkey

Serving: 14 servings. | Prep: 40mins | Cook: 02hours45mins | Ready in:

Ingredients

- 4 cartons (32 ounces each) vegetable broth
- 1 cup kosher salt
- 1/2 cup packed brown sugar
- 1 tablespoon whole peppercorns
- 1-1/2 teaspoons whole allspice
- 1-1/2 teaspoons minced fresh gingerroot

- 4 quarts cold water
- 2 turkey-size oven roasting bags
- 1 turkey (14 to 16 pounds)
- 1 cup water
- 1 medium apple, sliced
- 1 small onion, sliced
- 1 cinnamon stick (3 inches)
- 4 fresh rosemary sprigs
- 6 fresh sage leaves
- 1 tablespoon canola oil
- 1/2 teaspoon pepper

Direction

- Mix the first 6 ingredients in a stockpot. Boil. Stir and cook until brown sugar and salt dissolve. Take off from the heat. Pour in cold water to cool the brine to room temperature.
- Arrange a turkey-size oven roasting bag inside another roasting bag; put in turkey. Pour the cooled brine carefully into the bag. Squeeze to remove as much air as you can; seal and turn the bags to coat. Arrange into a roasting pan. Store in the fridge and turn from time to time for 18-24 hours.
- Mix cinnamon, onion, apple, and water in a microwave-safe bowl. Microwave on high heat until the apples become tender, for 3-4 minutes; drain off the water.
- Drain and discard the brine. Wash the turkey with cold water; pat it dry. Fill the turkey cavity with sage, rosemary, and the cooked apple mixture. Skewer the turkey openings; tie drumsticks together.
- On a rack set in a roasting pan, arrange the turkey with breast side up. Rub with pepper and oil. Bake with no cover at 325 degrees until a thermometer registers 170-175 degrees when inserted into the thickest part of the thigh, for 2.75 to 3.25 hours. If the turkey browns too fast, lightly cover it in foil. Before carving, cover the turkey and allow to stand for 15 minutes; discard herbs and the apple mixture.

Nutrition Information

- Calories: 538 calories
- Sodium: 240mg sodium
- Fiber: 0 fiber)
- Total Carbohydrate: 0 carbohydrate (0 sugars
- Cholesterol: 245mg cholesterol
- Protein: 72g protein.
- Total Fat: 25g fat (7g saturated fat)

383. Gourmet Deli Turkey Wraps

Serving: 6 servings. | Prep: 15mins | Cook: 0mins | Ready in:

Ingredients

- 2 tablespoons water
- 2 tablespoons red wine vinegar
- 1 tablespoon olive oil
- 1/8 teaspoon pepper
- 3/4 pound sliced deli turkey
- 6 flour tortillas (8 inches), room temperature
- 4 cups spring mix salad greens
- 2 medium pears, peeled and sliced
- 6 tablespoons crumbled blue cheese
- 6 tablespoons dried cranberries
- 1/4 cup chopped walnuts

Direction

- Whisk the pepper, oil, vinegar and water in a small bowl.
- Among the tortillas, distribute the turkey, then top with salad greens, pears, cheese, cranberries and walnuts. Drizzle it with dressing and roll it up tightly. Use toothpicks to secure.

Nutrition Information

- Calories: 330 calories
- Fiber: 3g fiber)
- Total Carbohydrate: 44g carbohydrate (10g sugars

- Cholesterol: 25mg cholesterol
- Protein: 17g protein.
- Total Fat: 11g fat (2g saturated fat)
- Sodium: 819mg sodium

384. Great Grandma's Italian Meatballs

Serving: 8 servings. | Prep: 30mins | Cook: 20mins | Ready in:

Ingredients

- 2 teaspoons olive oil
- 1 medium onion, chopped
- 3 garlic cloves, minced
- 3/4 cup seasoned bread crumbs
- 1/2 cup grated Parmesan cheese
- 2 large eggs, lightly beaten
- 1 teaspoon each dried basil, oregano and parsley flakes
- 3/4 teaspoon salt
- 1 pound lean ground turkey
- 1 pound lean ground beef (90% lean)
- Hot cooked pasta and pasta sauce, optional

Direction

- Start preheating the oven to 375°. Heat oil in a small skillet over medium-high heat. Put in onion; stir and cook until soft, about 3-4 minutes. Add garlic then cook for another 1 minute. Cool briefly.
- Mix onion mixture, seasonings, eggs, cheese, and bread crumbs together in a big bowl. Add beef and turkey, stirring gently but well. Form into balls, about 1-1/2-inch each ball.
- On a greased rack set over a 15x10x1-inch baking pan, put the meatballs. Bake until thoroughly cooked and turning light brown, about 18-22 minutes. Enjoy with pasta sauce and pasta if you want.

Nutrition Information

- Calories: 271 calories
- Protein: 27g protein. Diabetic Exchanges: 4 lean meat
- Total Fat: 13g fat (5g saturated fat)
- Sodium: 569mg sodium
- Fiber: 1g fiber)
- Total Carbohydrate: 10g carbohydrate (1g sugars
- Cholesterol: 125mg cholesterol

385. Grilled Turkey Tenderloin

Serving: 4 servings. | Prep: 5mins | Cook: 20mins | Ready in:

Ingredients

- 1/4 cup apple juice
- 1/4 cup reduced-sodium soy sauce
- 1/4 cup canola oil
- 2 tablespoons lemon juice
- 2 tablespoons dried minced onion
- 1 teaspoon vanilla extract
- 1/4 teaspoon ground ginger
- Dash each garlic powder and pepper
- 2 turkey breast tenderloins (1/2 pound each)

Direction

- In a large resealable plastic bag, blend pepper, garlic powder, ginger, vanilla, onion, lemon juice, oil, soy sauce, and apple juice; put in the turkey. Close the bag and shake to coat. Let cool in the refrigerator for a minimum of 2 hours.
- Drain turkey, discard marinade. Cover and grill turkey on medium heat, about 8 to 10 minutes per side, until a thermometer shows 170°.

Nutrition Information

- Calories: 157 calories

- Total Carbohydrate: 1g carbohydrate (1g sugars
- Cholesterol: 56mg cholesterol
- Protein: 27g protein. Diabetic Exchanges: 3 lean meat
- Total Fat: 5g fat (1g saturated fat)
- Sodium: 211mg sodium
- Fiber: 0 fiber)

- Calories: 431 calories
- Cholesterol: 121mg cholesterol
- Protein: 23g protein.
- Total Fat: 31g fat (14g saturated fat)
- Sodium: 999mg sodium
- Fiber: 1g fiber)
- Total Carbohydrate: 13g carbohydrate (5g sugars

386. Ground Turkey Stroganoff

Serving: 4 servings. | Prep: 25mins | Cook: 0mins | Ready in:

Ingredients

- 1 pound ground turkey
- 1 small onion, grated
- 1 cup sliced mushrooms
- 2 cans (10-3/4 ounces each) condensed cream of mushroom soup, undiluted
- 1/3 cup buttermilk
- 1 teaspoon garlic powder
- 1/2 teaspoon salt
- 1/4 to 1/2 teaspoon pepper
- 1 cup (8 ounces) sour cream
- Hot cooked noodles
- Minced fresh parsley, optional

Direction

- Cook onion and turkey in a skillet until the meat is not pink anymore; then drain. Put in mushrooms; stir and cook for a minute. Stir in pepper, salt, garlic powder, buttermilk, and soup. Boil; turn down the heat. Without the cover, simmer for 5-10 minutes. Mix in sour cream; gently heat by don't boil. Place over noodles to serve. If desired, add parsley to decorate.

Nutrition Information

387. Ground Turkey And Hominy

Serving: 8 servings. | Prep: 5mins | Cook: 15mins | Ready in:

Ingredients

- 1-1/2 pounds ground turkey
- 1 large onion, chopped
- 2 tablespoons olive oil
- 1 teaspoon minced garlic
- 2 cans (14-1/2 ounces each) diced tomatoes, undrained
- 1 tablespoon chili powder
- 1-1/2 teaspoons ground cumin
- 1 teaspoon salt
- 1/2 teaspoon ground mustard
- 1/2 teaspoon dried thyme
- 1/4 teaspoon ground cinnamon
- 1/4 teaspoon ground allspice
- 1/4 teaspoon pepper
- 2 cans (15-1/2 ounces each) hominy, rinsed and drained

Direction

- In a large skillet, cook onion and turkey in heated oil on medium heat until meat is no more pink. Put in garlic; cook for an extra 1 minute. Drain. Blend in seasonings and tomatoes; heat thoroughly. Include in hominy and heat thoroughly.

Nutrition Information

- Calories: 287 calories
- Fiber: 5g fiber)
- Total Carbohydrate: 20g carbohydrate (4g sugars
- Cholesterol: 58mg cholesterol
- Protein: 16g protein.
- Total Fat: 16g fat (4g saturated fat)
- Sodium: 989mg sodium

388. Hearty Chicken Club

Serving: 2 servings. | Prep: 15mins | Cook: 0mins | Ready in:

Ingredients

- 1/4 cup mayonnaise
- 2 tablespoons salsa
- 4 slices seven-grain sandwich bread
- 2 lettuce leaves
- 4 slices tomato
- 8 ounces sliced cooked chicken or turkey
- 4 bacon strips, cooked
- 4 slices cheddar cheese
- 1 ripe avocado, sliced

Direction

- Mix together salsa and mayonnaise, then spread on 2 bread slices. Put on slice with layer of lettuce, tomato, turkey or chicken, bacon, cheese and avocado, then place leftover bread on top.

Nutrition Information

- Calories: 926 calories
- Protein: 46g protein.
- Total Fat: 67g fat (21g saturated fat)
- Sodium: 2029mg sodium
- Fiber: 9g fiber)
- Total Carbohydrate: 36g carbohydrate (7g sugars
- Cholesterol: 133mg cholesterol

389. Herb Glazed Turkey

Serving: 18 servings. | Prep: 10mins | Cook: 04hours00mins | Ready in:

Ingredients

- 1 turkey (14 to 16 pounds)
- 1/4 cup olive oil
- 2 teaspoons dried thyme
- 1-1/2 teaspoons salt divided
- 1-1/4 teaspoons pepper, divided
- 1 cup honey
- 1 cup corn syrup
- 1/4 cup butter, melted
- 2 teaspoons dried rosemary, crushed
- 1 teaspoon rubbed sage
- 1 teaspoon dried basil

Direction

- Brush oil over the turkey; tie together drumsticks. In roasting pan, put the turkey breast side facing up, on rack. Combine one teaspoon of pepper, one teaspoon of salt and thyme; evenly sprinkle over the turkey. Bake at 325°, uncovered, about 120 mins.
- Combine remaining pepper and salt, basil, sage, rosemary, butter, corn syrup and honey in a small bowl. Brush over the turkey. Bake for 90 more mins, basting with the pan drippings frequently, until a thermometer reads 170°-175° when inserted in the thickest part of the thigh.
- If the turkey is browned too quickly, loosely wrap in foil. Allow to stand 15 mins with a cover before carving.

Nutrition Information

- Calories: 570 calories
- Fiber: 0 fiber)
- Total Carbohydrate: 30g carbohydrate (24g sugars

- Cholesterol: 197mg cholesterol
- Protein: 56g protein.
- Total Fat: 25g fat (8g saturated fat)
- Sodium: 380mg sodium

- Total Fat: 4g fat (1g saturated fat)
- Sodium: 570mg sodium
- Fiber: 0 fiber)
- Total Carbohydrate: 11g carbohydrate (8g sugars

390. Herb Glazed Turkey Slices

Serving: 4 servings. | Prep: 10mins | Cook: 10mins | Ready in:

Ingredients

- 1 package (17.6 ounces) turkey breast cutlets
- 1 tablespoon canola oil
- 1/2 cup chicken broth
- 1/2 cup apple juice
- 1 tablespoon honey
- 1 tablespoon Dijon mustard
- 1/2 teaspoon salt
- 1/4 teaspoon each dried basil, dried rosemary, crushed and garlic powder
- 1 tablespoon cornstarch
- 1 tablespoon water

Direction

- Brown each side of turkey slices in oil in a large skillet. Mix garlic powder, rosemary, basil, salt, mustard, honey, apple juice, and broth in a small bowl; add to the turkey. Boil. Turn down the heat; put on a cover and simmer until the turkey is not pink anymore, 8 minutes.
- Mix water and cornstarch until the mixture becomes smooth; then mix into the skillet. Boil; stir and cook until thick, 2 minutes.

Nutrition Information

- Calories: 213 calories
- Cholesterol: 78mg cholesterol
- Protein: 31g protein. Diabetic Exchanges: 4 lean meat

391. Herb Roasted Turkey

Serving: 12 | Prep: | Cook: 30mins | Ready in:

Ingredients

- 1 1 10- to 12-pound turkey
- ¼ cup fresh herbs, plus 20 whole sprigs, such as thyme, rosemary, sage, oregano and/or marjoram, divided
- 2 tablespoons canola, oil
- 1 teaspoon salt
- 1 teaspoon freshly ground pepper
- Aromatics, onion, apple, lemon and/or orange, cut into 2-inch pieces (1½ cups)
- 3 cups water, plus more as needed

Direction

- In the bottom third of oven, position a rack; preheat an oven to 475 °F.
- Take neck and giblets off turkey cavities and save for creating gravy. On rack in big roasting pan, put the turkey, breast-side facing up; pat it dry using paper towels. In a small bowl, mix pepper, salt, oil and minced herbs. Rub the entire turkey with herb mixture, beneath skin and on breast meat. In the cavity, put 10 of herb sprigs and aromatics. Fold wing tips beneath turkey. Using kitchen string, bind legs together. In the pan, put the leftover 10 herb sprigs and 3 cups of water.
- Let the turkey roast for 45 minutes, or till skin turn golden brown.
- Take turkey out of the oven. Insert remote digital thermometer into the deepest portion of thigh, near joint if using it. With double layers of foil, cover the breast, trimming as needed to fit the breast. Lower the oven heat

to 350 °and keep roasting for an additional of 1 1/4 to 1 3/4 hours. Tilt the turkey to allow the juices to flow out of cavity into pan and put in a cup water in case the pan dries. Turkey is done once thermometer or an instant-read thermometer inserted into the thickest portion of thigh but not reaching the bone reads 165°F.
- On serving platter, put the turkey and cover in foil. In case you're preparing Herbed Pan Gravy, begin here. Allow the turkey to sit for 20 minutes. Take off string and carve.

Nutrition Information

- Calories: 146 calories;
- Fiber: 0
- Protein: 25
- Total Fat: 4
- Saturated Fat: 1
- Sodium: 202
- Cholesterol: 82
- Total Carbohydrate: 0
- Sugar: 0

392. Herbed Roast Turkey Breast

Serving: 10-12 servings. | Prep: 10mins | Cook: 02hours00mins | Ready in:

Ingredients

- 1 bone-in turkey breast (5 to 6 pounds)
- 5 teaspoons lemon juice
- 1 tablespoon olive oil
- 1 to 2 teaspoons pepper
- 1 teaspoon dried rosemary, crushed
- 1 teaspoon dried thyme
- 1 teaspoon garlic salt
- 1 medium onion, cut into wedges
- 1 celery rib, cut into 2-inch pieces
- 1/2 cup white wine or chicken broth

Direction

- Set an oven to 325 degrees and start preheating. Loosen the skin gently with your fingers from both sides of the turkey breast. Blend oil and lemon juice; brush on the underside of the skin. Blend garlic salt, thyme, rosemary, and pepper; rub on top of the turkey.
- In a 3-quart baking dish, arrange celery and onion. Place the turkey breast with skin side up on top. Pour wine into the dish.
- Bake, uncovered, basting with pan drippings every half an hour, until a thermometer registers 170 degrees or 2-2 1/2 hours (If the turkey browns too fast, use foil to loosely cover). Before carving, allow to stand, covered, for 15 minutes.

Nutrition Information

- Calories: 285 calories
- Sodium: 241mg sodium
- Fiber: 0 fiber)
- Total Carbohydrate: 2g carbohydrate (1g sugars
- Cholesterol: 102mg cholesterol
- Protein: 40g protein. Diabetic Exchanges: 5 medium-fat meat.
- Total Fat: 11g fat (3g saturated fat)

393. Herbed Rubbed Turkey

Serving: 12-14 servings. | Prep: 10mins | Cook: 04hours00mins | Ready in:

Ingredients

- 2 tablespoons rubbed sage
- 1 tablespoon salt
- 2 teaspoons garlic powder
- 2 teaspoons celery seed
- 2 teaspoons dried parsley flakes
- 2 teaspoons curry powder
- 2 to 3 teaspoons pepper
- 1 teaspoon paprika

- 1/2 teaspoon ground mustard
- 1/4 teaspoon ground allspice
- 3 bay leaves
- 1 turkey (14 to 16 pounds)

Direction

- Blend the first 10 ingredients in a small bowl. Rub in the hole/cavity of the turkey with half of the seasoning mixture; put in the bay leaves. Rub over the turkey skin with the remaining mixture.
- Tie together the drumsticks, then arrange the turkey in a roasting pan. Using your chosen cooking method, roast until a thermometer inserted in the thickest part of the thigh registers 170-175 degrees. Before cutting, put a cover on the turkey and allow to stand for 15 minutes.

Nutrition Information

- Calories:
- Protein:
- Total Fat:
- Sodium:
- Fiber:
- Total Carbohydrate:
- Cholesterol:

394. Herbed Stuffed Green Peppers

Serving: 6 servings. | Prep: 25mins | Cook: 30mins | Ready in:

Ingredients

- 6 green peppers, tops and seeds removed
- 1 pound ground turkey
- 1 can (28 ounces) crushed tomatoes
- 1 medium onion, chopped
- 2 celery ribs, chopped
- 2 garlic cloves, minced
- 1 teaspoon dried oregano
- 1/2 teaspoon dried thyme
- 1/2 teaspoon dried rosemary, crushed
- 1/2 teaspoon dried basil
- 1/2 teaspoon rubbed sage
- 1/8 teaspoon pepper
- 1-1/2 cups cooked rice
- 1/3 cup shredded reduced-fat mozzarella cheese

Direction

- Blanch the peppers for 3 minutes in the boiling water in a large kettle. Drain the peppers and wash under cold water. Put aside.
- Brown the turkey in a large non-stick skillet. Take the turkey and put aside. Mix herbs, garlic, celery, onion, and tomato liquid in the same skillet. Let simmer until the mixture starts to thicken and vegetables become tender. Stir in rice, turkey, and tomatoes.
- Fill the peppers with the mixture and arrange in a baking pan. Bake for half an hour at 350 degrees. Add a tablespoon of cheese on top of each pepper. Place back into the oven until the cheese melts, for 3 minutes.

Nutrition Information

- Calories: 267 calories
- Sodium: 483mg sodium
- Fiber: 0 fiber)
- Total Carbohydrate: 29g carbohydrate (0 sugars
- Cholesterol: 51mg cholesterol
- Protein: 21g protein. Diabetic Exchanges: 2 meat
- Total Fat: 10g fat (0 saturated fat)

395. Herbed Turkey Breast

Serving: 12 servings. | Prep: 10mins | Cook: 01hours30mins | Ready in:

Ingredients

- 1/2 cup butter, cubed
- 1/4 cup lemon juice
- 2 tablespoons reduced-sodium soy sauce
- 2 tablespoons finely chopped green onions
- 1 tablespoon rubbed sage
- 1 teaspoon dried thyme
- 1 teaspoon dried marjoram
- 1/4 teaspoon pepper
- 1 bone-in turkey breast (5-1/2 to 6 pounds)

Direction

- Mix the first 8 ingredients in a small saucepan; then boil. Take off from the heat. In a shallow roasting pan, arrange the turkey; sprinkle butter mixture over.
- Bake with no cover at 325 degrees until a thermometer registers 165 degrees, for 1 1/2-2 hours and baste every half an hour. Before carving, allow to stand for 10 minutes.

Nutrition Information

- Calories: 291 calories
- Protein: 44g protein.
- Total Fat: 11g fat (3g saturated fat)
- Sodium: 192mg sodium
- Fiber: 0 fiber)
- Total Carbohydrate: 1g carbohydrate (0 sugars
- Cholesterol: 112mg cholesterol

396. Herbed Turkey Tetrazzini

Serving: 12 servings. | Prep: 30mins | Cook: 25mins | Ready in:

Ingredients

- 6 cups uncooked egg noodles
- 2 tablespoons olive oil
- 1/3 cup sliced green onions
- 1 pound sliced fresh mushrooms
- 3 tablespoons minced fresh parsley
- 1 tablespoon minced fresh thyme or 1 teaspoon dried thyme
- 2 bay leaves
- 1 garlic clove, minced
- 2 teaspoons grated lemon zest
- 1/4 cup butter, cubed
- 1/4 cup all-purpose flour
- 2 cups chicken broth
- 1 cup milk
- 1 large egg yolk, lightly beaten
- 4 cups cubed cooked turkey
- Salt and pepper to taste
- 1/3 cup dry bread crumbs
- 1/3 cup grated Parmesan cheese
- 1/2 cup sliced almonds, toasted

Direction

- Following the package instructions, cook the noodles. At the same time, heat the oil in a Dutch oven over medium heat. Put in green onions; stir and cook for 3 minutes. Add bay leaves, thyme, parsley, and mushrooms. Cook until the mushrooms are browned lightly. Put in garlic and cook for 1 more minute. Remove the bay leaves.
- Place the mushroom mixture into a small bowl; mix in lemon zest, then put aside. Drain the noodles.
- Set the oven to 350 degrees and start preheating. Melt the butter in the Dutch oven over medium heat. Mix in flour until it becomes smooth. Beat in broth. Boil; stir for 2 minutes until thick. Mix egg yolk and milk; then pour into the sauce. Cook and stir for 2 more minutes.
- Stir in turkey and the mushroom mixture; heat through. Then fold in the noodles. Flavor with pepper and salt.
- Add to a 13x9-inch baking dish coated with cooking spray. Toss cheese and breadcrumbs; dust on the top. Without the cover, bake for 25-30 minutes until lightly browned. Dust with almonds.

Nutrition Information

- Calories: 326 calories
- Protein: 22g protein.
- Total Fat: 14g fat (5g saturated fat)
- Sodium: 296mg sodium
- Fiber: 2g fiber)
- Total Carbohydrate: 28g carbohydrate (3g sugars
- Cholesterol: 91mg cholesterol

397. Herbed Turkey And Dressing

Serving: 14-16 servings (18 cups dressing). | Prep: 55mins | Cook: 05hours00mins | Ready in:

Ingredients

- BASTING SAUCE:
- 2-1/4 cups chicken broth
- 1/2 cup butter, cubed
- 1/2 teaspoon salt
- 1 teaspoon dried thyme
- 1/4 teaspoon each dried marjoram, rubbed sage and dried rosemary, crushed
- 1/4 cup minced fresh parsley
- 2 tablespoons minced chives
- DRESSING:
- 1 loaf (1 pound) sliced bread
- 1 pound Jones No Sugar Pork Sausage Roll
- 1/2 cup butter, cubed
- 4 cups thinly sliced celery
- 3 cups thinly sliced carrots
- 1/2 pound fresh mushrooms, chopped
- 1/2 pound cubed fully cooked ham
- 2 cups green onions
- 2 cups chopped pecans
- 1 large tart apple, chopped
- 1 cup chopped dried apricots
- 1 tablespoon rubbed sage
- 2 teaspoons dried marjoram
- 1 teaspoon dried rosemary, crushed
- 1 teaspoon salt
- 1/8 teaspoon ground nutmeg
- 1 cup egg substitute
- 1 turkey (16 to 18 pounds)
- 1 cup chicken broth

Direction

- Blend salt, butter, and broth in a small saucepan; boil. Put in herbs; then put aside.
- Toast the bread, then slice it into 1/2-inch cubes. Put in a bowl. Cook the sausage on medium heat in a skillet until it is not pink anymore; use a slotted spoon to take out and add to the bread. Put the butter into drippings; sauté onions, ham, mushrooms, carrots, and celery for 15 minutes.
- Put into the bread mixture; stir in seasonings, fruit, and nuts. Put in 3/4 cup of basting sauce and egg substitute; lightly combine.
- Fill about 8 cups of dressing in the turkey. Skewer the openings and tie together the drumsticks. Put it on a rack in the roasting pan. Baste it with some of the remaining basting sauce.
- Bake without cover at 325 degrees until a thermometer registers 165 degrees in the stuffing and 180° in the turkey or 5-5 1/2 hours and baste every half an hour. Use foil to lightly cover once turkey starts to brown.
- Pour the broth into the remaining dressing; toss it to coat. Arrange in a 2 1/2-quart baking dish that's greased and put in the fridge. Half an hour before baking, take out from the fridge. Put a cover on and bake for an hour at 325 degrees; bake, uncovered, for 10 minutes.

Nutrition Information

- Calories:
- Protein:
- Total Fat:
- Sodium:
- Fiber:
- Total Carbohydrate:
- Cholesterol:

398. Hickory Turkey

Serving: 12 servings. | Prep: 45mins | Cook: 02hours00mins | Ready in:

Ingredients

- 2 cups packed brown sugar
- 3/4 cup salt
- 1 jar (6 ounces) pickled ginger slices, drained
- 4 bay leaves
- 2 whole garlic bulbs, halved
- 2 tablespoons minced fresh marjoram or 2 teaspoons dried marjoram
- 2 tablespoons minced fresh thyme or 2 teaspoons dried thyme
- 2 tablespoons minced fresh sage
- 2 teaspoons crushed red pepper flakes
- 3 quarts water
- 1-1/2 cups reduced-sodium soy sauce
- 1 cup maple syrup
- 1 turkey (12 to 14 pounds)
- 4 cups soaked hickory wood chips
- 1 large onion, cut into wedges
- 1 large navel orange, cut into wedges
- 6 garlic cloves, peeled
- 1/4 cup canola oil
- 2 tablespoons sesame oil

Direction

- Boil the first 12 ingredients in a stockpot. Stir and cook until salt and sugar have dissolved. Take away from the heat; allow to cool to room temperature.
- Separate giblets from the turkey and discard. Put a turkey-size oven roasting bag into the second roasting bag; put in the turkey. Fill the bag with cooled brine gently. Squeeze to remove as much air as possible; seal closed and turn the bags to coat. Arrange in a roasting pan. Put in the fridge, turning from time to time, for 18-24 hours.
- Use a drip pan to prepare the grill over indirect heat. Following the manufacturer's instructions, put the wood chips onto the grill. Drain the turkey and remove brine. Wash the turkey with cold water; then pat it dry. Fill the cavity with garlic, orange, and onion. Tuck the wings under the turkey and tie together drumsticks. Mix oils and rub on the skin.
- Arrange the turkey on the drip pan. Put on a cover and grill for an hour over indirect medium heat. Use foil to cover the turkey; grill until a thermometer registers 170-175 degrees when inserted in the thickest part of the thigh, 1-2 more hours. Before carving, put on a cover and allow to stand for 20 minutes.

Nutrition Information

- Calories: 607 calories
- Fiber: 1g fiber)
- Total Carbohydrate: 4g carbohydrate (3g sugars
- Cholesterol: 245mg cholesterol
- Protein: 73g protein.
- Total Fat: 31g fat (8g saturated fat)
- Sodium: 235mg sodium

399. Honey Glazed Turkey

Serving: 14 servings (8 cups stuffing). | Prep: 25mins | Cook: 03hours45mins | Ready in:

Ingredients

- 1 turkey (14 to 16 pounds)
- GLAZE:
- 1/2 cup honey
- 1/2 cup Dijon mustard
- 1-1/2 teaspoons dried rosemary, crushed
- 1 teaspoon onion powder
- 1/2 teaspoon salt
- 1/4 teaspoon garlic powder
- 1/4 teaspoon pepper
- STUFFING:
- 1/2 cup butter, cubed
- 2 cups chopped onion
- 1-1/2 cups chopped celery

- 12 cups unseasoned stuffing cubes or dry bread cubes
- 1 tablespoon poultry seasoning
- 2 teaspoons chicken bouillon granules
- 1 teaspoon pepper
- 1 teaspoon dried rosemary, crushed
- 1 teaspoon lemon-pepper seasoning
- 3/4 teaspoon salt
- 3-1/4 to 3-3/4 cups boiling water

Direction

- On a rack set in a shallow roasting pan, put turkey with the breast-side up; tuck the wings underneath then tie the drumsticks as one. Bake for 2 hours in a 325 degrees oven.
- Combine the glaze ingredients in a small bowl then slather all over the turkey. Bake for another 1 3/4-2 1/4 hours more or until an inserted thermometer in the thickest thigh part registers 170 to 175 degrees. Use the pan dripping to baste from time to time. Tent the turkey with foil if it browns too fast. On medium high heat, heat butter in a Dutch oven to prepare the stuffing. Include in celery and onion and mix and stir till soft. Toss in seasonings and stuffing cubes to combine. Mix in enough boiling water until you get the preferred moistness; move to a greased 13x9-inch baking dish. Bake for an hour while covered; uncover then bake for another 10-15 minutes or until pale brown.
- Take the turkey out of the oven then loosely cover with foil; set aside for 15 minutes then carve. Remove the fat and thicken the pan drippings to make gravy, if desired. Serve the gravy with stuffing and turkey.

Nutrition Information

- Calories: 663 calories
- Total Fat: 20g fat (8g saturated fat)
- Sodium: 1129mg sodium
- Fiber: 3g fiber)
- Total Carbohydrate: 47g carbohydrate (13g sugars
- Cholesterol: 189mg cholesterol

- Protein: 73g protein.

400. Hot Brown Turkey Casserole

Serving: 12 servings. | Prep: 40mins | Cook: 20mins | Ready in:

Ingredients

- 1/4 cup butter
- 1/4 cup all-purpose flour
- 4 cups 2% milk
- 1 large egg
- 2/3 cup grated Parmesan cheese, divided
- 1/4 teaspoon salt
- 1/4 teaspoon pepper
- 12 slices bread, toasted and divided
- 2 pounds thinly sliced cooked turkey or chicken
- 1/4 teaspoon paprika
- 6 bacon strips, cooked and crumbled
- 1 cup tomatoes, chopped and seeded
- 1 teaspoon minced fresh parsley

Direction

- Set the oven at 350° and start preheating. Place a large saucepan on medium heat; melt butter. Mix in flour till smooth; slowly whisk in milk. Allow to boil while stirring constantly; cook for 6-8 minutes till slightly thickened. Take away from the heat.
- Lightly beat egg into a small bowl. Slowly whisk in 1/2 cup of sauce. Gradually put back all into the pan, whisking constantly. Put in pepper, salt and 1/2 cup of Parmesan. Cook while stirring till thickened. (Do not boil.) Layer 6 toast slices and turkey on a greased 13x9-in. baking dish; pour the sauce over. Sprinkle with the remaining Parmesan cheese, bacon and paprika.
- Bake for 20-25 minutes, till heated through. Place parsley and tomatoes on top. Cut the

remaining toast slices in half diagonally; serve on the side.

Nutrition Information

- Calories: 316 calories
- Sodium: 472mg sodium
- Fiber: 1g fiber)
- Total Carbohydrate: 19g carbohydrate (6g sugars
- Cholesterol: 117mg cholesterol
- Protein: 30g protein.
- Total Fat: 13g fat (6g saturated fat)

401. Italian Sausage Orzo

Serving: 6 servings. | Prep: 15mins | Cook: 25mins | Ready in:

Ingredients

- 8 cups water
- 3 teaspoons reduced-sodium chicken bouillon granules
- 1-1/2 cups uncooked whole wheat orzo pasta (about 8 ounces)
- 1 package (19-1/2 ounces) Italian turkey sausage links, casings removed
- 1/2 cup chopped sweet onion
- 2 garlic cloves, minced
- 3 plum tomatoes, chopped
- 1/2 cup chopped roasted sweet red pepper
- 1/8 teaspoon salt
- 1/8 teaspoon pepper
- 1/8 teaspoon crushed red pepper flakes
- 1/3 cup chopped fresh basil
- 1/4 cup grated Parmesan cheese

Direction

- Bring the bouillon and water in a large saucepan to a boil. Mix in orzo; bring to another boil. Cook for 8 to 10 minutes until al dente. Strain orzo, saving 3/4 cooking water.
- Crumble sausage with garlic and onion over medium heat in a large skillet greased with cooking spray, for 6 to 8 minutes or until meat is no longer pink. Mix in orzo, pepper flakes, pepper, salt, roasted pepper, and tomatoes. Cook over medium-low heat until thoroughly heated; mix in the reserved cooking water to moisten the mixture if desired. Turn off the heat; mix in cheese and basil.

Nutrition Information

- Calories: 265 calories
- Sodium: 623mg sodium
- Fiber: 7g fiber)
- Total Carbohydrate: 32g carbohydrate (2g sugars
- Cholesterol: 37mg cholesterol
- Protein: 16g protein. Diabetic Exchanges: 2 starch
- Total Fat: 7g fat (2g saturated fat)

402. Italian Turkey Meatballs

Serving: 8 | Prep: | Cook: | Ready in:

Ingredients

- 1 1/2 pounds ground lean turkey
- 1/4 cup shredded Parmesan cheese
- 2/3 cup dry Italian bread crumbs
- 1/3 cup chopped fresh parsley
- 3 tablespoons chopped fresh oregano
- 2 teaspoons chopped fresh rosemary
- 1 teaspoon dry mustard
- 1/4 cup tomato sauce
- 1/4 teaspoon salt
- 1/2 teaspoon crushed red pepper
- 3 garlic cloves, minced
- 2 teaspoons Melt® Organic Buttery Spread, softened

Direction

- Set the oven at 400° to preheat.
- In a bowl, mix all the ingredients except for the Melt(R); stir well. Roll out around 30 balls of the mixture. Use the melted Melt to coat a broiler pan, then put the balls on. Bake until the inside of a cut meatball is not pink anymore, for around 15 minutes. Server with sauce and pasta or place on a sandwich.

Nutrition Information

- Calories: 188 calories;
- Sodium: 351
- Total Carbohydrate: 8.1
- Cholesterol: 65
- Protein: 19.6
- Total Fat: 8.6

403. Juicy Roast Turkey

Serving: 10-12 servings. | Prep: 20mins | Cook: 03hours30mins | Ready in:

Ingredients

- 1/4 cup ground mustard
- 2 tablespoons Worcestershire sauce
- 2 tablespoons olive oil
- 1/2 teaspoon white vinegar
- 1 teaspoon salt
- 1/8 teaspoon pepper
- 1 turkey (10 to 12 pounds)
- 1 medium onion, quartered
- 2 celery ribs, quartered lengthwise
- Fresh parsley sprigs
- 2 bacon strips
- 1/4 cup butter, softened
- Additional olive oil
- 2 cups chicken broth
- 1 cup water

Direction

- In a small bowl, combine the first 6 ingredients; mix until a smooth paste is formed. Brush inside and outside of turkey. Cover and put into a 2-gallon resealable plastic bag; chill in the fridge for 1 to 24 hours.
- Arrange turkey on a rack in a large roasting pan. Fill inside of turkey cavity with parsley, celery, and onion. Place bacon across the breast. Spread between legs and body with butter. Tie drumsticks together. Brush oil over the turkey. Pour water and broth into the pan.
- Bake without covering for 3.5 to 4 hours at 325°, basting constantly, until a thermometer registers 185°. Take turkey out of the oven; discard the bacon. Allow turkey to rest for 20 minutes before carving. If desired, thicken juices in the pan for gravy.

Nutrition Information

- Calories: 541 calories
- Sodium: 596mg sodium
- Fiber: 1g fiber)
- Total Carbohydrate: 3g carbohydrate (1g sugars
- Cholesterol: 217mg cholesterol
- Protein: 62g protein.
- Total Fat: 30g fat (9g saturated fat)

404. Leftover Turkey Croquettes

Serving: 6 servings. | Prep: 20mins | Cook: 20mins | Ready in:

Ingredients

- 2 cups mashed potatoes (with added milk and butter)
- 1/2 cup grated Parmesan cheese
- 1/2 cup shredded Swiss cheese
- 1 shallot, finely chopped
- 2 teaspoons minced fresh rosemary or 1/2 teaspoon dried rosemary, crushed

- 1 teaspoon minced fresh sage or 1/4 teaspoon dried sage leaves
- 1/2 teaspoon salt
- 1/4 teaspoon pepper
- 3 cups finely chopped cooked turkey
- 1 large egg
- 2 tablespoons water
- 1-1/4 cups panko (Japanese) bread crumbs
- 1/4 cup butter, divided
- Sour cream, optional

Direction

- Combine pepper, salt, sage, rosemary, shallot, cheese, and mashed potatoes in a large bowl. Mix in turkey. Form mixture into 12 patties, about 1-inch thick.
- Stir together water and egg in a shallow bowl. Spread bread crumbs in a separate shallow bowl. Immerse croquettes in egg mixture, then in bread crumbs, patting to help coating adhere.
- Melt 2 tablespoons butter in a large skillet over medium heat. Cook half of croquettes until browned, for 4 to 5 minutes per side. Take out and keep warm. Repeat. Serve croquettes with sour cream, if desired.

Nutrition Information

- Calories: 383 calories
- Sodium: 734mg sodium
- Fiber: 2g fiber)
- Total Carbohydrate: 22g carbohydrate (2g sugars
- Cholesterol: 144mg cholesterol
- Protein: 29g protein.
- Total Fat: 19g fat (10g saturated fat)

405. Lemon Garlic Turkey Breast

Serving: 12 servings. | Prep: 15mins | Cook: 05hours00mins |Ready in:

Ingredients

- 2 medium lemons, sliced
- 1 bone-in turkey breast (6 to 7 pounds), skin removed
- 1/4 cup minced fresh parsley
- 8 garlic cloves, minced
- 4 teaspoons grated lemon peel
- 2 teaspoons salt-free lemon-pepper seasoning
- 1-1/2 teaspoons salt

Direction

- Line 3/4 lemon slices onto the bottom of a greased 6-quart slow cooker. Arrange the turkey atop of the lemons with the breast side up. Combine the salt, pepper seasoning, lemon peel, garlic, and parsley and rub over the turkey. Add the remaining lemon slices on top. Cook while covering for 5-6 hours on low until the turkey becomes soft.
- Take the turkey away from the slow cooker and cover with a foil-tent. Let it sit for 15 minutes before carving. You can skim the fat and thicken the drippings in the pan to make sauce if you want. Serve the turkey with the sauce.

Nutrition Information

- Calories: 197 calories
- Sodium: 371mg sodium
- Fiber: 0 fiber)
- Total Carbohydrate: 2g carbohydrate (0 sugars
- Cholesterol: 117mg cholesterol
- Protein: 43g protein. Diabetic Exchanges: 6 lean meat.
- Total Fat: 1g fat (0 saturated fat)

406. Low Sodium Herb Rubbed Turkey

Serving: 28 servings. | Prep: 30mins | Cook: 02hours00mins |Ready in:

Ingredients

- 6 garlic cloves, minced
- 2 tablespoons plus 2 teaspoons rubbed sage
- 1 tablespoon minced fresh thyme or 1 teaspoon dried thyme
- 2 teaspoons pepper
- 1/2 teaspoon each ground allspice, ginger and mustard
- 1/4 teaspoon cayenne pepper
- 1 tablespoon all-purpose flour
- 1 turkey-size oven roasting bag
- 2 celery ribs, chopped
- 2 small carrots, chopped
- 1 small onion, chopped
- 1 small potato, sliced
- 1 turkey (14 pounds)
- 1 tablespoon cornstarch
- 2 tablespoons cold water

Direction

- Set the oven at 350° and start preheating. Combine spices, herbs and garlic till well blended in a small bowl. Sprinkle flour into the oven bag; shake properly to coat. Arrange the bag in a roasting pan; put in vegetables; sprinkle with 5 teaspoons of the herb mixture.
- Pat turkey dry. Loosen the skin from the turkey breast carefully with fingers; rub the under of the skin with half of the remaining herb mixture. Use toothpicks to secure the skin to underside of the breast. Rub the inside of turkey with the leftover herb mixture. Tuck the wings under the turkey; tie drumsticks together.
- Place the turkey in the bag over the vegetables, breast side up; use nylon tie to close the bag. In the top of the bag, cut six 1/2-in. slits; use the tie provided to close. Bake till a thermometer reads 170°-175° when inserted into the thickest part of the thigh, 2-2 1/2 hours.
- Move the turkey from the oven bag to a serving platter; tent with foil. Allow to sit for 20 minutes before carving. Strain the contents of the oven bag into a small saucepan; remove and discard the vegetables; skim fat from the cooking juices. Combine water with cornstarch till smooth in a small bowl; slowly blend into the cooking juices. Boil; cook while stirring till thickened, 2 minutes. Serve with turkey.

Nutrition Information

- Calories: 198 calories
- Total Fat: 6g fat (2g saturated fat)
- Sodium: 80mg sodium
- Fiber: 0 fiber)
- Total Carbohydrate: 1g carbohydrate (0 sugars
- Cholesterol: 86mg cholesterol
- Protein: 33g protein. Diabetic Exchanges: 4 lean meat.

407. Make Ahead Turkey And Gravy

Serving: 16 servings (2-1/2 cups gravy). | Prep: 04hours15mins | Cook: 50mins | Ready in:

Ingredients

- 1 turkey (14 to 16 pounds)
- 2 teaspoons poultry seasoning
- 1 teaspoon pepper
- 3 cups chicken broth
- 1/2 cup minced fresh parsley
- 1 tablespoon minced fresh thyme or 1 teaspoon dried thyme
- 1 tablespoon minced fresh rosemary or 1 teaspoon dried rosemary, crushed
- 2 teaspoons grated lemon peel
- 1/4 cup lemon juice
- 2 garlic cloves, minced
- FOR SERVING:
- 1-1/2 cups chicken broth
- 1 tablespoon butter
- 1 tablespoon all-purpose flour

Direction

- Set an oven to 325 degrees and start preheating. In a roasting pan, arrange the turkey breast side up on a rack. Sprinkle with pepper and poultry seasoning. Tuck the wings under the turkey; tie together the drumsticks.
- Roast without cover for half an hour. Combine garlic, juice, lemon peel, herbs, and broth in a 4-cup measuring cup; add to the turkey. Roast, uncovered, basting with the broth mixture from time to time, for 3-3 1/2 hours until a thermometer inserted in the thickest part of the thigh registers 170-175 degrees. If the turkey browns too fast, use foil to cover loosely.
- Take the turkey out from the pan; before craving, allow to stand for at least 20 minutes. Remove the fat from the surface of the cooking juices.
- To freeze: Carve the turkey and arrange it in shallow freezer containers. Pour the cooking juices on top of the turkey; allow to cool slightly for about an hour. Put a cover on and freeze for up to 3 months.
- To serve: Put the turkey in the fridge overnight to thaw partially. Set an oven to 350 degrees and start preheating. Place the cooking juices and the turkey into a large baking dish. Pour with 1-1 1/2cups of broth on top. Cover and bake for 50-60 minutes until a thermometer inserted in the turkey registers 165 degrees.
- To make gravy: Transfer the turkey into a platter, save the broth mixture and keep it warm. In a saucepan, let the butter melt on medium heat; stir in flour until it becomes smooth. Slowly whisk in the broth mixture; boil and constantly stir. Stir and cook for about 2 minutes until thick. Serve together with turkey.

Nutrition Information

- Calories: 480 calories
- Total Carbohydrate: 2g carbohydrate (1g sugars
- Cholesterol: 218mg cholesterol
- Protein: 64g protein.
- Total Fat: 22g fat (7g saturated fat)
- Sodium: 434mg sodium
- Fiber: 0 fiber)

408. Maple Butter Turkey With Gravy

Serving: 14-16 servings (3-1/3 cups gravy). | Prep: 40mins | Cook: 03hours00mins | Ready in:

Ingredients

- 2 cups apple cider or juice
- 1/3 cup maple syrup
- 3/4 cup butter, cubed
- 2 tablespoons minced fresh thyme or 2 teaspoons dried thyme
- 1 tablespoon minced fresh sage or 1 teaspoon dried sage leaves
- 2 teaspoons dried marjoram
- 1 teaspoon salt
- 1 teaspoon pepper
- 1 turkey (14 to 16 pounds)
- 2 to 2-1/2 cups chicken broth
- 3 tablespoons all-purpose flour

Direction

- Boil syrup and cider in a small heavy saucepan for the maple butter. Cook for 20 minutes until it reduces to half a cup. Take away from the heat; then stir in pepper, salt, marjoram, sage, thyme, and butter. Place into a small bowl; put on a cover and put in the fridge until set.
- Loosen the skin gently from both sides of the turkey breasts using fingers. Rub under the turkey skin with 1/2 cup of maple butter. Put the remaining maple butter in the fridge. Fasten the turkey openings using a skewer and tie drumsticks together. In a roasting pan, arrange turkey on a rack. Use foil to cover and bake for 2 hours at 325 degrees.

- Brush 1/3 cup of the maple butter over the top. Without the cover, bake, basting with pan drippings from time to time, until a thermometer registers 180 degrees, 1-1 1/2 more hours (If the turkey browns too fast, use foil to loosely cover). Transfer the turkey to a serving platter and keep it warm. Before carving, put on a cover and allow to stand for 20 minutes.
- Add the loosened browned bits and the drippings to a 4-cup measuring cup. Remove the fat and discard. Pour sufficient broth into the drippings to make 3 cups. Mix the broth mixture and flour until the mixture becomes smooth. Mix in the remaining maple butter. Boil; stir and cook until thick, 2 minutes. Serve alongside turkey.

Nutrition Information

- Calories: 579 calories
- Fiber: 0 fiber)
- Total Carbohydrate: 10g carbohydrate (8g sugars
- Cholesterol: 237mg cholesterol
- Protein: 64g protein.
- Total Fat: 30g fat (12g saturated fat)
- Sodium: 506mg sodium

409. Maple Sage Brined Turkey

Serving: 20 servings. | Prep: 40mins | Cook: 02hours30mins | Ready in:

Ingredients

- 4 quarts water
- 1-1/2 cups packed brown sugar
- 1 cup sea salt
- 1 cup maple syrup
- 1 cup cider vinegar
- 24 fresh sage leaves
- 6 bay leaves
- 2 tablespoons yellow prepared mustard
- 2 tablespoons coarsely ground pepper
- 1 teaspoon ground cloves
- 4 quarts ice water
- 2 turkey-size oven roasting bags
- 1 turkey (14 to 16 pounds)
- TURKEY:
- 2 tablespoons olive oil
- 1/2 teaspoon pepper
- 1/2 teaspoon salt, optional

Direction

- In a large stockpot, blend the first 10 ingredients; heat to a boil. Cook and stir until dissolved. Take away from heat. Pour in 4-quart ice water to cool the brine to room temperature.
- Put 1 turkey-sized oven roasting bag inside the other; put in a large stockpot. Put turkey in both bags; transfer in cooled brine. Close bags, and press out as much air as possible. Put in the refrigerator for 18 to 24 hours.
- Start preheating the oven at 350°. Take turkey out from brine; wash and pat dry. Discard the brine. Arrange the turkey on a rack in a shallow roasting pan, with the breast side up. Tuck the wings under turkey; bind drumsticks together. Coat oil on the skin of turkey; scatter with salt, if needed, and pepper.
- Roast, without covering, until a thermometer shows 170° to 175° when inserted in the thickest part of thigh, about 2 1/2 to 3 hours. (If turkey turns brown too fast, cover loosely with foil) Take turkey out from the oven; tent with foil. Allow to stand before carving 20 minutes.

Nutrition Information

- Calories: 384 calories
- Fiber: 0 fiber)
- Total Carbohydrate: 0 carbohydrate (0 sugars
- Cholesterol: 172mg cholesterol
- Protein: 51g protein.
- Total Fat: 18g fat (5g saturated fat)

- Sodium: 168mg sodium

410. Marinated Thanksgiving Turkey

Serving: 12 servings. | Prep: 10mins | Cook: 02hours30mins | Ready in:

Ingredients

- 2 cups water
- 1-1/2 cups chicken broth
- 1 cup reduced-sodium soy sauce
- 2/3 cup lemon juice
- 2 garlic cloves, minced
- 1-1/2 teaspoons ground ginger
- 1 teaspoon pepper
- 2 large oven roasting bags
- 1 turkey (12 to 14 pounds)

Direction

- Blend the first 7 ingredients; put aside and place a cup in the fridge for basting. Put an oven roasting bag inside the other. Put inside both bags the turkey; add in the remaining marinade. Seal the bags and press as much air out as you can; then turn the bag to coat the turkey. Arrange in a shallow roasting pan. Put in the fridge overnight and turn a few times.
- Take the turkey out, then drain it and discard the marinade.
- Regular roasting method: Set an oven to 325 degrees and start preheating. In a large roaster, arrange a turkey on a rack. Bake without cover until a thermometer inserted in thigh registers 170 degrees or 3-3 1/2 hours. Baste regularly with the saved marinade. Use a tent of aluminum foil to lightly cover once the turkey starts to brown. Take the turkey out from the oven; use foil to tent it. Before carving, allow to stand for 20 minutes. Remove the fat from the surface and thicken the pan drippings for gravy, if desired. Serve together with turkey.
- Grill method: Set the grill on indirect medium heat. Tuck the wings under the turkey and place it on a grill rack, breast side down. Put a cover on and grill for an hour.
- Put ten briquettes to coals if you will be using a charcoal grill, then turn the turkey. Baste with the saved marinade. Put a cover, cook for 1-1/2 to 2 hours and add ten briquettes to keep the heat and brush with the marinade every half an hour until a thermometer inserted in the thigh registers 170 degrees. Take the turkey out from the grill; use foil to tent it. Before carving, allow to stand for 20 minutes.

Nutrition Information

- Calories: 407 calories
- Cholesterol: 171mg cholesterol
- Protein: 67g protein.
- Total Fat: 12g fat (4g saturated fat)
- Sodium: 383mg sodium
- Fiber: 1g fiber)
- Total Carbohydrate: 5g carbohydrate (0 sugars

411. Marinated Turkey

Serving: 8-10 servings. | Prep: 10mins | Cook: 01hours30mins | Ready in:

Ingredients

- 1 cup soy sauce
- 1 cup canola oil
- 1/4 cup honey
- 4 teaspoons Worcestershire sauce
- 2 teaspoons ground ginger
- 2 teaspoons ground mustard
- 2 teaspoons lemon juice
- 4 garlic cloves, minced
- 6 to 7 pounds fresh turkey parts
- 1/4 cup all-purpose flour, optional
- Salt and pepper, optional

Direction

- Mix the first 8 ingredients in a small bowl. In a large heavy-duty plastic bag, arrange the turkey; put in half of the marinade. Seal the bag, then put in the fridge, turning the bag from time to time, overnight. Put on a cover and place the remaining marinade in the fridge.
- Drain the marinade off the turkey and discard; in a large shallow roasting pan, place the turkey in a single layer. Add the saved marinade to the turkey. Without the cover, bake at 325 degrees until tender, 1 1/2-2 hours, and if desired, baste from time to time while baking. Transfer the turkey to a serving platter and keep it warm.
- Prepare gravy if desired: Strain the pan juices into a large measuring cup. Remove the fat and save 1/4 cup in a medium saucepan; then discard all the remaining fat. Stir the flour into a saucepan. Pour the water into the pan juices to measure 2 cups. Put into the saucepan; stir and cook until bubbling and thick. Stir and cook for 1 more minute. Flavor with pepper and salt. Serve alongside turkey.

Nutrition Information

- Calories:
- Protein:
- Total Fat:
- Sodium:
- Fiber:
- Total Carbohydrate:
- Cholesterol:

412. Marinated Turkey For Two

Serving: 2 servings. | Prep: 10mins | Cook: 50mins | Ready in:

Ingredients

- 2 turkey breast tenderloins (about 1 pound)
- 1-1/2 cups pineapple juice
- 1/3 cup sugar
- 3/4 teaspoon salt
- 1/8 teaspoon pepper
- 1/8 teaspoon ground ginger
- Dash ground cloves
- Dash garlic powder

Direction

- In a shallow glass dish, arrange the turkey. Mix the rest of the ingredients; combine thoroughly. Put 1/3 cup aside; put a cover on and store in the fridge. Pour over the turkey with the remaining marinade. Put a cover and store in the fridge for 4 hours or overnight.
- Drain off the marinade and discard. In an ungreased 11x7-inch baking dish, arrange the turkey. Pour over the turkey with the saved marinade. Put a cover and bake for half an hour at 350 degrees. Remove the cover and bake, basting 2 times, until not pink anymore, for 20-30 more minutes. Cut and serve right away.

Nutrition Information

- Calories:
- Total Carbohydrate:
- Cholesterol:
- Protein:
- Total Fat:
- Sodium:
- Fiber:

413. Meaty Spanish Rice

Serving: 4 servings. | Prep: 15mins | Cook: 30mins | Ready in:

Ingredients

- 2 tablespoons butter

- 1/2 pound ground turkey
- 1 medium onion, chopped
- 1 medium green pepper, chopped
- 2 cups water
- 1 can (8 ounces) tomato sauce
- 1 cup uncooked long grain rice
- 2 tablespoons Worcestershire sauce
- 1/2 teaspoon chili powder
- 1/2 teaspoon dried thyme
- 1/4 teaspoon hot pepper sauce
- 1/8 teaspoon cayenne pepper, optional
- Black pepper to taste

Direction

- Melt the butter in a skillet over medium heat. Put in green pepper, onion, and ground turkey; cook until the vegetables become tender and the meat turns brown. Put in the remaining ingredients and boil. Turn down the heat, put on a cover and simmer for half an hour until the rice becomes tender.

Nutrition Information

- Calories: 300 calories
- Fiber: 0 fiber)
- Total Carbohydrate: 27g carbohydrate (0 sugars
- Cholesterol: 52mg cholesterol
- Protein: 17g protein. Diabetic Exchanges: 2 meat
- Total Fat: 14g fat (0 saturated fat)
- Sodium: 379mg sodium

414. Mock Monte Cristos

Serving: 6 servings. | Prep: 15mins | Cook: 15mins | Ready in:

Ingredients

- 3 tablespoons mayonnaise
- 12 slices white bread
- 6 ounces fully cooked ham, thinly sliced
- 6 slices process Swiss cheese
- 6 ounces cooked turkey, thinly sliced
- 2 tablespoons Dijon mustard
- 3 large eggs, beaten
- 3/4 cup whole milk
- 2 tablespoons confectioners' sugar, optional
- 1/4 teaspoon salt, optional
- 2 cups crushed crisp rice cereal
- 1/2 cup sour cream
- 1/4 cup strawberry jam

Direction

- Spread 6 bread slices with mayonnaise. Place the ham, the cheese and the turkey on top of each. Spread the remaining bread with mustard; put over the turkey. Combine confectioners' sugar, milk, eggs and if desired, salt in a shallow dish. Dip every sandwich into the egg mixture, followed by crushed cereal.
- Put on an oiled 15x10x1 inches baking pan. Bake for 7 minutes at 425°. Flip then bake until golden brown, or for about 5 to 7 minutes longer. Mix jam and sour cream. Enjoy as dip with the hot sandwiches.

Nutrition Information

- Calories:
- Protein:
- Total Fat:
- Sodium:
- Fiber:
- Total Carbohydrate:
- Cholesterol:

415. Moist & Tender Turkey Breast

Serving: 12 servings. | Prep: 10mins | Cook: 04hours00mins | Ready in:

Ingredients

- 1 bone-in turkey breast (6 to 7 pounds)
- 4 fresh rosemary sprigs
- 4 garlic cloves, peeled
- 1/2 cup water
- 1 tablespoon brown sugar
- 1/2 teaspoon coarsely ground pepper
- 1/4 teaspoon salt

Direction

- In a 6-quart slow cooker, put water, garlic, rosemary, and turkey breast. Stir salt, pepper, and brown sugar; dust on the turkey. Put a cover and cook on low until the turkey becomes tender and a thermometer registers no less than 170 degrees when inserted into the turkey, for 4-6 hours.

Nutrition Information

- Calories: 318 calories
- Fiber: 0 fiber)
- Total Carbohydrate: 2g carbohydrate (1g sugars
- Cholesterol: 122mg cholesterol
- Protein: 47g protein.
- Total Fat: 12g fat (3g saturated fat)
- Sodium: 154mg sodium

416. Moist Italian Turkey Breast

Serving: 12 servings. | Prep: 25mins | Cook: 05hours00mins | Ready in:

Ingredients

- 1 pound carrots, cut into 2-inch pieces
- 2 medium onions, cut into wedges
- 3 celery ribs, cut into 2-inch pieces
- 1 can (14-1/2 ounces) chicken broth
- 1 bone-in turkey breast (6 to 7 pounds), thawed and skin removed
- 2 tablespoons olive oil
- 1-1/2 teaspoons seasoned salt
- 1 teaspoon Italian seasoning
- 1/2 teaspoon pepper

Direction

- In a 6- to 7-quart slow cooker, put the broth and vegetables; place turkey breast on top. Brush oil over the turkey; dust with the seasonings.
- Put a cover and cook for 5-6 hours on low until a thermometer registers at least 170 degrees when inserted into the turkey. Take the turkey out of the slow cooker; before carving, put a cover and allow to stand for 15 minutes. Serve along with vegetables. Filter and thicken cooking juices for the graving if desired.

Nutrition Information

- Calories: 360 calories
- Sodium: 477mg sodium
- Fiber: 2g fiber)
- Total Carbohydrate: 6g carbohydrate (3g sugars
- Cholesterol: 123mg cholesterol
- Protein: 48g protein.
- Total Fat: 15g fat (4g saturated fat)

417. Moist Turkey Breast

Serving: 12-14 servings. | Prep: 10mins | Cook: 02hours00mins | Ready in:

Ingredients

- 1 bone-in turkey breast (about 7 pounds)
- 1 teaspoon garlic powder
- 1/2 teaspoon onion powder
- 1/2 teaspoon salt
- 1/4 teaspoon pepper
- 1-1/2 cups Italian dressing

Direction

- In a 13x9-inch, greased baking dish, arrange the turkey breast. Mix the seasonings; dust on the turkey. Top with the dressing.
- Put a cover and bake at 325 degrees, basting with the pan drippings from time to time, until a thermometer registers 170 degrees, for 2-2 1/2 hours. Before cutting, allow to stand for 10 minutes.

Nutrition Information

- Calories: 406 calories
- Sodium: 621mg sodium
- Fiber: 0 fiber)
- Total Carbohydrate: 2g carbohydrate (1g sugars
- Cholesterol: 122mg cholesterol
- Protein: 47g protein.
- Total Fat: 22g fat (5g saturated fat)

418. Mushroom Meat Loaf

Serving: 6 servings. | Prep: 30mins | Cook: 03hours15mins | Ready in:

Ingredients

- 2 eggs, lightly beaten
- 1-1/3 cups soft bread crumbs
- 1/2 pound large portobello mushrooms, stems removed, finely chopped
- 1 small onion, finely chopped
- 2 garlic cloves, minced
- 3/4 teaspoon salt
- 1/2 teaspoon dried thyme
- 1/4 teaspoon pepper
- 1 pound lean ground turkey
- 1/4 cup chili sauce
- 2 teaspoons stone-ground mustard
- 1/8 teaspoon cayenne pepper

Direction

- Cut three 20x3-inch strips of heavy-duty foil; crisscross for them to resemble spokes of a wheel. Put strips on the bottom and up the sides of a 3-quart slow cooker. Grease the strips.
- Mix pepper, thyme, salt, garlic, onion, mushrooms, breadcrumbs, and eggs in a big bowl. Crumble turkey over the mixture and combine well. Form into a 7-1/2x4-inch loaf. Cook immediately or freeze with a cover for up to 3 months.
- Put meat loaf in the center of the strips. Cook with a cover until no longer pink and a thermometer reads 160 degrees, 3 to 4 hours on low. Mix cayenne, mustard, and chili sauce; drizzle over meat. Cook with a cover until heated through, 15 minutes more. Using foil strips as handles, transfer the meat loaf to a platter.
- To use frozen meat loaf: Defrost in the fridge overnight. Cook as instructed.

Nutrition Information

- Calories: 194 calories
- Sodium: 648mg sodium
- Fiber: 1g fiber)
- Total Carbohydrate: 12g carbohydrate (4g sugars
- Cholesterol: 130mg cholesterol
- Protein: 17g protein. Diabetic Exchanges: 2 lean meat
- Total Fat: 8g fat (2g saturated fat)

419. Mushroom Turkey Tetrazzini

Serving: 8 servings. | Prep: 35mins | Cook: 25mins | Ready in:

Ingredients

- 12 ounces uncooked multigrain spaghetti, broken into 2-inch pieces

- 2 teaspoons chicken bouillon granules
- 2 tablespoons butter
- 1/2 pound sliced fresh mushrooms
- 2 tablespoons all-purpose flour
- 1/4 cup sherry or additional pasta water
- 3/4 teaspoon salt-free lemon-pepper seasoning
- 1/2 teaspoon salt
- 1/8 teaspoon ground nutmeg
- 1 cup fat-free evaporated milk
- 2/3 cup grated Parmesan cheese, divided
- 4 cups cubed cooked turkey breast
- 1/4 teaspoon paprika, optional

Direction

- Set the oven at 375° to preheat. Cook spaghetti following the package directions until al dente. Drain, reserve 2-1/2 cups pasta water; then transfer the spaghetti to a 13x9-in. baking dish greased with cooking spray. Next, dissolve the bouillon in the retained pasta water. Over medium-high heat, heat butter in a large nonstick skillet; sauté mushrooms until softened. After that, stir in flour until well blended. Stir in the seasonings, reserved pasta water, and sherry gradually. Boil; cook and stir until thickened, for about 2 minutes.
- Reduce the heat to low; stir in 1/3 cup cheese and milk until blended. Put in the turkey, stirring constantly, heat through. Pour over the spaghetti and toss to combine. Dust with the leftover cheese and, paprika if desired.
- Cover and bake until bubbly, for 25-30 minutes.

Nutrition Information

- Calories: 357 calories
- Cholesterol: 71mg cholesterol
- Protein: 34g protein. Diabetic Exchanges: 3 starch
- Total Fat: 7g fat (3g saturated fat)
- Sodium: 717mg sodium
- Fiber: 3g fiber)
- Total Carbohydrate: 38g carbohydrate (5g sugars

420. Mushroom Onion Stuffed Turkey

Serving: 14 servings (9 cups stuffing). | Prep: 60mins | Cook: 03hours30mins | Ready in:

Ingredients

- 1 loaf (14 ounces) ciabatta bread, cubed
- 1-1/2 pounds sliced baby portobello mushrooms
- 4 small onions, finely chopped
- 2 celery ribs with leaves, finely chopped
- 6 tablespoons butter
- 4 garlic cloves, minced
- 1 cup white wine or reduced-sodium chicken broth
- 1 cup reduced-sodium chicken broth
- 1/4 cup minced fresh parsley
- 1 tablespoon minced fresh thyme or 1 teaspoon dried thyme
- 1/2 teaspoon salt
- 1/2 teaspoon pepper
- 1 cup heavy whipping cream
- 3/4 cup egg substitute
- 1 turkey (14 to 16 pounds)
- Melted butter

Direction

- Arrange bread on a baking sheet; bake at 250°, until lightly toasted, for 25 to 30 minutes.
- In a large skillet, sauté celery, onions, and mushrooms in melted butter until softened. Put in garlic; cook for an extra 1 minute. Pour in wine; heat to a boil. Lower the heat; simmer, without covering, until liquid evaporates. Combine in pepper, salt, thyme, parsley, and broth; heat thoroughly.
- In a large bowl, mix mushroom mixture and toasted bread. In a small bowl, beat egg

- substitute and cream; transfer over bread mixture and stir to coat.
- Before baking, loosely fill the turkey with 4 cups of stuffing. Arrange the remaining stuffing on an oiled 8-inch baking dish; let cool in the refrigerator until ready to bake. Skewer turkey openings; bind drumsticks together. Arrange the breast side up on a rack in a roasting pan. Coat with melted butter.
- Bake, without covering, at 325° for 3 1/2 to 4 hours, until a thermometer shows 180° when inserted the turkey and 165° when inserted in the stuffing, basting sometimes with pan drippings. Use foil to cover loosely if turkey turns brown too fast.
- Cover and bake additional stuffing in 20 minutes. Take out the cover; bake for an additional 20 minutes, until lightly browned. Cover turkey and allow to stand for 20 minutes before removing the stuffing and slicing turkey. If wanted, thicken pan drippings for the gravy.

Nutrition Information

- Calories: 758 calories
- Sodium: 510mg sodium
- Fiber: 2g fiber)
- Total Carbohydrate: 23g carbohydrate (3g sugars
- Cholesterol: 281mg cholesterol
- Protein: 78g protein.
- Total Fat: 37g fat (14g saturated fat)

421. Nutty Turkey Slices

Serving: 3-6 servings. | Prep: 20mins | Cook: 0mins | Ready in:

Ingredients

- 3/4 cup ground walnuts
- 1/4 cup grated Parmesan cheese
- 1/2 teaspoon Italian seasoning
- 1/2 teaspoon paprika
- 1 package (17.6 ounces) turkey breast cutlets
- 3 tablespoons butter
- 1 teaspoon cornstarch
- 1/2 cup chicken broth
- 2 teaspoons lemon juice

Direction

- Mix paprika, Italian seasoning, cheese, and walnuts in a large resealable plastic bag. Put in a few pieces of turkey at a time and shake the bag to coat.
- Working in batches, brown the turkey in butter in a large skillet over medium heat until it is not pink anymore, 3-4 minutes per side; then take the turkey out and keep it warm.
- Mix lemon juice, broth, and cornstarch until the mixture becomes smooth; then gradually place into the skillet. Remove the browned bits by stirring and boil; stir and cook until thick, about a minute. Serve alongside turkey.

Nutrition Information

- Calories: 232 calories
- Sodium: 241mg sodium
- Fiber: 1g fiber)
- Total Carbohydrate: 2g carbohydrate (1g sugars
- Cholesterol: 72mg cholesterol
- Protein: 25g protein.
- Total Fat: 14g fat (5g saturated fat)

422. Orange Barbecued Turkey

Serving: about 4 servings. | Prep: 10mins | Cook: 10mins | Ready in:

Ingredients

- 1/2 cup orange juice
- 1 teaspoon grated orange zest

- 1 tablespoon vegetable oil
- 2 teaspoons Worcestershire sauce
- 1 teaspoon ground mustard
- 1/2 teaspoon ground pepper
- 1/8 teaspoon garlic powder or 1 garlic clove, minced
- 4 turkey breast steaks (about 1-1/4 pounds)

Direction

- Mix the first 7 ingredients in a large resealable plastic bag; put in turkey. Seal closed and turn the bag to coat; put in the fridge, turning from time to time, overnight or for at least 4 hours.
- Drain the marinade and discard. Broil or grill the steaks until juices from the steak run clear, 3-5 minutes per side. Don't overcook.

Nutrition Information

- Calories:
- Cholesterol:
- Protein:
- Total Fat:
- Sodium:
- Fiber:
- Total Carbohydrate:

423. Orange Roasted Turkey

Serving: 16 servings. | Prep: 20mins | Cook: 03hours15mins | Ready in:

Ingredients

- 1 turkey (14 to 16 pounds)
- 1 tablespoon canola oil
- 1/2 teaspoon salt
- 1/4 teaspoon pepper
- Orange and onion wedges, optional
- GLAZE:
- 1/2 cup orange juice
- 1/2 cup orange marmalade
- 1/4 cup butter, cubed
- 2 teaspoons grated orange zest
- 2 teaspoons minced fresh thyme or 1/2 teaspoon dried thyme
- Fresh parsley sprigs, optional

Direction

- Set the oven at 325° and start preheating. Arrange turkey, breast side up, on a rack in a shallow roasting pan. Tuck the wings under the turkey; tie drumsticks together. Rub the turkey with oil; sprinkle pepper and salt over all. Put onion and orange wedges into the roasting pan if desired.
- Roast without a cover for 2 3/4 hours. Meanwhile, to prepare glaze, boil the mixture of butter, marmalade and orange juice in a small saucepan. Lower the heat; simmer while stirring occasionally without a cover till slightly thickened, 15-20 minutes. Mix in thyme and orange zest.
- Brush the turkey with some of the prepared glaze. Roast while basting occasionally with the remaining glaze, until a thermometer reads 170-175° when inserted into the thickest part of the thigh, 15-30 minutes. (Use foil to loosely cover if the turkey turns brown too quickly.) Take the turkey away from the oven; tent with foil. Allow to sit for 20 minutes before carving. Skim fat and thicken the pan drippings for gravy if desired. Serve with the turkey and parsley, onion and orange wedges if you like.

Nutrition Information

- Calories: 516 calories
- Sodium: 251mg sodium
- Fiber: 0 fiber)
- Total Carbohydrate: 8g carbohydrate (7g sugars
- Cholesterol: 222mg cholesterol
- Protein: 63g protein.
- Total Fat: 24g fat (8g saturated fat)

424. Orange Turkey Croissants

Serving: 6 servings. | Prep: 10mins | Cook: 0mins | Ready in:

Ingredients

- 6 tablespoons spreadable cream cheese
- 6 tablespoons orange marmalade
- 6 croissants, split
- 1/2 cup chopped pecans
- 1 pound thinly sliced deli turkey

Direction

- Smear marmalade and cream cheese onto the bottom half of croissants. Scatter with pecans. Place turkey atop pecans. Place top half over turkey to finish.

Nutrition Information

- Calories: 479 calories
- Cholesterol: 80mg cholesterol
- Protein: 21g protein.
- Total Fat: 25g fat (11g saturated fat)
- Sodium: 1165mg sodium
- Fiber: 3g fiber)
- Total Carbohydrate: 43g carbohydrate (19g sugars

425. Orange Turkey Stir Fry

Serving: 4 servings. | Prep: 30mins | Cook: 0mins | Ready in:

Ingredients

- 3/4 cup orange juice
- 1/4 cup orange marmalade
- 2 tablespoons soy sauce
- 2 tablespoons cornstarch
- 1/8 teaspoon ground ginger
- 1/8 teaspoon hot pepper sauce
- 1/4 cup all-purpose flour
- 1 pound turkey cutlets, cut into 1-inch strips
- 2 tablespoons vegetable oil, divided
- 4 green onions, cut into 1-inch pieces
- 1/2 cup coarsely chopped green pepper
- 1 seedless orange, peeled, sliced and halved
- Cooked rice

Direction

- Mix initial 6 ingredients in a small bowl; put aside. Put flour on waxed paper sheet. Coat turkey strips; shake excess off. Heat 1 tbsp. oil in 10-in. skillet on medium high heat. In 3 batches, cook turkey till all sides are lightly browned and strips are tender. Remove turkey; keep warm. Put leftover oil in skillet; mix and cook green pepper and green onions for 1 minute. Mix in orange juice mixture; boil. Lower heat; simmer for 3 minutes. Add orange slices and turkey; heat through. Serve on rice.

Nutrition Information

- Calories: 324 calories
- Protein: 29g protein.
- Total Fat: 9g fat (1g saturated fat)
- Sodium: 536mg sodium
- Fiber: 2g fiber)
- Total Carbohydrate: 34g carbohydrate (21g sugars
- Cholesterol: 56mg cholesterol

426. Orange Glazed Turkey

Serving: 18-20 servings. | Prep: 35mins | Cook: 04hours15mins | Ready in:

Ingredients

- 2 teaspoons salt
- 2 teaspoons pepper
- 2 teaspoons dried savory
- 2 teaspoons rubbed sage

- 1 turkey (18 to 20 pounds)
- 2 medium pears, thinly sliced
- 1 large onion, quartered
- 1 celery rib, quartered
- 1/2 cup butter, melted
- 3/4 cup orange marmalade
- 3/4 cup orange juice
- 1 tablespoon honey

Direction

- In a small bowl, blend sage, savory, pepper, and salt. Coat 1 tablespoon of the seasoning mixture on the turkey cavity. Put celery, onion, and pears in turkey cavity; bind drumsticks together. Arrange the breast side up on a rack in a roasting pan. Mix the seasoning mixture left and butter; coat over the turkey. Bake, without covering, at 325° for 3 1/4 to 3 1/2 hours.
- While baking, blend honey, orange juice, and orange marmalade in a saucepan. Heat to a boil. Lower the heat; simmer, without covering, in 15 minutes, or until thickened, stirring on occasion. Put aside and keep warm. When turkey turns brown, use a tent of foil to cover lightly. Bake for an additional 1 hour, or until thermometer shows 180°, covering on occasion with the orange glaze. Cover and allow to stand in 15 minutes before carving. For gravy, thicken the pan juices if wanted.

Nutrition Information

- Calories: 567 calories
- Fiber: 1g fiber)
- Total Carbohydrate: 13g carbohydrate (12g sugars
- Cholesterol: 233mg cholesterol
- Protein: 65g protein.
- Total Fat: 27g fat (9g saturated fat)
- Sodium: 447mg sodium

427. Peanutty Asian Lettuce Wraps

Serving: 6 servings. | Prep: 15mins | Cook: 15mins | Ready in:

Ingredients

- 1/3 cup reduced-sodium teriyaki sauce
- 1/4 cup hoisin sauce
- 3 tablespoons creamy peanut butter
- 1 tablespoon rice vinegar
- 1 tablespoon sesame oil
- 1-1/2 pounds lean ground turkey
- 1/2 cup shredded carrot
- 2 tablespoons minced fresh gingerroot
- 4 garlic cloves, minced
- 1 can (8 ounces) whole water chestnuts, drained and chopped
- 1/2 cup chopped fresh snow peas
- 4 green onions, chopped
- 12 Bibb lettuce leaves
- Additional hoisin sauce, optional

Direction

- Combine the first 5 ingredients until no lumps remain. Sauté carrot and turkey over medium high heat in a large skillet for 6 to 8 minutes until meat is no longer pink, crumbling turkey while cooking; drain well. Stir in garlic and ginger, sauté for another minute. Mix in green onions, snow peas, water chestnuts, and sauce mixture; cook until thoroughly heated.
- Spoon mixture into lettuce leaves to serve. Drizzle with more hoisin sauce, if desired.

Nutrition Information

- Calories: 313 calories
- Total Fat: 16g fat (4g saturated fat)
- Sodium: 613mg sodium
- Fiber: 3g fiber)
- Total Carbohydrate: 18g carbohydrate (9g sugars
- Cholesterol: 90mg cholesterol

- Protein: 24g protein. Diabetic Exchanges: 3 lean meat

428. Pepper Lover's BLT

Serving: 4 servings. | Prep: 15mins | Cook: 0mins | Ready in:

Ingredients

- 1/4 cup mayonnaise
- 1 tablespoon diced pimientos
- 1/8 teaspoon coarsely ground pepper
- 1/4 teaspoon hot pepper sauce
- 8 slices sourdough bread, toasted
- 4 teaspoons Dijon-mayonnaise blend
- 6 tablespoons shredded sharp cheddar cheese
- 4 pickled jalapeno peppers or green chilies, thinly sliced
- 12 bacon strips, cooked and drained
- 8 tomato slices
- 4 lettuce leaves
- 8 thin slices cooked turkey

Direction

- Mix together pepper sauce, pepper, pimientos and mayonnaise in a small bowl, then refrigerate for a minimum of an hour.
- Spread Dijon-mayonnaise blend on 4 toast slices, then use cheese to sprinkle over. Put turkey, lettuce, tomato, bacon and jalapenos on top. Spread on leftover toast with mayonnaise mixture and put over turkey.

Nutrition Information

- Calories: 485 calories
- Fiber: 3g fiber)
- Total Carbohydrate: 39g carbohydrate (3g sugars
- Cholesterol: 51mg cholesterol
- Protein: 23g protein.
- Total Fat: 26g fat (7g saturated fat)

- Sodium: 1469mg sodium

429. Pepperoni Pizza Casserole

Serving: 8 | Prep: 15mins | Cook: 45mins | Ready in:

Ingredients

- 1 pound ground beef
- 1 (8 ounce) package uncooked egg noodles
- 1 (16 ounce) jar spaghetti sauce, or as needed
- 1 (2.25 ounce) can sliced black olives, drained
- 1 (2.5 ounce) can sliced mushrooms, drained
- 1 (8 ounce) package sliced pepperoni, coarsely chopped
- 20 ounces shredded mozzarella cheese, divided

Direction

- Set oven temperature to 375* F or 190* C.
- In a frying pan, place ground beef and cook on medium heat until not pink. While the beef is cooking, break it into small pieces like crumbles. Should be done in 10 minutes.
- Place water and a little salt in a large saucepan and bring to a boil. Add the egg noodles and cook for 5 minutes. The noodles should be a little firm but cooked through. Drain the water from the noodles.
- In a large bowl, mix together noodles, pepperoni, spaghetti sauce, mushrooms, half the mozzarella cheese, and black olives. Transfer noodle mixture to a 9x13-inch pan and place rest of cheese on top. Use foil to cover.
- Place pan in heated oven for 30-45 minutes or until the mixture is bubbly.

Nutrition Information

- Calories: 586 calories;
- Protein: 38.2

- Total Fat: 33.9
- Sodium: 1276
- Total Carbohydrate: 30.6
- Cholesterol: 134

430. Posse Stew

Serving: 16 | Prep: 15mins | Cook: 45mins | Ready in:

Ingredients

- 1 pound ground beef
- 1 (20 ounce) can white or yellow hominy, rinsed and drained
- 2 (14.5 ounce) cans stewed tomatoes
- 1 (15.25 ounce) can whole kernel corn
- 1 (15 ounce) can kidney beans
- 2 (15 ounce) cans ranch-style beans
- 1 large yellow onion, chopped
- 2 green chile peppers, chopped

Direction

- In a large frying pan, cook ground beef over medium-high heat while stirring often to crumble, until evenly browned. Drain to remove grease, and shift to a soup pot. Pour in the ranch-style beans, kidney beans, corn, stewed tomatoes, hominy, then add green chilies and onion. Cook over medium heat while covered for 1 hour.

Nutrition Information

- Calories: 183 calories;
- Sodium: 594
- Total Carbohydrate: 26.3
- Cholesterol: 17
- Protein: 10.9
- Total Fat: 4.1

431. Pronto Pita Pizzas

Serving: 4 servings. | Prep: 10mins | Cook: 15mins | Ready in:

Ingredients

- 1 pound ground turkey breast
- 1 cup sliced fresh mushrooms
- 1/2 cup chopped onion
- 2 garlic cloves, minced
- 1 can (8 ounces) no-salt-added tomato sauce
- 1/2 teaspoon fennel seed
- 1/4 teaspoon dried oregano
- 4 pita breads, warmed
- 1/2 cup shredded part-skim mozzarella cheese

Direction

- Brown the turkey in a skillet; drain. Add garlic, onion, and mushrooms; cook until softened. Mix in oregano, fennel seed, and tomato sauce. Simmer for 10 to 15 minutes, covered, or until heated through.
- Put 1 cup meat mixture on each pita and spread; dust with cheese. Serve right away.

Nutrition Information

- Calories: 358 calories
- Fiber: 0 fiber)
- Total Carbohydrate: 41g carbohydrate (0 sugars
- Cholesterol: 63mg cholesterol
- Protein: 38g protein. Diabetic Exchanges: 4 lean meat
- Total Fat: 5g fat (0 saturated fat)
- Sodium: 187mg sodium

432. Quick And Easy Stromboli

Serving: 8 servings. | Prep: 10mins | Cook: 20mins | Ready in:

Ingredients

- 1 tube (13.80 ounces) refrigerated pizza crust
- 1/2 pound thinly sliced deli turkey
- 1/2 pound thinly sliced Muenster cheese
- 1/4 cup pickled pepper rings
- 2 teaspoons yellow mustard
- 2 teaspoons minced fresh herbs or 1/2 teaspoon dried herbs
- 1 large egg, beaten
- 1 tablespoon water

Direction

- Set oven to 350 degrees and start preheating. Spread out the pizza dough over the bottom of an oiled 15x10x1-inch baking pan. Arrange layers of deli meats, cheese, and your favorite vegetables over the dough (suggested layers: a layer of sliced turkey breast, a layer of Muenster cheese and a layer of pickled peppers). Spread yellow mustard over layers, then sprinkle with dried herbs (or fresh herbs).
- Roll dough again and brush oil over it. Bake for 20-25 minutes till crust is slightly browned. Cut into slices; serve.

Nutrition Information

- Calories: 271 calories
- Total Fat: 11g fat (6g saturated fat)
- Sodium: 965mg sodium
- Fiber: 1g fiber)
- Total Carbohydrate: 25g carbohydrate (3g sugars
- Cholesterol: 42mg cholesterol
- Protein: 19g protein.

---

433. Raspberry Turkey Tenderloins

Serving: 6 servings. | Prep: 20mins | Cook: 15mins | Ready in:

Ingredients

- 1/2 cup seedless raspberry jam
- 1/3 cup cider vinegar
- 1/4 cup Dijon mustard
- 1 teaspoon grated orange zest
- 1/2 teaspoon minced fresh thyme or 1/8 teaspoon dried thyme
- 4 turkey breast tenderloins (6 ounces each)
- 1/8 teaspoon salt

Direction

- Combine first 5 ingredients in small saucepan. Cook while stirring until heated through, about 2 to 3 minutes. Put aside a quarter cup for serving.
- Sprinkle salt over turkey. Use cooking oil to moisten paper towel. Coat grill rack lightly with long-handled tongs. Cover and grill turkey over medium heat or broil 4 inches from heat source, turning occasionally, until thermometer registers 170°, about 13 to 18 minutes. During the last 5 minutes of the cooking, baste with the remaining sauce.
- Allow to stand 5 minutes. Then slice. Enjoy with the reserved sauce.

Nutrition Information

- Calories: 199 calories
- Protein: 26g protein. Diabetic Exchanges: 3 lean meat
- Total Fat: 2g fat (0 saturated fat)
- Sodium: 351mg sodium
- Fiber: 0 fiber)
- Total Carbohydrate: 20g carbohydrate (16g sugars
- Cholesterol: 56mg cholesterol

434. Red Beans And Rice With Turkey Sausage

Serving: 10 servings. | Prep: 15mins | Cook: 15mins | Ready in:

Ingredients

- 3 celery ribs, chopped
- 1 medium onion, chopped
- 6 green onions, thinly sliced
- 2 garlic cloves, minced
- 1-3/4 cups water
- 1 can (16 ounces) light red kidney beans, rinsed and drained
- 1 can (16 ounces) dark red kidney beans, rinsed and drained
- 1/2 teaspoon dried oregano
- 1/2 teaspoon dried thyme
- 1/4 teaspoon crushed red pepper flakes
- 1/4 teaspoon pepper
- 1/4 pound fully cooked smoked turkey sausage, halved and cut into 1/2-inch pieces
- 4 cups hot cooked rice

Direction

- Using a cooking spray, coat a large skillet; sauté in garlic, onions and celery till tender. Include in pepper, red pepper flakes, thyme, oregano, beans and water. Allow the mixture to boil; lower the heat. Simmer while stirring occasionally without a cover for 10 minutes.
- Take out about 1 1/2 cups of bean mixture; use a fork to mash. Turn back to the skillet. Include in sausage; bring to boil. Keep boiling until the bean mixture is thickened to your preference, or for about 5 minutes. Serve over rice.

Nutrition Information

- Calories: 197 calories
- Fiber: 0 fiber)
- Total Carbohydrate: 35g carbohydrate (0 sugars
- Cholesterol: 7mg cholesterol
- Protein: 9g protein. Diabetic Exchanges: 2 starch
- Total Fat: 2g fat (0 saturated fat)
- Sodium: 116mg sodium

435. Roasted Citrus & Herb Turkey

Serving: 16 servings (2 cups gravy). | Prep: 30mins | Cook: 03hours30mins | Ready in:

Ingredients

- 1/4 cup butter, softened
- 2 tablespoons Italian seasoning
- 1 turkey (14 to 16 pounds)
- 2 teaspoons salt
- 2 teaspoons pepper
- 1 large onion, quartered
- 1 medium orange, quartered
- 1 medium lemon, quartered
- 3 fresh rosemary sprigs
- 3 fresh sage sprigs
- 3 cups chicken broth, divided
- 3 to 4 tablespoons all-purpose flour
- 1/8 teaspoon browning sauce, optional

Direction

- Set an oven to 325 degrees and start preheating. Combine Italian seasoning and butter.
- In a roasting pan, arrange the turkey on a rack with its breast side up; pat it dry. Gently remove the skin from the turkey breast using your fingers; rub under the skin with half of the butter. Use toothpicks to secure the skin to the underside of the breast. Rub with pepper and salt in the hole/cavity; stuff with herbs, lemon, orange, and onion. Tuck the wings under turkey and tie together the drumsticks.
- Let the remaining butter mixture melt; brush the outside of turkey. Pour in 2 cups of broth into the roasting pan.

- Roast, without cover, basting with pan drippings from time to time, for 3 1/2-4 hours until a thermometer inserted in the thickest part of the thigh registers 170-175 degrees (If the turkey browns too fast, use foil to loosely cover). Take the turkey out from the oven; use foil to tent it. Before carving, allow to stand for 20 minutes.
- Add the pan drippings into a small saucepan; remove the fat from the surface. Combine the remaining broth and flour and brown the sauce, if desired, until it becomes smooth; whisk into the pan. Boil; stir and cook for 1-2 minutes until thick. Serve along with the turkey.

Nutrition Information

- Calories: 500 calories
- Protein: 64g protein.
- Total Fat: 24g fat (8g saturated fat)
- Sodium: 653mg sodium
- Fiber: 0 fiber)
- Total Carbohydrate: 2g carbohydrate (0 sugars
- Cholesterol: 223mg cholesterol

436. Roasted Turkey Breast Tenderloins & Vegetables

Serving: 4 servings plus 16 ounces cooked turkey breast tenderloins. | Prep: 15mins | Cook: 35mins | Ready in:

Ingredients

- 1 teaspoon dill weed
- 1 teaspoon dried thyme
- 1 teaspoon dried oregano
- 1 teaspoon dried minced onion
- 3/4 teaspoon salt
- 1/4 teaspoon pepper
- 1/4 cup butter, melted
- 3 cups fresh baby carrots
- 4 celery ribs, cut into 2-inch pieces
- 2 medium onions, cut into wedges
- 1 tablespoon olive oil
- 8 turkey breast tenderloins (5 ounces each)
- 2 teaspoons cornstarch
- 1/4 cup water

Direction

- Start preheating the oven at 425°. In a small bowl, blend the first 6 ingredients. Mix 2 teaspoons of the seasoning mixture with butter; stir with vegetables. Place into a roasting pan. Bake, without covering, for 15 minutes.
- In the meantime, coat oil over turkey; scatter with the seasoning mixture left. Transfer vegetables to edges of pan; arrange the turkey in the center. Bake, without covering, about 20 to 25 minutes, until a thermometer shows 165° when inserted in turkey and vegetables are softened.
- Reserve 1/2 turkey for Buffalo Turkey with Linguine or save for next use. Transfer vegetables and the remaining turkey to a serving platter and save warm.
- Stream cooking juices into a small saucepan. Blend water and cornstarch until glossy; slowly mix into pan. Heat to a boil; cook and stir about 2 minutes, until thickened. Use with turkey and vegetables.

Nutrition Information

- Calories: 363 calories
- Protein: 35g protein.
- Total Fat: 17g fat (8g saturated fat)
- Sodium: 718mg sodium
- Fiber: 4g fiber)
- Total Carbohydrate: 19g carbohydrate (10g sugars
- Cholesterol: 100mg cholesterol

437. Roasted Turkey With Cornbread Dressing

Serving: 8-10 servings (10 cups dressing). | Prep: 01hours10mins | Cook: 04hours30mins | Ready in:

Ingredients

- CORNBREAD:
- 3 cups cornmeal
- 1 cup self-rising flour
- 4-1/2 teaspoons baking powder
- 1-1/2 teaspoons salt
- 1-1/4 cups chopped celery
- 1/3 cup chopped onion
- 1/2 teaspoon celery seed
- 2 cups milk
- 1/4 cup canola oil
- 1 large egg
- DRESSING:
- 1/2 cup chopped fresh parsley
- 1 to 2 tablespoons poultry seasoning
- 3/4 teaspoon pepper
- 3/4 cup egg substitute
- 1 cup butter, melted, divided
- 1 turkey (10 to 12 pounds)

Direction

- Mix the first 7 ingredients in a large bowl. Mix egg, oil and milk in a small bowl; pour over the cornmeal mixture and combine well. Pour the mixture to a greased 13x9-in. baking pan.
- Bake at 350° until the inserted toothpick in the center comes out clean or for 50 minutes. Allow to cool on a wire rack.
- Break cornbread to crumbles into a large bowl. Add pepper, poultry seasoning and parsley and toss. Mix 3/4 cup of butter and egg substitute; add them to the cornbread mixture; stir just until they are blended.
- Stuff the dressing in the turkey just before baking. Fasten or skewer openings. Tie together drumsticks. Put on a rack in a roasting pan. Brush the remaining butter over the turkey. Transfer the remaining dressing in a greased baking dish; refrigerate, covered, until ready to bake.
- Bake the turkey at 325° until thermometer reads 165° when thermometer inserted in the center of stuffing and the thigh reaches at least 170° or for 3-1/2 to 4-1/2 hours. When turkey starts turning brown, use a tent of aluminum foil to cover lightly.
- Bake extra dressing for 1 hour at 325°. When turkey is done, allow to stand for 20 minutes, then carve. Transfer all dressing to a serving bowl.

Nutrition Information

- Calories: 983 calories
- Total Fat: 51g fat (20g saturated fat)
- Sodium: 1120mg sodium
- Fiber: 4g fiber)
- Total Carbohydrate: 45g carbohydrate (3g sugars
- Cholesterol: 322mg cholesterol
- Protein: 81g protein.

438. Roasted Wild Turkey

Serving: 10-12 servings. | Prep: 10mins | Cook: 03hours30mins | Ready in:

Ingredients

- 1 wild turkey (10 to 15 pounds)
- 2 large apples, quartered
- 6 to 8 medium red potatoes, quartered
- 2 pound baby carrots
- 2 medium onions, sliced
- 2 cups water
- 1-1/2 teaspoons seasoned salt
- 1 teaspoon salt
- 1 teaspoon pepper
- 1/2 cup maple syrup
- 1/4 cup French salad dressing
- 1/4 cup barbecue sauce
- 2 tablespoons ketchup

- 2 tablespoons steak sauce
- 1 tablespoon lemon juice

Direction

- Prepare the turkey by stuffing it with apples, and position it on top of a rack in a roasting pan. Place vegetables such as onions, carrots and potatoes all around the turkey then add some water on the vegetables. For tasting, mix together pepper, salt, and seasoned salt and rub all over the turkey. Pour all over the turkey with the mixture of the remaining ingredients.
- Bake in the oven while covering for 3 and 1/2 hours at 325 degrees, or until internal temperature reaches 180 degrees and baste as per ones' taste. Additional browning can be done by removing the cover of the turkey on the last 30 minutes of cooking time.

Nutrition Information

- Calories: 615 calories
- Sodium: 766mg sodium
- Fiber: 4g fiber)
- Total Carbohydrate: 37g carbohydrate (22g sugars
- Cholesterol: 204mg cholesterol
- Protein: 63g protein.
- Total Fat: 23g fat (6g saturated fat)

439. Romano Basil Turkey Breast

Serving: 8 servings. | Prep: 15mins | Cook: 01hours30mins | Ready in:

Ingredients

- 4 ounces Romano cheese, shredded
- 1/2 cup fresh basil leaves, chopped
- 4 lemon slices
- 4 garlic cloves, minced

- 1 bone-in turkey breast (4 to 5 pounds)
- 2 tablespoons olive oil
- 1/2 teaspoon salt
- 1/4 teaspoon pepper

Direction

- Mix garlic, cheese, lemon slices, and basil. Loosen the turkey breast skin carefully with fingers then put the mixture beneath the skin. Secure the skin to underside the breast using toothpicks. Rub oil on the skin then scatter with pepper and salt.
- Use a drip pan to set the grill for indirect heat. Put the turkey on top of the drip pan. On indirect medium heat, grill the chicken for 1 1/2-2hrs while covering or until a thermometer registers 170 degrees F. Discard the toothpicks then cover. Let it sit for 10 mins then cut.

Nutrition Information

- Calories: 402 calories
- Cholesterol: 136mg cholesterol
- Protein: 53g protein.
- Total Fat: 20g fat (7g saturated fat)
- Sodium: 493mg sodium
- Fiber: 0 fiber)
- Total Carbohydrate: 1g carbohydrate (0 sugars

440. Rosemary Turkey Breast

Serving: 15 servings. | Prep: 10mins | Cook: 01hours30mins | Ready in:

Ingredients

- 2 tablespoons olive oil
- 8 to 10 garlic cloves, peeled
- 3 tablespoons chopped fresh rosemary or 3 teaspoons dried rosemary, crushed
- 1 teaspoon salt
- 1 teaspoon paprika

- 1/2 teaspoon coarsely ground pepper
- 1 bone-in turkey breast (5 pounds)

Direction

- Mix pepper, paprika, salt, rosemary, garlic, and oil in a food processor; put a cover and pulse until the garlic is chopped coarsely.
- Loose the skin from both sides of the turkey breast carefully using fingers. Spread on the meat under the skin with 1/2 of garlic mixture. Smooth the skin on the meat and use toothpicks to secure to the underside of the breast. Spread on the turkey skin with the rest of the garlic mixture.
- On a rack set in a shallow roasting pan, arrange the turkey breast. Bake with no cover at 325 degrees until a thermometer registers 170 degrees, for 1 1/2-2 hours. Before cutting, allow to stand for 15 minutes. Remove the toothpicks.

Nutrition Information

- Calories: 148 calories
- Protein: 29g protein. Diabetic Exchanges: 4 lean meat.
- Total Fat: 3g fat (0 saturated fat)
- Sodium: 207mg sodium
- Fiber: 0 fiber)
- Total Carbohydrate: 1g carbohydrate (0 sugars
- Cholesterol: 78mg cholesterol

441. Sausage & Rice Stew

Serving: 6 servings. | Prep: 20mins | Cook: 30mins | Ready in:

Ingredients

- 1 package (14 ounces) smoked turkey kielbasa, halved lengthwise and sliced
- 1 large sweet onion, chopped
- 2 shallots, chopped
- 1 tablespoon chopped pickled jalapeno slices
- 3 garlic cloves, minced
- 1 tablespoon canola oil
- 2 cups water
- 1 can (14-1/2 ounces) reduced-sodium chicken broth
- 2 cans (15 ounces each) white kidney or cannellini beans, rinsed and drained
- 1 cup uncooked long grain rice
- 1 teaspoon dried oregano
- 1 teaspoon dried thyme
- 1/2 teaspoon pepper
- 2 cups fresh baby spinach

Direction

- Stir-fry the onion, kielbasa, garlic, jalapeno and shallots in oil in a Dutch oven. Once the onion is tender, add water, beans, broth, seasonings and rice then boil.
- Lower the heat and let it simmer for 15 to 20 minutes with the cover on. Once the rice is tender, put it the spinach and cook for another 5 minutes or until the spinach gets wilted.

Nutrition Information

- Calories: 369 calories
- Total Carbohydrate: 52g carbohydrate (3g sugars
- Cholesterol: 47mg cholesterol
- Protein: 22g protein.
- Total Fat: 7g fat (2g saturated fat)
- Sodium: 1162mg sodium
- Fiber: 7g fiber)

442. Sausage And Pumpkin Pasta

Serving: 4 servings. | Prep: 20mins | Cook: 15mins | Ready in:

Ingredients

- 2 cups uncooked multigrain bow tie pasta

- 1/2 pound Italian turkey sausage links, casings removed
- 1/2 pound sliced fresh mushrooms
- 1 medium onion, chopped
- 4 garlic cloves, minced
- 1 cup reduced-sodium chicken broth
- 1 cup canned pumpkin
- 1/2 cup white wine or additional reduced-sodium chicken broth
- 1/2 teaspoon rubbed sage
- 1/4 teaspoon salt
- 1/4 teaspoon garlic powder
- 1/4 teaspoon pepper
- 1/4 cup grated Parmesan cheese
- 1 tablespoon dried parsley flakes

Direction

- Following the package instructions, cook the pasta.
- At the same time, cook onion, mushrooms, and sausage in a greased large non-stick skillet over medium heat until the meat is not pink anymore. Put in garlic and cook for 1 more minute. Stir in pepper, garlic powder, salt, sage, wine, pumpkin, and broth. Boil. Turn down the heat; without the cover, simmer until thick slightly, 5-6 minutes.
- Then drain the pasta; then place into the skillet and heat through. Dust with parsley and cheese just before serving.

Nutrition Information

- Calories: 348 calories
- Total Carbohydrate: 42g carbohydrate (7g sugars
- Cholesterol: 38mg cholesterol
- Protein: 23g protein. Diabetic Exchanges: 2-1/2 starch
- Total Fat: 9g fat (2g saturated fat)
- Sodium: 733mg sodium
- Fiber: 7g fiber)

443. Sesame Turkey Stir Fry

Serving: 4 servings. | Prep: 15mins | Cook: 10mins | Ready in:

Ingredients

- 1 teaspoon cornstarch
- 1/2 cup water
- 2 tablespoons reduced-sodium soy sauce
- 1 tablespoon honey
- 2 teaspoons curry powder
- 1/8 teaspoon crushed red pepper flakes
- 2 teaspoons sesame or canola oil
- 1 medium sweet red pepper, julienned
- 1 small onion, cut into thin wedges
- 1 garlic clove, minced
- 2 cups shredded cooked turkey breast
- 1 green onion, sliced
- 2 cups hot cooked brown rice
- Thinly sliced serrano pepper and toasted sesame seeds, optional

Direction

- Combine the first 6 ingredients in a small bowl until blended. Put oil onto the large skillet and heat it over medium-high heat. Add the onion and red pepper. Stir-fry the mixture until crisp-tender. Add the garlic and cook the mixture for 1 minute.
- Whisk the cornstarch mixture, and then pour it into the pan. Let the mixture boil. Cook for 2 minutes, stirring until the sauce is thick. Add the turkey and heat the mixture through. Mix in green onion. Serve the mixture together with the rice and top it with sesame seeds and serrano pepper if desired.

Nutrition Information

- Calories: 269 calories
- Sodium: 349mg sodium
- Fiber: 3g fiber)
- Total Carbohydrate: 32g carbohydrate (7g sugars
- Cholesterol: 60mg cholesterol

- Protein: 25g protein. Diabetic Exchanges: 3 lean meat
- Total Fat: 4g fat (1g saturated fat)

444. Skillet Tacos

Serving: 2 servings. | Prep: 15mins | Cook: 15mins | Ready in:

Ingredients

- 1/4 pound lean ground turkey
- 2 tablespoons chopped onion
- 2 tablespoons chopped green pepper
- 1 can (8 ounces) tomato sauce
- 1/2 cup uncooked elbow macaroni
- 1/2 cup water
- 1/4 cup picante sauce
- 2 tablespoons shredded fat-free cheddar cheese
- 1/4 cup crushed baked tortilla chip scoops
- 1/4 cup chopped avocado
- Iceberg lettuce wedges and fat-free sour cream, optional

Direction

- Coat a large non-stick skillet with cooking spray and cook the green pepper, onion, and turkey on medium heat until the turkey isn't pink.
- Mix in the macaroni, picante sauce, water, and tomato sauce and bring it up to a boil. Bring the heat down and cover it to simmer for 10-15 minutes or until the macaroni gets tender.
- Split it to two plates and sprinkle it with cheese, avocado, and tortilla chips. Eat it with sour cream and lettuce if you want.

Nutrition Information

- Calories: 267 calories
- Protein: 18g protein. Diabetic Exchanges: 2 lean meat
- Total Fat: 9g fat (2g saturated fat)
- Sodium: 795mg sodium
- Fiber: 3g fiber)
- Total Carbohydrate: 30g carbohydrate (5g sugars
- Cholesterol: 46mg cholesterol

445. Slow Cooker Turkey Breast

Serving: 12 | Prep: 10mins | Cook: 8hours | Ready in:

Ingredients

- 1 (6 pound) bone-in turkey breast
- 1 (1 ounce) envelope dry onion soup mix

Direction

- Wash breast of turkey and pat it dry. Remove any extra skin; however retain the skin covering the breast. Massage onion soup mix on the entire outside of turkey and beneath the skin. Put in slow cooker. Put cover on, and cook for an hour on High, then turn to Low, and let cook for 7 hours.

Nutrition Information

- Calories: 273 calories;
- Total Fat: 1.5
- Sodium: 309
- Total Carbohydrate: 1.5
- Cholesterol: 164
- Protein: 59.5

446. Slow Cooker Turkey Pesto Lasagna

Serving: 8 servings. | Prep: 25mins | Cook: 03hours00mins | Ready in:

Ingredients

- 1 pound ground turkey
- 1 small onion, chopped
- 2 teaspoons Italian seasoning
- 1/2 teaspoon salt
- 2 cups shredded part-skim mozzarella cheese, divided
- 1 container (15 ounces) whole-milk ricotta cheese
- 1/4 cup prepared pesto
- 1 jar (24 ounces) marinara sauce
- 9 no-cook lasagna noodles
- Grated Parmesan cheese

Direction

- Cut heavy-duty foil in three 25x3-inch strips then arrange in crisscross so that all three strips intersect in the middle. In a greased 5-quart slow cooker, put the crisscrossing strips at the bottom of the slow cooker extending up on the sides. Use cooking spray to grease the strips.
- Put onion and turkey in a large frying pan then cook for 6 to 8 minutes over medium heat or until turkey is not pink and crumble turkey as it cooks, drain excess oil. Put in salt and Italian seasoning.
- Combine ricotta cheese, pesto and 1 cup of mozzarella cheese in a small bowl. In the slow cooker with greased crisscross aluminum strips, put a layer of 1/3 of marinara sauce, 1/3 of lasagna noodles (cut noodles to fit in the slow cooker if needed), 1/3 of turkey mixture, and 1/3 of cheese mixture. Do the whole layering process 2 times more. Top with the remaining mozzarella cheese.
- Cover the slow cooker and cook for 3 to 4 hours on low heat setting or until noodles are soft. Switch off the slow cooker and remove the inner pot. Remove the lid and allow it to cool down for about 30 minutes. To remove and transfer the lasagna to the serving plate, use the foil strips. Top off with a sprinkle of Parmesan cheese then serve.

Nutrition Information

- Calories: 397 calories
- Sodium: 883mg sodium
- Fiber: 3g fiber)
- Total Carbohydrate: 28g carbohydrate (9g sugars
- Cholesterol: 79mg cholesterol
- Protein: 28g protein.
- Total Fat: 19g fat (8g saturated fat)

447. Slow Cooker Turkey Stuffed Peppers

Serving: 6 servings. | Prep: 35mins | Cook: 04hours00mins | Ready in:

Ingredients

- 2 medium sweet yellow or orange peppers
- 2 medium sweet red peppers
- 2 medium green peppers
- 1 pound lean ground turkey
- 1 small red onion, finely chopped
- 1 small zucchini, shredded
- 2 cups cooked brown rice
- 1 jar (16 ounces) spaghetti sauce, divided
- 1 tablespoon Creole seasoning
- 1/4 teaspoon pepper
- 2 tablespoons shredded Parmesan cheese

Direction

- Cut the tops from peppers and discard seeds. Chop enough tops finely to measure 1 cup for the filling.
- Over medium heat, cook the reserved chopped peppers, onion, and turkey in a large skillet until the turkey is not pink anymore and the greens are soft for 6-8 minutes while crumbling the turkey; drain.
- Add zucchini and stir; cook and stir for 2 minutes more. Put in pepper, Creole seasoning, 2/3 cup spaghetti sauce, and rice.

- Drizzle the bottom of a greased 6-qt. slow cooker with half cup spaghetti sauce. Fill the peppers with the turkey mixture and put over the sauce. Then, drizzle the peppers with the remaining spaghetti sauce; dust with cheese.
- Cover and cook on low for 4-5 hours or until the filling is heated through and the peppers are soft.

Nutrition Information

- Calories: 290 calories
- Cholesterol: 63mg cholesterol
- Protein: 19g protein. Diabetic Exchanges: 3 lean meat
- Total Fat: 10g fat (3g saturated fat)
- Sodium: 818mg sodium
- Fiber: 5g fiber)
- Total Carbohydrate: 31g carbohydrate (9g sugars

448. Slow Cooked Turkey With Berry Compote

Serving: 12 servings (3-1/4 cups compote). | Prep: 35mins | Cook: 03hours00mins | Ready in:

Ingredients

- 1 teaspoon salt
- 1/2 teaspoon garlic powder
- 1/2 teaspoon dried thyme
- 1/2 teaspoon pepper
- 2 boneless turkey breast halves (2 pounds each)
- 1/3 cup water
- COMPOTE:
- 2 medium apples, peeled and finely chopped
- 2 cups fresh raspberries
- 2 cups fresh blueberries
- 1 cup white grape juice
- 1/4 teaspoon crushed red pepper flakes
- 1/4 teaspoon ground ginger

Direction

- Combine the pepper, thyme, garlic powder, and salt, then rub the turkey breasts with the spices mixture. Add to a 5- or 6-quart slow cooker. Add water around the turkey. Cook while covering for 3-4 hours on low until the thermometer you insert into the turkey reaches a minimum of 165°.
- Take the turkey away from the slow cooker and make a tent with foil to cover. Let it sit for 10 minutes before cutting.
- At the same time, mix the compote ingredients in a big saucepan. Bring the mixture to a boil. Lower the heat to medium. Cook without covering for 15-20 minutes until the apples are softened and a bit thickened, whisking occasionally. Serve the compote with the turkey.

Nutrition Information

- Calories: 215 calories
- Sodium: 272mg sodium
- Fiber: 2g fiber)
- Total Carbohydrate: 12g carbohydrate (8g sugars
- Cholesterol: 94mg cholesterol
- Protein: 38g protein. Diabetic Exchanges: 5 lean meat
- Total Fat: 1g fat (0 saturated fat)

449. Slow Cooked Turkey With Herbed Stuffing

Serving: 8 servings. | Prep: 20mins | Cook: 03hours00mins | Ready in:

Ingredients

- 2 boneless skinless turkey breast halves (1 pound each) or 2 pounds turkey breast tenderloins
- 1 jar (12 ounces) turkey gravy, divided

- 1 can (10-1/2 ounces) reduced-fat reduced-sodium condensed cream of mushroom soup, undiluted
- 1/2 teaspoon salt
- 1/2 teaspoon poultry seasoning
- 1/4 teaspoon pepper
- 1 medium Granny Smith apple, finely chopped
- 2 celery ribs, thinly sliced
- 1 small onion, finely chopped
- 1 cup sliced fresh mushrooms, optional
- 6 cups seasoned stuffing cubes

Direction

- Arrange the turkey in a 5 or 6-quart slow cooker. Combine seasonings, condensed soup, and 1/4 cup of gravy. Cover and put in the refrigerator the remaining gravy. Blend mushrooms (if wanted), onion, celery, and apple into the gravy mixture. Mix in stuffing cubes; ladle over the turkey. Cover and cook on low until a thermometer shows 170° and meat is softened, about 3 to 4 hours.
- Take the turkey out from slow cooker; tent with foil. Allow to stand in 10 minutes before cutting. Warm the remaining gravy. Use with stuffing and turkey.

Nutrition Information

- Calories: 324 calories
- Total Carbohydrate: 38g carbohydrate (5g sugars
- Cholesterol: 70mg cholesterol
- Protein: 32g protein.
- Total Fat: 4g fat (1g saturated fat)
- Sodium: 1172mg sodium
- Fiber: 3g fiber)

450. Southern Barbecue Spaghetti Sauce

Serving: 12 servings. | Prep: 20mins | Cook: 04hours00mins | Ready in:

Ingredients

- 1 pound lean ground turkey
- 2 medium onions, chopped
- 1-1/2 cups sliced fresh mushrooms
- 1 medium green pepper, chopped
- 2 garlic cloves, minced
- 1 can (14-1/2 ounces) diced tomatoes, undrained
- 1 can (12 ounces) tomato paste
- 1 can (8 ounces) tomato sauce
- 1 cup ketchup
- 1/2 cup beef broth
- 2 tablespoons Worcestershire sauce
- 2 tablespoons brown sugar
- 1 tablespoon ground cumin
- 2 teaspoons chili powder
- 12 cups hot cooked spaghetti

Direction

- Cook the green pepper, mushrooms, onions, and the turkey in a big nonstick skillet over medium heat until the meat is not pink anymore. Put in garlic and cook for 1 more minute, then drain.
- Move to a 3-quart slow cooker. Whisk in chili powder, cumin, brown sugar, Worcestershire sauce, broth, ketchup, tomato sauce, tomato paste and the tomatoes. Cook while covering for 4-5 hours on low until the vegetables become soft. Serve with spaghetti.

Nutrition Information

- Calories: 342 calories
- Sodium: 491mg sodium
- Fiber: 5g fiber)
- Total Carbohydrate: 60g carbohydrate (0 sugars
- Cholesterol: 30mg cholesterol

- Protein: 17g protein.
- Total Fat: 4g fat (1g saturated fat)

451. Spaghetti With Homemade Turkey Sausage

Serving: 6 servings. | Prep: 10mins | Cook: 10mins | Ready in:

Ingredients

- 1 pound ground turkey
- 1 teaspoon fennel seed, crushed
- 1 teaspoon water
- 1/2 teaspoon salt
- 1/2 teaspoon pepper
- 1 jar (24 ounces) spaghetti sauce
- 12 ounces spaghetti, cooked and drained

Direction

- In a big bowl mix pepper, salt, water, fennel seed and the turkey together then cover it. Keep it in the fridge overnight. In a big skillet on medium heat, break the mixture up to bite-sized pieces and cook until it's not pink. Add spaghetti sauce, stirring until thoroughly heated. Serve over hot spaghetti.

Nutrition Information

- Calories: 467 calories
- Protein: 22g protein.
- Total Fat: 17g fat (5g saturated fat)
- Sodium: 917mg sodium
- Fiber: 4g fiber)
- Total Carbohydrate: 56g carbohydrate (10g sugars
- Cholesterol: 54mg cholesterol

452. Spatchcocked Herb Roasted Turkey

Serving: 16 servings. | Prep: 15mins | Cook: 01hours15mins | Ready in:

Ingredients

- 1 turkey (12 to 14 pounds)
- 3 tablespoons kosher salt
- 2 teaspoons coarsely ground pepper
- 1 tablespoon minced fresh rosemary
- 1 tablespoon minced fresh thyme
- 1 tablespoon minced fresh sage

Direction

- On a work surface, arrange the turkey with the tail end facing you and breast side down. Slice along each side of the backbone with kitchen shears; remove it and reserve for gravy. Flip the turkey over so that the breast side faces up. Firmly press the breastbone down to flatten until it cracks. Use a knife to slice through the joints to remove the wing tips; reserve for making the gravy.
- Combine the rest of the ingredients; rub the turkey on all sides. Place the turkey onto a rack set in a foil-lined rimmed baking pan. Store in the fridge overnight with no cover.
- Set an oven to 450 degrees and start preheating. While heating the oven, take the turkey out of the fridge. Roast for 1 1/4-1 1/2 hours until a thermometer registers 170-175 degrees when inserted into the thickest part of the thigh. Take the turkey out of the oven; before carving, allow to stand for 15 minutes.

Nutrition Information

- Calories: 399 calories
- Protein: 54g protein.
- Total Fat: 18g fat (5g saturated fat)
- Sodium: 1210mg sodium
- Fiber: 0 fiber)
- Total Carbohydrate: 0 carbohydrate (0 sugars
- Cholesterol: 184mg cholesterol

453. Special Roast Turkey

Serving: 8 servings. | Prep: 30mins | Cook: 04hours00mins | Ready in:

Ingredients

- 1 turkey (12 to 14 pounds)
- 2 cups water
- 2-1/2 cups chicken broth, divided
- 1-1/2 cups orange juice, divided
- 4 tablespoons soy sauce, divided
- 1 tablespoon chicken bouillon granules
- 1 teaspoon dried minced onion
- 1/2 teaspoon garlic powder
- ORANGE GIBLET GRAVY:
- 3/4 cup chicken broth
- 1/4 cup orange juice
- 2 teaspoons Worcestershire sauce
- 1/2 teaspoon dried thyme
- 1/2 teaspoon sugar
- 1/4 teaspoon pepper
- 3 tablespoons cornstarch
- 1/2 cup water

Direction

- On a greased rack set in a roasting pan, arrange the turkey. Add neck, giblets, and water into the pan. Mix 2 tablespoons of soy sauce. 3/4 cup of orange juice, and 1 1/4 cups of broth; add on the turkey. Mix the garlic powder, onion, and bouillon; scatter on the turkey. Bake with no cover at 325 degrees, basting every half an hour, for 3 1/2 hours. Cover the turkey loosely in foil once it starts to brown. Remove the neck and giblets once they are tender; put aside for gravy. Mix soy sauce, orange juice, and the remaining broth. Take the foil off turkey; pour on the turkey with the broth mixture. Bake until a thermometer registers 180 degrees, for half an hour more.
- Take the meat from the neck for gravy and discard bones. Chop the neck meat and giblets; then put aside. Mix the Worcestershire sauce, orange juice, broth, and 2 cups of pan juices in a saucepan; then stir thoroughly. Stir in pepper, sugar, and thyme. Mix water and cornstarch until smooth. Beat into the broth mixture; then boil. Stir and cook for 2 minutes. Stir in the saved neck meat and giblets. Carve the turkey; then serve along with the gravy.

Nutrition Information

- Calories: 846 calories
- Sodium: 1426mg sodium
- Fiber: 0 fiber)
- Total Carbohydrate: 10g carbohydrate (6g sugars
- Cholesterol: 368mg cholesterol
- Protein: 110g protein.
- Total Fat: 37g fat (11g saturated fat)

454. Spicy Chili Mac

Serving: 6 servings. | Prep: 10mins | Cook: 20mins | Ready in:

Ingredients

- 2 cups uncooked whole wheat elbow macaroni
- 1 pound lean ground turkey
- 1 small onion, chopped
- 2 to 3 jalapeno peppers, seeded and chopped
- 2 teaspoons olive oil
- 2 garlic cloves, minced
- 1 can (15 ounces) black beans, rinsed and drained
- 1 can (14-1/2 ounces) diced tomatoes, undrained
- 1 can (8 ounces) tomato sauce
- 1 to 2 tablespoons hot pepper sauce
- 2 to 3 teaspoons chili powder
- 1 teaspoon ground cumin
- 1/4 teaspoon cayenne pepper
- 1/4 teaspoon pepper
- 3/4 cup shredded reduced-fat cheddar cheese

Direction

- Cook macaroni based on the package directions. In the meantime, use cooking spray to coat a large nonstick skillet, then put oil and cook in the jalapenos, onion and turkey on medium heat until meat is not pink. Mix in garlic; cook for a minute longer. Strain.
- Stir in the seasonings, pepper sauce, tomato sauce, tomatoes and beans. Strain macaroni; add into turkey mixture. Then cook for 5 minutes over medium-low heat or until heated through.
- Dust with cheese. Separate from heat; then cover and allow to stand until cheese is dissolved.

Nutrition Information

- Calories: 396 calories
- Total Carbohydrate: 45g carbohydrate (5g sugars
- Cholesterol: 70mg cholesterol
- Protein: 28g protein. Diabetic Exchanges: 3 lean meat
- Total Fat: 12g fat (4g saturated fat)
- Sodium: 581mg sodium
- Fiber: 9g fiber)

455. Spicy Skillet Supper

Serving: 5 servings. | Prep: 15mins | Cook: 20mins | Ready in:

Ingredients

- 1 pound lean ground turkey
- 1 can (16 ounces) chili beans, undrained
- 1-1/2 cups cooked brown rice
- 1 cup salsa
- 1 tablespoon vinegar
- 2 to 3 teaspoons chili powder
- 1 teaspoon sugar
- 1 teaspoon ground cumin
- 1/4 teaspoon garlic powder
- 1/4 teaspoon pepper
- 1/4 cup shredded reduced-fat cheddar cheese, optional

Direction

- Over medium heat, brown turkey in a skillet coated with cooking spray; drain if needed. Add seasonings, vinegar, salsa, rice and chili beans; combine well. Bring to a boil. Lower the heat; simmer with a cover for 20 minutes. Top with cheese if preferred.

Nutrition Information

- Calories: 248 calories
- Protein: 28g protein. Diabetic Exchanges: 3 lean meat
- Total Fat: 3g fat (0 saturated fat)
- Sodium: 944mg sodium
- Fiber: 0 fiber)
- Total Carbohydrate: 32g carbohydrate (0 sugars
- Cholesterol: 45mg cholesterol

456. Spinach Turkey Meatballs

Serving: 4 servings. | Prep: 10mins | Cook: 20mins | Ready in:

Ingredients

- 1 package (10 ounces) frozen chopped spinach, thawed and squeezed dry
- 1 egg, beaten
- 1 cup soft bread crumbs
- 2 tablespoons grated onion
- 1 teaspoon seasoned salt
- 1 pound ground turkey
- Tomato wedges, optional

Direction

- Combine seasoned salt, onion, bread crumbs, egg, and spinach in a bowl. Add turkey, combine well. Form into 2-inch balls. Arrange meatballs on an oiled rack set in a shallow baking pan. Bake at 400 degrees without cover until meat is not pink anymore, about 20 minutes. Place on paper towels, drain. Put tomato wedge to garnish if wanted.

Nutrition Information

- Calories: 295 calories
- Fiber: 2g fiber)
- Total Carbohydrate: 10g carbohydrate (1g sugars
- Cholesterol: 130mg cholesterol
- Protein: 23g protein.
- Total Fat: 19g fat (6g saturated fat)
- Sodium: 626mg sodium

457. Spinach And Turkey Pinwheels

Serving: 8 servings. | Prep: 15mins | Cook: 0mins | Ready in:

Ingredients

- 8 flour tortillas (8 inches)
- 1 carton (8 ounces) spreadable garden vegetable cream cheese
- 4 cups fresh baby spinach
- 1 pound sliced deli turkey

Direction

- Spread over tortillas with cream cheese. Layer with spinach and turkey. Tightly roll-up. Use plastic wrap to wrap and chill until serving.
- Then unwrap, cut the rolls crosswise into 1-in. slices.

Nutrition Information

- Calories: 307 calories
- Fiber: 2g fiber)
- Total Carbohydrate: 31g carbohydrate (1g sugars
- Cholesterol: 52mg cholesterol
- Protein: 17g protein.
- Total Fat: 13g fat (6g saturated fat)
- Sodium: 866mg sodium

458. Stuffing Crust Turkey Potpie

Serving: 6 servings. | Prep: 35mins | Cook: 25mins | Ready in:

Ingredients

- 2 cups cooked corn bread stuffing
- 3 to 4 tablespoons chicken broth
- 1/4 cup cream cheese, softened
- 1/2 cup turkey gravy
- 2 cups cubed cooked turkey
- 1 cup frozen broccoli florets, thawed
- 1/2 cup shredded Swiss cheese
- 1/4 teaspoon salt
- 1/4 teaspoon pepper
- 2 cups mashed potatoes
- 1/4 cup half-and-half cream
- 2 tablespoons butter, melted
- French-fried onions, optional

Direction

- Start preheating the oven to 350°. Combine enough broth and stuffing in a small bowl until it reaches the preferred moistness. Then press up sides and onto bottom of an oiled 9 inches deep-dish pie plate. Bake for 10 to 15 mins or until browned lightly.
- Beat gravy and cream cheese in a large bowl until they become smooth. Stir in pepper, salt, Swiss cheese, broccoli and turkey. Add over the crust.
- Combine cream and potatoes in small bowl; spread over the turkey mixture. Then drizzle

butter over. Sprinkle onions over, if desired. Bake for 20 to 25 mins or until browned lightly and heated through.

Nutrition Information

- Calories: 389 calories
- Protein: 22g protein.
- Total Fat: 20g fat (9g saturated fat)
- Sodium: 910mg sodium
- Fiber: 2g fiber)
- Total Carbohydrate: 30g carbohydrate (2g sugars
- Cholesterol: 73mg cholesterol

459. Super Italian Sub

Serving: 10-12 servings. | Prep: 30mins | Cook: 0mins | Ready in:

Ingredients

- 1 loaf (1 pound) unsliced Italian bread
- 1/3 cup olive oil
- 1/4 cup cider vinegar
- 8 garlic cloves, minced
- 1 teaspoon dried oregano
- 1/4 teaspoon pepper
- 1/2 pound fully cooked ham, thinly sliced
- 1/2 pound thinly sliced cooked turkey
- 1/4 pound thinly sliced hard salami
- 1/4 pound sliced provolone cheese
- 1/4 pound sliced mozzarella cheese
- 1 medium green pepper, thinly sliced into rings

Direction

- Halve bread lengthways, then hollow out bottom and top to leave a shell of 1/2 inch. Get rid of removed bread or reserve for another use.
- Mix together pepper, oregano, garlic, vinegar and oil in a small bowl, then brush mixture on cut sides of both bread top and bottom. Layer 1/2 of meats, cheeses and green pepper on the bottom half, then repeat layers as same order. Replace top of bread and use plastic wrap to wrap bread tightly, then chill for a maximum of 24 hours.

Nutrition Information

- Calories: 309 calories
- Total Fat: 16g fat (6g saturated fat)
- Sodium: 701mg sodium
- Fiber: 1g fiber)
- Total Carbohydrate: 22g carbohydrate (1g sugars
- Cholesterol: 44mg cholesterol
- Protein: 19g protein.

460. Super Supper Hero

Serving: 6 servings. | Prep: 20mins | Cook: 10mins | Ready in:

Ingredients

- 1/4 cup olive oil
- 2-1/2 cups cubed eggplant
- 1 each medium green, sweet yellow and red peppers, julienned
- 1 large red onion, thinly sliced
- 1 medium tomato, chopped
- 1 teaspoon dried oregano
- 1/2 teaspoon salt
- 1/4 teaspoon pepper
- 1 loaf (1 pound) unsliced Italian bread
- Lettuce leaves
- 1/2 pound sliced fully cooked ham
- 1/2 pound sliced cooked turkey breast
- 1/4 pound sliced hard salami
- 8 slices part-skim mozzarella cheese

Direction

- Heat oil in a big skillet over moderately high heat. Put in onion, peppers and eggplant, then cook and stir until vegetables are tender yet still crispy, about 4 to 6 minutes. Put in pepper, salt, oregano and tomato, then take away from the heat.
- Halve bread lengthways, then hollow out bottom of loaf to leave a shell of 3/4 inch. Reserve removed bread for another use. Layer lettuce, ham, turkey, salami, and cheese on bottom, then put vegetables on top and replace top. Use toothpicks to secure and cut bread crosswise into 6 slices.

Nutrition Information

- Calories: 606 calories
- Sodium: 1650mg sodium
- Fiber: 5g fiber)
- Total Carbohydrate: 49g carbohydrate (8g sugars
- Cholesterol: 96mg cholesterol
- Protein: 42g protein.
- Total Fat: 27g fat (8g saturated fat)

461. Sweet And Sour Turkey Meat Loaf

Serving: 2 servings. | Prep: 15mins | Cook: 45mins | Ready in:

Ingredients

- 1/4 cup tomato sauce
- 1 tablespoon brown sugar
- 1 tablespoon cider vinegar
- 1/4 teaspoon prepared mustard
- 1 tablespoon beaten egg or egg substitute
- 2 tablespoons finely chopped onion
- 1 tablespoon crushed butter-flavored crackers
- 1 tablespoon minced fresh parsley
- 1/4 teaspoon salt
- Dash pepper
- 1/2 pound lean ground turkey

Direction

- Stir mustard, vinegar, brown sugar and tomato sauce together in a small bowl and put to the side. Mix 2 tablespoons of reserved tomato mixture, pepper, salt, parsley, crackers, onion and egg in a separate bowl. Sprinkle crumbled turkey on top and blend well. Form the mixture into a 4x3" oval.
- Grease an 8" square baking dish with cooking spray and transfer the loaf onto the dish; place the leftover tomato mixture on top. Bake without a cover for 45-50 minutes at 350 degrees or until no pink meat remains and a thermometer registers 165 degrees. Let sit for 10 minutes, then slice.

Nutrition Information

- Calories: 235 calories
- Protein: 22g protein. Diabetic Exchanges: 3 lean meat
- Total Fat: 11g fat (3g saturated fat)
- Sodium: 587mg sodium
- Fiber: 1g fiber)
- Total Carbohydrate: 11g carbohydrate (8g sugars
- Cholesterol: 122mg cholesterol

462. Taco Skillet Supper

Serving: 8 servings. | Prep: 10mins | Cook: 60mins | Ready in:

Ingredients

- 4 cups thinly sliced peeled potatoes
- 1 small onion, chopped, divided
- 1 teaspoon reduced-sodium chicken bouillon granules
- 1 cup hot water
- 1 pound lean ground turkey
- 1 envelope reduced-sodium taco seasoning
- 1/4 cup fat-free milk

- 1-1/4 cups salsa, divided
- 1/2 cup quick-cooking oats
- 1/4 cup egg substitute

Direction

- Use cooking spray to coat a 2-qt. baking dish; add a tablespoon onion and potatoes. Dissolve bouillon in water; place half cup over potatoes. Mix the rest of onion, egg substitute, oats, 1/4 cup salsa, milk and taco seasoning in a large bowl; break turkey into crumble over mixture; combine well.
- Place on top of potatoes and spread. Mix chicken broth with the rest of salsa; place over turkey mixture. Bake without a cover for an hour at 350° or until meat is no longer pink and the thermometer registers 165°.

Nutrition Information

- Calories: 206 calories
- Fiber: 3g fiber)
- Total Carbohydrate: 25g carbohydrate (5g sugars
- Cholesterol: 45mg cholesterol
- Protein: 13g protein. Diabetic Exchanges: 2 lean meat
- Total Fat: 5g fat (1g saturated fat)
- Sodium: 531mg sodium

463. Tasty Turkey Sub

Serving: 6 servings. | Prep: 20mins | Cook: 0mins | Ready in:

Ingredients

- 1 loaf (1 pound) French bread
- 1/3 cup blue cheese salad dressing
- 1/3 cup mayonnaise
- 2 tablespoons Dijon mustard
- 1 pound smoked or cooked turkey, thinly sliced
- 12 bacon strips, cooked and drained
- 1 avocado, thinly sliced
- 6 tomato slices (1/4 inch thick)
- Shredded lettuce

Direction

- Cut bread lengthwise in half. Spread on cut side of top of bread with blue cheese dressing. Mix mustard and mayonnaise together, then spread on cut side of bottom of bread. Put in layer of turkey, bacon, avocado, tomato and lettuce, then use top half of bread to cover. Serve instantly.

Nutrition Information

- Calories: 580 calories
- Fiber: 4g fiber)
- Total Carbohydrate: 44g carbohydrate (3g sugars
- Cholesterol: 45mg cholesterol
- Protein: 28g protein.
- Total Fat: 32g fat (6g saturated fat)
- Sodium: 1576mg sodium

464. Tasty Turkey And Mushrooms

Serving: 2 servings. | Prep: 5mins | Cook: 10mins | Ready in:

Ingredients

- 1 garlic clove, minced
- 1 tablespoon butter
- 1/2 pound boneless skinless turkey breast, cut into 2-inch strips
- 3/4 cup reduced-sodium beef broth
- 1 tablespoon tomato paste
- 2 cups sliced fresh mushrooms
- 1/8 teaspoon salt

Direction

- Sauté garlic in butter in a large nonstick skillet until tender. Mix in turkey; cook until turkey juices run clear. Take out of the pan; set aside to keep warm. Add salt, mushrooms, tomato paste, and broth to the skillet; cook until mushrooms are tender, stirring sometimes, for 3 to 5 minutes. Put turkey back into the pan; cook until thoroughly heated.

Nutrition Information

- Calories: 209 calories
- Sodium: 435mg sodium
- Fiber: 1g fiber)
- Total Carbohydrate: 5g carbohydrate (3g sugars
- Cholesterol: 88mg cholesterol
- Protein: 31g protein. Diabetic Exchanges: 3 lean meat
- Total Fat: 7g fat (4g saturated fat)

465. Terrific Turkey Enchiladas

Serving: 3 servings. | Prep: 35mins | Cook: 35mins | Ready in:

Ingredients

- 1-1/4 cups frozen corn, thawed
- 1 can (4 ounces) chopped green chilies
- 1 cup fresh cilantro leaves
- 1/3 cup heavy whipping cream
- 1/4 teaspoon salt
- 1/4 teaspoon pepper
- ENCHILADAS:
- 3/4 pound ground turkey
- 1/3 cup chopped onion
- 1 garlic clove, minced
- 1 tablespoon olive oil
- 3/4 cup salsa
- 1 tablespoon cornmeal
- 2 teaspoons chili powder
- 1-1/2 teaspoons ground cumin
- 1 teaspoon dried oregano
- 1/8 teaspoon salt
- 1/8 teaspoon pepper
- 6 flour tortillas (8 inches), warmed
- 1-1/4 cups shredded Mexican cheese blend, divided
- 1/4 cup sliced ripe olives

Direction

- Turn oven to 350° to preheat. Put the first 6 ingredients into a processor; cover and process until incorporated.
- In a large skillet over medium heat, cook garlic, onion, and turkey in oil until no pink remains. Turn off the heat; mix in seasonings, cornmeal, and salsa.
- In the center of each tortilla, place 1/3 cup turkey mixture; place 2 tablespoons cheese atop turkey on each serving. Roll up; arrange rolls in an oiled 11x7-inch baking dish, seam side down. Spread corn mixture over top; scatter with the rest of cheese and olives.
- Bake in the preheated oven, covered, for 30 minutes. Remove cover, bake until heated through, about 5 to 10 minutes.

Nutrition Information

- Calories: 968 calories
- Total Fat: 55g fat (23g saturated fat)
- Sodium: 1766mg sodium
- Fiber: 5g fiber)
- Total Carbohydrate: 81g carbohydrate (4g sugars
- Cholesterol: 155mg cholesterol
- Protein: 41g protein.

466. Thanksgiving Sandwiches

Serving: 6 servings. | Prep: 15mins | Cook: 0mins | Ready in:

Ingredients

- 2 cups cubed cooked turkey breast
- 1/2 cup mayonnaise
- 1/2 cup finely chopped fresh or frozen cranberries
- 1 orange, peeled and chopped
- 1 teaspoon sugar
- 1 teaspoon prepared mustard
- 1/2 teaspoon salt
- 1/4 cup chopped pecans
- Lettuce leaves
- 6 rolls or croissants, split

Direction

- Mix salt, mustard, sugar, orange, cranberries, mayonnaise, and turkey in a big-sized bowl. Just prior to serving, mix in pecans. Over each roll, add half cup of turkey mixture and lettuce.

Nutrition Information

- Calories: 458 calories
- Total Fat: 23g fat (5g saturated fat)
- Sodium: 679mg sodium
- Fiber: 3g fiber)
- Total Carbohydrate: 40g carbohydrate (9g sugars
- Cholesterol: 47mg cholesterol
- Protein: 22g protein.

467. Toasted Turkey Sandwiches

Serving: 6 servings. | Prep: 15mins | Cook: 10mins | Ready in:

Ingredients

- 6 thin slices cooked turkey
- 6 thin slices fully cooked ham
- 12 slices buttered French bread (1/2 inch thick)
- 2 large eggs, lightly beaten
- 1/2 cup 2% milk
- 2 tablespoons butter
- 1/2 cup mayonnaise
- 1/2 cup Miracle Whip
- 1/3 cup whole-berry cranberry sauce

Direction

- Arrange 1 slice of ham and 1 slice of turkey on 6 bread slices. Place the remaining bread on top. Whisk eggs and milk together in a shallow mixing bowl. Immerse sandwich into egg mixture, turning until evenly coated.
- Melt butter over medium heat in a large skillet. Sear sandwiches in melted butter until both sides are browned. Combine cranberry sauce and Miracle Whipped in a small mixing bowl. Serve the sauce with sandwiches.

Nutrition Information

- Calories: 300 calories
- Fiber: 1g fiber)
- Total Carbohydrate: 23g carbohydrate (6g sugars
- Cholesterol: 110mg cholesterol
- Protein: 14g protein.
- Total Fat: 17g fat (5g saturated fat)
- Sodium: 799mg sodium

468. Tropical Turkey Meat Loaf

Serving: 8 servings (2/3 cup sauce). | Prep: 10mins | Cook: 60mins | Ready in:

Ingredients

- 1/2 cup egg substitute
- 1 can (8 ounces) unsweetened crushed pineapple, undrained, divided

- 3 tablespoons reduced-sodium soy sauce
- 1 teaspoon sugar
- 3/4 teaspoon ground ginger
- 1/2 teaspoon ground mustard
- 1/4 teaspoon garlic powder
- 1 cup dry bread crumbs
- 1-1/2 pounds lean ground turkey
- 1 tablespoon finely chopped onion
- 1 green onion, finely chopped
- 2 teaspoons finely chopped jalapeno pepper
- 1 teaspoon honey
- 1 teaspoon lime juice
- Pinch pepper

Direction

- Mix together the seasonings, 1/3 cup of pineapple and egg substitute in a bowl. Put in breadcrumbs, then mix well. Add crumbled meat to the mixture then stir well. Push into an 8x4-in. loaf pan greased with cooking spray. Put 1 tablespoon of pineapple on top. Bake for 1 to 1-1/4 hours at 350°, until a thermometer shows 165°.
- Allow to sit for 5 minutes before serving. In the meantime, combine the rest of pineapple, pepper, lime juice, honey, jalapeno and onions in a small bowl. Well-served with the meat loaf.

Nutrition Information

- Calories: 174 calories
- Protein: 24g protein. Diabetic Exchanges: 3 lean meat
- Total Fat: 2g fat (0 saturated fat)
- Sodium: 387mg sodium
- Fiber: 0 fiber)
- Total Carbohydrate: 15g carbohydrate (0 sugars
- Cholesterol: 25mg cholesterol

469. Turkey & Cornbread Stuffing Rellenos

Serving: 6 servings. | Prep: 30mins | Cook: 5mins | Ready in:

Ingredients

- 6 large poblano peppers (about 1-1/2 pounds)
- 1-1/2 cups chopped cooked turkey
- 1-1/2 cups cooked cornbread stuffing
- 2 packages (8-1/2 ounces each) cornbread/muffin mix
- 1 carton (8 ounces) egg substitute
- Oil for deep-fat frying
- 1 can (14 ounces) whole-berry cranberry sauce
- 1 chipotle pepper in adobo sauce plus 1 tablespoon adobo sauce

Direction

- Arrange the peppers on a broiler pan. Broil 4 inches from the heat source for 5 minutes until the skins blister. Rotate the peppers 1/4 turn using tongs. Broil and rotate until all sides are blacken and blister. Transfer the peppers into a large bowl right away; put a cover and allow to stand for 10 minutes.
- Peel off the charred skin and discard. Slice and discard the tops of the peppers; then remove the seeds. Mix the stuffing and turkey in a small bowl. Place the turkey mixture into the peppers. In individual shallow bowls, put the egg substitute and corn muffin mix. Roll the filled peppers into the corn muffin mix first, then into the egg substitute, then back into the corn muffin mix.
- Heat 1/2 inch of oil in an electric skillet to 375 degrees. Fry several filled peppers at a time until brown, for 2-4 minutes per side. Transfer onto paper towels to drain.
- In a blender, place adobo sauce, pepper, and the cranberry sauce; put a cover and pulse for 10 seconds until combined. Serve along with peppers.

Nutrition Information

- Calories: 592 calories
- Fiber: 5g fiber)
- Total Carbohydrate: 60g carbohydrate (26g sugars
- Cholesterol: 36mg cholesterol
- Protein: 17g protein.
- Total Fat: 33g fat (4g saturated fat)
- Sodium: 632mg sodium

470. Turkey 'N' Beef Loaf

Serving: 8 servings. | Prep: 20mins | Cook: 40mins | Ready in:

Ingredients

- 1 large onion, chopped
- 3/4 cup chopped sweet red or green pepper
- 2 garlic cloves, minced
- 2 teaspoons vegetable oil
- 1 egg, lightly beaten
- 1/4 cup egg substitute
- 1 cup soft whole wheat bread crumbs (2 slices)
- 1/4 cup minced fresh parsley
- 1 tablespoon minced fresh marjoram or 1 teaspoon dried marjoram
- 1 tablespoon minced fresh thyme or 1 teaspoon dried thyme
- 1 teaspoon salt
- 1/4 teaspoon pepper
- 1 pound lean ground beef (90% lean)
- 1 pound lean ground turkey
- 1/4 cup ketchup
- Additional parsley, optional

Direction

- Sauté garlic, red pepper, and onion in oil in a nonstick skillet for 3 minutes. Pour into a bowl; allow to cool a bit. Add pepper, salt, thyme, marjoram, parsley, bread crumbs, egg substitute, and egg. Crumble turkey and beef over mixture and stir to combine.
- Form meat mixture into a 9x5-inch loaf; arrange the meatloaf in a 13x9-inch baking dish. Bake without covering for 40 minutes at 350°. Spoon ketchup over top.
- Bake until meatloaf's center is no longer pink and a thermometer registers 160°, for 35 to 40 minutes. Allow to rest for 15 minutes before cutting. Garnish with parsley if desired.

Nutrition Information

- Calories: 249 calories
- Total Fat: 12g fat (4g saturated fat)
- Sodium: 539mg sodium
- Fiber: 1g fiber)
- Total Carbohydrate: 9g carbohydrate (0 sugars
- Cholesterol: 92mg cholesterol
- Protein: 25g protein. Diabetic Exchanges: 3 lean meat

471. Turkey 'n' Stuffing Pie

Serving: 4-6 servings. | Prep: 30mins | Cook: 25mins | Ready in:

Ingredients

- 1 egg, lightly beaten
- 1 cup chicken broth
- 1/3 cup butter, melted
- 5 cups seasoned stuffing cubes
- FILLING:
- 1 can (4 ounces) mushroom stems and pieces, drained
- 1/2 cup chopped onion
- 1 tablespoon butter
- 1 tablespoon all-purpose flour
- 3 cups cubed cooked turkey
- 1 cup frozen peas
- 1 tablespoon minced fresh parsley
- 1 teaspoon Worcestershire sauce
- 1/2 teaspoon dried thyme
- 1 jar (12 ounces) turkey gravy
- 5 slices process American cheese, cut into strips

Direction

- Mix butter, broth, and egg in a large bowl. Add in the stuffing and stir. Press up the sides and on the bottom of a 9-inch, greased pie plate; put aside.
- For the filling: Sauté onion and mushrooms in butter in a large skillet until they are tender. Dust with the flour until combined thoroughly. Stir in thyme, Worcestershire sauce, parsley, peas, and turkey. Add in gravy and stir. Let come to a boil; stir and boil for 2 minutes.
- Scoop into the crust. Bake for 20 minutes at 375 degrees. Place the cheese strips over the filling in a lattice pattern. Bake until the cheese melts, for 5-10 more minutes.

Nutrition Information

- Calories: 511 calories
- Total Carbohydrate: 43g carbohydrate (6g sugars
- Cholesterol: 137mg cholesterol
- Protein: 32g protein.
- Total Fat: 23g fat (12g saturated fat)
- Sodium: 1560mg sodium
- Fiber: 4g fiber)

472. Turkey Asparagus Casserole

Serving: 4 servings. | Prep: 10mins | Cook: 30mins | Ready in:

Ingredients

- 1 package (10 ounces) frozen cut asparagus
- 2 cups cubed cooked turkey or chicken
- 1 can (10-3/4 ounces) condensed cream of chicken soup, undiluted
- 1/4 cup water
- 1 can (2.8 ounces) french-fried onions

Direction

- Cook asparagus for 2mins in a small pot with a small amount of water; drain then arrange in an oiled 11-in by 7-in baking dish. Place turkey on top. Mix water and soup together; spoon on top of the turkey. Bake for 25-30mins without cover in a 350°F oven. Scatter onions on top then bake for another 5mins until it turns golden brown.

Nutrition Information

- Calories: 328 calories
- Sodium: 800mg sodium
- Fiber: 2g fiber)
- Total Carbohydrate: 16g carbohydrate (2g sugars
- Cholesterol: 59mg cholesterol
- Protein: 24g protein.
- Total Fat: 18g fat (5g saturated fat)

473. Turkey BLT

Serving: 2 servings. | Prep: 5mins | Cook: 5mins | Ready in:

Ingredients

- 2 tablespoons mayonnaise
- 1 tablespoon spicy brown mustard
- 1 tablespoon honey
- 2 large pumpernickel rolls, split
- 4 slices cooked turkey
- 4 bacon strips, cooked and drained
- 2 slices Swiss cheese
- 4 slices tomato
- Lettuce leaves

Direction

- Mix together honey, mustard and mayonnaise in a small bowl, then spread mixture on cut sides of rolls. Layer turkey, bacon and cheese on the bottom halves of rolls, then broil 4 inches away from the heat until cheese starts to melt, about 2 to 3 minutes. Put lettuce and tomato on top, then replace roll tops.

Nutrition Information

- Calories:
- Total Fat:
- Sodium:
- Fiber:
- Total Carbohydrate:
- Cholesterol:
- Protein:

474. Turkey Biscuit Stew

Serving: 8 servings. | Prep: 15mins | Cook: 20mins | Ready in:

Ingredients

- 1/3 cup chopped onion
- 1/4 cup butter, cubed
- 1/3 cup all-purpose flour
- 1/2 teaspoon salt
- 1/8 teaspoon pepper
- 1 can (10-1/2 ounces) condensed chicken broth, undiluted
- 3/4 cup whole milk
- 2 cups cubed cooked turkey
- 1 cup cooked peas
- 1 cup cooked whole baby carrots
- 1 tube (10 ounces) refrigerated buttermilk biscuits

Direction

- Sauté the onion in butter in a 10-inch ovenproof skillet until it becomes tender. Stir in pepper, salt, and flour until combined. Pour in milk and broth gradually. Boil. Stir and cook until bubbling and thick, 2 minutes. Put in carrots, peas, and turkey; heat them through.

Separate the biscuits and place the biscuits on the stew.
- Bake at 375 degrees until biscuits turn golden brown, 20-25 minutes.

Nutrition Information

- Calories: 263 calories
- Protein: 17g protein.
- Total Fat: 10g fat (5g saturated fat)
- Sodium: 792mg sodium
- Fiber: 2g fiber)
- Total Carbohydrate: 27g carbohydrate (4g sugars
- Cholesterol: 45mg cholesterol

475. Turkey Bow Tie Skillet

Serving: 6 servings. | Prep: 15mins | Cook: 15mins | Ready in:

Ingredients

- 1/2 pound ground turkey breast
- 1-1/2 teaspoons canola oil
- 3/4 cup chopped celery
- 1/2 cup chopped onion
- 1/2 cup chopped green pepper
- 1 garlic clove, minced
- 1 can (14-1/2 ounces) chicken broth
- 2 cups uncooked bow tie pasta
- 1 can (14-1/2 ounces) stewed tomatoes
- 1 tablespoon white vinegar
- 3/4 teaspoon sugar
- 1/2 teaspoon chili powder
- 1/2 teaspoon garlic salt
- 2 tablespoons grated Parmesan cheese
- 1 tablespoon minced fresh parsley

Direction

- Cook the turkey in oil in a Dutch oven or a large skillet over medium heat until it is not pink anymore. Put in garlic, green pepper,

onion, and celery; then cook until the vegetables become tender. Using a slotted spoon, take the vegetables and turkey out using a slotted spoon and keep them warm.
- Pour the chicken broth into the pan; then boil. Put in the bow tie pasta and cook until tender, 10 minutes. Turn down the heat and stir in the turkey mixture, garlic salt, chili powder, sugar, vinegar, and stewed tomatoes. Simmer until heated through, 10 minutes. Dust with fresh parsley and Parmesan cheese.

Nutrition Information

- Calories:
- Protein:
- Total Fat:
- Sodium:
- Fiber:
- Total Carbohydrate:
- Cholesterol:

476. Turkey Burger Pie

Serving: 6 servings. | Prep: 10mins | Cook: 20mins | Ready in:

Ingredients

- 1 pound lean ground turkey
- 1 cup chopped onion
- 1 cup shredded reduced-fat cheddar cheese
- 1/2 cup egg substitute
- 1 cup fat-free milk
- 1/2 cup reduced-fat biscuit/baking mix

Direction

- Cook onion and turkey in a large skillet over medium heat until the meat is not pink anymore; then drain. Place into a greased 9-inch pie plate. Dust with cheese.
- Mix baking mix, milk, and egg substitute in a small bowl. Add to the cheese. Bake at 400 degrees until golden brown and a knife pierced in the center comes out clean, 20-25 minutes.

Nutrition Information

- Calories: 221 calories
- Total Fat: 6g fat (0 saturated fat)
- Sodium: 226mg sodium
- Fiber: 0 fiber)
- Total Carbohydrate: 12g carbohydrate (0 sugars
- Cholesterol: 51mg cholesterol
- Protein: 30g protein. Diabetic Exchanges: 3 lean meat

477. Turkey Burritos

Serving: 10-12 servings. | Prep: 30mins | Cook: 0mins | Ready in:

Ingredients

- 1 pound ground turkey
- 1/2 cup chopped onion
- 1 can (14-1/2 ounces) diced tomatoes, undrained
- 1 can (16 ounces) refried beans with green chilies
- 1 can (4 ounces) chopped green chilies
- 1 can (2-1/4 ounces) sliced ripe olives, drained
- 1 envelope taco seasoning
- 1/4 cup frozen corn
- 1/4 cup uncooked instant rice
- 10 to 12 flour tortillas (7 to 8 inches)
- Shredded cheddar or Monterey Jack cheese, optional

Direction

- Brown onion and turkey in a large nonstick saucepan; drain. Add corn, taco seasoning, olives, chilies, beans and tomatoes; bring to a boil. Lower the heat; simmer with a cover for 15 minutes. Return to a boil. Stir in rice; take out of the heat. Rest with a cover for 5 minutes. Put about half cup filling down the center of each tortilla; top with cheese if preferred. Fold in sides of tortilla.

Nutrition Information

- Calories: 267 calories
- Sodium: 865mg sodium
- Fiber: 3g fiber)
- Total Carbohydrate: 34g carbohydrate (2g sugars
- Cholesterol: 27mg cholesterol
- Protein: 12g protein.
- Total Fat: 9g fat (2g saturated fat)

478. Turkey Cranwich

Serving: 2 servings. | Prep: 15mins | Cook: 0mins | Ready in:

Ingredients

- 2 tablespoons cream cheese, softened
- 4 slices sourdough bread
- 1/4 cup chopped walnuts
- 1/3 pound thinly sliced cooked turkey
- 1/4 cup whole-berry cranberry sauce
- 2 slices Swiss cheese
- Lettuce leaves

Direction

- Spread on 2 bread slices with cream cheese, then use walnuts to sprinkle over. Put turkey on top and spread over turkey with cranberry sauce. Put lettuce, Swiss cheese and leftover bread on top.

Nutrition Information

- Calories: 589 calories
- Total Carbohydrate: 48g carbohydrate (10g sugars
- Cholesterol: 98mg cholesterol
- Protein: 39g protein.
- Total Fat: 27g fat (10g saturated fat)
- Sodium: 533mg sodium
- Fiber: 3g fiber)

479. Turkey Day Bake

Serving: 6-8 servings. | Prep: 10mins | Cook: 30mins | Ready in:

Ingredients

- 4 cups cooked stuffing
- 2-1/2 cups cubed cooked turkey
- 2 cups cooked broccoli florets
- 2 cups turkey gravy
- 4 slices process American cheese, halved

Direction

- Press the stuffing on the bottom of a 2 1/2-quart baking dish coated with cooking spray. Put broccoli and turkey on top. Spread gravy over all.
- Without the cover, bake at 350 degrees until the edges bubble, 25-30 minutes. Put cheese on top; bake until the cheese melts, 2-4 more minutes.

Nutrition Information

- Calories: 251 calories
- Total Fat: 6g fat (2g saturated fat)
- Sodium: 1002mg sodium
- Fiber: 1g fiber)
- Total Carbohydrate: 26g carbohydrate (4g sugars
- Cholesterol: 45mg cholesterol
- Protein: 20g protein.

480. Turkey Dressing Pie

Serving: 6 servings. | Prep: 25mins | Cook: 20mins | Ready in:

Ingredients

- 3-1/2 to 4 cups leftover cooked turkey dressing
- 1/2 cup turkey or chicken broth
- 2 tablespoons butter, melted
- 1 egg, beaten
- 1/2 cup chopped onion
- 1 tablespoon canola oil
- 3 cups diced leftover cooked turkey
- 1 cup leftover turkey gravy
- 1 cup peas, optional
- 2 tablespoons dried parsley flakes
- 2 tablespoons diced pimientos
- 1 teaspoon Worcestershire sauce
- 1/2 teaspoon dried thyme
- 4 slices process American cheese, optional

Direction

- Mix egg, butter, broth, and dressing in a large bowl. Press on sides and bottom of an ungreased 10-inch pie plate; then put aside.
- Sauté onion in oil in a large skillet until it becomes tender. Stir in thyme, Worcestershire sauce, pimientos, parsley, peas (if desired), gravy, and turkey; then heat completely. Pour on the turkey.
- Bake at 375 degrees until golden, for 20 minutes. Top with cheese slices if desired; bake until the cheese melts, for 5 minutes.

Nutrition Information

- Calories: 422 calories
- Sodium: 1041mg sodium
- Fiber: 4g fiber)
- Total Carbohydrate: 30g carbohydrate (3g sugars
- Cholesterol: 102mg cholesterol
- Protein: 26g protein.
- Total Fat: 21g fat (6g saturated fat)

481. Turkey Dumpling Stew

Serving: 6 servings. | Prep: 20mins | Cook: 50mins | Ready in:

Ingredients

- 4 bacon strips, finely chopped
- 1-1/2 pounds turkey breast tenderloins, cut into 1-inch pieces
- 4 medium carrots, sliced
- 2 small onions, quartered
- 2 celery ribs, sliced
- 1 bay leaf
- 1/4 teaspoon dried rosemary, crushed
- 2 cups water, divided
- 1 can (14-1/2 ounces) reduced-sodium chicken broth
- 3 tablespoons all-purpose flour
- 1/2 teaspoon salt
- 1/8 to 1/4 teaspoon pepper
- 1 cup reduced-fat biscuit/baking mix
- 1/3 cup plus 1 tablespoon fat-free milk
- Coarsely ground pepper and chopped fresh parsley, optional

Direction

- In a Dutch oven, cook while stirring bacon occasionally over medium heat till crisp. Use a slotted spoon to take away; drain on paper towels. Set aside 2 teaspoons of drippings.
- Sauté turkey in the drippings over medium heat till slightly browned. Pour in broth, 1 3/4 cups of water, herbs and vegetables; boil. Lower the heat; simmer with a cover for 20-30 minutes, or till the vegetables become tender.
- Combine the remaining water and flour till smooth; mix into the turkey mixture. Boil; cook while stirring for around 2 minutes, or till thickened. Remove and discard bay leaf. Mix in bacon, pepper and salt.
- Combine milk and biscuit mix in a small bowl so that a soft dough forms; drop six mounds

on top of the simmering stew. Simmer with a cover till a toothpick comes out clean when inserted into the dumplings, 15 minutes. Sprinkle with parsley and pepper if desired. Serve.

Nutrition Information

- Calories: 284 calories
- Protein: 34g protein. Diabetic exchanges: 4 lean meat
- Total Fat: 6g fat (1g saturated fat)
- Sodium: 822mg sodium
- Fiber: 2g fiber)
- Total Carbohydrate: 24g carbohydrate (6g sugars
- Cholesterol: 52mg cholesterol

482. Turkey Hero

Serving: 6 servings. | Prep: 15mins | Cook: 0mins | Ready in:

Ingredients

- 3 ounces cream cheese, softened
- 2 tablespoons ranch salad dressing
- 1 teaspoon poppy seeds
- Pinch garlic powder
- 1 loaf (1 pound) French bread, split lengthwise
- Shredded lettuce
- 3/4 pound thinly sliced cooked turkey
- 1/4 pound thinly sliced Swiss cheese
- 2 medium tomatoes, sliced

Direction

- Beat the first 4 ingredients together in a small bowl until smooth, then spread mixture on both cut surfaces of bread. On bottom half of bread, layer lettuce, turkey, cheese, and tomatoes, then place another half on top. Slice bread into serving-size pieces.

Nutrition Information

- Calories: 467 calories
- Fiber: 3g fiber)
- Total Carbohydrate: 43g carbohydrate (3g sugars
- Cholesterol: 80mg cholesterol
- Protein: 30g protein.
- Total Fat: 19g fat (9g saturated fat)
- Sodium: 620mg sodium

483. Turkey Lasagna Roll Ups

Serving: 4 servings. | Prep: 20mins | Cook: 45mins | Ready in:

Ingredients

- 4 lasagna noodles
- 6 ounces lean ground turkey
- 1 small onion, chopped
- 1 cup chopped fresh broccoli
- 1/4 cup water
- 1 cup (8 ounces) reduced-fat ricotta cheese
- 1 egg, lightly beaten
- 1 tablespoon fat-free milk
- 1-1/2 teaspoons minced fresh thyme or 1/2 teaspoon dried thyme
- 1/4 teaspoon salt
- 2 cups meatless spaghetti sauce, divided
- 1/4 cup shredded Parmesan cheese

Direction

- Prepare the lasagna noodles as specified on the box. Rinse noodles and drain. Over medium heat sauté the onion and turkey in a non-stick skillet until the turkey is not pink.
- Boil the broccoli in water in a separate saucepan. Decrease the heat. Put a lid on and let it simmer for 5 minutes. Drain once the broccoli has a crisp-tender texture.
- In the turkey mixture, add milk, egg, ricotta cheese, salt, thyme and the cooked broccoli. Spread the mixture on each noodle and add

1/4 cup of spaghetti sauce over each. Roll the noodles jelly roll style carefully.
- Coat an 8-inch square dish with cooking spray. Carefully place each noodle roll with its seam side down in dish. Put the remaining spaghetti sauce on top.
- Cover the dish. Bake at 375°F until the thermometer registers 160°F, 45-50 minutes. Top with Parmesan cheese before serving.

Nutrition Information

- Calories: 347 calories
- Total Carbohydrate: 33g carbohydrate (0 sugars
- Cholesterol: 110mg cholesterol
- Protein: 23g protein. Diabetic Exchanges: 3 lean meat
- Total Fat: 13g fat (6g saturated fat)
- Sodium: 853mg sodium
- Fiber: 4g fiber)

484. Turkey Legs With Mushroom Gravy

Serving: 4 servings. | Prep: 5mins | Cook: 01hours45mins | Ready in:

Ingredients

- 4 turkey drumsticks (12 ounces each)
- 1/4 cup lemon juice
- 2 tablespoons canola oil
- 1 teaspoon garlic powder
- 1 teaspoon dried oregano
- 1 teaspoon dried basil
- 1/4 teaspoon pepper
- MUSHROOM GRAVY:
- 1 tablespoon cornstarch
- 1 cup cold water
- 1 can (10-1/2 ounces) mushroom gravy
- 1 can (4 ounces) sliced mushrooms, drained
- 1 tablespoon minced fresh parsley
- 1 teaspoon garlic powder
- 1 teaspoon finely chopped onion
- Hot cooked noodles, optional

Direction

- In roasting pan, put turkey legs. Combine seasonings, oil and lemon juice in small bowl. Add over the turkey legs.
- Bake at 375°, uncovered, until lightly browned, about 45 mins. Flip the legs 2 times and occasionally baste the pan drippings over. Discard from oven.
- For gravy, combine water and cornstarch in a small saucepan until they become smooth. Boil over the medium heat. Cook while stirring until bubbly and thickened, about 1 to 2 mins. Stir in onion, garlic powder, parsley, mushrooms and gravy; heat through. Place over the turkey legs.
- Loosely wrap in foil. Bake until a thermometer registers 180° when inserted in the turkey, about 60 mins, basting with the pan drippings frequently. Enjoy with noodles, if desired.

Nutrition Information

- Calories: 467 calories
- Total Carbohydrate: 10g carbohydrate (2g sugars
- Cholesterol: 177mg cholesterol
- Protein: 57g protein.
- Total Fat: 21g fat (7g saturated fat)
- Sodium: 714mg sodium
- Fiber: 1g fiber)

485. Turkey Lime Kabobs

Serving: 8 servings. | Prep: 20mins | Cook: 20mins | Ready in:

Ingredients

- 3 cans (6 ounces each) orange juice concentrate, thawed
- 1-1/4 cups lime juice

- 1 cup honey
- 4 to 5 jalapeno peppers, seeded and chopped
- 10 garlic cloves, minced
- 3 tablespoons ground cumin
- 2 tablespoons grated lime zest
- 1 teaspoon salt
- 2 pounds boneless turkey, chicken or pork, cut into 1-1/4-inch cubes
- 4 medium sweet red or green peppers, cut into 1-inch pieces
- 1 large red onion, cut into 1-inch pieces
- 3 small zucchini, cut into 3/4-inch slices
- 8 ounces fresh mushrooms
- 3 medium limes, cut into wedges

Direction

- Combine the first eight ingredients in a bowl. Place meat into a large zip-top bag and pour in half of the marinade. Seal the bag and turn to coat. Pour the other half of the marinade into another large zip-top bag, add the vegetables and turn to coat. Seal both bags and marinate in the fridge for at least 8 hours, or even overnight, turning the bag occasionally. Drain the meat and discard its marinade. Save the marinade when draining the vegetables; to be used for basting later. Alternately cue meat, vegetables, and lime wedges onto metal or pre-soaked wooden skewers. Cook on an open grill at medium heat for 4-5 minutes per side, basting with reserved marinade. Turn and baste for another 10-12 minutes, until meat juices are clear and the vegetables are tender.

Nutrition Information

- Calories:
- Protein:
- Total Fat:
- Sodium:
- Fiber:
- Total Carbohydrate:
- Cholesterol:

486. Turkey Linguine

Serving: 4 servings. | Prep: 5mins | Cook: 15mins | Ready in:

Ingredients

- 1 pound boneless turkey breast, cut into 1/2-inch strips
- 1 tablespoon olive oil
- 1/2 cup chopped onion
- 2 garlic cloves, minced
- 1 cup broccoli florets
- 1 cup thinly sliced carrots
- 1 tablespoon minced fresh basil or 1 teaspoon dried basil
- 1 teaspoon minced fresh tarragon or 1/4 teaspoon dried tarragon
- 1 teaspoon minced fresh thyme or 1/4 teaspoon dried thyme
- 1/8 teaspoon pepper
- 2 tablespoons cornstarch
- 1-1/2 cups chicken broth
- 8 ounces linguini or pasta of your choice, cooked
- 1/2 cup grated Parmesan cheese

Direction

- Stir-fry the turkey in a wok or large skillet with oil for 2 minutes. Add the garlic and onion. Cook and stir the mixture for 1 minute. Add the pepper, tarragon, broccoli, thyme, basil, and carrots. Stir-fry the vegetables for 3-4 minutes until crisp-tender.
- Mix the broth and cornstarch until smooth, and then pour it into the turkey mixture. Cook for 2 minutes, stirring until the mixture comes to boil. Serve the mixture over linguine that is sprinkled with Parmesan cheese.

Nutrition Information

- Calories: 331 calories
- Total Fat: 8g fat (3g saturated fat)
- Sodium: 608mg sodium
- Fiber: 3g fiber)

- Total Carbohydrate: 27g carbohydrate (5g sugars
- Cholesterol: 78mg cholesterol
- Protein: 37g protein.

487. Turkey Manicotti

Serving: 6-8 servings. | Prep: 25mins | Cook: 25mins | Ready in:

Ingredients

- 2 slices bread
- 1-1/2 pounds ground turkey
- 1/4 cup chopped onion
- 2 garlic cloves, minced
- 1/2 teaspoon salt
- 1/4 teaspoon pepper
- 1 cup shredded mozzarella cheese
- 1/2 cup grated Parmesan cheese
- 14 manicotti shells (8 ounces), cooked and drained
- 3-3/4 cups spaghetti sauce

Direction

- Soak bread in water; squeeze to remove any excess water. Tear into small pieces; put aside. Cook pepper, salt, garlic, onion and turkey in a skillet until onion becomes tender and meat is no longer pink; drain. Stir in cheeses and bread; combine well. Scoop into manicotti shells. Transfer 1/2 of the spaghetti sauce into a greased 13x9-in. baking dish. Place shells over sauce; pour the rest of the sauce on top. Bake with a cover at 350° until heated through or for 25-30 minutes.

Nutrition Information

- Calories: 440 calories
- Total Fat: 22g fat (8g saturated fat)
- Sodium: 947mg sodium
- Fiber: 3g fiber)

- Total Carbohydrate: 36g carbohydrate (9g sugars
- Cholesterol: 75mg cholesterol
- Protein: 25g protein.

488. Turkey Meat Loaf

Serving: 10 servings. | Prep: 15mins | Cook: 60mins | Ready in:

Ingredients

- 1 cup quick-cooking oats
- 1 medium onion, chopped
- 1/2 cup shredded carrot
- 1/2 cup fat-free milk
- 1/4 cup egg substitute
- 2 tablespoons ketchup
- 1 teaspoon garlic powder
- 1/4 teaspoon pepper
- 2 pounds lean ground turkey
- TOPPING:
- 1/4 cup ketchup
- 1/4 cup quick-cooking oats

Direction

- Set oven to 350 degrees and start preheating. Mix together first 8 ingredients. Put in turkey, then lightly mix yet thoroughly.
- Move the mixture into a greased 9x5" loaf pan. Combine topping ingredients, then spread on top of the meat loaf. Bake for 60-65 minutes until it reaches 165 degrees on a meat thermometer. Allow the loaf to stand for 10 minutes, then slice.

Nutrition Information

- Calories: 195 calories
- Fiber: 1g fiber)
- Total Carbohydrate: 12g carbohydrate (4g sugars
- Cholesterol: 63mg cholesterol

- Protein: 20g protein. Diabetic Exchanges: 3 lean meat
- Total Fat: 8g fat (2g saturated fat)
- Sodium: 188mg sodium

489. Turkey Minute Steaks

Serving: 6-8 servings. | Prep: 10mins | Cook: 15mins | Ready in:

Ingredients

- 3/4 cup Italian-seasoned bread crumbs
- 1/4 cup grated Parmesan cheese
- 1/2 teaspoon dried basil
- Salt and pepper to taste
- 1 egg, beaten
- 1-1/2 pounds uncooked sliced turkey breast
- 3 tablespoons butter

Direction

- Combine pepper, salt, basil, Parmesan cheese and bread crumbs together in a shallow bowl. Place egg into another shallow bowl. Dip turkey in egg, coat both sides in crumbs.
- Place a large skillet on medium-high heat; melt butter. Cook in turkey for 2-3 minutes per side, or till the juices run clear and the meat turns golden brown.

Nutrition Information

- Calories: 194 calories
- Sodium: 301mg sodium
- Fiber: 0 fiber)
- Total Carbohydrate: 8g carbohydrate (1g sugars
- Cholesterol: 93mg cholesterol
- Protein: 24g protein.
- Total Fat: 7g fat (3g saturated fat)

490. Turkey Mushroom Tetrazzini

Serving: 6 | Prep: 20mins | Cook: 45mins | Ready in:

Ingredients

- 8 ounces uncooked linguine pasta
- 2 tablespoons butter
- 2 cups fresh mushrooms, quartered
- 1/2 cup sliced green onion
- 1/4 cup chopped red bell pepper
- 1/4 cup all-purpose flour
- 1/8 teaspoon black pepper
- 2 tablespoons garlic spread seasoning (such as Johnny's® Great Caesar! Garlic Spread & Seasoning)
- 1 1/4 cups chicken broth
- 1 1/4 cups heavy cream
- 2 cups chopped cooked turkey
- 3/4 cup grated Parmesan cheese, divided
- 1/4 cup sliced almonds
- 2 tablespoons chopped fresh parsley (optional)

Direction

- Preheat the oven to 175°C or 350°F. Oil a rectangular baking dish, 2 quarts in size.
- Fill slightly salted water into a big pot and bring to a rolling boil. When boiling, mix in linguine, and bring back to a boil. Let the pasta cook without a cover for 11 minutes, mixing from time to time, till pasta has cooked completely yet still firm to the bite. Drain thoroughly in a colander placed in sink.
- In a big skillet, heat the butter; cook and mix bell pepper, green onion and mushrooms for 5 minutes till vegetables are softened and onion is translucent. Mix in garlic spread seasoning, black pepper and flour. Add cream and chicken broth, beating the mixture till thickened and smooth, 5 to 8 minutes longer. Mix in cooked linguine, 1/2 the Parmesan cheese and turkey, and gently mix to coat every ingredient in sauce.
- Into the prepped baking dish, scatter the mixture, and scatter the rest of the Parmesan

cheese and almonds on top. In the prepped oven, bake for 20 minutes till mixture is bubbling and surface has started to brown, and scatter parsley on top prior to serving.

Nutrition Information

- Calories: 515 calories;
- Protein: 25.6
- Total Fat: 30.3
- Sodium: 676
- Total Carbohydrate: 37
- Cholesterol: 123

491. Turkey Noodle Casserole

Serving: 2 casseroles (6 serving each). | Prep: 30mins | Cook: 30mins | Ready in:

Ingredients

- 2 pounds ground turkey
- 2 cups chopped celery
- 1/4 cup chopped green pepper
- 1/4 cup chopped onion
- 1 can (10-3/4 ounces) condensed cream of mushroom soup, undiluted
- 1 can (8 ounces) sliced water chestnuts, drained
- 1 jar (4-1/2 ounces) sliced mushrooms, drained
- 1 jar (4 ounces) diced pimientos, drained
- 1/4 cup soy sauce
- 1/2 teaspoon salt
- 1/2 teaspoon lemon-pepper seasoning
- 1 cup sour cream
- 8 ounces cooked wide egg noodles

Direction

- Cook the turkey in a large skillet over medium heat until it is not pink anymore. Put in onion, green pepper, and celery; cook until they become tender. Stir in lemon-pepper, salt, soy sauce, pimientos, mushrooms, water chestnuts, and soup. Turn down the heat; simmer for 20 minutes.
- Take away from the heat; add noodles and sour cream. Store half in a freezer container; put on a cover and freeze for up to 3 months. In a 2-quart baking dish coated with cooking spray, arrange the remaining mixture. Put on a cover and bake at 350 degrees until heated through, 30-35 minutes.
- Put in the fridge to thaw to use the frozen casserole. Place into a 2-quart baking dish coated with cooking spray, then bake following the instructions.

Nutrition Information

- Calories: 307 calories
- Total Carbohydrate: 22g carbohydrate (2g sugars
- Cholesterol: 84mg cholesterol
- Protein: 17g protein.
- Total Fat: 17g fat (6g saturated fat)
- Sodium: 760mg sodium
- Fiber: 2g fiber)

492. Turkey Pasta Primavera

Serving: 6 servings. | Prep: 30mins | Cook: 0mins | Ready in:

Ingredients

- 8 ounces fettuccine or spaghetti
- 1 cup broccoli florets
- 1 cup julienned carrots
- 1/2 cup chopped sweet red pepper
- 2 tablespoons all-purpose flour
- 1-3/4 cups fat-free milk
- 1 package (8 ounces) cream cheese, cubed
- 1/2 cup chopped green onions
- 3/4 teaspoon Italian seasoning
- 1/4 teaspoon garlic powder
- 1/8 teaspoon pepper

- 1/2 teaspoon salt, optional
- 2 cups julienned cooked turkey
- 1/2 cup grated Parmesan cheese

Direction

- Following package directions to cook pasta while putting in red pepper, carrots and broccoli during the final 5 minutes of cooking process.
- Meantime, stir milk and flour in a medium saucepan until smooth. Put in seasonings, onions and cream cheese, then bring to a boil on medium low heat. Cook and stir about 1 to 2 minutes, then put in Parmesan cheese and turkey, heat through. Drain pasta and toss with the cheese sauce.

Nutrition Information

- Calories: 333 calories
- Total Fat: 8g fat (0 saturated fat)
- Sodium: 348mg sodium
- Fiber: 0 fiber)
- Total Carbohydrate: 40g carbohydrate (0 sugars
- Cholesterol: 50mg cholesterol
- Protein: 23g protein. Diabetic Exchanges: 2 starch

493. Turkey Penne With Lemon Cream Sauce

Serving: 4 servings. | Prep: 20mins | Cook: 10mins | Ready in:

Ingredients

- 2 cups uncooked penne pasta
- 1/2 pound turkey breast cutlets, cut into 3/4-inch pieces
- 3 tablespoons butter, divided
- 2 cups fresh broccoli florets
- 3 small carrots, thinly sliced
- 2 garlic cloves, minced
- 2 tablespoons all-purpose flour
- 1-1/2 teaspoons chicken bouillon granules
- 1/2 teaspoon dried thyme
- 1/4 teaspoon pepper
- 1/8 teaspoon salt
- 2-1/2 cups half-and-half cream
- 1/4 cup lemon juice
- 2 plum tomatoes, seeded and chopped

Direction

- Follow the directions on the package to cook the pasta. While waiting, put 1 tablespoon of butter in a large frying pan and sauté turkey until not pink. Remove the turkey and keep warm. Put the rest of the butter in the same pan and sauté carrots and broccoli until tender and crispy. Add the garlic and cook 1 more minute. Mix in salt, bouillon granules, flour, pepper, and thyme until combined. In a separate bowl, mix lemon juice and cream. Slowly stir cream mixture into the frying pan with broccoli mixture. Heat to a boil. Stirring constantly, cook until thick, 2-3 minutes. Drain water from pasta. Add the pasta to the frying pan. Finally, mix in tomatoes and turkey and heat until completely hot.

Nutrition Information

- Calories: 528 calories
- Protein: 28g protein.
- Total Fat: 25g fat (16g saturated fat)
- Sodium: 594mg sodium
- Fiber: 4g fiber)
- Total Carbohydrate: 43g carbohydrate (10g sugars
- Cholesterol: 136mg cholesterol

494. Turkey Piccata

Serving: 4 | Prep: | Cook: 30mins | Ready in:

Ingredients

- 1 lemon
- ⅓ cup all-purpose flour
- ½ teaspoon salt
- ½ teaspoon freshly ground pepper
- 4 turkey cutlets, (about 1 pound), each cutlet sliced in half across the grain
- 2 teaspoons extra-virgin olive oil
- 1 clove garlic, minced
- ½ cup reduced-sodium chicken broth
- 1 tablespoon drained capers, rinsed
- ½ teaspoon sugar
- 2 teaspoons butter
- 1 tablespoon chopped fresh parsley
- 12 caper berries, for garnish (optional)

Direction

- Use a sharp knife to take skin and white pith out of the lemon. Cut the lemon segments from their surrounding membranes, working over a bowl to collect juice coming out. Coarsely chop the segments and save the juice.
- Mix pepper, salt, and flour together in a shallow dish. Gently press turkey into flour, patting off excess. Heat oil over medium-high heat in a large nonstick skillet. Cook turkey in heated oil for 2 to 3 minutes on each side, until inside is no longer pink and outside turns golden brown. Remove browned turkey to a platter and keep it warm.
- Cook garlic in the same pan for a couple of seconds, stirring. Add broth and bring to a boil, stirring to dissolve any browned bits from the pan. Boil mixture for 1 minute. Mix in sugar, capers, the reserved lemon segments and juice; cook for half a minute. Put in butter, tilting the pan to melt the butter.
- Ladle sauce over the cutlets; scatter with pepper and parsley. If desired, garnish with caper berries.

Nutrition Information

- Calories: 206 calories;
- Saturated Fat: 2
- Fiber: 1
- Total Carbohydrate: 10
- Sugar: 1
- Sodium: 483
- Cholesterol: 50
- Protein: 30
- Total Fat: 5

495. Turkey Pita Tacos

Serving: 5 servings. | Prep: 25mins | Cook: 5mins | Ready in:

Ingredients

- 1 tablespoon canola oil
- 1 tablespoon cider or red wine vinegar
- 1 teaspoon chili powder
- 1 teaspoon ground cumin
- 1/4 teaspoon salt
- 1/4 teaspoon pepper
- 1 cup cubed cooked turkey or chicken
- 1 medium green pepper, chopped
- 1 medium sweet red pepper, chopped
- 1 small tomato, chopped
- 1 cup chunky salsa
- 3 green onions, thinly sliced
- 1 can (2-1/4 ounces) sliced ripe olives, drained
- 1 garlic clove, minced
- 1 cup shredded cheddar cheese
- 5 pita breads (6 inches), halved

Direction

- Mix the first six ingredients together in a small bowl; set aside. Combine garlic, olives, onions, salsa, tomato, peppers and turkey in a large bowl. Mix in the oil mixture; spread over the turkey mixture; stir properly. Mix in cheese. Heat pita breads on both sides on a lightly greased griddle. Using a spoon, place around 1/2 cup of the turkey mixture into each half.

Nutrition Information

- Calories:
- Protein:
- Total Fat:
- Sodium:
- Fiber:
- Total Carbohydrate:
- Cholesterol:

496. Turkey Pitas With Creamy Slaw

Serving: 4 servings. | Prep: 10mins | Cook: 0mins | Ready in:

Ingredients

- 3 cups coleslaw mix
- 1/4 cup golden raisins
- 3 tablespoons chopped red onion
- 1/3 cup reduced-fat mayonnaise
- 3 tablespoons mango chutney
- 8 pita pocket halves
- 1/2 pound sliced deli turkey
- 8 ready-to-serve fully cooked bacon strips, warmed
- 1 medium cucumber, thinly sliced

Direction

- Mix together onion, raisins and coleslaw mix in a big bowl, then put in chutney and mayonnaise, tossing to coat well. Use turkey, cucumber and bacon to line pita halves, then fill in coleslaw mixture.

Nutrition Information

- Calories: 427 calories
- Fiber: 3g fiber)
- Total Carbohydrate: 57g carbohydrate (18g sugars
- Cholesterol: 27mg cholesterol
- Protein: 21g protein.
- Total Fat: 12g fat (2g saturated fat)

- Sodium: 1257mg sodium

497. Turkey Potato Meatballs

Serving: 10 servings. | Prep: 20mins | Cook: 30mins | Ready in:

Ingredients

- 2 medium potatoes, peeled and shredded
- 1 small onion, grated
- 2 medium carrots, grated
- 1/2 cup dry bread crumbs
- 1/4 cup egg substitute
- 1/8 teaspoon pepper
- 1-1/2 pounds ground turkey
- 1 tablespoon shortening
- 1 can (10-3/4 ounces) reduced-fat reduced-sodium condensed cream of mushroom soup, undiluted
- 1-1/3 cups fat-free milk
- 1/2 cup uncooked instant rice

Direction

- In a big bowl, whisk the first six ingredients. Put in turkey; stir properly. Roll into 1-in. balls. In a frying pan, brown meatballs in shortening then put aside. In an ungreased 13x9-in. baking dish, mix rice, milk and soup together; combine in meatballs. Bake, covered, at 350° for 30-35 minutes till meatballs are not pink anymore.

Nutrition Information

- Calories: 218 calories
- Total Fat: 8g fat (0 saturated fat)
- Sodium: 263mg sodium
- Fiber: 0 fiber)
- Total Carbohydrate: 20g carbohydrate (0 sugars
- Cholesterol: 55mg cholesterol

- Protein: 16g protein. Diabetic Exchanges: 1-1/2 meat

498. Turkey Potato Pancakes

Serving: 12 pancakes. | Prep: 10mins | Cook: 30mins | Ready in:

Ingredients

- 3 cups shredded peeled potatoes
- 1-1/2 cups finely chopped cooked turkey
- 1/4 cup sliced green onions with tops
- 2 tablespoons all-purpose flour
- 1-1/2 teaspoons salt
- 3 large eggs, lightly beaten
- Canola oil
- Cranberry sauce, optional

Direction

- Place the potato in a colander or sieve, pressing to get rid of excess liquid. Then pat dry and set aside. Mix salt, flour, onions, and turkey in a large bowl. Mix in eggs until incorporated. Stir in the reserved potatoes; toss to coat. In a large nonstick skillet over medium heat, add about 2 tablespoons of oil. Pour batter by 1/3 cupfuls into the oil. Cook in batches until both sides are golden brown, using the rest of the oil as necessary. Place to a paper towel to drain on. Pair with cranberry sauce to serve, if desired.

Nutrition Information

- Calories: 262 calories
- Total Fat: 7g fat (2g saturated fat)
- Sodium: 976mg sodium
- Fiber: 2g fiber)
- Total Carbohydrate: 27g carbohydrate (2g sugars
- Cholesterol: 199mg cholesterol
- Protein: 23g protein.

499. Turkey Primavera

Serving: 4-6 servings. | Prep: 25mins | Cook: 20mins | Ready in:

Ingredients

- 1/4 cup all-purpose flour
- 2 teaspoons minced fresh parsley
- 1-1/2 pounds turkey breast tenderloins, cubed
- 2 tablespoons olive oil
- 1/2 cup chicken broth
- 1 cup sliced fresh mushrooms
- 1 medium onion, chopped
- 4 garlic cloves, minced
- 1/2 medium green pepper, chopped
- 1 can (14-1/2 ounces) beef broth
- 3/4 cup tomato puree
- 1/2 teaspoon dried thyme
- 1/2 teaspoon dried rosemary, crushed
- 1/2 teaspoon dried basil
- 1 bay leaf
- 1/4 teaspoon salt
- 1/8 teaspoon pepper
- Hot cooked fettuccine or spaghetti
- Parmesan cheese, optional

Direction

- Combine parsley and flour. Put in turkey; toss to coat. Brown turkey in oil in a skillet until no longer pink. Use a slotted spoon to take them out. Put aside.
- Combine green pepper, garlic, onion, mushrooms and chicken broth in the same skillet. Cook while stirring about 3 to 4 minutes. Put in seasonings, tomato puree and beef broth. Cook while stirring until sauce reaches the consistency you desire, about 20 to 25 minutes.
- Put in turkey and heat through. Discard bay leaf. Add over the pasta; if desired, sprinkle Parmesan over and serve.

Nutrition Information

- Calories: 215 calories
- Total Fat: 7g fat (1g saturated fat)
- Sodium: 494mg sodium
- Fiber: 1g fiber)
- Total Carbohydrate: 11g carbohydrate (3g sugars
- Cholesterol: 56mg cholesterol
- Protein: 29g protein.

500. Turkey Ranch Wraps

Serving: 4 servings. | Prep: 10mins | Cook: 0mins | Ready in:

Ingredients

- 8 thin slices cooked turkey
- 4 flour tortillas (6 inches), room temperature
- 1 large tomato, thinly sliced
- 1 medium green pepper, cut into thin strips
- 1 cup shredded lettuce
- 1 cup shredded cheddar cheese
- 1/3 cup ranch salad dressing

Direction

- On each tortilla, put 2 turkey slices, then layer tomato, green pepper, lettuce and cheese on top. Drizzle salad dressing over top then roll up tortilla tightly.

Nutrition Information

- Calories: 403 calories
- Total Fat: 25g fat (9g saturated fat)
- Sodium: 601mg sodium
- Fiber: 1g fiber)
- Total Carbohydrate: 19g carbohydrate (3g sugars
- Cholesterol: 76mg cholesterol
- Protein: 26g protein.

501. Turkey Ravioli Lasagna

Serving: 12 servings. | Prep: 30mins | Cook: 35mins | Ready in:

Ingredients

- 1 pound ground turkey
- 1/2 teaspoon garlic powder
- Salt and pepper to taste
- 1 cup grated carrots
- 1 cup sliced fresh mushrooms
- 1 tablespoon olive oil
- 3-1/2 cups spaghetti sauce
- 1 package (25 ounces) frozen cheese ravioli, cooked and drained
- 3 cups shredded part-skim mozzarella cheese
- 1/2 cup grated Parmesan cheese
- Minced fresh parsley, optional

Direction

- Cook the turkey in a large pan over moderate heat. Cook until it is no longer pink and then drain. Add in some salt, pepper and garlic powder then set aside for later use.
- Sauté the mushrooms and carrots in a large skillet with oil until already soft. Add the spaghetti sauce in the pan; stir. Grease your 13x9-inch baking pan and lay half cup of the sauce. Arrange 1/2 of the ravioli, spaghetti sauce mixture, turkey, and cheeses to form layers twice. You can top it with parsley if you want.
- Let it bake covered for 25-30 minutes at a temperature of 375°F until bubbling. Remove the cover and bake it again for another 10 more minutes. Let it rest for 15 minutes before serving it.

Nutrition Information

- Calories:
- Protein:
- Total Fat:
- Sodium:
- Fiber:

- Total Carbohydrate:
- Cholesterol:

502. Turkey Sausage Stew

Serving: 8 servings. | Prep: 10mins | Cook: 35mins | Ready in:

Ingredients

- 1 package (16 ounces) frozen vegetables for stew
- 1 can (10-3/4 ounces) reduced-sodium condensed tomato soup, undiluted
- 2 cups water
- 1 pound low-fat smoked turkey sausage, sliced 1/4 inch thick
- 1/4 cup ketchup
- 2 garlic cloves, minced
- 1/2 teaspoon dried basil
- 1/4 teaspoon pepper

Direction

- Mix together water, soup and vegetables in a big saucepan, then bring to a boil. Lower heat; put in remaining ingredients and simmer until vegetables are softened, about 35 to 45 minutes.

Nutrition Information

- Calories: 190 calories
- Cholesterol: 25mg cholesterol
- Protein: 11g protein. Diabetic Exchanges: 1-1/2 meat
- Total Fat: 8g fat (0 saturated fat)
- Sodium: 622mg sodium
- Fiber: 0 fiber
- Total Carbohydrate: 17g carbohydrate (0 sugars

503. Turkey Sausage Stuffed Acorn Squash

Serving: 8 servings. | Prep: 30mins | Cook: 50mins | Ready in:

Ingredients

- 4 medium acorn squash (about 1-1/2 pounds each)
- 1 cup cherry tomatoes, halved
- 1 pound Italian turkey sausage links, casings removed
- 1/2 pound sliced fresh mushrooms
- 1 medium apple, peeled and finely chopped
- 1 small onion, finely chopped
- 2 teaspoons fennel seed
- 2 teaspoons caraway seeds
- 1/2 teaspoon dried sage leaves
- 3 cups fresh baby spinach
- 1 tablespoon minced fresh thyme
- 1/4 teaspoon salt
- 1/8 teaspoon pepper
- 8 ounces fresh mozzarella cheese, chopped
- 1 tablespoon red wine vinegar

Direction

- Turn oven to 400° to preheat. Cut squash in half vertically; pick out and discard seeds. Cut a thin slice from the bottom of each half using a sharp knife so they can lay flat. Arrange squash with hollow side down in a shallow roasting pan, add halved tomatoes and pour in 1/4 inch of hot water. Bake without covering for 45 minutes.
- In the meantime, sauté dried seasonings, onion, apple, mushrooms and sausage in a large skillet over medium heat until sausage is no longer pink, for 8 to 10 minutes, crumbling sausage; drain well. Add pepper, salt, thyme, and spinach; sauté for 2 more minutes. Put off from the heat.
- Gently take squash out of the roasting pan. Drain cooking juices, retaining tomatoes. Place squash with hollow side up back into the pan.

- Mix the reserved tomatoes, vinegar, and cheese into the sausage mixture. Fill mixture into squash cavities. Bake until squash is fork-tender and thoroughly heated, for 5 to 10 minutes more.

Nutrition Information

- Calories: 302 calories
- Sodium: 370mg sodium
- Fiber: 7g fiber)
- Total Carbohydrate: 42g carbohydrate (11g sugars
- Cholesterol: 43mg cholesterol
- Protein: 15g protein. Diabetic Exchanges: 2-1/2 starch
- Total Fat: 10g fat (5g saturated fat)

504. Turkey Scallopini

Serving: 4 servings. | Prep: 10mins | Cook: 10mins | Ready in:

Ingredients

- 1 package (17.6 ounces) turkey breast cutlets
- 1/4 cup all-purpose flour
- 1/8 teaspoon salt
- 1/8 teaspoon pepper
- 1 large egg
- 2 tablespoons water
- 1 cup soft bread crumbs
- 1/2 cup grated Parmesan cheese
- 1/4 cup butter, cubed
- Minced fresh parsley

Direction

- Pound the turkey to 1/4 inch in thickness. Mix pepper, salt, and flour in a shallow bowl. Whisk water and egg in a different bowl. Mix cheese and breadcrumbs in a third shallow bowl.
- Dredge the turkey in the flour mixture, plunge into the egg mixture and coat in crumbs. Allow to stand for 5 minutes.
- In a large skillet, melt the butter on medium-high heat; cook the turkey until the coating turns golden brown and the meat is not pink anymore, for 2-3 minutes per side. Scatter with parsley.

Nutrition Information

- Calories: 358 calories
- Protein: 38g protein.
- Total Fat: 17g fat (10g saturated fat)
- Sodium: 463mg sodium
- Fiber: 0 fiber)
- Total Carbohydrate: 12g carbohydrate (1g sugars
- Cholesterol: 169mg cholesterol

505. Turkey Scallopini With Marsala Sauce

Serving: 4 servings. | Prep: 10mins | Cook: 20mins | Ready in:

Ingredients

- 1/2 cup all-purpose flour
- 1/2 teaspoon salt
- 1/2 teaspoon pepper
- 1 package (17.6 ounces) turkey breast cutlets
- 2 tablespoons olive oil
- 1-1/2 cups Marsala wine
- 3 tablespoons butter
- 3 tablespoons shredded Parmesan cheese
- Hot cooked linguine, optional

Direction

- In a large resealable plastic bag, blend pepper, salt, and flour. Put in turkey cutlets, one each time, close the bag and turn to coat.

- Heat oil over medium heat in a large skillet. Add in turkey; cook for 3 to 4 minutes per side, or until meat is no more pink. Take out from the pan. Blend in wine. Heat to a boil; cook about 8 to 10 minutes, or until liquid is evaporated to about 1/2 cup. Mix in butter until it is melted. Bring turkey back to the pan; heat through. Serve alongside cheese and, if wanted, linguine.

Nutrition Information

- Calories: 459 calories
- Sodium: 341mg sodium
- Fiber: 0 fiber)
- Total Carbohydrate: 18g carbohydrate (7g sugars
- Cholesterol: 103mg cholesterol
- Protein: 33g protein.
- Total Fat: 17g fat (7g saturated fat)

506. Turkey Stew With Dumplings

Serving: 10-12 servings. | Prep: 30mins | Cook: 45mins | Ready in:

Ingredients

- 8 medium carrots, cut into 1-inch chunks
- 4 celery ribs, cut into 1-inch chunks
- 1 cup chopped onion
- 1/2 cup butter, cubed
- 2 cans (10-1/2 ounces each) condensed beef consomme, undiluted
- 4-2/3 cups water, divided
- 2 teaspoons salt
- 1/4 teaspoon pepper
- 3 cups cubed cooked turkey
- 2 cups frozen cut green beans
- 1/2 cup all-purpose flour
- 2 teaspoons Worcestershire sauce
- DUMPLINGS:
- 1-1/2 cups all-purpose flour
- 2 teaspoons baking powder
- 1 teaspoon salt
- 2 tablespoons minced parsley
- 1/8 teaspoon poultry seasoning
- 3/4 cup 2% milk
- 1 egg

Direction

- Sauté onion, celery, and carrots in butter in a Dutch oven for 10 minutes. Add pepper, salt, 4 cups water, and consomme. Bring to a boil. Lower the heat; cook over low heat, covered until vegetables are tender, for 15 minutes.
- Add beans and turkeys; cook for 5 minutes. Stir together remaining water, Worcestershire sauce, and flour until smooth; mix into the turkey mixture. Bring to a boil. Lower the heat; simmer, covered until thickened, for 5 minutes.
- To make dumplings, combine salt, baking powder, and flour in a large bowl. Mix in poultry seasonings and parsley. Whisk egg and milk together; mix into the flour mixture until just moistened. Drop by tablespoonfuls onto the simmering stew. Simmer, covered until a toothpick comes out clean when inserted in a dumpling, for 20 minutes (do not open the pan during simmering time).

Nutrition Information

- Calories: 255 calories
- Total Carbohydrate: 24g carbohydrate (6g sugars
- Cholesterol: 68mg cholesterol
- Protein: 15g protein.
- Total Fat: 11g fat (6g saturated fat)
- Sodium: 995mg sodium
- Fiber: 3g fiber)

507. Turkey Stir Fry

Serving: 6 servings. | Prep: 10mins | Cook: 20mins | Ready in:

Ingredients

- 1-1/2 pounds boneless turkey breast halves, cut into strips
- 1 tablespoon canola oil
- 1 small onion, chopped
- 1 carrot, julienned
- 1/2 medium green pepper, sliced
- 2 cups fresh mushrooms, sliced
- 1 cup chicken broth
- 3 tablespoons cornstarch
- 3 tablespoons reduced-sodium soy sauce
- 1/2 teaspoon ground ginger
- 2 cups pea pods, trimmed
- Cooked rice, optional
- 1/3 cup cashews, optional

Direction

- Stir-fry turkey with oil in a big skillet or wok over medium-high heat for 5 to 6 minutes till not pink anymore. Take turkey out and retain warmth. Stir-fry the mushrooms, green pepper, carrot and onion for 5 minutes till crisp-tender.
- Mix the ginger, soy sauce, cornstarch and chicken broth in a small bowl. Put to skillet; cook and mix till bubbly and thickened.
- Put turkey back to skillet together with pea pods; cook and mix till heated through. If desired, serve with rice. Scatter cashews on top.

Nutrition Information

- Calories: 277 calories
- Total Fat: 7g fat (0 saturated fat)
- Sodium: 200mg sodium
- Fiber: 0 fiber)
- Total Carbohydrate: 11g carbohydrate (0 sugars
- Cholesterol: 84mg cholesterol
- Protein: 40g protein. Diabetic Exchanges: 4 lean meat

508. Turkey Stir Fry Supper

Serving: 14 servings. | Prep: 15mins | Cook: 20mins | Ready in:

Ingredients

- 2-1/4 pounds boneless skinless turkey breast
- 2 tablespoons canola oil
- 3/4 cup uncooked long grain rice
- 2 cans (14-1/2 ounces each) chicken broth, divided
- 5 tablespoons soy sauce
- 2 garlic cloves, minced
- 1/2 teaspoon ground ginger
- 1/4 teaspoon pepper
- 1 package (10 ounces) frozen broccoli spears, thawed
- 1 pound carrots, thinly sliced
- 3 bunches green onions, sliced
- 3 tablespoons cornstarch
- 1 can (14 ounces) bean sprouts, drained

Direction

- Slice turkey into 2-in. strips. Stir-fry turkey in batches in oil in a Dutch oven or wok until juices run clear, 5-7 minutes. Put turkey aside.
- Combine pepper, ginger, garlic, soy sauce, 3-1/2 cups broth and rice to pan; bring to a boil. Lower the heat; cover up and let simmer until rice is tender, 15 minutes.
- Slice broccoli into 3 in. pieces. Put onions, carrots and the broccoli to rice mixture; let simmer for 3-5 minutes. Mix together the rest of broth and cornstarch; pour into pan. Bring to a boil; cook while stirring until thickened, 2 minutes. Mix in bean sprouts and turkey; cook through.

Nutrition Information

- Calories: 233 calories
- Protein: 22g protein. Diabetic Exchanges: 2 meat
- Total Fat: 8g fat (0 saturated fat)
- Sodium: 345mg sodium
- Fiber: 0 fiber)
- Total Carbohydrate: 19g carbohydrate (0 sugars
- Cholesterol: 46mg cholesterol

509. Turkey Stroganoff With Spaghetti Squash

Serving: 6 servings. | Prep: 25mins | Cook: 15mins | Ready in:

Ingredients

- 1 medium spaghetti squash (about 4 pounds)
- 1 pound lean ground turkey
- 2 cups sliced fresh mushrooms
- 1 medium onion, chopped
- 2 garlic cloves, minced
- 1/2 cup white wine or beef stock
- 3 tablespoons cornstarch
- 2 cups beef stock
- 2 tablespoons Worcestershire sauce
- 1 tablespoon Montreal steak seasoning
- 1 teaspoon minced fresh thyme or 1/4 teaspoon dried thyme
- 1/4 cup half-and-half cream
- Grated Parmesan cheese and minced fresh parsley, optional

Direction

- Lengthwise, halve squash; discard seeds. Put squash on microwave-safe plate, cut side down. Microwave on high, uncovered, till tender for 15-18 minutes.
- Meanwhile, cook onion, mushrooms and turkey in big nonstick skillet on medium heat till turkey isn't pink; drain. Put garlic in; cook for a minute. Mix wine in.
- Mix stock and cornstarch till smooth; put into pan. Mix thyme, steak seasoning and Worcestershire sauce in; boil. Mix and cook till thick for 2 minutes. Lower heat; mix cream in and heat through.
- Use fork to separate strands when squash is cool to handle. Serve with the turkey mixture. If desired, sprinkle parsley and cheese.

Nutrition Information

- Calories: 246 calories
- Total Fat: 9g fat (3g saturated fat)
- Sodium: 677mg sodium
- Fiber: 4g fiber)
- Total Carbohydrate: 25g carbohydrate (4g sugars
- Cholesterol: 65mg cholesterol
- Protein: 17g protein. Diabetic Exchanges: 2 lean meat

510. Turkey Stuffing Roll Ups

Serving: 6 servings. | Prep: 15mins | Cook: 25mins | Ready in:

Ingredients

- 1 package (6 ounces) stuffing mix
- 1 can (10-3/4 ounces) condensed cream of chicken soup, undiluted
- 3/4 cup 2% milk
- 1 pound sliced deli smoked turkey
- 1 can (2.8 ounces) french-fried onions, crushed

Direction

- Prepare stuffing mix as directed on package. In the meantime, combine milk and soup in a small bowl; put to one side. Spread each turkey slice with about 1/4 cup of stuffing.
- Roll up; arrange in an oiled 13x9-inch baking dish. Stream soup mixture over the roll-ups. Bake without covering for 20 minutes at 350°.

Sprinkle with onions. Bake until thoroughly heated, for 5 more minutes.

Nutrition Information

- Calories:
- Sodium:
- Fiber:
- Total Carbohydrate:
- Cholesterol:
- Protein:
- Total Fat:

511. Turkey Tenderloins With Shallot Berry Sauce

Serving: 8 servings. | Prep: 15mins | Cook: 25mins | Ready in:

Ingredients

- 4 turkey breast tenderloins (12 ounces each)
- 1/2 teaspoon salt
- 1/2 teaspoon pepper
- 1 tablespoon olive oil
- 1/4 cup chicken broth
- SAUCE:
- 1 tablespoon olive oil
- 5 shallots, thinly sliced
- 1/4 teaspoon salt
- 1/4 teaspoon pepper
- 1/2 cup chicken broth
- 1/4 cup balsamic vinegar
- 3 tablespoons seedless raspberry jam

Direction

- Sprinkle pepper and salt to turkey. Heat oil over medium heat in a large skillet; cook tenderloins in batches until browned. Cover and cook for another 8 to 10 minutes until a thermometer registers 165 degrees. Take tenderloins out of the pan and keep warm.
- Pour broth into the skillet, then raise heat to medium-high heat. Cook and stir to loosen browned bits from pan; turn off the heat.
- In the meantime, heat oil over medium-high heat in a separate skillet. Add in pepper, salt and shallots; cook, stirring, until shallots are softened. Pour in broth and stir to loosen browned bits from pan. Whisk in jam and vinegar. Boil; cook and stir occasionally for 4 to 5 minutes until thickened a little.
- Cut up tenderloins and drizzle with pan juices. Serve alongside berry sauce.

Nutrition Information

- Calories: 258 calories
- Sodium: 414mg sodium
- Fiber: 0 fiber)
- Total Carbohydrate: 12g carbohydrate (8g sugars
- Cholesterol: 68mg cholesterol
- Protein: 43g protein. Diabetic Exchanges: 5 lean meat
- Total Fat: 6g fat (0 saturated fat)

512. Turkey Thyme Risotto

Serving: 4 servings. | Prep: 10mins | Cook: 35mins | Ready in:

Ingredients

- 2-3/4 to 3-1/4 cups reduced-sodium chicken broth
- 1 tablespoon olive oil
- 2 cups sliced fresh mushrooms
- 1 small onion, chopped
- 1 garlic clove, minced
- 1 cup uncooked arborio rice
- 1 teaspoon minced fresh thyme or 1/4 teaspoon dried thyme
- 1/2 cup white wine or additional broth
- 1-1/2 cups cubed cooked turkey breast
- 2 tablespoons shredded Romano cheese

- 1/4 teaspoon salt
- 1/4 teaspoon pepper

Direction

- Simmer the broth in a small saucepan; then keep it hot. Heat the oil in a large non-stick skillet on medium-high heat; sauté garlic, onion, and mushrooms for 3 minutes. Add thyme and rice; stir and cook for 2 minutes.
- Add in wine and stir. Lower the heat to keep a simmer; cook while mixing until the wine absorbs. Add 1/2 cup of the hot broth at a time, stir and cook for 20 minutes until the risotto becomes creamy, the rice becomes tender yet al dente, and broth has been absorbed after every addition, for approximately 20 minutes. Add the rest of the ingredients; stir and cook until they are heated fully. Serve right away.

Nutrition Information

- Calories: 337 calories
- Protein: 24g protein. Diabetic Exchanges: 3 starch
- Total Fat: 6g fat (2g saturated fat)
- Sodium: 651mg sodium
- Fiber: 1g fiber)
- Total Carbohydrate: 44g carbohydrate (2g sugars
- Cholesterol: 43mg cholesterol

513. Turkey Turnovers

Serving: 12 turnovers. | Prep: 40mins | Cook: 15mins | Ready in:

Ingredients

- FILLING:
- 1 cup chopped celery
- 1/4 cup chopped onion
- 1/4 cup butter, cubed
- 1/3 cup all-purpose flour
- 1 to 2 teaspoons salt
- 1/4 teaspoon pepper
- 1-1/4 cup whole milk
- 4 cups cubed cooked turkey
- 1/4 cup minced fresh parsley
- DOUGH:
- 4 cups all-purpose flour
- 1 teaspoon salt
- 1-1/2 cups cold butter
- 2 cups shredded sharp cheddar cheese
- 2 cups sour cream

Direction

- Sauté the onion and celery in butter in a large skillet until they are tender. Combine in pepper, salt, and flour. Add milk gradually. Boil; stir and cook until thicken, for 2 minutes. Add parsley and turkey. Then put aside.
- Blend salt and flour in a large bowl; mash in the butter until the mixture looks like coarse crumbs. Add in cheese and stir. Add the sour cream and mix until the dough shapes into a ball. Split the dough in half. Roll 1/2 of the dough out to an 18x12-inch rectangle. Slice into six 6-inch squares. Repeat the process with the second dough half.
- On each square, arrange 1/3 cup of the turkey filling. Fold on diagonal to shape into a triangle; press down the fork tines to seal the edges. Make slits in the top of the turnovers. Arrange on the baking sheet.
- Bake for 10 minutes at 450 degrees; lower the heat to 400 degrees. Bake until the crust turns golden brown, for 5-8 more minutes.

Nutrition Information

- Calories: 644 calories
- Sodium: 852mg sodium
- Fiber: 2g fiber)
- Total Carbohydrate: 38g carbohydrate (4g sugars
- Cholesterol: 157mg cholesterol
- Protein: 25g protein.
- Total Fat: 42g fat (27g saturated fat)

514. Turkey Vegetable Skillet

Serving: 6 servings. | Prep: 15mins | Cook: 5mins | Ready in:

Ingredients

- 1 pound ground turkey breast
- 1 small onion, chopped
- 1 teaspoon canola oil
- 1 garlic clove, minced
- 1 pound fresh tomatoes, chopped
- 1/4 pound zucchini, diced
- 1/4 cup chopped dill pickle
- 1 teaspoon dried basil
- 1/2 teaspoon pepper

Direction

- Cook the onion and turkey in a big skillet in oil on medium heat, until the turkey has no visible pink color anymore. Add the garlic and let it cook for 1 minute more. Let it drain if needed. Add the leftover ingredients. Lower the heat and let it simmer for 5-10 minutes without a cover or until it is heated through.

Nutrition Information

- Calories: 135 calories
- Protein: 21g protein. Diabetic Exchanges: 3 lean meat
- Total Fat: 3g fat (0 saturated fat)
- Sodium: 104mg sodium
- Fiber: 0 fiber)
- Total Carbohydrate: 5g carbohydrate (0 sugars
- Cholesterol: 47mg cholesterol

515. Turkey Wafflewiches

Serving: 4 servings. | Prep: 10mins | Cook: 5mins | Ready in:

Ingredients

- 3 ounces cream cheese, softened
- 1/4 cup whole-berry cranberry sauce
- 1 tablespoon maple pancake syrup
- 1/4 teaspoon pepper
- 8 slices white bread
- 3/4 pound sliced deli turkey
- 2 tablespoons butter, softened

Direction

- Beat pepper, syrup, cranberry sauce and cream cheese until combined in a small bowl. Spread over 4 slices of bread; put turkey and the leftover bread on top. Over both sides of sandwiches, spread butter.
- According to directions of manufacturer, cook in a preheated indoor grill or waffle iron for 2-3 minutes or until turning golden brown.

Nutrition Information

- Calories: 407 calories
- Sodium: 1179mg sodium
- Fiber: 2g fiber)
- Total Carbohydrate: 41g carbohydrate (10g sugars
- Cholesterol: 67mg cholesterol
- Protein: 23g protein.
- Total Fat: 17g fat (8g saturated fat)

516. Turkey With Rye Dressing

Serving: 10-12 servings (11 cups stuffing). | Prep: 20mins | Cook: 04hours30mins | Ready in:

Ingredients

- 1 pound day-old light rye bread, cubed
- 1/2 pound day-old dark rye bread, cubed
- 1-1/2 cups chopped onion
- 2 large tart apples, peeled and chopped
- 1 cup chopped celery
- 4 garlic cloves, minced
- 1/2 cup butter, cubed
- 3/4 cup chopped salted mixed nuts
- 2 tablespoons dried parsley flakes
- 2 teaspoons salt
- 2 teaspoons dried thyme
- 1-1/2 teaspoons rubbed sage
- 3/4 teaspoon dried rosemary, crushed
- 1/2 teaspoon pepper
- 1/4 teaspoon ground nutmeg
- 3 to 3-1/2 cups chicken broth
- 1 turkey (12 to 14 pounds)
- 2 tablespoons canola oil

Direction

- In a large bowl, toss the bread cubes. Sauté garlic, celery, apples, and onion in butter in a skillet until the vegetables and apples become tender; add to the bread. Add seasonings, nuts, and sufficient broth to moisten.
- Fill the turkey just before baking. Fasten the openings using a skewer and tie the drumsticks together. In a roasting pan, arrange turkey on a rack. Brush with some oil. Use a tent of foil to lightly cover.
- Bake at 325 degrees, brushing with oil from to time, until a thermometer registers 185 degrees, 4 1/2-5 hours. Take all the stuffing away.

Nutrition Information

- Calories:
- Sodium:
- Fiber:
- Total Carbohydrate:
- Cholesterol:
- Protein:
- Total Fat:

---

517. Turkey A La King With Rice

Serving: 4 servings. | Prep: 15mins | Cook: 15mins | Ready in:

Ingredients

- 2 tablespoons butter
- 1-3/4 cups sliced fresh mushrooms
- 1 celery rib, chopped
- 1/4 cup chopped onion
- 1/4 cup chopped green pepper
- 1/4 cup all-purpose flour
- 1 cup reduced-sodium chicken broth
- 1 cup fat-free milk
- 2 cups cubed cooked turkey breast
- 1 cup frozen peas
- 1/2 teaspoon salt
- 2 cups hot cooked rice

Direction

- In a large nonstick skillet over medium-high heat, heat butter. Put in pepper, onion, celery and mushrooms; cook while stirring till tender.
- Mix broth with flour till smooth in a small bowl; mix into the vegetable mixture. Mix in milk. Allow to boil; cook while stirring till thickened, 1-2 minutes. Put in salt, peas and turkey; heat through. Serve over rice.

Nutrition Information

- Calories: 350 calories
- Protein: 30g protein. Diabetic Exchanges: 3 lean meat
- Total Fat: 7g fat (4g saturated fat)
- Sodium: 594mg sodium
- Fiber: 3g fiber)
- Total Carbohydrate: 40g carbohydrate (7g sugars
- Cholesterol: 76mg cholesterol

518. Turkey And Mushroom Potpies

Serving: 8 servings. | Prep: 40mins | Cook: 20mins | Ready in:

Ingredients

- 4-1/3 cups sliced baby portobello mushrooms
- 1 large onion, chopped
- 1 tablespoon olive oil
- 2-1/2 cups cubed cooked turkey
- 1 package (16 ounces) frozen peas and carrots
- 1/4 teaspoon salt
- 1/4 teaspoon pepper
- 1/4 cup cornstarch
- 2-1/2 cups chicken broth
- 1/4 cup sour cream
- TOPPING:
- 1-1/2 cups all-purpose flour
- 2 teaspoons sugar
- 1-1/2 teaspoons baking powder
- 1 teaspoon dried thyme
- 1/4 teaspoon baking soda
- 1/4 teaspoon salt
- 2 tablespoons cold butter
- 1 cup buttermilk
- 1 tablespoon canola oil

Direction

- Set oven to 400° to preheat. Sauté onion and mushrooms in oil in a Dutch oven until softened. Mix in pepper, salt, carrots, peas, and turkey. Stir together broth and cornstarch until smooth; slowly mix into the pan. Bring everything in the pan to a boil. Lower heat; cook for 2 minutes, stirring, until thickened. Mix in sour cream, pour mixture into 8 greased 8-ounce ramekins.
- Mix salt, baking soda, thyme, baking powder, sugar, and flour together in a large mixing bowl. Cut in butter until mixture is coarse and crumbly. Stir oil and buttermilk together in a small mixing bowl; mix into dry ingredients just until moistened. Drop mixture over filling by heaping teaspoonfuls.
- Bake without a cover for 20 to 25 minutes in the preheated oven until filling is bubbly and topping turns golden brown. Allow to cool for 5 minutes before serving.

Nutrition Information

- Calories: 314 calories
- Sodium: 701mg sodium
- Fiber: 3g fiber)
- Total Carbohydrate: 34g carbohydrate (8g sugars
- Cholesterol: 49mg cholesterol
- Protein: 20g protein. Diabetic Exchanges: 2 starch
- Total Fat: 11g fat (4g saturated fat)

519. Turkey In Cream Sauce

Serving: 8 servings. | Prep: 20mins | Cook: 07hours00mins | Ready in:

Ingredients

- 1-1/4 cups white wine or chicken broth
- 1 medium onion, chopped
- 2 garlic cloves, minced
- 2 bay leaves
- 2 teaspoons dried rosemary, crushed
- 1/2 teaspoon pepper
- 3 turkey breast tenderloins (3/4 pound each)
- 3 tablespoons cornstarch
- 1/2 cup half-and-half cream or whole milk
- 1/2 teaspoon salt

Direction

- Mix bay leaves, garlic, onion, and wine together in a 3-quart slow cooker. Mix together pepper and rosemary; rub onto the turkey. Put in the slow cooker. Put the lid on and cook on low until the turkey is soft, about 7-9 hours.

- Transfer the turkey to a serving dish, keep warm. Strain and remove the fat from the cooking juices; transfer to a small saucepan. Boil the liquid. Mix together salt, cream, and cornstarch until smooth. Slowly mix into the pan. Boil it, stir and cook until thickened, about 2 minutes. Enjoy with the turkey.

Nutrition Information

- Calories: 205 calories
- Total Carbohydrate: 6g carbohydrate (1g sugars
- Cholesterol: 58mg cholesterol
- Protein: 32g protein. Diabetic Exchanges: 4 lean meat
- Total Fat: 3g fat (1g saturated fat)
- Sodium: 231mg sodium
- Fiber: 0 fiber)

520. Turkey In Mushroom Sauce

Serving: 6 servings. | Prep: 20mins | Cook: 01hours30mins | Ready in:

Ingredients

- 3/4 cup all-purpose flour
- 2 teaspoons salt
- 1/4 teaspoon pepper
- 6 turkey thighs (4 to 5 pounds)
- 3 tablespoons vegetable oil
- 2 cups chopped fresh mushrooms
- 3 green onions, sliced
- 1-1/2 teaspoons dried thyme
- 2 cups turkey or chicken broth
- 1/3 cup tomato paste
- 1 cup (8 ounces) sour cream
- Hot cooked noodles

Direction

- Mix pepper, salt, and flour in a resealable plastic bag or bowl. Add 1 piece of turkey at a time; shake or dredge to coat.
- Brown the turkey in the oil in a skillet. Add thyme, onions, and mushrooms. Mix tomato paste and broth until smooth; pour on the turkey.
- Put a cover and let simmer until juices from the turkey run clear, for 1 1/2 hours; then remove the fat. Add in sour cream and stir; heat fully without bringing to a boil. Serve on top of noodles.

Nutrition Information

- Calories: 464 calories
- Protein: 49g protein.
- Total Fat: 20g fat (7g saturated fat)
- Sodium: 1252mg sodium
- Fiber: 2g fiber)
- Total Carbohydrate: 19g carbohydrate (5g sugars
- Cholesterol: 205mg cholesterol

521. Turkey In The Strawganoff

Serving: 6-8 servings. | Prep: 5mins | Cook: 25mins | Ready in:

Ingredients

- 1 cup chopped onion
- 1/2 cup butter
- 2 garlic cloves, minced
- 1/4 cup all-purpose flour
- 1 to 2 teaspoons salt
- 1/2 teaspoon pepper
- 2 cans (10-3/4 ounces each) condensed cream of chicken soup, undiluted
- 4 cups cubed cooked turkey
- 1 can (8 ounces) mushroom stems and pieces, drained
- 2 cups sour cream

- 1/4 cup plus 2 tablespoons minced fresh parsley, divided
- 1 pound fine noodles, cooked
- 1 tablespoon diced pimientos, drained

Direction

- Sauté onion in butter in a large skillet. Stir in garlic; sauté for 2 more minutes. Mix in pepper, salt, and flour until well combined. Add mushrooms, turkey, and soup. Bring to a boil. Lower the heat; simmer without covering for 10 minutes. Mix in 1/4 cup parsley and sour cream; cook, stirring constantly, for 6 minutes. Spoon mixture over noodles. Sprinkle with remaining parsley and pimientos to garnish.

Nutrition Information

- Calories:
- Total Fat:
- Sodium:
- Fiber:
- Total Carbohydrate:
- Cholesterol:
- Protein:

522. Turkey With Cornbread Dressing

Serving: 8-10 servings. | Prep: 20mins | Cook: 03hours30mins | Ready in:

Ingredients

- 2 cups chopped celery
- 1 cup chopped onion
- 1/2 cup butter
- 6 cups cubed day-old cornbread
- 2 cups fresh bread crumbs
- 1 tablespoon dried sage
- 1 tablespoon poultry seasoning
- 1/2 cup egg substitute
- 1 cup chicken broth
- 1 turkey (10 to 12 pounds)
- Melted butter

Direction

- Stir-fry the celery and onion with butter in a frying pan until tender. Combine crumbs, cornbread, poultry seasoning and sage in a big bowl. Mix together the egg substitute and broth. Mix in the corn bread mixture while stirring gently.
- Just before baking, fill the inside of the neck and body cavity with the dressing. Fasten or skewer the openings then tie the drumstick together. Place on a rack in a roasting pan. Apply melted butter. Let it cook in the oven for about 3 and a half to 4 hours at 350°F or if the turkey reaches 180°F using a thermometer and the stuffing reads 165°F. Use an aluminum foil to tent lightly the turkey when it begins to turn brown. Once the turkey is cooked, let it sit for about 20 minutes before serving and transfer all the dressing into a serving bowl.

Nutrition Information

- Calories: 663 calories
- Total Carbohydrate: 34g carbohydrate (3g sugars
- Cholesterol: 202mg cholesterol
- Protein: 72g protein.
- Total Fat: 25g fat (11g saturated fat)
- Sodium: 845mg sodium
- Fiber: 3g fiber)

523. Turkey With Country Ham Stuffing

Serving: 10-12 servings. | Prep: 45mins | Cook: 04hours30mins | Ready in:

Ingredients

- 3 cups cubed day-old white bread, crust removed
- 3 cups cubed day-old whole wheat bread, crust removed
- 1-1/2 cups cubed fully cooked ham
- 1/2 cup butter, cubed
- 3 cups chopped onion
- 2 cups chopped celery
- 1-1/2 teaspoons rubbed sage
- 1-1/2 teaspoons dried thyme
- 1/2 teaspoon pepper
- 1 to 1-1/2 cups chicken broth
- 1 turkey (12 to 14 pounds)

Direction

- In a 13x 9-inch baking pan, arrange bread cubes in a single layer. Bake at 325 degrees, stirring once in a while, until they turn golden brown or 20-25 minutes. Arrange in a large bowl; then put aside.
- Cook the ham in butter in a large skillet until the edges become crisp or 5-10 minutes. Use a slotted spoon to take it out and put on top of the bread cubes.
- Sauté pepper, thyme, sage, celery, and onion in the same skillet until the vegetables become tender; toss together with ham and bread. Pour in enough broth and stir to moisten.
- Fill the turkey just before baking. Secure the openings with skewer and tie together the drumsticks. In a roasting pan, arrange it on a rack. Bake at 325 degrees until thermometer registers 185 degrees or 4 1/2-5 hours.
- Use a tent of aluminum foil to cover lightly and baste if necessary, once the turkey starts to brown. Before removing the filling and carving the turkey, put a cover on the turkey and allow to stand for 20 minutes.

Nutrition Information

- Calories: 691 calories
- Total Carbohydrate: 14g carbohydrate (4g sugars
- Cholesterol: 275mg cholesterol
- Protein: 78g protein.

- Total Fat: 34g fat (12g saturated fat)
- Sodium: 666mg sodium
- Fiber: 2g fiber)

524. Turkey With Cranberry Sauce

Serving: 4 servings. | Prep: 10mins | Cook: 25mins | Ready in:

Ingredients

- 2 turkey breast tenderloins (1 to 1-1/2 pounds)
- 1/2 teaspoon poultry seasoning
- 1 tablespoon vegetable oil
- 1 tablespoon butter
- 1 cup whole-berry cranberry sauce
- 3 tablespoons apple jelly
- 3/4 teaspoon Dijon mustard
- 1/4 teaspoon ground allspice

Direction

- Slice tenderloins in half along the width. Cut each half in half along the length, but don't slice all the way through. Open each piece and flatten. Dust the poultry seasoning over both sides. Cook the turkey in butter and oil in a large skillet on medium-high heat for 3-4 minutes per side. Lower the heat to medium-low; put a cover and cook until juices run clear, for 12-15 minutes. Transfer the turkey onto a platter and keep it warm. Add allspice, mustard, jelly, and the cranberry sauce into the skillet; let simmer for 2-3 minutes. Scoop on the turkey.

Nutrition Information

- Calories: 314 calories
- Sodium: 128mg sodium
- Fiber: 1g fiber)
- Total Carbohydrate: 36g carbohydrate (26g sugars

- Cholesterol: 63mg cholesterol
- Protein: 27g protein.
- Total Fat: 8g fat (3g saturated fat)

525. Turkey With Herbed Rice Dressing

Serving: 8-10 servings. | Prep: 25mins | Cook: 04hours00mins | Ready in:

Ingredients

- 1/2 pound Jones No Sugar Pork Sausage Roll sausage
- 1/2 pound ground beef
- 1/2 cup chopped onion
- 1/2 cup egg substitute
- 1 tablespoon poultry seasoning
- 2 tablespoons chopped fresh parsley
- 2 tablespoons chopped celery leaves
- 2 teaspoons salt, divided
- 2 teaspoons pepper, divided
- 3/4 teaspoon garlic powder, divided
- 4 cups cooked white rice, cooled
- 3 garlic cloves, minced
- 1 teaspoon each dried thyme, tarragon and marjoram
- 1 turkey (10 to 12 pounds)
- 2 cans (14-1/2 ounces each) chicken broth
- 3 tablespoons butter

Direction

- Cook onion, beef, and pork in a large skillet on medium heat until the meat is not pink anymore; then drain. Mix 1/2 teaspoon of garlic powder, a teaspoon of pepper, a teaspoon of salt, celery leaves, parsley, poultry seasoning, and egg substitute in a large bowl. Add rice and the meat mixture.
- Stuff the turkey just before baking. Skewer the openings; then tie together the drumsticks. Arrange onto a rack set in a roasting pan. Mix remaining garlic powder, remaining pepper, remaining salt, marjoram, tarragon, thyme, and garlic; rub on the turkey. Add butter and broth into the pan.
- Bake at 325 degrees, basting often, until a thermometer registers 165 degrees for stuffing and 180 degrees for the turkey, for 4-4 1/2 hours. Cover the turkey loosely in a tent of aluminum foil if it starts to brown. Then remove all of the dressing.

Nutrition Information

- Calories: 749 calories
- Protein: 82g protein.
- Total Fat: 35g fat (12g saturated fat)
- Sodium: 974mg sodium
- Fiber: 1g fiber)
- Total Carbohydrate: 21g carbohydrate (2g sugars
- Cholesterol: 278mg cholesterol

526. Turkey With Mushroom Sauce

Serving: 8 servings. | Prep: 20mins | Cook: 03hours00mins | Ready in:

Ingredients

- 1 boneless skinless turkey breast half (2-1/2 pounds)
- 2 tablespoons butter, melted
- 2 tablespoons dried parsley flakes
- 1/2 teaspoon salt
- 1/2 teaspoon dried tarragon
- 1/8 teaspoon pepper
- 1 jar (4-1/2 ounces) sliced mushrooms, drained, or 1 cup sliced fresh mushrooms
- 1/2 cup white wine or chicken broth
- 2 tablespoons cornstarch
- 1/4 cup cold water

Direction

- Use a five-quart slow cooker, put in turkey then brush it with melted butter; sprinkle the seasonings on the turkey. Add mushrooms on top then pour wine over the turkey. Cook for 3-4hrs on low with a cover on until an inserted thermometer in the turkey registers 165 degrees F at least.
- Move to a serving platter then tent the turkey with foil. Before slicing and serving, let it rest for 10 minutes.
- Pour the cooking juices into a small pot and boil. Combine water and cornstarch in a small bowl until smooth; stir in the cooking juices gradually then boil. Cook for 2 minutes while stirring constantly for 2mins until it thickened. Serve sauce with the turkey.

Nutrition Information

- Calories:
- Fiber:
- Total Carbohydrate:
- Cholesterol:
- Protein:
- Total Fat:
- Sodium:

527. Turkey With Sausage Stuffing

Serving: 10-14 servings. | Prep: 30mins | Cook: 02hours00mins | Ready in:

Ingredients

- 1 bone-in turkey breast (5 to 7 pounds)
- 1/4 cup butter, melted
- 1-1/2 pounds Jones No Sugar Pork Sausage Roll sausage
- 2 cups sliced celery
- 2 medium onions, chopped
- 4 cups dry bread cubes
- 2 cups pecan halves
- 1 cup raisins
- 2/3 cup chicken broth
- 2 eggs, beaten
- 1 teaspoon salt
- 1/2 teaspoon rubbed sage
- 1/4 teaspoon pepper

Direction

- In a shallow roasting pan, arrange the turkey breast side up. Use butter to brush it. Bake uncovered at 325 degrees until a thermometer registers 170 degrees or 2-2 1/2 hours (if needed, use foil to loosely cover to avoid over-browning).
- At the same time, cook onions, celery, and sausage in a large skillet on medium heat until the meat is not pink anymore; let drain. Place into a bowl; stir in pepper, sage, salt, eggs, broth, raisins, pecans, and bread cubes.
- Scoop into a 3-quart baking dish that's greased. Put a cover on and bake for an hour at 325 degrees.
- Before cutting, allow the turkey to stand for 10 minutes. Serve together with filling.

Nutrition Information

- Calories:
- Cholesterol:
- Protein:
- Total Fat:
- Sodium:
- Fiber:
- Total Carbohydrate:

528. Turkey With Sausage Pecan Stuffing

Serving: 12 servings (12 cups stuffing). | Prep: 25mins | Cook: 03hours30mins | Ready in:

Ingredients

- 4 medium onions

- 1 pound Jones No Sugar Pork Sausage Roll
- 2 packages (6 ounces each) herb stuffing mix
- 1 package (15 ounces) golden raisins
- 1 cup pecan halves
- 6 celery ribs, diced
- 1/4 teaspoon each dried basil, oregano, curry powder, caraway seeds, poultry seasoning, garlic powder, salt and pepper
- 2-1/2 cups chicken broth
- 1 turkey (12 to 14 pounds)

Direction

- Set an oven to 325 degrees and start preheating. Cut 2 onions; then put aside. Chop the rest of the onions.
- Cook the chopped onions and sausage in a large skillet on medium heat, crumbling the sausages, until the sausage is not pink anymore. Add the herb packets from the stuffing mixes. Stir in the seasonings, celery, pecans, and raisins. Boil. Lower the heat; let simmer with no cover for 10 minutes. Add broth and the stuffing mixes; stir thoroughly. Stir and cook for 5 minutes.
- Fill the turkey with the saved onions. Stuff the turkey lightly with 6-7 cups of the stuffing. In a greased 1 1/2-quart baking dish, put the rest of the stuffing; store in the fridge until it is ready to bake. Tuck the wings under the turkey; tie together drumsticks. Arrange, breast side up, onto a rack set in a shallow roasting pan.
- Roast with no cover until a thermometer inserted into the center of the stuffing registers 165 degrees and at least 170 degrees for the thigh, for 3 1/2-4 hours. If the turkey browns too fast, cover lightly in foil. Put a cover on the rest of the stuffing and bake for an hour. Remove the cover and bake for 10 minutes.
- Take the turkey out of oven; cover in foil. Before carving, allow to stand for 20 minutes. Thicken the pan drippings and remove the fat for the gravy if desired. Serve along with the stuffing and turkey.

Nutrition Information

- Calories:
- Sodium:
- Fiber:
- Total Carbohydrate:
- Cholesterol:
- Protein:
- Total Fat:

529. Turkey Stuffed Peppers

Serving: 4 | Prep: 20mins | Cook: 35mins | Ready in:

Ingredients

- 2 large red bell peppers, tops and seeds removed and halved lengthwise
- 2 tablespoons olive oil
- 1 pound ground turkey
- 2 small onions, chopped
- 1 (4 ounce) package sliced fresh mushrooms
- 6 cloves garlic, minced
- 2 tablespoons butter
- 2 tablespoons all-purpose flour
- 1 teaspoon salt
- 1/4 teaspoon ground black pepper
- 1 cup milk
- 1 teaspoon half-and-half, or to taste
- 1 cup chopped tomatoes
- 1/2 cup shredded Cheddar cheese, divided
- 1/2 cup shredded Parmesan cheese
- 1/2 cup panko (Japanese bread crumbs)

Direction

- Set the oven to 350°F (175°C) for preheating. Grease the 1-qt baking dish.
- Boil water in a large saucepan. Cook the peppers in boiling water for 3 minutes until they are slightly tender. Drain the peppers and wash them with cold water until cooled.
- Put oil in a skillet and heat it over medium heat. Cook the ground turkey, garlic, onions, and mushrooms in hot oil until the turkey is

evenly browned; strain grease from the turkey blend. Pour the drained turkey mixture in a bowl. Place the skillet back into the medium heat.
- In the skillet, melt the butter and add the salt, black pepper, and flour; stir until smooth. Pour the half-and-half and milk into the flour mixture while stirring it. Bring the mixture to a boil. Cook and stir the mixture for 1-2 minutes until thickened. Place the turkey mixture back into the skillet. Add 2 tbsp. of Cheddar cheese and tomatoes. Cook and stir the turkey mixture for 3 minutes until the cheese is completely melted and hot. Spoon the mixture into the bell pepper halves. Arrange the stuffed pepper halves into the prepared baking dish and top them with the Parmesan cheese, panko, and remaining Cheddar cheese. Use an aluminum foil to cover the dish.
- Let it bake inside the preheated oven for 25-30 minutes until the filling is hot and the peppers are tender.
- Switch the oven to broil. Remove the foil from the dish. Cook the peppers under the broiler for 5 minutes until the panko is browned.

Nutrition Information

- Calories: 519 calories;
- Sodium: 1028
- Total Carbohydrate: 28.3
- Cholesterol: 128
- Protein: 36.5
- Total Fat: 30.9

530. Upside Down Frito Pie

Serving: 6 servings. | Prep: 15mins | Cook: 02hours00mins | Ready in:

Ingredients

- 2 pounds ground turkey or beef
- 1 medium onion, chopped
- 2 envelopes chili seasoning mix
- 1 can (10 ounces) diced tomatoes and green chilies, undrained
- 1 can (8 ounces) tomato sauce
- 1 can (15 ounces) pinto beans, rinsed and drained
- 1 cup shredded cheddar cheese
- 3 cups corn chips
- Sour cream, minced fresh cilantro and additional chopped onion, optional

Direction

- Cook onion along with turkey on medium heat for 8-10 minutes in a big skillet, until it isn't pink anymore. Break into crumbles and stir in chili seasoning. Turn it to 3- or 4-qt. slow cooker. Add tomato sauce and tomatoes over turkey.
- Cook with a cover on low for 2-3 hours until heated through. Combine turkey mixture by stirring it. Put beans on top. Dredge in cheese. Cover and cook for 5-10 minutes until cheese is melted. Add chips on top. If wanted, serve with additional onion, minced cilantro and sour cream.

Nutrition Information

- Calories: 524 calories
- Total Carbohydrate: 33g carbohydrate (5g sugars
- Cholesterol: 118mg cholesterol
- Protein: 41g protein.
- Total Fat: 26g fat (8g saturated fat)
- Sodium: 1662mg sodium
- Fiber: 6g fiber)

531. Waffle Monte Cristos

Serving: 4 servings. | Prep: 10mins | Cook: 10mins | Ready in:

Ingredients

- 1/2 cup apricot preserves
- 8 frozen waffles
- 4 slices deli turkey
- 4 slices deli ham
- 4 slices Havarti cheese (about 3 ounces)
- 4 bacon strips, cooked
- 2 tablespoons butter, softened
- Maple syrup

Direction

- Set the griddle over moderate heat. Spread over 4 waffles with the preserves, then layer with turkey, ham, cheese and bacon. Put the leftover waffles on top and spread outsides of waffles slightly with butter.
- Put on the griddle and cook until heated through and golden brown, about 4 to 5 minutes per side. Serve together with syrup as dipping.

Nutrition Information

- Calories: 511 calories
- Protein: 21g protein.
- Total Fat: 23g fat (10g saturated fat)
- Sodium: 1163mg sodium
- Fiber: 2g fiber)
- Total Carbohydrate: 57g carbohydrate (22g sugars
- Cholesterol: 70mg cholesterol

532. Waldorf Turkey Sandwiches

Serving: 4 servings. | Prep: 15mins | Cook: 0mins | Ready in:

Ingredients

- 1/4 cup finely chopped celery
- 3 tablespoons fat-free mayonnaise
- 2 tablespoons fat-free plain yogurt
- 2 tablespoons chopped walnuts
- 1 tablespoon raisins
- 1/8 teaspoon ground nutmeg
- 1/8 teaspoon ground cinnamon
- 1-1/4 cups cubed cooked turkey breast
- 1 small apple, chopped
- 8 slices cinnamon-raisin bread, toasted
- 4 lettuce leaves

Direction

- Mix the first 7 ingredients together in a large bowl. Add apple and turkey, mix to combine. Put a cover on and put in the fridge to chill for a minimum of 1 hour. Put 3/4 cup of turkey mixture on 4 slices of bread, put lettuce leaf and the rest of the bread on top.

Nutrition Information

- Calories: 127 calories
- Fiber: 0 fiber)
- Total Carbohydrate: 9g carbohydrate (0 sugars
- Cholesterol: 26mg cholesterol
- Protein: 12g protein. Diabetic Exchanges: 1-1/2 lean meat
- Total Fat: 5g fat (0 saturated fat)
- Sodium: 114mg sodium

533. Zesty Turkey

Serving: 6 servings. | Prep: 15mins | Cook: 02hours00mins | Ready in:

Ingredients

- 2 tablespoons rubbed sage
- 1 tablespoon pepper
- 2 teaspoons curry powder
- 2 teaspoons garlic powder
- 2 teaspoons dried parsley flakes
- 2 teaspoons celery seed
- 1 teaspoon paprika
- 1/2 teaspoon ground mustard
- 1/4 teaspoon ground allspice

- 3 to 4 bay leaves, crumbled
- 1 turkey breast (4 to 4-1/2 pounds)
- 2 cups reduced-sodium chicken broth

Direction

- Mix spices together and combine well in a small bowl. Position turkey on a rack in a roasting pan; rub roast with spice mixture. Pour broth into the pan. Bake for 2 to 3 hours at 350° or until a thermometer reaches 170°, basting after each 30 minutes.

Nutrition Information

- Calories: 187 calories
- Fiber: 0 fiber)
- Total Carbohydrate: 3g carbohydrate (0 sugars
- Cholesterol: 69mg cholesterol
- Protein: 32g protein. Diabetic Exchanges: 3-1/2 lean meat.
- Total Fat: 4g fat (0 saturated fat)
- Sodium: 85mg sodium

534. Zippy Turkey Tortilla Bake

Serving: 8 | Prep: 10mins | Cook: 25mins | Ready in:

Ingredients

- 1 small onion, finely chopped
- 1/2 teaspoon garlic powder
- 1 teaspoon vegetable oil
- 1 pound lean ground turkey
- 1 tablespoon vinegar
- 2 teaspoons chili powder
- 1 1/2 teaspoons dried oregano
- 1/2 teaspoon ground cumin
- 1/4 teaspoon cayenne pepper
- 1 (15 ounce) can black beans, rinsed and drained
- 1 (16 ounce) jar salsa
- 3/4 cup reduced-sodium chicken broth
- 8 (8 inch) fat-free tortillas
- 1/2 cup shredded reduced-fat Monterey Jack cheese
- 1/3 cup reduced-fat sour cream

Direction

- Sauté garlic powder and onion in oil in a skillet until onion is softened. Add cayenne, cumin, oregano, chili powder, vinegar and turkey; cook over medium heat until pink color no longer remains, remember to stir while cooking. Stir in beans. Remove from the heat. Coat a 2-1/2qt baking dish with nonstick cooking spray. Combine broth and salsa and pour in the prepared baking dish to create a thin layer. Slice tortillas into 1 inch strips then into thirds; place half of them on top of salsa mixture. Arrange half of the turkey mixture and half of remaining salsa mixture on top. Repeat layering with remaining ingredients. Add cheese on top. Bake at 350°F, covered, for 25 minutes or until bubbles appear on top. Serve with sour cream on top.

Nutrition Information

Chapter 4: Turkey Appetizer Recipes

***

535. After Christmas Empanadas

Serving: about 1-1/2 dozen. | Prep: 30mins | Cook: 15mins | Ready in:

Ingredients

- 1 cup cubed cooked turkey
- 1/2 cup cooked stuffing
- 2 tablespoons whole-berry cranberry sauce
- 2 tablespoons turkey gravy
- 2 packages (14.1 ounces each) refrigerated pie pastry
- 1 large egg
- 1 tablespoon water
- Rubbed sage, optional
- Additional turkey gravy or whole-berry cranberry sauce, optional

Direction

- Preheat an oven to 400°. Mix gravy, cranberry sauce, stuffing and turkey in small bowl.
- Unroll a pastry on lightly floured surface. Roll out to 12-in. circle. Use 4-in. floured biscuit cutter to cut. Repeat with leftover pastry.
- Whisk water and egg in small bowl; brush on pastry circles' edges. On 1 side, put 1 tablespoon filing. Fold dough on filling. Use fork to press edges to seal.
- Put on greased baking sheets, 2-in. apart. Brush leftover egg mixture on tops. If desired, sprinkle sage. Bake till golden brown or for 12-15 minutes. Serve warm with cranberry sauce/gravy if desired. Freezing: In resealable plastic freezer bags, freeze cooled pastries. Using: On greased baking sheet, reheat pastries in preheated 400° oven till heated through and lightly browned or for 8-10 minutes.

Nutrition Information

- Calories:
- Total Carbohydrate:
- Cholesterol:
- Protein:
- Total Fat:
- Sodium:
- Fiber:

536. Appetizer Roll Ups

Serving: 6-7 dozen. | Prep: 20mins | Cook: 0mins | Ready in:

Ingredients

- ROAST BEEF ROLL-UPS:
- 4 ounces cream cheese, softened
- 1/4 cup minced fresh cilantro
- 2 to 3 tablespoons minced banana peppers
- 1 garlic clove, minced
- 1/2 pound thinly sliced cooked roast beef
- HAM AND TURKEY ROLL-UPS:
- 12 ounces cream cheese, softened
- 1/2 cup shredded carrot
- 1/2 cup shredded zucchini
- 4 teaspoons dill weed
- 1/2 pound thinly sliced fully cooked ham
- 1/2 pound thinly sliced cooked turkey

Direction

- Mix garlic, peppers, cilantro and cream cheese in a small bowl. On every beef slice, spread 2 tbsp. Tightly roll up; use plastic to wrap.
- Ham and turkey rolls: mix dill, zucchini, carrot and cream cheese in another bowl. On every slice of turkey and ham, spread 2 tbsp. Tightly roll up. Use plastic to wrap. Refrigerate overnight.
- Cut rollups to 1 – 1/2-in. pieces.

Nutrition Information

- Calories: 96 calories
- Sodium: 213mg sodium
- Fiber: 0 fiber)
- Total Carbohydrate: 1g carbohydrate (0 sugars
- Cholesterol: 33mg cholesterol
- Protein: 7g protein.
- Total Fat: 7g fat (4g saturated fat)

537. Asparagus Pepperoni Triangles

Serving: 3 dozen. | Prep: 30mins | Cook: 10mins | Ready in:

Ingredients

- 2/3 cup part-skim ricotta cheese
- 1 large egg yolk
- 1-1/2 ounces sliced turkey pepperoni, chopped
- 6 tablespoons grated Parmesan cheese
- 1/4 cup minced fresh basil or 4 teaspoons dried basil
- 4-1/2 teaspoons minced chives
- 4-1/2 teaspoons minced fresh parsley
- Dash pepper
- 1 cup water
- 1/2 pound fresh asparagus, trimmed and cut into 1/2-inch pieces
- 1 green onion, chopped
- 3 garlic cloves, minced
- 2 teaspoons plus 3 tablespoons butter, divided
- 12 sheets phyllo dough (14x9 inches)
- Butter-flavored cooking spray

Direction

- Mix initial 8 ingredients in big bowl; put aside. Boil water in small saucepan. Add asparagus; cover. Boil for 3 minutes and drain. Put asparagus in ice water immediately. Drain. Pat dry.
- Cook garlic and onion in 2 teaspoons butter in small nonstick skillet on medium heat till just tender or for 2 minutes. Add into ricotta mixture; mix asparagus in. Melt leftover butter; put aside.
- On work surface, put 1 phyllo dough sheet, short end facing you. Cover leftover phyllo with plastic wrap to avoid drying out. Spray butter-flavored spray on sheet; cut to 3 14x3-in. strips. On lower corner of every strip, put scant tablespoon asparagus mixture. Fold dough on filling, making a triangle. Fold the triangle up; fold triangle over, making another triangle. Keep folding like a flag till you reach strip's end.
- Brush butter on dough's end. Press on triangle to seal. Flip triangle. Brush melted butter on top; repeat with leftover filling and phyllo.
- Put triangles onto baking sheets coated in cooking spray. Bake for 10-12 minutes or till golden brown at 375°. Serve warm

Nutrition Information

- Calories: 36 calories
- Protein: 2g protein. Diabetic Exchanges: 1/2 fat.
- Total Fat: 2g fat (1g saturated fat)
- Sodium: 71mg sodium
- Fiber: 0 fiber)
- Total Carbohydrate: 3g carbohydrate (0 sugars
- Cholesterol: 13mg cholesterol

538. BBQ Turkey Meatballs

Serving: about 4 dozen. | Prep: 45mins | Cook: 03hours00mins | Ready in:

Ingredients

- 1 large egg, lightly beaten
- 2/3 cup soft bread crumbs
- 1/4 cup finely chopped onion
- 1/2 teaspoon pepper
- 2 pounds ground turkey
- SAUCE:
- 1 bottle (20 ounces) ketchup
- 1/4 cup packed brown sugar
- 2 tablespoons Worcestershire sauce
- 1 teaspoon garlic salt
- 1/2 to 1 teaspoon hot pepper sauce

Direction

- Preheat an oven to 375°. Mix pepper, onion, breadcrumbs and eggs; add turkey. Lightly but thoroughly mix. Form to 1-inch balls. Put

on a 15x10x1-inch greased pan. Bake for 15-20 minutes till lightly browned.
- Put meatballs in a 3-quart slow cooker. Stir sauce ingredients; put on top. Cook on low, covered, for 3-4 hours till meatballs cook through.

Nutrition Information

- Calories:
- Sodium:
- Fiber:
- Total Carbohydrate:
- Cholesterol:
- Protein:
- Total Fat:

539. Berry 'n' Smoked Turkey Twirls

Serving: 40 appetizers. | Prep: 20mins | Cook: 5mins | Ready in:

Ingredients

- 1 package (8 ounces) reduced-fat cream cheese
- 1 cup shredded reduced-fat Mexican cheese blend
- 1/4 pound thinly sliced deli smoked turkey, finely chopped
- 2 tablespoons chopped dried cranberries
- 2 tablespoons chopped pimiento-stuffed olives
- 2 tablespoons salsa
- 3/4 teaspoon chili powder
- 4 flour tortillas (10 inches), room temperature

Direction

- Beat cream cheese till smooth in a small bowl. Mix chili powder, salsa, olives, cranberries, turkey and cheese blend in. On each tortilla, spread 1/2 cup mixture; tightly roll up then wrap in plastic. Refrigerate till firm for 2 hours.

- Unwrap. Slice to scant 1-in. slices. Serve this on a baking sheet that's been coated with cooking spray, 1-in. apart and baked for 5-7 minutes till heated through at 400° or serve chilled.

Nutrition Information

- Calories: 49 calories
- Protein: 3g protein.
- Total Fat: 2g fat (1g saturated fat)
- Sodium: 117mg sodium
- Fiber: 1g fiber)
- Total Carbohydrate: 4g carbohydrate (0 sugars
- Cholesterol: 7mg cholesterol

540. Bone Crunching Meatballs

Serving: 5 dozen. | Prep: 30mins | Cook: 10mins | Ready in:

Ingredients

- 1 can (8 ounces) sliced water chestnuts, drained
- 1 large egg, lightly beaten
- 3 tablespoons reduced-sodium soy sauce
- 1/2 cup chopped green onions (green part only)
- 1/4 cup dry bread crumbs
- 2 tablespoons minced fresh cilantro
- 1-1/2 teaspoons grated lime zest
- 1-1/2 teaspoons minced fresh gingerroot
- 1 garlic clove, minced
- 1/4 teaspoon salt
- 1/4 teaspoon pepper
- 1-1/2 pounds lean ground turkey
- 2 tablespoons canola oil
- Plum sauce

Direction

- Halve water chestnut slices to get 60 pieces; put aside. Keep leftover water chestnut slices for later.
- Mix initial 10 ingredients in big bowl. Crumble turkey on mixture; stir well. Divide to 60 portions; form each portion around water chestnut piece.
- Preheat an oven to 350°. Sauté meatballs in oil in big nonstick skillet for 5 minutes or till browned in batches. Put in 13x9-in. baking dish.
- Cover. Bake till meat isn't pink anymore or for 10-15 minutes; drain. Serve it with plum sauce.

Nutrition Information

- Calories: 27 calories
- Total Carbohydrate: 1g carbohydrate (0 sugars
- Cholesterol: 12mg cholesterol
- Protein: 2g protein.
- Total Fat: 2g fat (0 saturated fat)
- Sodium: 71mg sodium
- Fiber: 0 fiber)

541. Butter Chicken Meatballs

Serving: about 3 dozen. | Prep: 30mins | Cook: 03hours00mins | Ready in:

Ingredients

- 1-1/2 pounds ground chicken or turkey
- 1 large egg, lightly beaten
- 1/2 cup soft bread crumbs
- 1 teaspoon garam masala
- 1/2 teaspoon tandoori masala seasoning
- 1/2 teaspoon salt
- 1/4 teaspoon cayenne pepper
- 3 tablespoons minced fresh cilantro, divided
- 1 jar (14.1 ounces) butter chicken sauce

Direction

- Lightly yet thoroughly mix initial 7 ingredients plus 2 tablespoons cilantro. Form to 1-in. balls with wet hands. In 3-qt. slow cooker coated in cooking spray, put meatballs. Put butter sauce on meatballs.
- Cook on low, covered, for 3-4 hours till meatballs are cooked through. Use leftover cilantro to top.
- Freezing: Freeze cooled meatball mixture, omitting leftover cilantro, in freezer containers. Using: Thaw partially overnight in the fridge. Microwave on high in microwave-safe dish, covered, gently mixing and adding a bit of water if needed, till heated through. Serving: Sprinkle leftover cilantro.

Nutrition Information

- Calories: 40 calories
- Total Fat: 2g fat (1g saturated fat)
- Sodium: 87mg sodium
- Fiber: 0 fiber)
- Total Carbohydrate: 1g carbohydrate (1g sugars
- Cholesterol: 18mg cholesterol
- Protein: 3g protein.

542. Cabbage Bowl Nibbler Dip

Serving: 24 servings. | Prep: 50mins | Cook: 0mins | Ready in:

Ingredients

- 1 small head cabbage
- 2 cups cubed cheddar cheese
- 3 small cucumbers, cut into 1/4-inch pieces
- 1 pound thickly sliced deli turkey, cut into 1/4-inch pieces
- 1 pint grape tomatoes
- Frilled toothpicks
- 1 carton (8 ounces) sour cream ranch dip

Direction

- Serving bowl: Peel back outer cabbage's leaves gently. Slice 1/2-in. from cabbage's bottom to sit flat. Slice 3-in. circle in cabbage's top; hollow out 1/3 cabbage to make a bowl; put aside.
- On toothpicks, thread tomatoes, turkey, cucumbers and cheese. Insert in cabbage, beginning at bottom. Refrigerate till serving time. Use dip to fill cabbage bowl right before serving.

Nutrition Information

- Calories:
- Protein:
- Total Fat:
- Sodium:
- Fiber:
- Total Carbohydrate:
- Cholesterol:

543. Crab Stuffed Jalapenos

Serving: 2 dozen. | Prep: 25mins | Cook: 40mins | Ready in:

Ingredients

- 24 large jalapeno peppers
- 6 ounces fat-free cream cheese
- 2 teaspoons Worcestershire sauce
- 1/4 teaspoon garlic powder
- 1 package (8 ounces) imitation crabmeat, chopped
- 1/4 cup shredded reduced-fat cheddar cheese
- 12 turkey bacon strips, halved widthwise

Direction

- Cut jalapenos' stems off. Remove membranes and seeds; put aside. Beat garlic powder, Worcestershire sauce and cream cheese till blended in small bowl. Mix cheese and crab in.
- Put in resealable plastic bag. In corner of bag, cut small hole. Pipe filling in jalapenos. Use bacon's piece to wrap each; secure using toothpicks.
- Put on ungreased baking sheet and bake till peppers are crisp-tender or for 40-50 minutes at 350°.

Nutrition Information

- Calories: 41 calories
- Protein: 3g protein. Diabetic Exchanges: 1/2 lean meat.
- Total Fat: 2g fat (1g saturated fat)
- Sodium: 188mg sodium
- Fiber: 0 fiber)
- Total Carbohydrate: 3g carbohydrate (0 sugars
- Cholesterol: 9mg cholesterol

544. Cranberry Turkey Crostini

Serving: 2-1/2 dozen. | Prep: 20mins | Cook: 10mins | Ready in:

Ingredients

- 1 package (12 ounces) fresh or frozen cranberries
- 1 medium tangerine, peeled and seeded
- 1/2 cup red wine vinegar
- 1/4 cup chopped shallots
- 1/2 cup sugar
- 1/4 cup chopped seeded jalapeno peppers
- 1/4 teaspoon pepper
- 30 slices French bread (1/4 inch thick)
- Cooking spray
- 1 package (8 ounces) reduced-fat cream cheese
- 1/2 pound shaved deli smoked turkey

Direction

- In food processor, process tangerine and

cranberries till chopped coarsely, covered. Put aside.
- Boil shallots and vinegar in small saucepan. Lower heat; simmer for 5 minutes, uncovered, occasionally mixing, or till mixture reduces to 1/3 cup. Mix reserved cranberry mixture, pepper, jalapenos and sugar in. Cook on medium heat, frequently mixing, for 5 minutes. Put in small bowl; refrigerate till chilled.
- Put bread onto ungreased baking sheets. Spray both sides of bread lightly using cooking spray. Broil 3-4-in. away from heat, 1-2 minutes per side or till lightly browned. Spread 1 1/2 teaspoons cream cheese on each slice. Top with 1 tablespoon cranberry mixture and turkey.

Nutrition Information

- Calories: 79 calories
- Total Fat: 3g fat (1g saturated fat)
- Sodium: 131mg sodium
- Fiber: 1g fiber)
- Total Carbohydrate: 11g carbohydrate (5g sugars
- Cholesterol: 8mg cholesterol
- Protein: 3g protein. Diabetic Exchanges: 1 starch

545. Deli Sandwich Party Platter

Serving: 24 servings. | Prep: 30mins | Cook: 0mins | Ready in:

Ingredients

- 1 bunch green leaf lettuce
- 2 pounds sliced deli turkey
- 2 pounds sliced deli roast beef
- 1 pound sliced deli ham
- 1 pound thinly sliced hard salami
- 2 cartons (7 ounces each) roasted red pepper hummus
- 2 cartons (6-1/2 ounces each) garden vegetable cheese spread
- Assorted breads and mini bagels

Direction

- On serving platter, put lettuce leaves; top using deli meats; if desired, rolled up. Serve with bagels, breads, cheese spread and hummus.

Nutrition Information

- Calories: 205 calories
- Cholesterol: 75mg cholesterol
- Protein: 25g protein.
- Total Fat: 10g fat (4g saturated fat)
- Sodium: 1235mg sodium
- Fiber: 1g fiber)
- Total Carbohydrate: 4g carbohydrate (1g sugars

546. Festive Holiday Sliders

Serving: 2 dozen. | Prep: 30mins | Cook: 0mins | Ready in:

Ingredients

- 1 package (8 ounces) cream cheese, softened
- 1/2 cup mayonnaise
- 1/4 cup Creole mustard
- 2 tablespoons minced fresh gingerroot
- 1 tablespoon grated orange zest
- 1-1/2 teaspoons prepared horseradish
- 1 cup whole-berry cranberry sauce
- 4 green onions, sliced
- 2 packages (12 ounces each) Hawaiian sweet rolls or 24 dinner rolls, split
- 1-1/2 pounds thinly sliced cooked turkey

Direction

- Beat mayonnaise and cream cheese till smooth. Beat horseradish, orange zest, ginger and mustard in. Mix green onions and cranberry sauce in another bowl.
- On roll bottoms, spread cream cheese mixture. Top with cranberry mixture, turkey and roll tops.

Nutrition Information

- Calories: 231 calories
- Protein: 13g protein.
- Total Fat: 10g fat (4g saturated fat)
- Sodium: 221mg sodium
- Fiber: 1g fiber)
- Total Carbohydrate: 22g carbohydrate (10g sugars
- Cholesterol: 54mg cholesterol

547. Festive Turkey Meatballs

Serving: about 3-1/2 dozen. | Prep: 25mins | Cook: 30mins | Ready in:

Ingredients

- 1 large egg, beaten
- 1/2 cup dry bread crumbs
- 1/4 cup finely chopped onion
- 1/2 teaspoon curry powder
- 1/4 teaspoon ground ginger
- 1/4 teaspoon ground cinnamon
- 1/4 teaspoon salt
- 1/4 teaspoon pepper
- 1 pound ground turkey
- SAUCE:
- 1 cup honey
- 1/4 cup Dijon mustard
- 1/2 teaspoon curry powder
- 1/2 teaspoon ground ginger
- OPTIONAL ADDITIONS:
- Fresh basil leaves
- Fresh cilantro leaves
- Fresh mint leaves
- Lime wedges

Direction

- Preheat an oven to 350°. Mix initial 8 ingredients. Put in turkey; stir well. Form to 1-in. balls. On greased rack in 15x10-in. baking pan, put meatballs in. Bake for 20-25 minutes till juices are clear and cooked through, uncovered.
- Meanwhile, mix sauce ingredients in small saucepan; whisk till heated through on medium heat. Brush 1/4 cup sauce on meatballs; put back in oven for 10 minutes. Serve leftover sauce for dipping with meatballs and, optional, lime wedges and fresh herbs.

Nutrition Information

- Calories: 46 calories
- Total Carbohydrate: 7g carbohydrate (6g sugars
- Cholesterol: 11mg cholesterol
- Protein: 2g protein.
- Total Fat: 1g fat (0 saturated fat)
- Sodium: 61mg sodium
- Fiber: 0 fiber)

548. Flavorful Turkey Meatballs

Serving: 2 servings. | Prep: 15mins | Cook: 20mins | Ready in:

Ingredients

- 2 tablespoons dry bread crumbs
- 2 tablespoons chopped green pepper
- 1 egg white
- 1 garlic clove, minced
- 2 drops Louisiana-style hot sauce
- 1/3 pound lean ground turkey
- 1 teaspoon canola oil

- SAUCE:
- 1/4 cup ketchup
- 2 tablespoons water
- 4 teaspoons lemon juice
- 4 teaspoons red wine vinegar
- 2 teaspoons brown sugar
- 2 teaspoons molasses
- 1/2 teaspoon ground mustard
- 1/4 to 1/2 teaspoon chili powder
- 1/8 to 1/4 teaspoon cayenne pepper
- 1/8 teaspoon pepper

Direction

- Mix hot sauce, garlic, egg white, green pepper and breadcrumbs in big bowl. Crumble turkey on mixture; stir well. Form to 1-inch balls. Brown meatballs in oil in small nonstick skillet; drain.
- Mix sauce ingredients; put on meatballs. Boil. Lower heat. Cover. Simmer till heated through for 10 minutes.

Nutrition Information

- Calories: 63 calories
- Total Fat: 2g fat (0 saturated fat)
- Sodium: 134mg sodium
- Fiber: 0 fiber)
- Total Carbohydrate: 6g carbohydrate (4g sugars
- Cholesterol: 15mg cholesterol
- Protein: 4g protein. Diabetic Exchanges: 2 lean meat

549. Game Day Miniature Peppers

Serving: 2 dozen. | Prep: 55mins | Cook: 20mins | Ready in:

Ingredients

- 8 each miniature sweet red, orange and yellow peppers
- 4 ounces ground turkey
- 1/2 cup finely chopped fresh mushrooms
- 1/4 cup chopped sweet onion
- 1 garlic clove, minced
- 1 can (15 ounces) tomato sauce, divided
- 1/4 cup cooked brown rice
- 1 tablespoon grated Parmesan cheese
- 1 tablespoon shredded part-skim mozzarella cheese
- 1/2 teaspoon dried basil
- 1/4 teaspoon salt
- 1/4 teaspoon cayenne pepper
- 1/4 teaspoon pepper

Direction

- Cut and keep tops off peppers; remove the seeds. From pepper's bottoms, cut thin slices to level; put aside the peppers.
- Cook garlic, onion, mushrooms and turkey in big skillet on medium heat till meat isn't pink. Take off heat; let stand for five minutes.
- Mix seasonings, cheeses, rice and 1/4 cup of tomato sauce in; spoon in peppers. Put in 11x7-inch greased baking dish, upright. Put leftover tomato sauce on peppers; put on pepper tops. Cover. Bake for 18-22 minutes till peppers are crisp-tender and heated through at 400°.

Nutrition Information

- Calories: 23 calories
- Sodium: 116mg sodium
- Fiber: 1g fiber)
- Total Carbohydrate: 3g carbohydrate (1g sugars
- Cholesterol: 4mg cholesterol
- Protein: 1g protein.
- Total Fat: 1g fat (0 saturated fat)

550. Gooey Pizza Dip

Serving: 3 cups. | Prep: 10mins | Cook: 25mins | Ready in:

Ingredients

- 1 cup (8 ounces) reduced-fat ricotta cheese
- 1 cup fat-free mayonnaise
- 1-1/2 cups shredded part-skim mozzarella cheese, divided
- 1/4 cup grated Parmesan cheese
- 3/4 cup diced seeded plum tomatoes, divided
- 1 can (2-1/2 ounces) sliced ripe olives, drained, divided
- 1/4 cup sliced turkey pepperoni
- 1 teaspoon garlic powder
- 1 teaspoon Italian seasoning
- 1/8 teaspoon crushed red pepper flakes
- Assorted crackers

Direction

- Mix pepper flakes, Italian seasoning, garlic powder, pepperoni, 6 tablespoons olives, 1/2 cup tomatoes, parmesan cheese, 1 cup mozzarella, mayonnaise and ricotta in big bowl.
- Spread in 9-in. pie plate coated in cooking spray. Sprinkle leftover mozzarella on.
- Bake for 25-30 minutes at 350° or till top is golden brown and edges are bubbly. Sprinkle leftover olives and tomatoes. Serve with crackers.

Nutrition Information

- Calories: 124 calories
- Sodium: 493mg sodium
- Fiber: 1g fiber)
- Total Carbohydrate: 7g carbohydrate (4g sugars
- Cholesterol: 25mg cholesterol
- Protein: 9g protein. Diabetic Exchanges: 1 lean meat
- Total Fat: 7g fat (3g saturated fat)

551. Greek Party Pitas

Serving: 2 dozen. | Prep: 25mins | Cook: 0mins | Ready in:

Ingredients

- 4 whole wheat pita pocket halves
- 1/3 cup Greek vinaigrette
- 1/2 pound thinly sliced deli turkey
- 1 jar (7-1/2 ounces) roasted sweet red peppers, drained and patted dry
- 2 cups fresh baby spinach
- 24 pitted Greek olives
- 24 frilled toothpicks

Direction

- Brush vinaigrette insides of pita pockets. Fill with spinach, peppers and turkey. Cut every pita pocket to 6 wedges.
- On toothpicks, thread olives then use to secure the wedges.

Nutrition Information

- Calories: 48 calories
- Sodium: 239mg sodium
- Fiber: 0 fiber)
- Total Carbohydrate: 4g carbohydrate (0 sugars
- Cholesterol: 3mg cholesterol
- Protein: 2g protein.
- Total Fat: 3g fat (0 saturated fat)

552. Healthy House

Serving: 1 serving | Prep: 10mins | Cook: 0mins | Ready in:

Ingredients

- 1 slice whole wheat bread, crust removed
- 1 tablespoon peanut butter

- 1 thin slice deli turkey
- 1 raisin
- 5 pieces Rice Chex
- 1 slice American cheese
- 1 celery stick

Direction

- Spread peanut butter on bread. Cut turkey to 1 – 1/2-in.x1 – 1/4-in. rectangle for door; put on bread. For doorknob, add raisin. For windows, add cereal.
- Diagonally, cut cheese slice in half. Put a piece above bread for the roof. Keep leftover piece for another time. For chimney, add celery stick.

Nutrition Information

- Calories:
- Total Carbohydrate:
- Cholesterol:
- Protein:
- Total Fat:
- Sodium:
- Fiber:

553. Healthy Steamed Dumplings

Serving: 50 dumplings. | Prep: 45mins | Cook: 10mins | Ready in:

Ingredients

- 1 cup finely shredded Chinese or napa cabbage
- 1/4 cup minced fresh cilantro
- 1/4 cup minced chives
- 1 large egg, lightly beaten
- 3 tablespoons rice vinegar
- 1 tablespoon sesame oil
- 4 garlic cloves, minced
- 1 teaspoon salt
- 1 teaspoon ground ginger
- 1 teaspoon Chinese five-spice powder
- 1/2 teaspoon grated lemon peel
- 1/2 teaspoon pepper
- 1-3/4 pounds lean ground turkey
- 50 pot sticker or gyoza wrappers
- 6 cabbage leaves
- Sweet chili sauce, optional

Direction

- Mix initial 12 ingredients in big bowl. Add turkey; mix thoroughly but lightly.
- In middle of every pot sticker wrapper, put 1 tablespoon filling. Use damp paper towel to cover leftover wrappers till using time. Use water to moisten wrapper edge. Fold wrapper on filling; pleat front side a few times to make a pleated pouch to seal edges. On work surface, stand dumplings to flatten bottoms. Slightly curve to make crescent shapes (optional).
- Line 6 cabbage leaves in steamer basket. Put dumplings on cabbage in batches, 1-in. apart. Put in big saucepan above 1-in. water; boil. Steam for 6-8 minutes or till cooked through, covered. Throw cabbage away. Serve with chili sauce if desired. Freezing: Cover. Freeze cooled dumplings over waxed-paper lined baking sheets till firm. Put in big resealable plastic freezer bag. Using: Microwave dumplings for 30-45 seconds or till heated through, covered.

Nutrition Information

- Calories: 44 calories
- Fiber: 0 fiber)
- Total Carbohydrate: 3g carbohydrate (0 sugars
- Cholesterol: 17mg cholesterol
- Protein: 3g protein.
- Total Fat: 2g fat (0 saturated fat)
- Sodium: 79mg sodium

554. Hearty Poppers

Serving: 2 dozen. | Prep: 35mins | Cook: 20mins | Ready in:

Ingredients

- 12 jalapeno peppers
- 1/2 pound lean ground turkey
- 1/4 cup finely chopped onion
- 4 ounces fat-free cream cheese
- 1-1/3 cups shredded part-skim mozzarella cheese, divided
- 1 tablespoon minced fresh cilantro
- 1 teaspoon chili powder
- 1/2 teaspoon garlic powder
- 1/2 teaspoon ground cumin
- 1/8 teaspoon salt
- 1/8 teaspoon pepper

Direction

- Lengthwise, cut jalapenos in half; leaves stems intact. Throw seeds; put aside. Cook onion and turkey in small nonstick skillet on medium heat till meat isn't pink anymore; drain.
- Mix pepper, salt, cumin, garlic powder, chili powder, cilantro, 1/3 cup cheese and cream cheese in small bowl. Mix turkey mixture in; generously spoon in pepper halves.
- Put in 15x10x1-in. baking pan coated in cooking spray then sprinkle leftover cheese. Bake at 350°, uncovered, 40 minutes for mild, 30 minutes for medium and 20 minutes for hot (spicy).

Nutrition Information

- Calories: 38 calories
- Protein: 4g protein. Diabetic Exchanges: 1 lean meat.
- Total Fat: 2g fat (1g saturated fat)
- Sodium: 78mg sodium
- Fiber: 0 fiber)
- Total Carbohydrate: 1g carbohydrate (0 sugars
- Cholesterol: 11mg cholesterol

555. Honey Mustard Turkey Meatballs

Serving: 2-1/2 dozen. | Prep: 20mins | Cook: 30mins | Ready in:

Ingredients

- 1 pound ground turkey
- 1 egg, lightly beaten
- 3/4 cup crushed butter-flavored crackers
- 1/2 cup shredded part-skim mozzarella cheese
- 1/4 cup chopped onion
- 1/2 teaspoon ground ginger
- 6 tablespoon Dijon mustard, divided
- 1 tablespoon cornstarch
- 1/4 teaspoon onion powder
- 1-1/4 cups unsweetened pineapple juice
- 1/4 cup chopped green pepper
- 2 tablespoons honey

Direction

- Mix 3 tablespoons of mustard, ginger, onion, cheese, cracker crumbs and egg in big bowl. Crumble turkey on mixture; stir well. Form to 30 1-inch balls.
- Put meatballs on greased rack in shallow baking pan. Bake for 20-25 minutes, uncovered, till juices are clear at 350°; drain.
- Mix onion powder and cornstarch in a small saucepan. Mix pineapple juice in till smooth. Add honey and pepper; boil. Mix and cook till thick for 2 minutes; lower heat. Mix leftover mustard in till smooth.
- Brush 1/4 cup of sauce on meatballs. Bake for 10 more minutes. Serve leftover sauce for meatball dip.

Nutrition Information

- Calories: 187 calories
- Sodium: 364mg sodium
- Fiber: 0 fiber)

- Total Carbohydrate: 15g carbohydrate (8g sugars
- Cholesterol: 55mg cholesterol
- Protein: 10g protein.
- Total Fat: 10g fat (3g saturated fat)

556. Horseradish Meatballs

Serving: 3 dozen. | Prep: 30mins | Cook: 35mins | Ready in:

Ingredients

- 2 large eggs
- 1/2 cup dry bread crumbs
- 1/4 cup chopped green onions
- 1 tablespoon prepared horseradish
- 1/2 teaspoon salt
- 1/4 teaspoon pepper
- 1-1/2 pounds lean ground beef (90% lean)
- 1/2 pound ground pork or turkey
- SAUCE:
- 1 small onion, finely chopped
- 1/2 cup water
- 1/2 cup chili sauce
- 1/2 cup ketchup
- 1/4 cup packed brown sugar
- 1/4 cup cider vinegar
- 1 tablespoon Worcestershire sauce
- 1 tablespoon prepared horseradish
- 1 garlic clove, minced
- 1 teaspoon ground mustard
- 1/4 teaspoon hot pepper sauce

Direction

- Preheat an oven to 350°. Mix initial 6 ingredients. Add pork and beef; lightly yet thoroughly mix. Form to 1 1/2-in. balls. Put on greased rack in 15x10x1-in. pan. Bake for 35-40 minutes till thermometer reads 160° or 165° for ground turkey (if used).
- Meanwhile, boil sauce ingredients in big saucepan, frequently mixing. Lower heat. Simmer for 10 minutes, uncovered. Mix meatballs in gently.

Nutrition Information

- Calories:
- Protein:
- Total Fat:
- Sodium:
- Fiber:
- Total Carbohydrate:
- Cholesterol:

557. Hot Mexican Dip

Serving: 32 | Prep: 10mins | Cook: 20mins | Ready in:

Ingredients

- 1 (15 ounce) can chili without beans
- 1 (8 ounce) jar salsa
- 1 (8 ounce) jar taco sauce
- 2 chopped green chile peppers
- crushed red pepper to taste
- 2 pounds processed cheese, cubed

Direction

- Put processed cheese, crushed red pepper, green chile peppers, taco sauce and chili without beans in slow cooker set on low heat. Occasionally mixing, heat till all ingredients are blended well and processed cheese melts.

Nutrition Information

- Calories: 110 calories;
- Cholesterol: 25
- Protein: 6.3
- Total Fat: 7.5
- Sodium: 497
- Total Carbohydrate: 4.4

558. Italian Pizza Bread

Serving: 2 servings. | Prep: 5mins | Cook: 15mins | Ready in:

Ingredients

- 1 French or Italian sandwich roll (about 4 to 5 inches long)
- 2 to 3 tablespoons pizza sauce
- 8 slices slices turkey pepperoni
- 1/4 cup shredded part-skim mozzarella cheese

Direction

- Lengthwise, cut roll in half; put on baking sheet. Over each half, spread pizza sauce. Put pepperoni on top. Sprinkle mozzarella cheese on.
- Bake for 10 minutes or till heated through at 350°. Broil 4-in. away from heat till cheese is golden brown and bubbly or for 2 minutes.

Nutrition Information

- Calories: 427 calories
- Total Fat: 18g fat (5g saturated fat)
- Sodium: 2410mg sodium
- Fiber: 1g fiber)
- Total Carbohydrate: 23g carbohydrate (3g sugars
- Cholesterol: 147mg cholesterol
- Protein: 43g protein.

559. Italian Sausage Stuffed Mushrooms

Serving: 32 appetizers. | Prep: 35mins | Cook: 25mins | Ready in:

Ingredients

- 32 large fresh mushrooms
- 1/2 pound Italian turkey sausage links, casings removed
- 4 ounces reduced-fat cream cheese
- 1/2 cup shredded reduced-fat cheddar cheese
- 1/4 cup thinly sliced green onions
- 2 bacon strips, cooked and crumbled

Direction

- Remove mushroom's stems; chop. Put aside mushroom caps. Cook sausage and mushroom stems in small nonstick skillet coated in cooking spray till meat isn't pink anymore; drain. Cool down to room temperature.
- Beat cream cheese till smooth in small bowl. Add sausage mixture, onions and cheddar cheese; put in mushroom caps.
- Put in 15x10x1-in. baking pan that's coated in cooking spray. Bake for 20 minutes at 400°. Sprinkle bacon on. Bake till heated through or for 3-5 more minutes. Serve warm and refrigerate leftovers.

Nutrition Information

- Calories: 68 calories
- Sodium: 155mg sodium
- Fiber: 1g fiber)
- Total Carbohydrate: 3g carbohydrate (1g sugars
- Cholesterol: 16mg cholesterol
- Protein: 6g protein. Diabetic Exchanges: 1 vegetable
- Total Fat: 4g fat (2g saturated fat)

560. Layered Three Cheese Spread

Serving: 10-15 servings. | Prep: 25mins | Cook: 0mins | Ready in:

Ingredients

- 3 ounces cream cheese, softened

- 1/2 cup sour cream
- 1/2 cup mayonnaise
- 1/2 teaspoon chicken bouillon granules
- 1/8 teaspoon cayenne pepper
- 2 tablespoons grated Parmesan cheese
- 3 bacon strips, cooked and crumbled
- 1 medium tomato, seeded and chopped
- 1/2 cup shredded Swiss cheese
- 1/2 cup cubed cooked chicken or turkey
- 2 tablespoons minced fresh parsley
- Crackers or tortilla chips

Direction

- Beat cayenne, bouillon, mayonnaise, cream cheese and sour cream till smooth in a small bowl; cover. Refrigerate it overnight.
- Spread on a 10-inch serving plate. Sprinkle parsley, chicken, Swiss cheese, tomato, bacon and Parmesan cheese. Serve with chips/crackers.

Nutrition Information

- Calories: 124 calories
- Protein: 4g protein.
- Total Fat: 11g fat (4g saturated fat)
- Sodium: 136mg sodium
- Fiber: 0 fiber)
- Total Carbohydrate: 1g carbohydrate (1g sugars
- Cholesterol: 23mg cholesterol

561. Leftover Turkey Turnovers

Serving: 1 dozen. | Prep: 40mins | Cook: 5mins | Ready in:

Ingredients

- 1-1/4 cups all-purpose flour
- 1/4 teaspoon salt
- 1/2 cup shortening
- 1 large egg
- 2 tablespoons ice water, divided
- FILLING:
- 2 tablespoons canola oil
- 1/3 cup finely chopped onion
- 1/4 teaspoon ground turmeric
- 1/4 teaspoon ground cinnamon
- 1 garlic clove, minced
- 1 cup finely chopped cooked turkey
- 1/4 cup raisins
- 1/4 teaspoon salt
- 1/8 teaspoon pepper
- Oil for frying

Direction

- Mix salt and flour in big bowl; cut shortening in till crumbly. Whisk 1 tablespoon of ice water and egg; add to flour with leftover water as needed slowly; tossing using fork till dough can hold together while pressing. Turn on a lightly floured surface; gently knead 6-8 times. Form to disk; use plastic to wrap. Refrigerate for 1 hour to overnight.
- Heat oil in big skillet on medium high heat. Add cinnamon, turmeric and onion; mix and cook till tender for 1-2 minutes. Add garlic and cook for 30 more seconds. Mix pepper, salt, raisins and turkey in.
- Roll dough to 1/8-inch thick on a lightly floured surface. Use a 4-inch floured round cookie cutter to cut. In middle of every circle, put a heaping tablespoon of filling. Use water to moisten edges; fold in half. Use a fork to press edges to seal then repeat with leftover filling and dough.
- Heat 1/2-inch of oil in an electric skillet/deep skillet to 375°. A few at a time, fry turnovers till golden brown, 2-3 minutes per side. Drain on paper towels.

Nutrition Information

- Calories: 212 calories
- Total Carbohydrate: 13g carbohydrate (2g sugars
- Cholesterol: 27mg cholesterol

- Protein: 5g protein.
- Total Fat: 15g fat (3g saturated fat)
- Sodium: 117mg sodium
- Fiber: 1g fiber)

562. Lemon Marinated Antipasto

Serving: 12 servings (1/2 cup each). | Prep: 20mins | Cook: 15mins | Ready in:

Ingredients

- 1 package (19-1/2 ounces) Italian turkey sausage links
- 2 teaspoons grated lemon peel
- 1/3 cup lemon juice
- 1/3 cup olive oil
- 2 tablespoons minced fresh basil
- 2 teaspoons Italian seasoning
- 3 garlic cloves, minced
- 1 jar (12 ounces) roasted sweet red peppers, drained and thinly sliced
- 1 cup pitted Greek olives
- 1 pound fresh mozzarella cheese, cut into 1/2-inch cubes

Direction

- Following package directions, cook the sausages then set aside to cool a bit. While it cools, beat together garlic, oil, lemon peel, lemon juice, basil and Italian seasoning.
- Cut the sausages and place in a big bowl. Toss in peppers and olives. Pour dressing over sausages. Cover the bowl and refrigerate overnight.
- Take sausage mixture and mix in cheese. Let it stand before serving, about 30 minutes.

Nutrition Information

- Calories: 250 calories
- Protein: 12g protein.

- Total Fat: 20g fat (7g saturated fat)
- Sodium: 533mg sodium
- Fiber: 0 fiber)
- Total Carbohydrate: 4g carbohydrate (2g sugars
- Cholesterol: 47mg cholesterol

563. Makeover Hot Pizza Dip

Serving: about 4 cups. | Prep: 20mins | Cook: 5mins | Ready in:

Ingredients

- 1 package (8 ounces) fat-free cream cheese
- 1-1/2 teaspoons Italian seasoning
- 1 cup shredded part-skim mozzarella cheese, divided
- 1/2 cup grated Parmigiano-Reggiano cheese, divided
- 1 small sweet red pepper, chopped
- 1/4 cup chopped sweet onion
- 1 teaspoon olive oil
- 1 garlic clove, minced
- 1 can (8 ounces) pizza sauce
- 4 ounces sliced turkey pepperoni, chopped
- 1 can (2-1/4 ounces) sliced ripe olives, drained
- 1 French bread baguette (10-1/2 ounces), cut into 1/4-inch slices, toasted

Direction

- Beat Italian seasoning and cream cheese till smooth in small bowl; spread in microwave-safe 9-in. pie plate. Sprinkle 1/4 cup Parmigiano-Reggiano cheese and 1/2 cup mozzarella cheese.
- Sauté onion and pepper in oil in small nonstick skillet till tender; add garlic. Cook for 1 more minute. Put cheese on using a spoon; spread pizza sauce on pepper mixture. Sprinkle olives, pepperoni and leftover cheeses.
- Microwave at 70% powder, uncovered, till

cheese melts or for 5-7 minutes. Serve with toasted baguette slices.

Nutrition Information

- Calories: 154 calories
- Total Fat: 6g fat (2g saturated fat)
- Sodium: 466mg sodium
- Fiber: 2g fiber)
- Total Carbohydrate: 17g carbohydrate (1g sugars
- Cholesterol: 16mg cholesterol
- Protein: 9g protein.

564. Mandarin Turkey Pinwheels

Serving: 2-1/2 dozen. | Prep: 15mins | Cook: 0mins | Ready in:

Ingredients

- 1 package (8 ounces) reduced-fat cream cheese
- 1/2 teaspoon curry powder
- 1/2 cup mandarin oranges, drained and chopped
- 3 flour tortillas (12 inches), room temperature
- 1/2 pound sliced deli smoked turkey
- 3 cups fresh baby spinach
- 2 green onions, chopped

Direction

- Beat curry powder and cream cheese till blended in a small bowl. Mix oranges in. Spread on tortillas. Layer with green onions, spinach and turkey; tightly roll up. Wrap in plastic. Refrigerate till firm enough to slice for 2 hours.
- Unwrap. Slice every roll to 10 slices.

Nutrition Information

- Calories: 50 calories
- Sodium: 149mg sodium
- Fiber: 1g fiber)
- Total Carbohydrate: 4g carbohydrate (1g sugars
- Cholesterol: 8mg cholesterol
- Protein: 3g protein.
- Total Fat: 2g fat (1g saturated fat)

565. Meatballs With Cranberry Sauce

Serving: 6 dozen. | Prep: 30mins | Cook: 20mins | Ready in:

Ingredients

- 1/2 cup egg substitute
- 1 cup crushed cornflakes
- 1/3 cup ketchup
- 2 tablespoons reduced-sodium soy sauce
- 1 tablespoon dried parsley flakes
- 2 tablespoons dried minced onion
- 1/4 teaspoon pepper
- 2 pounds lean ground turkey
- SAUCE:
- 1 can (14 ounces) jellied cranberry sauce
- 1 cup ketchup
- 3 tablespoons brown sugar
- 1 tablespoon lemon juice

Direction

- Mix initial 7 ingredients in big bowl. Crumble turkey on mixture; stir well. Form to 72 meatballs; put meatballs on racks coated in cooking spray inside shallow baking pans. Bake till not pink for 20-25 minutes at 350°.
- Mix sauce ingredients in a Dutch oven. Cook, frequently mixing, till cranberry sauce melts on low heat. Mix meatballs in gently till coated.

Nutrition Information

- Calories: 40 calories
- Total Carbohydrate: 5g carbohydrate (3g sugars
- Cholesterol: 10mg cholesterol
- Protein: 2g protein. Diabetic Exchanges: 1/2 starch.
- Total Fat: 1g fat (0 saturated fat)
- Sodium: 99mg sodium
- Fiber: 0 fiber)

566. Meaty Salsa Dip

Serving: 12 servings. | Prep: 20mins | Cook: 0mins | Ready in:

Ingredients

- 1 pound lean ground turkey
- 1 can (15 ounces) black beans, rinsed and drained
- 1 package (10 ounces) frozen white corn, thawed
- 1 jar (16 ounces) chunky salsa
- Tortilla chips

Direction

- Cook turkey in nonstick skillet on medium till not pink anymore; drain. Mix salsa, corn, beans and turkey in serving bowl. Serve with tortilla chips.

Nutrition Information

- Calories: 118 calories
- Fiber: 3g fiber)
- Total Carbohydrate: 11g carbohydrate (2g sugars
- Cholesterol: 30mg cholesterol
- Protein: 9g protein. Diabetic Exchanges: 1 lean meat
- Total Fat: 3g fat (1g saturated fat)
- Sodium: 280mg sodium

567. Mediterranean Pockets

Serving: 1 dozen. | Prep: 20mins | Cook: 15mins | Ready in:

Ingredients

- 1/3 pound lean ground turkey
- 1 small garlic clove, minced
- 1/3 cup crumbled feta cheese
- 1/4 cup frozen peas, thawed
- 1/4 cup chopped roasted sweet red pepper
- 1 green onion, chopped
- 2 tablespoons minced fresh parsley
- 1-1/2 teaspoons lemon juice
- 1/2 teaspoon grated lemon peel
- 1/2 teaspoon dried oregano
- 1/4 teaspoon salt
- 1/4 teaspoon pepper
- 2 tubes (8 ounces each) refrigerated reduced-fat crescent rolls

Direction

- Coat a big nonstick skillet with cooking spray. Cook garlic and turkey until meat isn't pink on medium heat; drain.
- Take off from heat. Mix in pepper, salt, oregano, lemon peel and juice, parsley, onion, red pepper, peas and cheese.
- Unroll crescent dough to 2 rectangles. Seal perforations and seams. Cut every rectangle to 6 squares. In the middle of every square, put 2 tbsp. turkey mixture. Fold dough on filling to make a triangle. Seal edges.
- Put to an ungreased baking sheet. Bake for 12-14 minutes at 375 degrees until golden brown.

Nutrition Information

- Calories: 167 calories
- Total Carbohydrate: 17g carbohydrate (4g sugars
- Cholesterol: 12mg cholesterol
- Protein: 6g protein.

- Total Fat: 8g fat (2g saturated fat)
- Sodium: 424mg sodium
- Fiber: 0 fiber)

568. Mexican Fiesta Dip

Serving: 18 servings, 2 Tbsp. each | Prep: 20mins | Cook: | Ready in:

Ingredients

- 1 onion , chopped
- 1 jalapeño pepper , finely chopped
- 1/3 cup milk
- 1 pkg. (16 oz.) KRAFT Singles
- 1 tomatoes , chopped
- 2 Tbsp. chopped fresh cilantro

Direction

- Cook peppers and onions in skillet sprayed in cooking spray over medium high heat till onions are tender, frequently mixing, or for 5 minutes.
- Mix milk in on low heat. Add singles slowly, cooking after every addition till melted, constantly mixing.
- Use cilantro and tomatoes to top.

Nutrition Information

- Calories: 80
- Total Fat: 6 g
- Saturated Fat: 3.5 g
- Total Carbohydrate: 3 g
- Protein: 5 g
- Sodium: 270 mg
- Fiber: 0 g
- Sugar: 3 g
- Cholesterol: 20 mg

569. Microwave Texas Nachos

Serving: 2 servings. | Prep: 25mins | Cook: 0mins | Ready in:

Ingredients

- 2 ounces uncooked chorizo or bulk spicy pork sausage
- 1 garlic clove, minced
- 1/4 cup refried beans
- 2 cups tortilla chips
- 1/2 cup shredded Colby-Monterey Jack cheese
- 1/2 cup shredded lettuce
- 1 small tomato, seeded and diced
- 3 tablespoons chopped onion
- 1/4 cup sour cream
- 1/4 cup guacamole
- 2 tablespoons sliced jalapeno pepper

Direction

- Crumble chorizo in small skillet; add garlic and cook for 6-8 minutes or till fully cooked on medium heat; drain. Mix beans and chorizo mixture in microwave-safe dish; cover. Microwave for 1-2 minutes or till heated through on high; mix.
- On microwave-safe serving plate, put tortilla chips. Sprinkle cheese on. Heat on high, uncovered, till cheese melts or for 1 minute. Put chorizo mixture on cheese and chips using a spoon. Top with jalapeno, guacamole, sour cream, onion, tomato and lettuce. Immediately serve.

Nutrition Information

- Calories: 388 calories
- Sodium: 871mg sodium
- Fiber: 7g fiber)
- Total Carbohydrate: 41g carbohydrate (5g sugars
- Cholesterol: 45mg cholesterol
- Protein: 21g protein.
- Total Fat: 17g fat (7g saturated fat)

570. Mini Hot Browns

Serving: 1-1/2 dozen. | Prep: 20mins | Cook: 10mins | Ready in:

Ingredients

- 1 teaspoon chicken bouillon granules
- 1/4 cup boiling water
- 3 tablespoons butter
- 2 tablespoons all-purpose flour
- 3/4 cup half-and-half cream
- 1 cup shredded Swiss cheese
- 18 slices snack rye bread
- 6 ounces sliced deli turkey
- 1 small onion, thinly sliced and separated into rings
- 5 bacon strips, cooked and crumbled
- 2 tablespoons minced fresh parsley

Direction

- Preheat an oven to 350°. Melt bouillon in water; put aside.
- Melt butter in a small saucepan on medium heat. Mix flour in till smooth; add bouillon and cream. Boil. Mix and cook for 1-2 minutes till thick. Mix cheese in till melted. Take off heat.
- Put bread on 2 baking sheets. Layer cheese mixture, onion and turkey on each slice. Bake for 10-12 minutes till heated through/preheat broiler then broil for 3-5 minutes till sauce is bubbly and bread's edges are crisp. Sprinkle parsley and bacon.

Nutrition Information

- Calories: 98 calories
- Sodium: 246mg sodium
- Fiber: 1g fiber)
- Total Carbohydrate: 5g carbohydrate (1g sugars
- Cholesterol: 21mg cholesterol
- Protein: 5g protein.
- Total Fat: 6g fat (3g saturated fat)

571. Mini Pizza Cups

Serving: 32 appetizers. | Prep: 25mins | Cook: 15mins | Ready in:

Ingredients

- 2 tubes (8 ounces each) refrigerated round crescent rolls
- 1 can (8 ounces) pizza sauce
- 1/4 cup finely chopped onion
- 1/3 cup finely chopped green pepper
- 2 ounces sliced turkey pepperoni, chopped
- 1 cup shredded part-skim mozzarella cheese

Direction

- Separate dough tubes to 8 rolls each then halve the rolls. Up the sides and bottom of miniature muffin cups that has been coated with cooking spray, press dough.
- In each cup, spoon pizza sauce on. Sprinkle cheese, pepperoni, green pepper and onion. Bake for 15-18 minutes or until cheese melts and crusts are browned at 375°.

Nutrition Information

- Calories: 75 calories
- Sodium: 193mg sodium
- Fiber: trace fiber)
- Total Carbohydrate: 7g carbohydrate (1g sugars
- Cholesterol: 4mg cholesterol
- Protein: 3g protein.
- Total Fat: 4g fat (2g saturated fat)

572. Mini Sausage Bundles

Serving: 1 dozen. | Prep: 25mins | Cook: 10mins | Ready in:

Ingredients

- 1/2 pound turkey Italian sausage links, casings removed
- 1 small onion, finely chopped
- 1/4 cup finely chopped sweet red pepper
- 1 garlic clove, minced
- 1/2 cup shredded cheddar cheese
- 12 sheets phyllo dough (14x9-inch size)
- Cooking spray
- 12 whole chives, optional

Direction

- Preheat an oven to 425°. Crumble and cook sausage, garlic, red pepper and onion in big skillet on medium high heat for 4-6 minutes till not pink. Mix cheese in; slightly cool.
- On a work surface, put 1 phyllo dough sheet. Spritz cooking spray. Layer using 2 extra phyllo sheets, spritzing every layer. Cover leftover phyllo in plastic wrap and a damp towel to avoid it from drying out. Crosswise, cut phyllo to 3 strips, 4 1/2-inch wide.
- Near end of each strip, put a rounded tablespoon of sausage mixture. Fold strip's end over filling; fold sides in. Roll up. Put, seam side down, on ungreased baking sheet. Repeat with leftover filling and phyllo.
- Bake for 8-10 minutes till lightly browned. Tie bundles with chives if desired. Serve warm.

Nutrition Information

- Calories: 74 calories
- Fiber: 0 fiber)
- Total Carbohydrate: 7g carbohydrate (1g sugars
- Cholesterol: 12mg cholesterol
- Protein: 4g protein. Diabetic Exchanges: 1 lean meat
- Total Fat: 3g fat (1g saturated fat)
- Sodium: 154mg sodium

573. Mongolian Fondue

Serving: 8 servings. | Prep: 15mins | Cook: 20mins | Ready in:

Ingredients

- 1/2 cup soy sauce
- 1/4 cup water
- 1 teaspoon white wine vinegar
- 1-1/2 teaspoons minced garlic, divided
- 1 cup sliced carrots (1/4 inch thick)
- 2 cans (14-1/2 ounces each) beef broth
- 1 teaspoon minced fresh gingerroot
- 2 pounds boneless beef sirloin steak, cut into 2-1/2-inch x 1/4-inch strips
- 1 pound turkey breast, cut into 2-1/2-inch x 1/4-inch strips
- 1 pound uncooked large shrimp, peeled and deveined
- 3 small zucchini, cut into 1/2-inch slices
- 1 each medium sweet red, yellow and green pepper, cut into 1-inch chunks
- 1 to 2 cups whole fresh mushrooms
- 1 cup cubed red onion (1-inch pieces)
- 1 jar (7 ounces) hoisin sauce
- 1 jar (4 ounces) Chinese hot mustard

Direction

- Boil 1/2 teaspoon garlic, vinegar, water and soy sauce in saucepan. Take off heat; cover. Refrigerate for 1 hour minimum.
- Cook carrots in small amount of water in small saucepan till crisp-tender or for 3 minutes; drain. Pat dry. Boil leftover garlic, ginger and broth in saucepan. Put in fondue pot; keep warm. Use paper towels to pat dry shrimp, turkey and steak.
- Cook beef to preferred doneness with fondue forks. Cook turkey till juices are clear. Cook shrimp till pink. Cook veggies till you get

desired doneness. Serve with reserved garlic-soy sauce, mustard sauce and hoisin sauce.

Nutrition Information

- Calories: 364 calories
- Cholesterol: 184mg cholesterol
- Protein: 50g protein.
- Total Fat: 8g fat (2g saturated fat)
- Sodium: 1826mg sodium
- Fiber: 3g fiber)
- Total Carbohydrate: 21g carbohydrate (5g sugars

574. Party Cranberry Meatballs

Serving: 4-1/2 dozen. | Prep: 30mins | Cook: 20mins | Ready in:

Ingredients

- 2 eggs, beaten
- 1/3 cup dry bread crumbs
- 1 teaspoon salt
- 1/2 teaspoon onion powder
- 1/2 teaspoon garlic powder
- 1/2 teaspoon dried thyme
- 1/2 teaspoon pepper
- 2 pounds ground turkey
- 1 can (14 ounces) jellied cranberry sauce
- 1 bottle (12 ounces) chili sauce
- 1/4 cup water
- 1/4 cup orange marmalade
- 2 tablespoons red wine vinegar
- 2 tablespoons reduced-sodium soy sauce

Direction

- Mix initial 7 ingredients in big bowl. Crumble turkey on mixture; stir well. Form to 1-inch balls.
- In batches, cook meatballs in big skillet till not pink; drain.
- Mix leftover ingredients in a Dutch oven. Mix and cook for 5 minutes on medium low heat. Add meatballs; boil. Lower heat. Simmer for 10 minutes, uncovered, till heated through; cool. Put in freezer containers then freeze for up to three months.
- Using frozen meatballs: in the fridge, thaw. Heat in a microwave/Dutch oven.

Nutrition Information

- Calories: 61 calories
- Protein: 3g protein.
- Total Fat: 3g fat (1g saturated fat)
- Sodium: 196mg sodium
- Fiber: 0 fiber)
- Total Carbohydrate: 6g carbohydrate (4g sugars
- Cholesterol: 19mg cholesterol

575. Party Pinwheels

Serving: 15 | Prep: 10mins | Cook: 5mins | Ready in:

Ingredients

- 2 (8 ounce) packages cream cheese, softened
- 1 (1 ounce) package ranch dressing mix
- 2 green onions, minced
- 4 (12 inch) flour tortillas
- 1/2 cup red bell pepper, diced
- 1/2 cup diced celery
- 1 (2 ounce) can sliced black olives
- 1/2 cup shredded Cheddar cheese

Direction

- Mix green onions, ranch dressing mix and cream cheese in a medium-sized mixing bowl. On each tortilla, spread mixture. Sprinkle cheese (optional), black olives, celery and red pepper on cream cheese mixture then roll up tortillas. Tightly wrap in aluminum foil.

- Chill for 2 hours to overnight. Cut roll ends off. Slice chilled rolls to 1-in. slices.

Nutrition Information

- Calories: 229 calories;
- Total Carbohydrate: 18.6
- Cholesterol: 37
- Protein: 5.9
- Total Fat: 14.5
- Sodium: 477

576. Pepperoni Pizza Bread

Serving: 12 | Prep: | Cook: | Ready in:

Ingredients

- 1 3/8 cups water
- 3 cups bread flour
- 2 tablespoons dry milk powder
- 2 tablespoons white sugar
- 1 1/2 teaspoons salt
- 2 tablespoons butter
- 1/2 cup pepperoni sausage, chopped
- 1/3 cup shredded mozzarella cheese
- 1 tablespoon grated Parmesan cheese
- 1/3 cup canned mushrooms
- 1/4 cup dried minced onion
- 3/4 teaspoon garlic powder
- 2 1/2 teaspoons active dry yeast

Direction

- In order recommended by manufacturer, put ingredients in bread machine pan. Choose basic bread setting and start.
- Baking bread in oven: Choose manual/dough cycle. Form dough, when cycle is completed, put in greased loaf pan. Let rise till doubled in size in a warm area. In preheated 175°C/350°F oven, bake for 35-45 minutes or till inserted thermometer in middle of load reads 95°C/200°F.

Nutrition Information

- Calories: 94 calories;
- Cholesterol: 18
- Protein: 4.1
- Total Fat: 6.8
- Sodium: 512
- Total Carbohydrate: 4.5

577. Pepperoni Pizza Pita

Serving: 1 serving. | Prep: 5mins | Cook: 5mins | Ready in:

Ingredients

- 2 tablespoons pizza sauce
- 1 whole pita bread (6 inches)
- 6 pepperoni slices
- 2 fresh mushrooms, sliced
- 1/4 cup shredded part-skim mozzarella cheese

Direction

- Spread pizza sauce on pita bread. Top with cheese, mushrooms and pepperoni. Put on ungreased baking sheet. Bake for 4-6 minutes or till cheese melts at 400°.

Nutrition Information

- Calories: 275 calories
- Total Carbohydrate: 38g carbohydrate (0 sugars
- Cholesterol: 25mg cholesterol
- Protein: 16g protein. Diabetic Exchanges: 2 starch
- Total Fat: 6g fat (3g saturated fat)
- Sodium: 756mg sodium
- Fiber: 2g fiber)

578. Phyllo Turkey Egg Rolls

Serving: 16 egg rolls. | Prep: 30mins | Cook: 30mins | Ready in:

Ingredients

- 1 pound ground turkey breast
- 4 cups coleslaw mix (about 8 ounces)
- 1/4 cup chopped green onions
- 3 tablespoons reduced-sodium soy sauce
- 2 garlic cloves, minced
- 1/2 teaspoon Chinese five-spice powder
- 1 teaspoon grated fresh gingerroot
- 24 sheets phyllo dough, (14 inches x 9 inches)
- Refrigerated butter-flavored spray
- Sweet-and-sour sauce and/or hot mustard, optional

Direction

- In big nonstick skillet, crumble turkey. Cook on medium heat till not pink anymore; drain. Add ginger, five-spice powder, garlic, soy sauce, onions and coleslaw mix. Cook till coleslaw wilts or about 2-3 minutes. Take off heat.
- On work surface, put 1 phyllo dough sheet, long side facing you then spritz butter spray. Brush to distribute evenly. Repeat with 2 extra phyllo sheets, spritzing and brushing every layer. Cover leftover phyllo dough using waxed paper to keep from drying out. Widthwise, cut stack to 2 14x4 – 1/2-in. strips. Put 1/4 cup turkey mixture along a short side of every rectangle. Fold long sides in, beginning at filling edge, tightly roll up. Put on ungreased baking sheets, seam side down. Spritz butter spray on top; repeat with leftover filling and phyllo.
- Bake for 25-30 minutes at 350°. Broil for 5 minutes or till golden brown 6-in. away from heat. Serve warm with mustard and/or sweet-and-sour sauce if you want.

Nutrition Information

- Calories: 108 calories
- Protein: 7g protein. Diabetic Exchanges: 1 starch
- Total Fat: 4g fat (1g saturated fat)
- Sodium: 236mg sodium
- Fiber: 1g fiber)
- Total Carbohydrate: 12g carbohydrate (0 sugars
- Cholesterol: 22mg cholesterol

579. Pistachio Turkey Meatballs In Orange Sauce

Serving: 4-1/2 dozen. | Prep: 25mins | Cook: 20mins | Ready in:

Ingredients

- 2/3 cup chopped pistachios
- 2 green onions, finely chopped
- 1/4 cup dry bread crumbs
- 1 large egg, lightly beaten
- 1 teaspoon grated orange zest
- 1/2 teaspoon salt
- 1/8 teaspoon pepper
- 1 pound ground turkey
- 1 Johnsonville® Mild Italian Sausage Links (4 ounces), casing removed
- SAUCE:
- 3 tablespoons butter
- 1 tablespoon olive oil
- 1/4 cup finely chopped sweet red pepper
- 1/8 teaspoon crushed red pepper flakes
- 2 tablespoons white wine
- 4 teaspoons cornstarch
- 1 cup orange juice
- 1/2 cup reduced-sodium chicken broth
- 1 tablespoon honey
- 1/2 teaspoon grated orange zest
- 1 tablespoon minced fresh basil
- 2 tablespoons chopped pistachios

Direction

- Preheat an oven to 375°. Mix initial 7 ingredients in big bowl. Add sausage and turkey; lightly but thoroughly mix. Form to 1-in. balls.
- On greased racks inside shallow baking pans, put meatballs. Bake till cooked through or for 18-22 minutes.
- Heat oil and butter on medium heat in big skillet. Add pepper flakes and red pepper; mix and cook till red pepper is tender or for 2-3 minutes. Add wine and cook for 1 minute more.
- Whisk orange zest, honey, broth, orange juice and cornstarch till blended in small bowl. Mix into pan; boil. Mix and cook till thickened or for 1-2 minutes. Mix meatballs and basil in. Sprinkle pistachios on.

Nutrition Information

- Calories: 49 calories
- Protein: 2g protein.
- Total Fat: 4g fat (1g saturated fat)
- Sodium: 66mg sodium
- Fiber: 0 fiber)
- Total Carbohydrate: 2g carbohydrate (1g sugars
- Cholesterol: 12mg cholesterol

580. Polynesian Kabobs

Serving: 14 kabobs | Prep: 30mins | Cook: 0mins | Ready in:

Ingredients

- 1 can (8 ounces) unsweetened pineapple chunks
- 1 package (14 ounces) breakfast turkey sausage links, cut in half
- 1 can (8 ounces) whole water chestnuts, drained
- 1 large sweet red pepper, cut into 1-inch chunks
- 2 tablespoons honey
- 2 teaspoons reduced-sodium soy sauce
- 1/8 teaspoon ground nutmeg
- Dash pepper

Direction

- Separate pineapples from its juice. Reserve 1 tablespoon of the juice, and either discard or keep the remaining juice for another use. Alternately skewer the sausages, pineapples, water chestnuts, and red peppers onto 14 metal or water-soaked wooden skewers. Get a small bowl and mix together the reserved tablespoon of pineapple juice, soy sauce, honey, pepper, and nutmeg. Cook the skewers on an open grill at medium heat for 6-7 minutes per side or until sausages are nicely browned, occasionally brushing the skewers with the pineapple juice mixture.

Nutrition Information

- Calories: 95 calories
- Sodium: 199mg sodium
- Fiber: 1g fiber)
- Total Carbohydrate: 7g carbohydrate (5g sugars
- Cholesterol: 23mg cholesterol
- Protein: 5g protein.
- Total Fat: 6g fat (2g saturated fat)

581. Pomegranate Glazed Turkey Meatballs

Serving: 3 dozen. | Prep: 30mins | Cook: 10mins | Ready in:

Ingredients

- 1 large egg, beaten
- 1/2 cup soft bread crumbs
- 1/2 cup minced fresh parsley
- 1 teaspoon salt

- 1 teaspoon smoked paprika
- 1 teaspoon coarsely ground pepper
- 1/4 teaspoon garlic salt
- 1-1/4 pounds ground turkey
- 3 cups plus 1 tablespoon pomegranate juice, divided
- 1/2 cup sugar
- 1 tablespoon cornstarch

Direction

- Mix garlic salt, pepper, paprika, salt, parsley, bread crumbs and egg in big bowl. Crumble turkey on mixture; stir well. Form to 1-in. balls.
- Distribute to two 15x10x1-in. ungreased baking pans. Bake for 10-15 minutes at 375° or till juices are clear and thermometer reads 165°.
- Meanwhile, boil sugar and 3 cups pomegranate juice in big skillet; cook till liquid reduces to 1 cup. Mix leftover juice and cornstarch; mix into skillet. Mix and cook till thickened or for 1 minute.
- Mix meatballs in gently; heat through. Serve in chafing dish/slow cooker.

Nutrition Information

- Calories:
- Cholesterol:
- Protein:
- Total Fat:
- Sodium:
- Fiber:
- Total Carbohydrate:

582. Pronto Mini Pizzas

Serving: 4 servings. | Prep: 20mins | Cook: 0mins | Ready in:

Ingredients

- 1 pound ground beef or turkey
- 1 cup sliced fresh mushrooms
- 1/2 cup chopped green pepper
- 1/2 cup chopped onion
- 2 garlic cloves, minced
- 1 can (8 ounces) tomato sauce
- 1 teaspoon fennel seed
- 1/2 teaspoon salt
- 1/2 teaspoon dried oregano
- 4 pita breads
- 1 cup shredded part-skim mozzarella cheese

Direction

- Cook garlic, onion, green pepper, mushroom and meat in skillet till veggies are tender and meat is browned. Drain. Mix oregano, salt, fennel and tomato sauce in. Simmer for 1-2 minutes.
- Meanwhile, in microwave, warm pitas. Top each using meat mixture; sprinkle cheese on. Broil/microwave till cheese melts. Cut to quarters.

Nutrition Information

- Calories: 456 calories
- Fiber: 3g fiber)
- Total Carbohydrate: 41g carbohydrate (4g sugars
- Cholesterol: 77mg cholesterol
- Protein: 33g protein.
- Total Fat: 17g fat (8g saturated fat)
- Sodium: 1059mg sodium

583. Quesadilla

Serving: 1 serving. | Prep: 5mins | Cook: 5mins | Ready in:

Ingredients

- 1 to 2 teaspoons canola oil
- 2 flour tortillas (6 inches)

- 1/2 cup shredded cheddar cheese, divided
- 1/2 cup cubed cooked chicken, turkey, pork or beef
- 1/4 cup sliced fresh mushrooms
- 1/2 cup shredded Monterey Jack cheese, divided
- Sour cream and salsa, optional

Direction

- In nonstick skillet, heat oil; add a tortilla. Layer with 1/2 cheddar cheese, 1/2 Monterey Jack cheese and all of mushrooms and chicken. Top with 2nd tortilla and cover. Heat till bottom tortilla is golden brown and crisp and cheese melts.
- Flip; sprinkle leftover cheese on top. Cook till cheese melts and bottom tortilla is golden brown and crisp. Slice to wedges. Serve with salsa and sour cream if desired.

Nutrition Information

- Calories: 768 calories
- Total Fat: 49g fat (25g saturated fat)
- Sodium: 1152mg sodium
- Fiber: 0 fiber)
- Total Carbohydrate: 29g carbohydrate (1g sugars
- Cholesterol: 173mg cholesterol
- Protein: 53g protein.

584. Quick Turkey Nachos Snack

Serving: 6-8 servings. | Prep: 25mins | Cook: 5mins | Ready in:

Ingredients

- 1 pound ground turkey
- 1 package (1-1/4 ounces) taco seasoning
- 3/4 cup water
- Tortilla chips
- 1/2 cup sour cream
- 1/2 cup salsa
- 1/2 cup shredded Monterey Jack cheese
- 1/2 cup shredded cheddar cheese
- Shredded lettuce, chopped
- Tomatoes and/or green onions, optional

Direction

- Brown turkey in skillet; drain. Add water and taco seasoning; simmer for 15 minutes. On greased baking sheet, put tortilla chips. Layer with salsa, sour cream and turkey. Sprinkle cheeses on.
- Broil/microwave till cheese melts or for a few minutes. Top with onions (optional), tomatoes and lettuce.

Nutrition Information

- Calories:
- Protein:
- Total Fat:
- Sodium:
- Fiber:
- Total Carbohydrate:
- Cholesterol:

585. Roasted Vegetable Turkey Pinwheels

Serving: 64 appetizers. | Prep: 20mins | Cook: 25mins | Ready in:

Ingredients

- 2 medium yellow summer squash, cut into 1/2-inch slices
- 1 large sweet yellow pepper, cut into 1-inch pieces
- 1 large sweet red pepper, cut into 1-inch pieces
- 2 large carrots, cut into 1/2-inch slices
- 3 garlic cloves, peeled
- 2 tablespoons olive oil

- 2 packages (8 ounces each) cream cheese, cubed
- 1/2 teaspoon salt
- 1/2 teaspoon pepper
- 8 flavored tortillas of your choice (10 inches), room temperature
- 1 pound thinly sliced deli turkey
- 4 cups torn Bibb or Boston lettuce

Direction

- In a 15x10x1-in. baking pan that's coated with cooking spray, put garlic, carrots, peppers and squash. Drizzle oil on; toss till coated. Bake for 25-30 minutes till tender and light brown at 425°, mixing once. Slightly cool.
- In food processor, process pepper, salt, cream cheese and veggies, covered, till blended. Put into a big bowl. Refrigerate till thick, covered, for 2-3 hours.
- On each tortilla, spread 1/2 cup of cream cheese mixture. Layer with lettuce and turkey; tightly roll up. Wrap each using plastic wrap. Refrigerate for 1 hour minimum; unwrap. Slice each to 8 slices.

Nutrition Information

- Calories: 61 calories
- Total Fat: 3g fat (2g saturated fat)
- Sodium: 141mg sodium
- Fiber: 0 fiber)
- Total Carbohydrate: 6g carbohydrate (1g sugars
- Cholesterol: 11mg cholesterol
- Protein: 3g protein. Diabetic Exchanges: 1/2 starch

586. Rustic Antipasto Tart

Serving: 12 servings. | Prep: 15mins | Cook: 25mins | Ready in:

Ingredients

- 1 sheet refrigerated pie pastry
- 2 tablespoons prepared pesto
- 1 cup shredded part-skim mozzarella cheese, divided
- 4 ounces sliced turkey pepperoni
- 1 jar (7 ounces) roasted sweet red peppers, drained and thinly sliced
- 1 jar (7-1/2 ounces) marinated quartered artichoke hearts, drained
- 1 tablespoon water

Direction

- On a baking sheet that is lined with parchment paper, unfold the pastry. Scatter pesto to within 2-inch of edges; sprinkle on 1/2 cup cheese. Layer with 1/4 cup cheese and pepperoni. Place artichokes and red peppers on top; sprinkle on left of cheese.
- Over filling, turn up edges of pastry, keep the middle uncovered. Brush the folded pastry with some water. Place inside the oven and bake for 25-30 minutes at 425°F or until cheese has melted and crust is golden in color. Present warm.

Nutrition Information

- Calories: 173 calories
- Protein: 6g protein.
- Total Fat: 11g fat (4g saturated fat)
- Sodium: 427mg sodium
- Fiber: 0 fiber)
- Total Carbohydrate: 11g carbohydrate (1g sugars
- Cholesterol: 21mg cholesterol

587. Saucy Asian Meatballs

Serving: about 3 dozen. | Prep: 20mins | Cook: 20mins | Ready in:

Ingredients

- 1 pound lean ground turkey

- 2 garlic cloves, minced
- 1 teaspoon plus 1/4 cup reduced-sodium soy sauce, divided
- 1/2 teaspoon ground ginger
- 1/4 cup rice vinegar
- 1/4 cup tomato paste
- 2 tablespoons molasses
- 1 teaspoon hot pepper sauce

Direction

- Preheat an oven to 350°. Put turkey in big bowl. Sprinkle ginger, 1 teaspoon soy sauce and garlic. Lightly but thoroughly mix. Form to 1-in. balls; put in 15x10-1-in. baking pan. Bake for 20-25 minutes till cooked through.
- Mix and cook leftover soy sauce, pepper sauce, molasses, tomato paste and vinegar in big saucepan for 3-5 minutes on medium heat. Add meatballs and heat through, gently mixing to coat.

Nutrition Information

- Calories: 26 calories
- Sodium: 87mg sodium
- Fiber: 0 fiber)
- Total Carbohydrate: 2g carbohydrate (1g sugars
- Cholesterol: 10mg cholesterol
- Protein: 2g protein.
- Total Fat: 1g fat (0 saturated fat)

588. Saucy Turkey Meatballs

Serving: 15 servings. | Prep: 20mins | Cook: 30mins | Ready in:

Ingredients

- 1 cup old-fashioned oats
- 3/4 cup fat-free evaporated milk
- 1 medium onion, chopped
- 1 teaspoon salt
- 1 teaspoon chili powder
- 1/4 teaspoon garlic salt
- 1/4 teaspoon pepper
- 1-1/2 pounds lean ground turkey
- SAUCE:
- 2 cups ketchup
- 1-1/2 cups packed brown sugar
- 1/4 cup chopped onion
- 2 tablespoons Liquid Smoke, optional
- 1/2 teaspoons garlic salt

Direction

- Mix initial 7 ingredients in big bowl. Crumble turkey on mixture; stir well. Form to 1-inch balls. Put on rack coated in cooking spray in a shallow baking pan. Bake for 10-15 minutes, uncovered, at 350°.
- Meanwhile, mix sauce ingredients; put on meatballs. Bake till meat isn't pink for 30-35 minutes more.

Nutrition Information

- Calories: 217 calories
- Sodium: 695mg sodium
- Fiber: 1g fiber)
- Total Carbohydrate: 36g carbohydrate (0 sugars
- Cholesterol: 36mg cholesterol
- Protein: 10g protein. Diabetic Exchanges: 2 starch
- Total Fat: 4g fat (1g saturated fat)

589. Sausage Stuffed Red Potatoes

Serving: 16 appetizers. | Prep: 25mins | Cook: 10mins | Ready in:

Ingredients

- 8 small red potatoes

- 1 pound Italian turkey sausage links, casings removed
- 1/2 cup chopped sweet red pepper
- 4 green onions, chopped
- 9 teaspoons minced fresh parsley, divided
- 1/3 cup shredded reduced-fat cheddar cheese

Direction

- Scrub then pierce potatoes; put in microwave-safe plate. Microwave on high, uncovered, till tender, turning once, or for 8-9 minutes.
- Meanwhile, cook pepper and sausage in big skillet on medium heat till sausage isn't pink anymore. Add 4 1/2 teaspoons parsley and onions; cook for 1-2 minutes more. Take off heat. Mix cheese in. Lengthwise, cut every potato in half. Scoop 1 tablespoon pulp out for another use.
- In each half, put 2 tablespoons sausage mixture. Put on microwave-safe plate. Microwave for 1-2 minutes on high or till cheese melts. Sprinkle with extra parsley.

Nutrition Information

- Calories: 63 calories
- Sodium: 186mg sodium
- Fiber: 1g fiber)
- Total Carbohydrate: 3g carbohydrate (1g sugars
- Cholesterol: 19mg cholesterol
- Protein: 5g protein. Diabetic Exchanges: 1 lean meat.
- Total Fat: 3g fat (1g saturated fat)

590. Silly Snake Sub

Serving: 12 servings. | Prep: 15mins | Cook: 15mins | Ready in:

Ingredients

- 12 frozen bread dough dinner rolls
- 1/4 cup mayonnaise
- 10 slices cheddar cheese
- 1/2 pound thinly sliced deli turkey
- 1/2 pound thinly sliced deli ham
- 2 cups shredded lettuce
- 1 plum tomato, thinly sliced
- 1/4 cup yellow mustard
- 2 pimiento-stuffed olives
- 2-inch piece thinly sliced deli ham, optional

Direction

- On greased baking sheet, put rolls in S-shape, 1/2-in. apart. Use plastic wrap coated in cooking spray to cover. Let rise for 3 hours till doubled in a warm place.
- Preheat an oven to 350°. Bake rolls till golden brown or for 15-20 minutes. On pan on wire rack, completely cool.
- Crosswise, cut rolls in half with a serrated knife; leave halves intact. Spread mayonnaise on bun bottoms. Keep 1 cheese slice for later; layer tomato, lettuce, ham, turkey and leftover cheese on bottoms. Spread mustard on bun tops; replace tops. Attach olive to front of the snake for each eye with a frilly toothpick. Slice reserved cheese to decorative shapes; put on back of the snake. Cut snake tongue from ham if desired; attach to snake. Before serving, discard toothpicks.

Nutrition Information

- Calories:
- Cholesterol:
- Protein:
- Total Fat:
- Sodium:
- Fiber:
- Total Carbohydrate:

591. Southwest Turkey Spirals

Serving: 1 dozen. | Prep: 15mins | Cook: 0mins | Ready in:

Ingredients

- 1/2 cup shredded cooked turkey
- 3 tablespoons chopped green chilies, drained
- 2 ounces cream cheese, softened
- 1 tablespoon diced pimientos, drained
- 1 tablespoon minced fresh cilantro
- 1 tablespoon chopped ripe olives
- 2 teaspoons prepared ranch salad dressing
- 2 flour tortillas (6 inches), room temperature

Direction

- Mix initial 7 ingredients till blended in a small bowl. Spread on tortillas. Tightly roll up like a jellyroll. Use plastic to wrap. Refrigerate till firm for 2-3 hours. Slice to 1-in. slices.

Nutrition Information

- Calories: 47 calories
- Fiber: 0 fiber)
- Total Carbohydrate: 3g carbohydrate (0 sugars
- Cholesterol: 10mg cholesterol
- Protein: 3g protein. Diabetic Exchanges: 1/2 vegetable
- Total Fat: 3g fat (1g saturated fat)
- Sodium: 77mg sodium

592. Spinach Bacon Tartlets

Serving: 2-1/2 dozen. | Prep: 25mins | Cook: 15mins | Ready in:

Ingredients

- 1 package (8 ounces) reduced-fat cream cheese
- 1 egg white
- 1/2 cup frozen chopped spinach, thawed and squeezed dry
- 3 tablespoons chopped green onions (white part only)
- 1 teaspoon salt-free seasoning blend
- 1/4 teaspoon ground nutmeg
- 2 packages (1.9 ounces each) frozen miniature phyllo tart shells
- 3 turkey bacon strips, diced and cooked

Direction

- Beat initial 6 ingredients till blended in small bowl. Put filling in tart shells using a spoon. Put on ungreased baking sheet.
- Bake for 10 minutes at 350°. Sprinkle bacon. Bake till shells are lightly browned and filling sets for 2-5 more minutes. Serve warm.

Nutrition Information

- Calories: 46 calories
- Fiber: 0 fiber)
- Total Carbohydrate: 3g carbohydrate (0 sugars
- Cholesterol: 7mg cholesterol
- Protein: 2g protein.
- Total Fat: 3g fat (1g saturated fat)
- Sodium: 63mg sodium

593. Steamed Turkey Dumplings

Serving: 20 appetizers (1/3 cup sauce). | Prep: 30mins | Cook: 10mins | Ready in:

Ingredients

- 2 green onions, thinly sliced
- 2 tablespoons cornstarch
- 2 tablespoons minced fresh gingerroot
- 1 tablespoon reduced-sodium soy sauce
- 1 teaspoon sesame oil
- 1/2 pound lean ground turkey
- 20 wonton wrappers
- 9 lettuce leaves
- DIPPING SAUCE:
- 1/4 cup reduced-sodium soy sauce
- 1-1/2 teaspoons finely chopped green onion
- 1-1/2 teaspoons sesame oil
- 1 garlic clove, minced

Direction

- Mix oil, soy sauce, ginger, cornstarch and onions in big bowl. Crumble turkey on mixture; stir well.
- In middle of wonton wrapper, put 1 tablespoon turkey mixture. Use a damp paper towel to keep leftover wrappers covered till you use it. Use water to moisten edges. Diagonally, fold a corner on filling; to seal, press edges.
- Line 3 lettuce leaves on steamer basket. Put 1/3 dumplings on lettuce, 1-in. apart. Put in big saucepan above 1-in. water. Boil; cover. Steam till thermometer reads 165° or for 10-12 minutes. Discard lettuce and repeat two times.
- Mix sauce ingredients then serve with dumplings.

Nutrition Information

- Calories: 52 calories
- Total Carbohydrate: 6g carbohydrate (0 sugars
- Cholesterol: 10mg cholesterol
- Protein: 3g protein. Diabetic Exchanges: 1/2 starch.
- Total Fat: 2g fat (0 saturated fat)
- Sodium: 208mg sodium
- Fiber: 0 fiber)

594. Stromboli Ladder Loaf

Serving: 1 loaf (2 pounds). | Prep: 25mins | Cook: 20mins | Ready in:

Ingredients

- 1-1/2 cups water (70° to 80°)
- 2 tablespoons canola oil
- 1 teaspoon lemon juice
- 2 tablespoons nonfat dry milk powder
- 2 tablespoons sugar
- 1 teaspoon salt
- 4 cups bread flour
- 3 teaspoons active dry yeast
- FILLING:
- 3/4 cup pizza sauce
- 1 package (3-1/2 ounces) sliced pepperoni
- 2 cups shredded part-skim mozzarella cheese
- 1/2 cup grated Parmesan cheese
- 1 large egg white
- 1 tablespoon water

Direction

- In order recommended by manufacturer, put initial 8 ingredients in bread machine pan. Choose dough setting, check the dough after 5 minutes of stirring. If needed, add 1-2 tablespoons of flour/water. Turn dough on lightly floured surface when cycle is completed. Roll to 15x12-inch rectangle; put on a greased baking sheet.
- In 3-inch-wide strip, spread pizza sauce lengthwise down the middle of dough within 2-inch of the ends. Put pepperoni on sauce; sprinkle cheese. Cut 1-inch-wide strips, 2 1/2-inch into middle, on each long side. Fold alternating strips, beginning at one end, at angle across the filling. Seal by pinching ends.
- Beat water and egg white; brush on dough. Bake till golden brown at 425 degrees for 20-25 minutes. Before cutting, let stand for 10 minutes.

Nutrition Information

- Calories: 259 calories
- Protein: 15g protein. Diabetic Exchanges: 2 starch
- Total Fat: 7g fat (3g saturated fat)
- Sodium: 554mg sodium
- Fiber: 1g fiber)
- Total Carbohydrate: 34g carbohydrate (4g sugars
- Cholesterol: 24mg cholesterol

595. Stuffed Turkey Spirals

Serving: about 30 servings. | Prep: 20mins | Cook: 01hours15mins | Ready in:

Ingredients

- 2 boneless skinless turkey breast halves (1 pound each)
- 1/4 cup olive oil, divided
- 4 teaspoons dried basil, divided
- 1 pound thinly sliced deli ham
- 1 pound thinly sliced Swiss cheese
- 1 teaspoon salt
- 1 teaspoon pepper
- BASIL SAUCE:
- 2 cups mayonnaise
- 1/2 cup milk
- 1 to 2 tablespoons dried basil
- 1 teaspoon sugar

Direction

- Horizontally, cut every turkey breast from long side within 1/2-inch of opposing side then open flat. Use plastic wrap to cover. Flatten to 12x10-inch rectangles.
- Discard plastic; put 1 teaspoon of basil and 1 teaspoon of oil on each. Within 1-inch of edges, layer with cheese and ham. Roll up, starting with long side, jellyroll style. Use kitchen string to tie. Put on rack in a roasting pan.
- Mix basil, leftover oil, pepper and salt in small bowl; put some on turkey.
- Bake for 75-90 minutes at 325° till thermometer reads 170°, occasionally basting with leftover oil mixture.
- In a blender, process sauce ingredients, covered, till blended. Before slicing, cool turkey for 5 minutes then serve with basil sauce.

Nutrition Information

- Calories: 218 calories
- Fiber: 0 fiber)
- Total Carbohydrate: 1g carbohydrate (1g sugars
- Cholesterol: 38mg cholesterol
- Protein: 11g protein.
- Total Fat: 19g fat (5g saturated fat)
- Sodium: 336mg sodium

596. Sun Dried Tomato Turkey Pinwheels

Serving: 40 appetizers. | Prep: 20mins | Cook: 0mins | Ready in:

Ingredients

- 2/3 cup sun-dried tomato pesto
- 4 flour tortillas (8 inches)
- 1/2 cup crumbled goat cheese
- 1/3 cup pitted Greek olives, chopped
- 1/4 cup minced fresh basil
- 8 slices deli turkey
- 1 cup fresh baby spinach

Direction

- Spread pesto on tortillas. Sprinkle basil, olives and cheese on each. Layer with spinach and turkey. Tightly roll up; use plastic to wrap. Refrigerate for 2 hours minimum.
- Unwrap. Slice each to 10 slices.

Nutrition Information

- Calories: 33 calories
- Protein: 2g protein.
- Total Fat: 1g fat (0 saturated fat)
- Sodium: 131mg sodium
- Fiber: 0 fiber)
- Total Carbohydrate: 3g carbohydrate (0 sugars
- Cholesterol: 3mg cholesterol

597. Sweet & Sour Turkey Meatballs

Serving: about 5 dozen. | Prep: 30mins | Cook: 02hours00mins | Ready in:

Ingredients

- 4 thick-sliced peppered bacon strips
- 1 large egg, beaten
- 1/2 cup seasoned bread crumbs
- 3 tablespoons minced fresh cilantro
- 1 teaspoon salt
- 1 teaspoon white pepper
- 2 pounds ground turkey
- 1 jar (18 ounces) apricot preserves
- 1 can (14-1/2 ounces) diced tomatoes, undrained
- 1 bottle (8 ounces) taco sauce
- 1/2 cup pomegranate juice

Direction

- Preheat an oven to 400°. In food processor, pulse bacon till finely chopped, covered. Mix pepper, salt, cilantro, bread crumbs and egg. Crumble bacon and turkey on egg mixture; lightly yet thoroughly mix. Form to 1-in. balls.
- Put in 2 15x10x1-in. ungreased baking pans. Bake for 8-10 minutes till not pink anymore.
- Mix juice, taco sauce, tomatoes and preserves in 4-qt. slow cooker. Mix meatballs in. Cook on high, covered, for 2-3 hours till inserted thermometer in a few meatballs reads 165°.

Nutrition Information

- Calories: 67 calories
- Sodium: 113mg sodium
- Fiber: 0 fiber)
- Total Carbohydrate: 7g carbohydrate (5g sugars
- Cholesterol: 15mg cholesterol
- Protein: 4g protein.
- Total Fat: 3g fat (1g saturated fat)

598. Tangy BBQ Meatballs

Serving: 3 dozen. | Prep: 15mins | Cook: 01hours20mins | Ready in:

Ingredients

- 1 egg white, lightly beaten
- 3/4 cup graham cracker crumbs (about 12 squares)
- 3 tablespoons milk
- 2 teaspoons prepared mustard
- 1/4 teaspoon salt
- 3/4 pound lean ground beef (90% lean)
- 3/4 pound ground turkey
- SAUCE:
- 1 cup barbecue sauce
- 1 can (6 ounces) frozen orange juice concentrate, thawed
- 1/4 cup water

Direction

- Mix salt, mustard, milk, cracker crumbs and egg white in big bowl. Crumble turkey and beef on mixture; stir well. Form to 1 1/2-inch balls. Put meatballs on greased rack in shallow baking pan. Bake for 20 minutes till meat isn't pink at 375°; drain.
- Put meatballs in a 2-quart greased baking dish. Mix sauce ingredients; put on meatballs. Cover. Bake for 1 hour at 350°.

Nutrition Information

- Calories: 109 calories
- Protein: 8g protein.
- Total Fat: 5g fat (2g saturated fat)
- Sodium: 210mg sodium
- Fiber: 0 fiber)
- Total Carbohydrate: 8g carbohydrate (6g sugars
- Cholesterol: 22mg cholesterol

599. Tangy Turkey Meatballs

Serving: about 5 dozen. | Prep: 10mins | Cook: 50mins | Ready in:

Ingredients

- 2 cups soft bread crumbs
- 1/2 cup finely chopped onion
- 2 pounds ground turkey
- 1 jar (12 ounces) currant jelly
- 1 bottle (12 ounces) chili sauce

Direction

- Mix onion and crumbs in a big bowl. Crumble turkey on mixture; mix well. Form to 1-inch balls. Put in 13x9-inch lightly greased baking dish. Mix chili sauce and jelly; put on meatballs.
- Cover. Bake for 40 minutes at 350°F. Uncover. Bake till meat isn't pink for 10 more minutes.

Nutrition Information

- Calories: 162 calories
- Total Fat: 7g fat (2g saturated fat)
- Sodium: 301mg sodium
- Fiber: 0 fiber
- Total Carbohydrate: 18g carbohydrate (14g sugars
- Cholesterol: 31mg cholesterol
- Protein: 8g protein.

600. Tender Turkey Meatballs

Serving: 6 servings. | Prep: 25mins | Cook: 20mins | Ready in:

Ingredients

- 1/2 cup chopped onion
- 1/4 cup egg substitute
- 1/4 cup toasted wheat germ
- 1/4 cup chopped green pepper
- 1/4 cup ketchup
- 1 teaspoon chili powder
- 1/2 teaspoon dried marjoram
- 1/2 teaspoon pepper
- 1 pound lean ground turkey
- 1 package (12 ounces) spaghetti
- 5 cups meatless spaghetti sauce

Direction

- Mix initial 8 ingredients in a bowl. Crumble turkey on mixture; stir well. Form to 30 balls, 1-inch each. Put meatballs on a rack coated in cooking spray in a shallow baking pan. Bake for 13-16 minutes till juices are clear at 400°. Drain.
- Meanwhile, follow package directions to cook spaghetti. Put meatballs in big saucepan; add spaghetti sauce and heat through. Drain the spaghetti. Put sauce and meatballs on top.

Nutrition Information

- Calories: 312 calories
- Sodium: 1047mg sodium
- Fiber: 5g fiber
- Total Carbohydrate: 40g carbohydrate (0 sugars
- Cholesterol: 60mg cholesterol
- Protein: 22g protein. Diabetic Exchanges: 2-1/2 starch
- Total Fat: 7g fat (2g saturated fat)

601. Thanksgiving Wontons

Serving: 3 dozen. | Prep: 15mins | Cook: 10mins | Ready in:

Ingredients

- 1-1/2 cups finely chopped cooked turkey breast

- 2/3 cup dried cranberries, finely chopped
- 1/3 cup whipped cream cheese
- 1/3 cup jellied cranberry sauce
- 36 wonton wrappers
- Oil for deep-fat frying

Direction

- Mix cranberry sauce, cream cheese, cranberries and turkey in a small bowl.
- In middle of wonton wrapper, put 1 tablespoon filling. Use damp paper towel to cover leftover wrappers till you use it. Use water to moisten edges. Diagonally, fold a corner over filling to make a triangle. Seal by pressing edges. Repeat with leftover wonton wrappers and filling.
- Heat oil to 375° in electric skillet. A few at a time, fry wontons till golden brown or 30-60 seconds per side. On paper towels, drain. Serve warm.

Nutrition Information

- Calories: 65 calories
- Sodium: 56mg sodium
- Fiber: 0 fiber)
- Total Carbohydrate: 8g carbohydrate (2g sugars
- Cholesterol: 8mg cholesterol
- Protein: 3g protein.
- Total Fat: 3g fat (1g saturated fat)

602. Turkey & Swiss Biscuit Sliders

Serving: 16 servings. | Prep: 35mins | Cook: 5mins | Ready in:

Ingredients

- 1 package (1/4 ounce) active dry yeast
- 2/3 cup warm buttermilk (110° to 115°)
- 2 tablespoons warm water (110° to 115°)
- 2 cups bread flour
- 3 tablespoons sugar
- 1-1/2 teaspoons baking powder
- 1/2 teaspoon salt
- 1/2 cup shortening
- 3/4 pound thinly sliced deli smoked turkey
- 1/2 pound sliced Swiss cheese
- Dijon mustard, optional

Direction

- Melt yeast in water and warm buttermilk in small bowl. In food processor, pulse salt, baking powder, sugar and flour till blended. Add shortening and pulse till shortening is pea-sized. Add yeast mixture slowly while processing then process just till dough becomes a ball.
- Turn dough on lightly floured surface and knead 8-10 times. Roll/pat to 1/2-in. thickness. Use floured 2-in. biscuit cutter to cut. Put on greased baking sheets, 2-in. apart. Rise for 30 minutes till nearly doubled.
- Preheat an oven to 425°. Bake biscuits till golden brown or for 7-9 minutes. Transfer to wire racks; slightly cool. Preheat the broiler.
- Split biscuits to half. Put bottoms onto greased baking sheets. Layer with cheese and turkey. Broil for 2-3 minutes or till cheese melts for 3-4-in. away from heat. Replace tops. Serve with mustard if desired.

Nutrition Information

- Calories: 198 calories
- Cholesterol: 23mg cholesterol
- Protein: 11g protein.
- Total Fat: 11g fat (5g saturated fat)
- Sodium: 306mg sodium
- Fiber: 0 fiber)
- Total Carbohydrate: 14g carbohydrate (3g sugars

603. Turkey Bolognese Polenta Nests

Serving: 2 dozen. | Prep: 40mins | Cook: 25mins | Ready in:

Ingredients

- 3-1/2 cups chicken stock, divided
- 1 cup yellow cornmeal
- 3/4 cup grated Parmigiano-Reggiano cheese, divided
- 1/2 cup heavy whipping cream
- 1/4 teaspoon salt
- 1/4 teaspoon pepper
- 1 tablespoon olive oil
- 1 cup chopped onion
- 3 garlic cloves, minced
- 1/2 pound ground turkey
- 1/3 cup tomato paste
- 1-1/2 teaspoons Italian seasoning

Direction

- Preheat an oven to 350°. Use cooking spray to coat 24 mini muffin cups; put aside.
- Boil 3 cups chicken stock in big heavy saucepan. Lower heat to gently boil; whisk cornmeal in slowly. Mix and cook with wooden spoon for 15-20 minutes till mixture is very thick and polenta cleanly pulls away from pans sides and thickens. Mix pepper, salt, cream and 1/2 cup cheese in. Put 2 tablespoons polenta mixture in every mini muffin cup. Press indentation in middle of each using wooden spoon handle's end as polenta cools to make a nest shape; put aside. Wipe pan out.
- Heat oil in same saucepan on medium high heat. Add onion; sauté for 2-3 minutes till translucent. Add garlic; cook for 1 more minute. Add turkey; sauté till not pink anymore. Mix leftover chicken stock, Italian seasoning and tomato paste in. Cook, occasionally mixing, for 5 minutes till thickened.
- Fill every polenta indention with 2 teaspoons turkey mixture. Sprinkle leftover cheese; bake for 25-30 minutes till edges are golden. Take out of oven. Before removing from muffin cups, cool for 10 minutes minimum. You can freeze for later use or refrigerate.

Nutrition Information

- Calories: 80 calories
- Total Carbohydrate: 7g carbohydrate (1g sugars
- Cholesterol: 14mg cholesterol
- Protein: 4g protein.
- Total Fat: 4g fat (2g saturated fat)
- Sodium: 154mg sodium
- Fiber: 0 fiber)

604. Turkey Cheese Ball

Serving: 24 servings, 2 Tbsp. each | Prep: 20mins | Cook: | Ready in:

Ingredients

- 1 cup PLANTERS Pecan Halves, divided
- 2 pkg. (8 oz. each) PHILADELPHIA Cream Cheese, softened
- 1 pkg. (8 oz.) KRAFT Finely Shredded Sharp Cheddar Cheese
- 4 slices cooked OSCAR MAYER Bacon, crumbled
- 2 green onions, chopped
- 1 Tbsp. (about half of 0.7-oz. env.) GOOD SEASONS Italian Dressing Mix
- 1 Tbsp. LEA & PERRINS Worcestershire Sauce
- 1 each orange, red and yellow pepper, cut into 1/2-inch-wide strips, divided

Direction

- Chop nuts to get 1/2 cup; put in big bowl. Add Worcestershire sauce, dressing mix,

onions, bacon, cheddar and cream cheese; beat using mixer till blended.
- Refrigerate till firm for 45 minutes.
- Keep 1 teaspoon of cream cheese mixture. Form leftover cream cheese mixture to oblong-shaped ball for turkey body.
- Cut off small piece from 1 yellow pepper strip; reserve with 2 red pepper strips for turkey's waddle and beak. Insert ends of 1/2 leftover pepper strips, starting at cheese ball's back end, into cheese ball for turkey's tail feathers. Fan leftover pepper strips around the back of bottom edge of the cheese ball for the 2nd feather row, inserting pepper ends into cheese ball so it is secure.
- Insert leftover nuts in top of cheese balls. Insert leftover red pepper strips in front of the cheese ball for turkey's waddle. Use leftover cream cheese mixture so you can attach leftover yellow pepper piece to 1 pepper strip's top for turkey's beak.

Nutrition Information

- Calories: 150
- Total Fat: 14 g
- Sodium: 220 mg
- Total Carbohydrate: 3 g
- Sugar: 2 g
- Cholesterol: 30 mg
- Protein: 4 g
- Saturated Fat: 6 g
- Fiber: 1 g

605. Turkey Crescents

Serving: 2 dozen. | Prep: 20mins | Cook: 10mins | Ready in:

Ingredients

- 1/2 cup finely chopped celery
- 1/4 cup finely chopped onion
- 1 teaspoon butter
- 2 cups finely chopped cooked turkey
- 1 can (10-3/4 ounces) condensed cream of mushroom soup, undiluted
- 3 packages (8 ounces each) refrigerated crescent rolls
- Dill weed

Direction

- Sauté onion and celery in butter in a nonstick skillet until tender for 3-4 minutes. Add soup and turkey; stir well. Take off from heat.
- Separate crescent dough to 24 triangles. On each triangle's wide end, put 1 tbsp. turkey mixture. Roll it up from the wide end. Put on greased baking sheets, 2-in. apart, pointed side down. Curve the ends to make a crescent shape. Sprinkle with dill.
- Bake for 8-9 minutes or until golden brown at 350 degrees. Immediately serve.

Nutrition Information

- Calories: 70 calories
- Fiber: 0 fiber)
- Total Carbohydrate: 5g carbohydrate (1g sugars
- Cholesterol: 10mg cholesterol
- Protein: 4g protein.
- Total Fat: 3g fat (1g saturated fat)
- Sodium: 175mg sodium

606. Turkey Croquettes With Cranberry Salsa

Serving: 16 croquettes (2 cups salsa). | Prep: 30mins | Cook: 5mins | Ready in:

Ingredients

- 2 tablespoons butter
- 1/3 cup chopped onion
- 1/4 cup all-purpose flour
- 1/4 cup 2% milk

- 1/4 cup chicken broth
- 2 cups finely chopped cooked turkey
- 1/2 cup mashed sweet potato
- 1/2 teaspoon salt
- 1/4 teaspoon pepper
- 1/8 teaspoon cayenne pepper
- SALSA:
- 3/4 cup chopped tart apple
- 1 tablespoon lemon juice
- 1/2 cup chopped cranberries
- 2 jalapeno peppers, seeded and chopped
- 2 green onions, chopped
- 3 tablespoons golden raisins, chopped
- 1 tablespoon honey
- CROQUETTES:
- 2 eggs
- 1 tablespoon water
- 1/2 cup all-purpose flour
- 1/2 cup dry bread crumbs
- Oil for deep-fat frying

Direction

- Heat butter in big saucepan on medium heat; add onion. Mix and cook till tender for 3-4 minutes.
- Mix flour in till blended. Add broth and milk slowly; boil. Mix and cook till thick for 2 minutes. Take off heat. Mix cayenne, pepper, salt, sweet potato and turkey in. Refrigerate for 2 hours till firm, covered.
- Meanwhile, toss lemon juice and apple in a small bowl. Mix leftover salsa ingredients in; refrigerate for 1 hour minimum, covered.
- Croquettes: Beat water and eggs in shallow bowl. Put bread crumbs and flour in different shallow bowls. Form turkey mixture to 1 1/2-inch balls. Roll flour in; shake excess off. Roll into egg mixture then into crumbs. Pat to adhere coating.
- Heat oil to 375° in deep-fat fryer/electric skillet. A few at a time, fry croquettes till golden brown, 1-2 minutes per side. On paper towels, drain. Serve with cranberry salsa.

Nutrition Information

- Calories: 317 calories
- Sodium: 315mg sodium
- Fiber: 2g fiber)
- Total Carbohydrate: 27g carbohydrate (8g sugars
- Cholesterol: 90mg cholesterol
- Protein: 15g protein.
- Total Fat: 17g fat (4g saturated fat)

607. Turkey Egg Rolls

Serving: 10 egg rolls. | Prep: 15mins | Cook: 15mins | Ready in:

Ingredients

- 1/2 pound ground turkey
- 2 cups coleslaw mix
- 1 tablespoon soy sauce
- 1/2 teaspoon ground ginger
- 1/4 teaspoon onion salt
- 1/4 teaspoon garlic powder
- 10 egg roll wrappers
- Oil for deep-fat frying
- Sweet-and-sour sauce

Direction

- Cook turkey in big skillet on medium heat till not pink anymore; drain. Mix garlic powder, onion salt, ginger, soy sauce and coleslaw mix in. In middle of every egg roll wrapper, put 1/4 cup. Fold bottom corner on filling; fold sides toward middle. Use water to moisten leftover wrapper's corner. Tightly roll up to seal then repeat.
- Heat oil to 375° in deep-fat fryer/electric skillet. A few at a time, fry egg rolls for 3-4 minutes or till golden brown, flipping often. On paper towels, drain. Serve it with sweet-and-sour sauce.

Nutrition Information

- Calories: 287 calories
- Sodium: 694mg sodium
- Fiber: 2g fiber)
- Total Carbohydrate: 39g carbohydrate (1g sugars
- Cholesterol: 37mg cholesterol
- Protein: 14g protein.
- Total Fat: 8g fat (2g saturated fat)

608. Turkey Nachos

Serving: Makes 6 to 8 hors d'oeuvre servings | Prep: | Cook: | Ready in:

Ingredients

- 1/2 lb leftover roast turkey meat, shredded
- 1 1/2 tablespoons fresh lime juice
- 2 tablespoons vegetable oil
- 3 bell peppers (preferably red and orange), finely chopped
- 1 garlic clove, finely chopped
- 1/4 teaspoon ground cumin
- 1 teaspoon dried oregano, crumbled
- 1 (15- to 16-oz) can black beans, rinsed and drained
- 4 oz corn tortilla chips (not low-fat)
- 2 cups grated jalapeño Jack cheese (8 oz)
- 1/4 cup chopped scallion greens
- 1/2 cup chopped fresh cilantro
- 1 cup sour cream
- 2 to 3 teaspoons finely chopped pickled jalapeño
- Accompaniment: tomato salsa

Direction

- Preheat an oven to 450°.
- Toss lime juice and turkey; season with pepper and salt.
- In 10-inch heavy skillet, heat 1 1/2 tablespoon of oil on moderately high heat till hot yet not smoking. Sauté bell peppers, mixing, for 3 minutes till crisp-tender. Put in bowl. Heat leftover 1/2 tablespoon of oil in skillet on medium heat. Cook oregano, cumin and garlic, mixing, for a minute. Mix beans in; cook, mixing, for 1 minute till heated through. Season with pepper and salt.
- Make 2 layers each of cilantro, scallion, cheese, turkey, beans, sautéed peppers and corn chips in a 3-quart shallow baking dish. In middle of oven, bake nachos for 6-10 minutes till cheese melts.
- Mix jalapeno to taste and sour cream. Serve along side with salsa.

Nutrition Information

- Calories: 481
- Total Carbohydrate: 31 g(10%)
- Cholesterol: 79 mg(26%)
- Protein: 25 g(50%)
- Total Fat: 29 g(45%)
- Saturated Fat: 13 g(63%)
- Sodium: 453 mg(19%)
- Fiber: 7 g(30%)

609. Turkey Quesadillas

Serving: 4 quesadillas (8 wedges each). | Prep: 15mins | Cook: 5mins | Ready in:

Ingredients

- 1 pound lean ground turkey
- 1 cup chopped red onion
- 1 to 2 garlic cloves, minced
- 2 cups julienned zucchini
- 1 cup salsa
- 1 cup frozen corn
- 1 cup julienned sweet red pepper
- 1 can (4 ounces) chopped green chilies
- 2 tablespoons minced fresh cilantro
- 1/2 teaspoon dried oregano
- 1/2 teaspoon ground cumin
- 1/4 teaspoon salt
- 1/8 teaspoon cayenne pepper
- 8 flour tortillas (8 inches)

- 2 cups shredded reduced-fat Mexican cheese blend

Direction

- Cook garlic, onion and turkey in big nonstick skillet on medium heat till meat isn't pink anymore; drain. Add chilies, red pepper, corn, salsa and zucchini. Lower heat. Cover. Simmer till veggies are tender; mix seasonings in.
- For each quesadilla: In ungreased nonstick skillet, put a tortilla. Sprinkle 1/4 cup cheese on. Put 1/2 cup filling on top. Sprinkle 1/4 cup cheese more. Cover with 2nd tortilla. Cook on medium heat, turning once carefully, till cheese starts to melt and quesadilla is lightly browned on both sides. Cut to 8 wedges.

Nutrition Information

- Calories: 179 calories
- Cholesterol: 32mg cholesterol
- Protein: 12g protein. Diabetic Exchanges: 2 starch
- Total Fat: 7g fat (2g saturated fat)
- Sodium: 388mg sodium
- Fiber: 1g fiber)
- Total Carbohydrate: 18g carbohydrate (2g sugars

610. Turkey Sandwiches With Red Pepper Hummus

Serving: 4 servings. | Prep: 20mins | Cook: 5mins | Ready in:

Ingredients

- 1/3 cup mayonnaise
- 1 tablespoon lime juice
- 1 can (15 ounces) garbanzo beans or chickpeas, rinsed and drained
- 1/4 cup chopped roasted sweet red peppers, drained
- 2 garlic cloves, peeled
- 1/2 teaspoon chili powder
- 1/4 teaspoon ground cumin
- 2 tablespoons butter, softened
- 8 slices rye bread
- 4 slices Muenster cheese
- 8 thin slices cooked turkey
- 1 small red onion, sliced
- 2 medium tomatoes, sliced

Direction

- Hummus: In blender, process initial 7 ingredients till smooth, covered. Put in small bowl; cover. Refrigerate for an hour.
- Spread butter on a side of every bread slice. Spread hummus on opposite side. Put 4 slices on griddle, buttered side down. Layer with leftover bread, hummus side down, tomatoes, onion, turkey and cheese. Toast till cheese melts and bread browns lightly or for 2-3 minutes per side.

Nutrition Information

- Calories:
- Total Fat:
- Sodium:
- Fiber:
- Total Carbohydrate:
- Cholesterol:
- Protein:

611. Turkey Sliders With Chili Cheese Mayo

Serving: 1 dozen. | Prep: 25mins | Cook: 10mins | Ready in:

Ingredients

- 4 bacon strips

- 1 medium onion, finely chopped
- 2 garlic cloves, minced
- 2 tablespoons Worcestershire sauce
- 1/2 teaspoon salt
- 1/4 teaspoon pepper
- 1 pound ground turkey
- 2 tablespoons olive oil
- 12 heat-and-serve rolls
- MAYO:
- 1 cup mayonnaise
- 1 jar (5 ounces) sharp American cheese spread
- 1 teaspoon onion powder
- 1 teaspoon garlic powder
- 1 teaspoon chili powder
- TOPPINGS:
- 12 small lettuce leaves
- 2 plum tomatoes, thinly sliced

Direction

- Cook bacon in big skillet till crisp on medium heat. Transfer to paper towels; drain. Crumble bacon; put aside. Sauté onion in drippings in same skillet till tender. Add garlic, cook for 1 more minute.
- Put into big bowl. Add pepper, salt, Worcestershire sauce and bacon. Crumble turkey on mixture; stir well. Form to 12 patties.
- In big skillet, cook in oil on medium heat, 3-4 minutes per side, or till juices are clear and thermometer reads 165°. Meanwhile, follow package directions to bake rolls.
- Mayo: Mix chili powder, garlic powder, onion powder, cheese spread and mayonnaise in small bowl. Split rolls then spread mayo on. Top tomato and lettuce on each burger.

Nutrition Information

- Calories: 420 calories
- Sodium: 686mg sodium
- Fiber: 2g fiber)
- Total Carbohydrate: 17g carbohydrate (3g sugars
- Cholesterol: 49mg cholesterol
- Protein: 11g protein.
- Total Fat: 33g fat (9g saturated fat)

612. Turkey Sliders With Sesame Slaw

Serving: 12 servings. | Prep: 20mins | Cook: 10mins | Ready in:

Ingredients

- 2/3 cup mayonnaise
- 2 tablespoons hoisin sauce
- 2 teaspoons Sriracha Asian hot chili sauce
- 1-1/2 pounds ground turkey
- 1/2 cup panko (Japanese) bread crumbs
- 2 green onions, finely chopped
- 2 tablespoons reduced-sodium soy sauce, divided
- 2 teaspoons minced fresh gingerroot
- 2 tablespoons rice vinegar
- 2 teaspoons sugar
- 2 teaspoons sesame oil
- 6 small carrots, grated (about 1-1/2 cups)
- 1/3 cup thinly sliced red onion
- 3 tablespoons chopped fresh cilantro
- 1 teaspoon sesame seeds, toasted
- 12 slider buns or dinner rolls, split and toasted

Direction

- Mix chili sauce, hoisin sauce and mayonnaise in small bowl; refrigerate till serving.
- Lightly yet thoroughly, mix ginger, 1 tablespoon soy sauce, green onions, panko and turkey in a big bowl. Form to 12 patties, 1/2-in. thick.
- Whisk leftover soy sauce, oil, sugar and vinegar in small bowl. Add sesame seeds, cilantro, onion and carrots; toss till combined.
- Use cooking oil to moisten paper towel. Rub on grill rack to lightly coat with long-handled tongs. Grill sliders on medium heat, covered or broil, 3 minutes per side, 4-in. away from heat till thermometer registers 165°. Spread

mayonnaise mixture on cut sides of buns. Layer with slaw and burger; replace tops.

Nutrition Information

- Calories:
- Total Carbohydrate:
- Cholesterol:
- Protein:
- Total Fat:
- Sodium:
- Fiber:

---

613. Turkey Sliders With Sweet Potato "Buns"

Serving: 10 servings. | Prep: 25mins | Cook: 45mins | Ready in:

Ingredients

- 4 applewood-smoked bacon strips, finely chopped
- 1 pound ground turkey
- 1/2 cup panko (Japanese) bread crumbs
- 2 large eggs
- 1/2 cup grated Parmesan cheese
- 4 tablespoons chopped fresh cilantro
- 1 teaspoon dried basil
- 1/2 teaspoon ground cumin
- 1 tablespoon soy sauce
- 2 large sweet potatoes
- Shredded Colby-Monterey Jack cheese
- Honey Dijon mustard

Direction

- Cook bacon in big skillet on medium heat till crisp; drain on paper towels. Throw all but 2 tablespoons of drippings. Put aside skillet. Mix bacon with next 8 ingredients till mixed well; cover. Refrigerate for 30 minutes minimum.
- Preheat an oven to 425°. Slice sweet potatoes to 20 slices, 1/2-inch thick. Put slices on ungreased baking sheet; bake for 30-35 minutes till tender yet not mushy. Remove slices. On wire rack, cool.
- Heat skillet with leftover drippings on medium high heat. Form turkey mixture to slider-sized patties. In batches, cook sliders, 3-4 minutes per side. Don't crowd skillet. After flipping every slider the 1st time, add pinch of shredded cheddar. Cook till juices are clear and thermometer reads 165°.
- Serving: On sweet potato slice, put each slider. Dab using honey Dijon mustard. Use 2nd sweet potato slice to cover. Use toothpick to pierce.

Nutrition Information

- Calories: 226 calories
- Protein: 14g protein.
- Total Fat: 10g fat (3g saturated fat)
- Sodium: 293mg sodium
- Fiber: 2g fiber)
- Total Carbohydrate: 20g carbohydrate (7g sugars
- Cholesterol: 78mg cholesterol

---

614. Turkey Taco Dip

Serving: Makes 3 cups dip or 24 servings, 2 Tbsp. dip and 16 crackers. | Prep: 5mins | Cook: | Ready in:

Ingredients

- 1/2 lb. ground turkey
- 1 pkg. (1-1/4 oz.) TACO BELL® Taco Seasoning Mix
- 1/2 cup water
- 1 can (16 oz.) black beans, drained
- 1/2 cup KRAFT Shredded Fat Free Cheddar Cheese
- 1 cup chopped tomato
- thin wheat snack crackers

Direction

- In nonstick skillet, mix and cook turkey, mixing to break turkey up, till not pink anymore. Add water and seasoning mix; boil. Cook for 2-3 minutes on medium heat.
- Mix beans in; cook for 5 more minutes, constantly mixing and slightly mashing with fork. Mix 1/4 cup cheese in.
- Put in serving bowl using a spoon. Put tomato and leftover cheese on top. Serve as dip with crackers.

Nutrition Information

- Calories: 190
- Total Fat: 7 g
- Saturated Fat: 1.5 g
- Fiber: 2 g
- Sugar: 4 g
- Total Carbohydrate: 25 g
- Cholesterol: 5 mg
- Protein: 7 g
- Sodium: 440 mg

615. Turkey Tea Sandwiches With Basil Mayonnaise

Serving: 20 tea sandwiches. | Prep: 15mins | Cook: 0mins | Ready in:

Ingredients

- 1/2 cup mayonnaise
- 1/3 cup loosely packed basil leaves
- 10 slices white bread, crusts removed
- 10 ounces thinly sliced deli turkey
- 5 slices provolone cheese

Direction

- In food processor, process basil and mayonnaise till basil is chopped finely, scraping sides down if needed. Over each bread slice, spread mayonnaise mixture. With cheese and turkey, layer 5 bread slices. Put leftover bread on top. Cut every sandwich to 4 triangles.

Nutrition Information

- Calories:
- Cholesterol:
- Protein:
- Total Fat:
- Sodium:
- Fiber:
- Total Carbohydrate:

616. Turkey Wonton Cups

Serving: 4 dozen. | Prep: 30mins | Cook: 5mins | Ready in:

Ingredients

- 48 wonton wrappers
- 1-1/4 pounds lean ground turkey
- 2 cups shredded reduced-fat cheddar cheese
- 1 cup fat-free ranch salad dressing
- 1/2 cup chopped green onions
- 1/4 cup chopped ripe olives

Direction

- In miniature muffin cups coated in cooking spray, press wonton wrappers. Cover wrappers with damp paper towel till baking time. Bake till lightly browned or for 5 minutes at 375°. Before transferring from pans onto wire racks, cool for 2 minutes.
- Cook turkey in big nonstick skillet coated in cooking spray on medium heat till not pink anymore; drain. Mix olives, onions, ranch dressing, cheese and turkey in big bowl. By rounded tablespoonfuls using a spoon, put in wonton cups.
- Put on ungreased baking sheet. Bake till heated through or for 5-6 minutes at 375°. Serve warm.

Nutrition Information

- Calories: 154 calories
- Sodium: 366mg sodium
- Fiber: 0 fiber)
- Total Carbohydrate: 14g carbohydrate (1g sugars
- Cholesterol: 34mg cholesterol
- Protein: 11g protein. Diabetic Exchanges: 1 starch
- Total Fat: 7g fat (3g saturated fat)

617. Turkey Cranberry Minis

Serving: 2-1/2 dozen. | Prep: 25mins | Cook: 10mins | Ready in:

Ingredients

- 1/3 cup mayonnaise
- 4 teaspoons minced fresh parsley
- 4 teaspoons honey mustard
- 1/2 teaspoon chopped seeded jalapeno pepper
- 1/8 teaspoon pepper
- 2 cups cubed cooked turkey breast
- 1/3 cup chopped celery
- 1/3 cup dried cranberries, chopped
- 1/3 cup shredded Swiss cheese
- 1/4 cup chopped pecans, toasted
- 30 frozen miniature phyllo tart shells

Direction

- Mix initial 5 ingredients in big bowl. Add pecans, cheese, cranberries, celery and turkey; toss to coat.
- On ungreased baking sheet, put tart shells. Fill using turkey mixture. Bake till heated through or for 10-12 minutes at 375°. Serve warm.

Nutrition Information

- Calories: 71 calories
- Sodium: 38mg sodium
- Fiber: 0 fiber)
- Total Carbohydrate: 4g carbohydrate (1g sugars
- Cholesterol: 10mg cholesterol
- Protein: 4g protein.
- Total Fat: 4g fat (1g saturated fat)

618. Turkey Mushroom Egg Rolls

Serving: 3-1/2 dozen. | Prep: 01hours15mins | Cook: 04hours00mins | Ready in:

Ingredients

- 1-1/2 pounds ground turkey
- 1/2 pound sliced fresh mushrooms
- 2 medium leeks (white portion only), thinly sliced
- 3 celery ribs, thinly sliced
- 1/2 cup hoisin sauce
- 2 tablespoons minced fresh gingerroot
- 2 tablespoons rice vinegar
- 2 tablespoons reduced-sodium soy sauce
- 1 tablespoon packed brown sugar
- 1 tablespoon sesame oil
- 2 garlic cloves, minced
- 1/2 cup sliced water chestnuts, chopped
- 3 green onions, thinly sliced
- 42 egg roll wrappers
- Oil for frying
- Sweet-and-sour sauce or Chinese-style mustard, optional

Direction

- Cook turkey in big skillet on medium heat till not pink anymore or for 8-10 minutes, breaking to crumbles. Put in 5-qt. slow cooker.
- Mix garlic, sesame oil, brown sugar, soy sauce, vinegar, ginger, hoisin sauce, celery, leeks and mushrooms in. Cook for 4-5 hours on low or till veggies are tender, covered. Mix green onions and water chestnuts into turkey mixture; slightly cool.

- Put 2 tablespoons filling right below middle of wrapper with a corner of egg roll wrapper facing you. Use damp paper towel to cover leftover wrappers till you use it. Fold the bottom corner over the filling. Use water to moisten leftover wrapper edges. Fold side corners toward middle over filling then tightly egg roll up, pressing tip to seal; repeat.
- Heat 1/4-in. oil in electric skillet to 375°. A few at a time, fry egg rolls till golden brown or for 3-4 minutes, occasionally turning. On paper towels, drain. Serve with sweet-and-sour sauce if desired. Freezing: Cover then freeze unfried egg rolls over waxed paper-lined baking sheets till firm. Put in resealable plastic freezer bags and put back to freezer. Using: As recipe says, fry egg rolls, increasing the cooking time to 4-5 minutes.

Nutrition Information

- Calories: 196 calories
- Protein: 7g protein.
- Total Fat: 9g fat (1g saturated fat)
- Sodium: 284mg sodium
- Fiber: 1g fiber)
- Total Carbohydrate: 22g carbohydrate (2g sugars
- Cholesterol: 14mg cholesterol

619. Whole Wheat Pepperoni Pizzas

Serving: 2 pizzas. | Prep: 15mins | Cook: 15mins | Ready in:

Ingredients

- 1-2/3 cups water
- 2 tablespoons olive oil
- 2 tablespoons sugar
- 2 tablespoons nonfat dry milk powder
- 1 teaspoon salt
- 1 teaspoon lemon juice
- 2-1/2 cups bread flour
- 2 cups whole wheat flour
- 2 teaspoons active dry yeast
- TOPPINGS:
- 4 teaspoons olive oil
- 1 can (15 ounces) pizza sauce
- 2 teaspoons dried oregano
- 4 cups shredded part-skim mozzarella cheese
- 2 ounces turkey pepperoni, diced
- 1/4 cup grated Parmesan cheese
- 2/3 cup chopped onion
- 2/3 cup chopped green pepper

Direction

- In order recommended by manufacturer, put initial 9 ingredients in bread machine pan. Choose dough setting. After 5 minutes of mixing, check dough. If needed, add 1-2 tablespoons flour/water. Turn dough on lightly floured surface when cycle is completed; halve dough. Cover. Let stand for ten minutes.
- Roll to 2 14-in. circles. Put in 2 14-in. pizza pans coated in cooking spray. Spread oil on each crust. Put green pepper, onion, parmesan cheese, pepperoni, mozzarella cheese, oregano and pizza sauce on top. Bake for 15-20 minutes or till crust is golden brown at 450°.

Nutrition Information

- Calories: 343 calories
- Fiber: 4g fiber)
- Total Carbohydrate: 43g carbohydrate (0 sugars
- Cholesterol: 29mg cholesterol
- Protein: 19g protein. Diabetic Exchanges: 2-1/2 starch
- Total Fat: 11g fat (5g saturated fat)
- Sodium: 611mg sodium

Chapter 5: Turkey Side Dish Recipes

***

620. After Thanksgiving Salad

Serving: 6 servings. | Prep: 15mins | Cook: 0mins | Ready in:

Ingredients

- 3-1/2 cups diced cooked turkey
- 4 celery ribs, sliced
- 4 green onions, sliced
- 1/2 cup chopped pecans, toasted
- 1/2 cup chopped sweet red pepper
- 1/2 cup mayonnaise
- 1 tablespoon lemon juice
- 1/4 teaspoon dill weed or dried tarragon
- 1/4 teaspoon salt
- 1/8 teaspoon pepper
- Lettuce leaves, optional

Direction

- Mix the red pepper, pecans, onions, celery, and turkey in a big bowl. Mix pepper, salt, dill, lemon juice and mayonnaise; mix into the turkey mixture. Keep in the refrigerator till serving. Serve over lettuce if you want.

Nutrition Information

- Calories: 352 calories
- Protein: 25g protein.
- Total Fat: 26g fat (4g saturated fat)
- Sodium: 281mg sodium
- Fiber: 2g fiber)
- Total Carbohydrate: 4g carbohydrate (1g sugars
- Cholesterol: 69mg cholesterol

621. After Thanksgiving Turkey Soup

Serving: 16 servings (about 4 quarts). | Prep: 15mins | Cook: 02hours30mins | Ready in:

Ingredients

- 1 leftover turkey carcass (from a 12- to 14-pound turkey)
- 3 medium onions, chopped
- 2 large carrots, diced
- 2 celery ribs, diced
- 1 cup butter, cubed
- 1 cup all-purpose flour
- 2 cups half-and-half cream
- 1 cup uncooked long grain rice
- 2 teaspoons salt
- 1 teaspoon chicken bouillon granules
- 3/4 teaspoon pepper

Direction

- Place the turkey carcass into a Dutch oven or soup kettle and cover with water, then set to boil. Lower the heat and simmer while covered for 1 hour. Remove the carcass and allow to cool. Set aside 3 quarts of broth and remove the turkey meat from the bones, then cut the turkey into bite-sized pieces, setting it aside.
- Use a soup kettle or Dutch oven to sauté celery, carrots, and onion with butter until tender. Turn the heat down and stir in the flour until combined. Slowly add 1 quart of the reserved broth, then boil. Cook while stirring for 2 minutes or until the mixture thickens.
- Add the reserved turkey meat, the remaining broth, pepper, bouillon, salt, rice, and cream. Lower the heat then simmer while covered until the rice becomes tender, or for 30 - 35 minutes.

Nutrition Information

- Calories:
- Sodium:
- Fiber:
- Total Carbohydrate:
- Cholesterol:
- Protein:
- Total Fat:

622. After The Holidays Salad

Serving: 4 servings. | Prep: 10mins | Cook: 0mins | Ready in:

Ingredients

- 2 cups diced cooked turkey
- 1 cup diced celery
- 1 cup green grapes
- 1 cup pineapple chunks, well drained
- 1/2 cup sliced green onions
- 2/3 cup mayonnaise
- 2 tablespoons chutney
- 1 tablespoon lime juice
- 1/2 teaspoon curry powder
- 1/4 teaspoon salt
- 1/4 cup dry roasted peanuts
- Lettuce leaves, optional

Direction

- Combine initial 5 ingredients. Mix 5 next ingredients in a small bowl. Put on top of turkey mixture and mix lightly; put peanuts on top. Keep it chilled. If you want, serve over a bed of lettuce.

Nutrition Information

- Calories: 528 calories
- Sodium: 501mg sodium
- Fiber: 3g fiber)
- Total Carbohydrate: 25g carbohydrate (19g sugars
- Cholesterol: 67mg cholesterol
- Protein: 24g protein.
- Total Fat: 38g fat (6g saturated fat)

623. Antipasto Tossed Salad

Serving: 16 servings. | Prep: 20mins | Cook: 0mins | Ready in:

Ingredients

- 1-3/4 cups thinly sliced halved zucchini
- 1-1/2 cups fresh cauliflowerets
- 1/4 cup thinly sliced green onions
- 1 cup reduced-fat Italian salad dressing
- 1 tablespoon lemon juice
- 12 cups torn romaine
- 2 medium tomatoes, cut into wedges
- 4 large fresh mushrooms, thinly sliced
- 4 ounces sliced turkey salami, julienned
- 4 ounces reduced-fat provolone cheese, julienned
- 1 can (2-1/4 ounces) sliced ripe olives, drained
- 1 cup fat-free Italian croutons
- 1/4 cup shredded Parmesan cheese

Direction

- Mix onions, cauliflower and zucchini in a big bowl. Whisk the lemon juice and salad dressing; put on top of the veggies and coat by tossing. Keep it covered and let chill in the fridge for a minimum of 4 hours.
- Just prior to serve, in a serving bowl, mix together the olives, provolone, salami, mushrooms, tomatoes and romaine. Pour in marinated vegetables; coat by tossing. Put the croutons and Parmesan cheese on top.

Nutrition Information

- Calories: 86 calories
- Fiber: 1g fiber)
- Total Carbohydrate: 7g carbohydrate (0 sugars
- Cholesterol: 12mg cholesterol

- Protein: 6g protein. Diabetic Exchanges: 1/2 starch
- Total Fat: 5g fat (2g saturated fat)
- Sodium: 329mg sodium

624. Artichoke Turkey Salami Salad

Serving: 8 servings. | Prep: 20mins | Cook: 0mins | Ready in:

Ingredients

- 4 cups cooked elbow macaroni
- 2 cups shredded part-skim mozzarella cheese
- 2 cups cherry tomatoes, halved
- 8 ounces turkey salami, cut into thin strips
- 1 cup roasted sweet red pepper strips, drained
- 1 jar (7-1/2 ounces) marinated artichoke hearts, drained and chopped
- 1 can (2-1/4 ounces) sliced ripe olives, drained
- 1/3 cup Italian salad dressing
- 1/4 cup minced fresh basil
- 1/2 teaspoon pepper

Direction

- Mix the olives, artichokes, red peppers, salami, tomatoes, mozzarella and macaroni together in a big salad bowl. Put in the pepper, basil and dressing; coat it by tossing.
- Keep it covered and chilled in the refrigerator for 2 hours to overnight. Toss prior to serve.

Nutrition Information

- Calories: 303 calories
- Sodium: 754mg sodium
- Fiber: 2g fiber)
- Total Carbohydrate: 23g carbohydrate (3g sugars
- Cholesterol: 44mg cholesterol
- Protein: 13g protein.
- Total Fat: 18g fat (6g saturated fat)

625. Autumn Acorn Squash

Serving: 4 servings. | Prep: 15mins | Cook: 45mins | Ready in:

Ingredients

- 2 medium acorn squash
- 1/2 pound ground turkey
- 1 egg
- 1/2 cup cooked wild rice
- 1/2 cup chopped peeled tart apple
- 1/2 cup chopped fresh or frozen cranberries
- 1/4 cup chopped celery
- 1/2 teaspoon salt
- 1/2 teaspoon dried parsley flakes
- 1/4 teaspoon ground allspice
- 1/4 teaspoon ground cardamom

Direction

- Halve squash; discard seeds. Put aside squash. Cook turkey in skillet on medium heat till not pink; drain. Add cardamom, allspice, parsley, salt, celery, cranberries, apple, rice and egg. Put in squash halves; put in 13x9-in. ungreased baking dish. Put 1/2-in. depth of hot water in dish. Cover; bake for 25 minutes at 350°. Uncover; bake till squash is tender for 20-25 minutes.

Nutrition Information

- Calories: 262 calories
- Total Carbohydrate: 33g carbohydrate (9g sugars
- Cholesterol: 92mg cholesterol
- Protein: 13g protein.
- Total Fat: 10g fat (3g saturated fat)
- Sodium: 384mg sodium
- Fiber: 5g fiber)

626. Autumn Pumpkin Chili

Serving: 4 servings. | Prep: 20mins | Cook: 07hours00mins | Ready in:

Ingredients

- 1 medium onion, chopped
- 1 small green pepper, chopped
- 1 small sweet yellow pepper, chopped
- 1 tablespoon canola oil
- 1 garlic clove, minced
- 1 pound ground turkey
- 1 can (15 ounces) solid-pack pumpkin
- 1 can (14-1/2 ounces) diced tomatoes, undrained
- 4-1/2 teaspoons chili powder
- 1/4 teaspoon pepper
- 1/4 teaspoon salt
- Optional toppings: shredded cheddar cheese, sour cream and sliced green onions

Direction

- In a large pan, sauté yellow peppers, green peppers, and onions until tender. Add garlic and cook for another minute, then crumble the turkey into the skillet. Cook on medium heat until the turkey meat is no longer pink.
- Transfer the mixture into a 3-quart slow cooker and stir in salt, pepper, chili powder, tomatoes, and pumpkin. Cook, covered, on a low setting for 7 - 9 hours. Serve with your choice of toppings.

Nutrition Information

- Calories: 281 calories
- Total Carbohydrate: 20g carbohydrate (9g sugars
- Cholesterol: 75mg cholesterol
- Protein: 25g protein. Diabetic Exchanges: 3 lean meat
- Total Fat: 13g fat (3g saturated fat)
- Sodium: 468mg sodium
- Fiber: 7g fiber)

627. Avocado Turkey Salad

Serving: 6 servings. | Prep: 15mins | Cook: 0mins | Ready in:

Ingredients

- 1/4 cup canola oil
- 2 tablespoons sour cream
- 1 tablespoon heavy whipping cream
- 1/4 teaspoon salt
- 1/8 to 1/4 teaspoon minced garlic
- 3 cups torn mixed salad greens
- 2 cups cubed cooked turkey breast
- 1 medium ripe avocado, peeled and chopped
- 1 cup grape tomatoes, halved
- Coarsely ground pepper

Direction

- Combine the first five ingredients in a large bowl and mix until smooth. Stir in tomatoes, avocado, turkey and greens; mix well to coat. Sprinkle coarse ground pepper (optional). Ready to serve immediately.

Nutrition Information

- Calories: 225 calories
- Sodium: 141mg sodium
- Fiber: 2g fiber)
- Total Carbohydrate: 4g carbohydrate (1g sugars
- Cholesterol: 47mg cholesterol
- Protein: 16g protein.
- Total Fat: 17g fat (3g saturated fat)

628. BLT Turkey Salad

Serving: 12 servings (1-1/4 cups each). | Prep: 35mins | Cook: 0mins | Ready in:

Ingredients

- 1/2 cup (4 ounces) plain yogurt
- 1/2 cup mayonnaise
- 2 tablespoons sugar
- 2 tablespoons red wine vinegar
- 1/2 teaspoon garlic powder
- 6 cups torn romaine or leaf lettuce
- 4 cups cubed cooked turkey
- 1-1/2 cups chopped tomatoes
- 1-1/2 cups shredded part-skim mozzarella cheese
- 1-1/2 cups shredded cheddar cheese
- 10 bacon strips, cooked and crumbled
- 1/2 cup chopped green pepper
- 1/2 cup chopped red onion
- 1/2 cup chopped cucumber

Direction

- Put the first five ingredients in a big salad bowl then whisk to mix. Add the rest of the ingredients to the bow; toss everything to coat.

Nutrition Information

- Calories: 294 calories
- Total Fat: 19g fat (7g saturated fat)
- Sodium: 410mg sodium
- Fiber: 1g fiber)
- Total Carbohydrate: 7g carbohydrate (4g sugars
- Cholesterol: 79mg cholesterol
- Protein: 23g protein.

629. Basic Turkey Soup

Serving: 10 servings. | Prep: 45mins | Cook: 15mins | Ready in:

Ingredients

- TURKEY BROTH:
- 1 leftover turkey carcass (from a 12-14 pound turkey)
- 8 cups water
- 1 teaspoon chicken bouillon granules
- 1 celery rib with leaves
- 1 small onion, halved
- 1 medium carrot
- 3 whole peppercorns
- 1 garlic clove
- 1 teaspoon seasoned salt
- 1 teaspoon dried thyme
- TURKEY VEGETABLE SOUP:
- 8 cups turkey broth
- 2 teaspoons chicken bouillon granules
- 1/2 to 3/4 teaspoon pepper
- 1-1/2 cups sliced fresh carrots
- 1-1/2 cups sliced celery
- 1 cup sliced fresh green beans
- 3/4 cup chopped onion
- 4 cups diced cooked turkey

Direction

- In a large stockpot, mix all the broth ingredients and cover. Bring the mixture to a boil. Reduce the heat and simmer the mixture for 25 minutes. Strain the broth, discarding the vegetables and bones. Let it cool, skimming off the fat. You can use it immediately for the turkey vegetable soup or you can store it inside the refrigerator. Make sure to use it within 24 hours.
- In making the soup, mix the vegetables, broth, pepper, and bouillon in a large stockpot. Cover the pot and let it simmer for 15-20 minutes until the vegetables are tender. Add the turkey and heat the mixture through.

Nutrition Information

- Calories: 136 calories
- Fiber: 2g fiber)
- Total Carbohydrate: 7g carbohydrate (5g sugars
- Cholesterol: 43mg cholesterol
- Protein: 19g protein.
- Total Fat: 3g fat (1g saturated fat)
- Sodium: 1024mg sodium

630. Beefy Vegetable Soup

Serving: 8 | Prep: | Cook: |Ready in:

Ingredients

- 10 cups beef broth
- 1 (15 ounce) can tomato sauce
- 1 (14.5 ounce) can diced tomatoes
- 1 1/2 cups diced carrots
- 1 1/2 cups diced potatoes
- 1 cup chopped celery
- 1/2 cup chopped onion
- 1 cup frozen corn kernels
- 1 cup chopped fresh green beans
- 1/4 tablespoon ground black pepper
- 1/2 teaspoon salt
- 1 1/2 cups seashell pasta
- 1 cup shredded Cheddar cheese

Direction

- Combine salt, pepper, green beans, corn, onion, celery, potatoes, carrots, chopped tomatoes along with its juice, tomato sauce, and broth in a big saucepan, then set to boil over high heat. Decrease the heat to medium-low; simmer, covered, for 15 minutes.
- Stir in pasta and cook for another 15 - 25 minutes or until the pasta becomes tender. Adjust the seasoning and serve the soup hot with a sprinkling of Cheddar cheese.

Nutrition Information

- Calories: 237 calories;
- Total Fat: 6.2
- Sodium: 1634
- Total Carbohydrate: 34.1
- Cholesterol: 15
- Protein: 12.7

631. Big Batch Turkey Salad

Serving: 185 (1-cup) servings. | Prep: 35mins | Cook: 0mins |Ready in:

Ingredients

- 25 quarts cubed cooked turkey or chicken
- 20 cans (20 ounces each) pineapple chunks, drained
- 20 cans (15 ounces each) mandarin oranges, drained
- 20 cans (2-1/4 ounces each) sliced ripe olives, drained
- 5 bunches celery, thinly sliced
- 10 large green peppers, chopped
- 5 to 6 quarts mayonnaise
- 3 large onions, grated
- 1-1/2 cups prepared mustard
- 5 tablespoons salt
- 1 to 2 tablespoons lemon-pepper seasoning, optional
- 8 cans (5 ounces each) chow mein noodles

Direction

- Combine the first six ingredients in several large bowls. In several other large bowls, combine mustard, onions, mayonnaise, lemon-pepper and salt (these two are optional).
- Cover and keep the dressing and chicken mixture separately cold in refrigerator for a minimum of 2 hours. Pour dressing on top of chicken mixture; toss until well coated. Add a sprinkle of chow mein noodles on top and serve.

Nutrition Information

- Calories: 316 calories
- Total Fat: 23g fat (4g saturated fat)
- Sodium: 420mg sodium
- Fiber: 1g fiber)
- Total Carbohydrate: 3g carbohydrate (1g sugars
- Cholesterol: 66mg cholesterol
- Protein: 23g protein.

632. Black Bean 'n' Pumpkin Chili

Serving: 10 servings (2-1/2 quarts). | Prep: 20mins | Cook: 04hours00mins | Ready in:

Ingredients

- 2 tablespoons olive oil
- 1 medium onion, chopped
- 1 medium sweet yellow pepper, chopped
- 3 garlic cloves, minced
- 2 cans (15 ounces each) black beans, rinsed and drained
- 1 can (15 ounces) solid-pack pumpkin
- 1 can (14-1/2 ounces) diced tomatoes, undrained
- 3 cups chicken broth
- 2-1/2 cups cubed cooked turkey
- 2 teaspoons dried parsley flakes
- 2 teaspoons chili powder
- 1-1/2 teaspoons ground cumin
- 1-1/2 teaspoons dried oregano
- 1/2 teaspoon salt
- Cubed avocado and thinly sliced green onions, optional

Direction

- In a big pan, heat oil on medium-high heat and add pepper, and onion, then cook, stirring, until tender. Add in garlic and cook for another minute.
- Move to a 5-quart slow cooker and stir in the next 10 ingredients. Cook while covered on a low setting for 4 - 5 hours. Top with green onions and avocado, if desired.

Nutrition Information

- Calories: 192 calories
- Fiber: 7g fiber)
- Total Carbohydrate: 21g carbohydrate (5g sugars
- Cholesterol: 28mg cholesterol
- Protein: 16g protein. Diabetic Exchanges: 2 lean meat
- Total Fat: 5g fat (1g saturated fat)
- Sodium: 658mg sodium

633. Broccoli Turkey Salad

Serving: 10 servings. | Prep: 20mins | Cook: 0mins | Ready in:

Ingredients

- 1 can (8 ounces) unsweetened pineapple chunks
- 2 cups torn salad greens
- 2 cups torn fresh spinach
- 2 cups broccoli florets
- 1 green pepper, julienned
- 1/2 cup thinly sliced red onion
- 2 cups cubed cooked turkey
- 1/4 cup olive oil
- 2 tablespoons balsamic vinegar
- 1 tablespoon poppy seeds
- 2 teaspoons sugar
- 2 teaspoons Dijon mustard

Direction

- Drain the pineapple, saving 2 tablespoon of juice; set aside (throw away remaining juice or reserve for later).
- Combine pineapple, turkey, onion, green pepper, broccoli, spinach and greens in a large bowl. In a small bowl, combine reserved pineapple juice, mustard, sugar, poppy seeds, vinegar and oil. Pour dressing over salad and toss until well coated.

Nutrition Information

- Calories: 111 calories

- Protein: 6g protein. Diabetic Exchanges: 1 vegetable
- Total Fat: 7g fat (1g saturated fat)
- Sodium: 46mg sodium
- Fiber: 1g fiber)
- Total Carbohydrate: 7g carbohydrate (0 sugars
- Cholesterol: 17mg cholesterol

634. Cabbage Parsley Slaw

Serving: 10 servings. | Prep: 15mins | Cook: 0mins | Ready in:

Ingredients

- 1 medium head cabbage, shredded (about 6 cups)
- 2 cups minced fresh parsley
- 1 celery rib, chopped
- 6 bacon strips, cooked and crumbled
- 1-1/2 cups Miracle Whip
- 2 tablespoons plus 1 teaspoon Worcestershire sauce
- 3/4 teaspoon onion powder

Direction

- Toss the bacon, celery, parsley and cabbage in a big bowl. Mix the onion powder, Worcestershire sauce and Miracle Whip in a small bowl. Put into the cabbage mixture and coat by tossing. Once done, cover it. For at least 2 hours, leave it in the refrigerator.

Nutrition Information

- Calories: 75 calories
- Total Carbohydrate: 12g carbohydrate (0 sugars
- Cholesterol: 7mg cholesterol
- Protein: 3g protein. Diabetic Exchanges: 2-1/2 vegetable
- Total Fat: 2g fat (0 saturated fat)
- Sodium: 428mg sodium

- Fiber: 3g fiber)

635. California Burger Bowls

Serving: 4 servings. | Prep: 15mins | Cook: 10mins | Ready in:

Ingredients

- 3 tablespoons fat-free milk
- 2 tablespoons quick-cooking oats
- 3/4 teaspoon salt
- 1/2 teaspoon ground cumin
- 1/2 teaspoon chili powder
- 1/2 teaspoon pepper
- 1 pound lean ground turkey
- 4 cups baby kale salad blend
- 1-1/2 cups cubed fresh pineapple (1/2 inch)
- 1 medium mango, peeled and thinly sliced
- 1 medium ripe avocado, peeled and thinly sliced
- 1 medium sweet red pepper, cut into strips
- 4 tomatillos, husks removed, thinly sliced
- 1/4 cup reduced-fat chipotle mayonnaise

Direction

- Combine seasonings, milk, and oats in a big bowl. Toss in turkey and lightly but thoroughly stir. Mold mixture into 4 patties with 1/2 inch thickness.
- On medium heat, cook burgers on greased grill rack. For 4 to 5 minutes a side, grill with cover until meat thermometer reaches 165°. Serve grilled patties over salad mixture with the rest of the ingredients.

Nutrition Information

- Calories: 390 calories
- Sodium: 666mg sodium
- Fiber: 7g fiber)
- Total Carbohydrate: 33g carbohydrate (22g sugars

- Cholesterol: 83mg cholesterol
- Protein: 26g protein. Diabetic Exchanges: 3 lean meat
- Total Fat: 19g fat (4g saturated fat)

636. Cannellini Comfort Soup

Serving: 4 servings. | Prep: 15mins | Cook: 35mins | Ready in:

Ingredients

- 1/2 pound reduced-fat fully cooked smoked sausage, cut into bite-size pieces
- 1 tablespoon olive oil
- 1/2 cup chopped green pepper
- 1/3 cup chopped onion
- 2 garlic cloves, minced
- 1 can (14-1/2 ounces) reduced-sodium chicken broth
- 1/3 cup white wine or chicken broth
- 1/2 teaspoon Italian seasoning
- 1/4 teaspoon pepper
- 1 can (15 ounces) white kidney or cannellini beans, rinsed and drained
- 3 cups coleslaw mix

Direction

- Cook sausage in oil in a big saucepan for 2 minutes. Add onion and green pepper. Stir and cook until the vegetables are soft, about 2-3 minutes. Add garlic, cook for another 1 minute. Mix in pepper, Italian seasoning, wine, and broth. Boil it. Lower the heat, put a cover on and simmer for 15 minutes.
- Mix in coleslaw mix and beans. Boil again. Lower the heat, put a cover on and simmer until the cabbage is soft and the beans are fully heated.

Nutrition Information

- Calories: 251 calories
- Protein: 14g protein. Diabetic Exchanges: 2 lean meat
- Total Fat: 7g fat (1g saturated fat)
- Sodium: 939mg sodium
- Fiber: 7g fiber)
- Total Carbohydrate: 31g carbohydrate (0 sugars
- Cholesterol: 25mg cholesterol

637. Cantaloupe Salami Salad

Serving: 4 servings. | Prep: 30mins | Cook: 0mins | Ready in:

Ingredients

- 2 medium cantaloupe
- 1 cup cubed salami
- 1 medium cucumber, halved, seeded and sliced
- 3 tablespoons lemon juice
- 2 tablespoons honey
- 1/4 teaspoon minced fresh marjoram

Direction

- Halve each cantaloupe, dispose the seeds and take out the melon. Cube the melon and put in a big bowl. From the bottom of each cantaloupe half, cut off a thin slice so that the shell can sit balance; blot dry and put aside.
- Add cucumber and salami to the melon cubes. In a tightly-fitting lidded jar, mix together marjoram, honey, and lemon juice; shake well. Sprinkle over the cantaloupe mixture and mix to coat. Enjoy in cantaloupe shells.

Nutrition Information

- Calories: 196 calories
- Sodium: 386mg sodium
- Fiber: 3g fiber)
- Total Carbohydrate: 35g carbohydrate (31g sugars

- Cholesterol: 27mg cholesterol
- Protein: 9g protein. Diabetic Exchanges: 2-1/2 fruit
- Total Fat: 4g fat (1g saturated fat)

638. Cashew Turkey Pasta Salad

Serving: 12 servings. | Prep: 20mins | Cook: 50mins | Ready in:

Ingredients

- 2 bone-in turkey breast (5 to 6 pounds each)
- 3 cups uncooked tricolor spiral pasta
- 2 celery ribs, diced
- 6 green onions, chopped
- 1/2 cup diced green pepper
- 1-1/2 cups mayonnaise
- 3/4 cup packed brown sugar
- 1 tablespoon cider vinegar
- 1-1/2 teaspoons salt
- 1-1/2 teaspoons lemon juice
- 2 cups salted cashew halves

Direction

- Grill turkey, while covered, for 25 to 30 minutes per side on medium heat until a thermometer reaches 170 degrees. Let it cool off a bit. Keep the cover on and let chill in the refrigerator till cooled down. At the same time, cook pasta based on package instructions; drain off and wash under cold water.
- Remove skin out of turkey; chop the turkey meat and transfer into a big bowl. Put in the green pepper, onions, celery and pasta. Mix lemon juice, salt, vinegar, brown sugar and mayonnaise in a small bowl; add on top of the pasta mixture and coat by mixing.
- Keep it covered and let chill in the refrigerator for no less than 2 hours. Just prior to serving, mix in cashews.

Nutrition Information

- Calories: 0
- Total Fat: 37 g fat (6 g saturated fat)
- Sodium: 732 mg sodium
- Fiber: 2 g fiber
- Total Carbohydrate: 37 g carbohydrate
- Cholesterol: 176 mg cholesterol
- Protein: 68 g protein.

639. Chef's Spinach Salad

Serving: 4 servings. | Prep: 25mins | Cook: 0mins | Ready in:

Ingredients

- 1 small red onion, thinly sliced
- 2 tablespoons white wine vinegar
- 1 teaspoon sugar
- 1 package (6 ounces) fresh baby spinach
- 1 cup quartered cherry tomatoes
- 1 cup fresh or frozen corn, thawed
- 4 ounces fully cooked lean ham, cut into thin strips
- 4 ounces sliced cooked turkey, cut into thin strips
- 1 piece (2 ounces) reduced-fat cheddar cheese, cut into thin strips
- DRESSING:
- 1/2 cup buttermilk
- 2 tablespoons minced chives
- 1 tablespoon reduced-fat mayonnaise
- 2 teaspoons white wine vinegar
- 2 teaspoons Dijon mustard
- 1/4 teaspoon minced garlic
- 1/4 teaspoon salt
- 1/4 teaspoon pepper

Direction

- Combine sugar, vinegar and onion in a small bowl; allow to stand for 15 minutes. On a serving platter, lay out cheese, turkey, ham, corn, tomatoes and spinach. Drain off excess water in onion mixture and put onions on top of salad. Whisk the dressing ingredients together in a bowl. Serve with salad.

Nutrition Information

- Calories: 172 calories
- Sodium: 783mg sodium
- Fiber: 2g fiber)
- Total Carbohydrate: 10g carbohydrate (0 sugars
- Cholesterol: 44mg cholesterol
- Protein: 21g protein. Diabetic Exchanges: 2 lean meat
- Total Fat: 6g fat (3g saturated fat)

640. Chili With Potato Dumplings

Serving: 8 servings (2 quarts). | Prep: 25mins | Cook: 55mins | Ready in:

Ingredients

- 1 pound ground beef
- 1 pound ground turkey
- 1/2 cup chopped onion
- 1 can (16 ounces) kidney beans, rinsed and drained
- 1 can (16 ounces) mild chili beans, undrained
- 1/2 cup chopped green pepper
- 4 teaspoons chili powder
- 1 teaspoon salt
- 1 teaspoon paprika
- 1 teaspoon cumin seeds
- 1/2 teaspoon garlic salt
- 1/2 teaspoon dried oregano
- 1/4 teaspoon crushed red pepper flakes
- 3 cups V8 juice
- DUMPLINGS:
- 1 cup mashed potato flakes
- 1 cup all-purpose flour
- 1 tablespoon minced fresh parsley
- 2 teaspoons baking powder
- 1/2 teaspoon salt
- 1 cup milk
- 1 egg, beaten

Direction

- Cook onion, turkey, and beef in a Dutch oven until the meat is not anymore pinkish. Add the next eleven ingredients. Bring the mixture to a boil. Lower the heat and cover the pot. Simmer for 30 minutes while stirring the mixture occasionally.
- For the dumplings, mix the first 5 ingredients in a large bowl. Add the egg and milk and mix until moistened. Let the mixture stand for 3 minutes.
- In a simmering chili, add tablespoonfuls on the mixture. Cover the pot and cook for 15 more minutes.

Nutrition Information

- Calories: 449 calories
- Protein: 30g protein.
- Total Fat: 16g fat (6g saturated fat)
- Sodium: 1333mg sodium
- Fiber: 7g fiber)
- Total Carbohydrate: 45g carbohydrate (7g sugars
- Cholesterol: 97mg cholesterol

641. Chinese Turkey Pasta Salad

Serving: 4-6 servings. | Prep: 20mins | Cook: 0mins | Ready in:

Ingredients

- 2 cups uncooked spiral pasta
- 2 cups cubed cooked turkey
- 1-1/2 cups fresh or frozen snow peas, thawed
- 1/2 cup chopped sweet red pepper
- 1/2 cup chopped green pepper

- 1/4 cup thinly sliced green onions
- 1/4 cup diced celery
- 1 can (8 ounces) sliced water chestnuts, drained
- 1 jar (2 ounces) diced pimientos, drained
- 1 cup mayonnaise
- 2 tablespoons soy sauce
- 1 teaspoon sugar
- 1 teaspoon ground ginger
- 1/4 to 1/2 teaspoon hot pepper sauce
- 1 cup salted cashews halves, divided

Direction

- Cook pasta following package directions; drain and run pasta under cold water. Place in a large bowl; add vegetables and turkey.
- Combine hot pepper sauce, ginger, sugar, soy sauce and mayonnaise in a small bowl. Add 1/2 cup cashews, stir well. Pour dressing on top of salad mixture and toss until well coated. Cover and keep cold in refrigerator for a minimum of 1 hour before serving. Add a sprinkle of remaining cashews on top.

Nutrition Information

- Calories:
- Protein:
- Total Fat:
- Sodium:
- Fiber:
- Total Carbohydrate:
- Cholesterol:

642. Chunky Turkey Chili

Serving: 24 servings (6 quarts). | Prep: 30mins | Cook: 02hours00mins | Ready in:

Ingredients

- 5 pounds ground turkey
- 6 cups chopped celery
- 2 medium green peppers, chopped
- 2 large onions, chopped
- 2 cans (28 ounces each) crushed tomatoes
- 2 cups water
- 2 envelopes (1-3/4 ounces each) chili seasoning
- 1 to 2 tablespoons chili powder
- 2 cans (16 ounces each) kidney beans, rinsed and drained

Direction

- Brown turkey in a Dutch oven over medium heat; drain. Add onions, peppers, and celery; stir and cook for 5 minutes. Add the next 4 ingredients, boil it. Lower the heat, put a cover on and simmer for 2 hours. Add beans, heat completely.

Nutrition Information

- Calories: 234 calories
- Sodium: 349mg sodium
- Fiber: 3g fiber)
- Total Carbohydrate: 10g carbohydrate (2g sugars
- Cholesterol: 64mg cholesterol
- Protein: 18g protein.
- Total Fat: 14g fat (4g saturated fat)

643. Chutney Turkey Salad

Serving: 4 servings. | Prep: 15mins | Cook: 0mins | Ready in:

Ingredients

- 3 cups cubed cooked turkey breast
- 1 cup chopped celery
- 1 cup golden raisins
- 4 ounces Monterey Jack cheese, cut into 1/2-inch cubes
- 3 tablespoons chopped green onions
- 1/3 cup mayonnaise

- 1/4 cup mango chutney
- 1/2 teaspoon ground ginger
- 1/4 teaspoon pepper
- Lettuce leaves, optional

Direction

- Combine onions, cheese, raisins, celery and turkey in a large bowl. In a small bowl, combine pepper, ginger, chutney and mayonnaise until blended. Pour dressing over turkey mixture and toss until well coated. Cover the mixture and keep in refrigerator for 1 hour. Serve on a lettuce-covered plate if desired.

Nutrition Information

- Calories: 567 calories
- Total Fat: 25g fat (7g saturated fat)
- Sodium: 520mg sodium
- Fiber: 11g fiber)
- Total Carbohydrate: 46g carbohydrate (24g sugars
- Cholesterol: 127mg cholesterol
- Protein: 39g protein.

644. Cincinnati Style Chili

Serving: 4 | Prep: | Cook: | Ready in:

Ingredients

- 8 ounces spaghetti
- 1 tablespoon olive oil
- 1 (12 ounce) package frozen burger-style crumbles
- 1 onion, chopped
- 1 tablespoon minced garlic
- 1 cup tomato sauce
- 1 cup water
- 1 (14.5 ounce) can diced tomatoes
- 2 tablespoons red wine vinegar
- 2 tablespoons chili powder
- 1/2 teaspoon ground cinnamon
- 1/2 teaspoon paprika
- 1/2 teaspoon ground allspice
- 1 tablespoon light brown sugar
- 1 tablespoon unsweetened cocoa powder
- 1 teaspoon hot pepper sauce
- 1 cup kidney beans, drained and rinsed
- 1 cup shredded Cheddar cheese (optional)

Direction

- In a large frying pan, heat olive oil and then sauté onion until tender. Stir in garlic and burger-style crumbles and then cook until the crumbles turn brown.
- Mix in tomato sauce, hot sauce, water, paprika, light brown sugar, chopped tomatoes, cocoa, vinegar, cinnamon, allspice, and chili powder. Heat over medium-high heat until the mixture starts to boil. Decrease the heat to low, cover the pan and let to simmer for about 15 to 20 minutes until the sauce thickens.
- As the sauce is thickening, bring to boil salted water in a large pot and add in spaghetti in the boiling water. Return to a boil and cook until al dente. Drain thoroughly.
- Mix the beans into the chili and combine lightly.
- Ladle the cooked spaghetti into bowls and add chili on top. Drizzle with cheese if desired.

Nutrition Information

- Calories: 769 calories;
- Total Carbohydrate: 74.8
- Cholesterol: 30
- Protein: 88.4
- Total Fat: 17.7
- Sodium: 1787

645. Classic Turkey Noodle Soup

Serving: 14 servings (3-1/2 quarts). | Prep: 20mins | Cook: 01hours30mins | Ready in:

Ingredients

- 1 leftover turkey carcass (from a 12- to 14-pound turkey)
- 3-1/2 quarts water
- 4 chicken bouillon cubes
- 1 large onion, halved
- 4 whole peppercorns
- 2 bay leaves
- 1 teaspoon poultry seasoning
- 1 teaspoon seasoned salt
- 1/2 to 3/4 teaspoon pepper
- 1 cup chopped carrots
- 1 cup chopped celery
- 1 medium potato, peeled and diced
- 1/2 cup chopped onion
- 1 medium turnip, peeled and diced, optional
- 1 cup uncooked egg noodles

Direction

- Place the first 9 of the ingredients into a stockpot, then boil. Lower the heat then simmer while covered for 1 hour.
- Strain the broth, discarding the bay leaves, peppercorns, and onion. Remove the carcass and cool. Remove the turkey meat from the bones, cutting into bite-sized pieces, then set aside.
- Add the vegetables into the broth and set to boil. Turn down the heat and simmer, covered, for 20 minutes or until tender. Add the reserved turkey meat and noodles, then bring back to a boil. Cook without a cover for 10 minutes or until the noodles become tender.

Nutrition Information

- Calories: 88 calories
- Cholesterol: 15mg cholesterol
- Protein: 7g protein.
- Total Fat: 2g fat (0 saturated fat)
- Sodium: 522mg sodium
- Fiber: 1g fiber)
- Total Carbohydrate: 8g carbohydrate (2g sugars

646. Club Sandwich Salad

Serving: 8-10 servings. | Prep: 20mins | Cook: 0mins | Ready in:

Ingredients

- 1 cup mayonnaise
- 1/4 cup ketchup
- 1 tablespoon chopped green onion
- Salt and pepper to taste
- 1 large head iceberg lettuce, torn
- 2 large tomatoes, cut into wedges
- 2 hard-boiled large eggs, chopped
- 10 bacon strips, cooked and crumbled
- 2 cups cubed cooked turkey or chicken
- Croutons, optional

Direction

- Mix pepper, salt, onion, ketchup and mayonnaise in a small bowl. Keep it covered and let chill in the refrigerator.
- Just prior to serving, in a big bowl, mix turkey, bacon, eggs, tomatoes and lettuce. If you want, put in croutons. Serve alongside dressing.

Nutrition Information

- Calories: 280 calories
- Total Carbohydrate: 5g carbohydrate (2g sugars
- Cholesterol: 77mg cholesterol
- Protein: 12g protein.
- Total Fat: 23g fat (4g saturated fat)
- Sodium: 332mg sodium
- Fiber: 1g fiber)

647. Contest Winning Turkey Meatball Soup

Serving: 5 servings. | Prep: 25mins | Cook: 30mins | Ready in:

Ingredients

- 2 cans (14-1/2 ounces each) chicken broth
- 1 celery rib with leaves, thinly sliced
- 1 medium carrot, thinly sliced
- 1/4 cup chopped onion
- 1 tablespoon butter
- 1 egg, lightly beaten
- 1/2 cup dry bread crumbs
- 2 tablespoons dried parsley flakes
- 1 tablespoon Worcestershire sauce
- 1/4 teaspoon pepper
- 1/2 pound lean ground turkey
- 1 cup uncooked egg noodles

Direction

- Boil the carrot, celery, and broth in a large saucepan. Reduce the heat and cover the pan. Simmer the mixture for 10 minutes.
- Sauté onion in a small skillet with butter until it's tender. Transfer the sautéed onion in a large bowl. Add the parsley, pepper, Worcestershire sauce, bread crumbs, and egg. Crumble the turkey over the mixture and mix well. Form the mixture into balls with a size of 1-inch.
- In a simmering broth, add the meatballs and bring the mixture to a boil. Decrease heat, then cover the pan and simmer for 15 minutes until the meat is no longer pink. Add the noodles and recover. Simmer for 5 more minutes until the noodles are tender.

Nutrition Information

- Calories: 193 calories
- Sodium: 545mg sodium
- Fiber: 1g fiber)
- Total Carbohydrate: 17g carbohydrate (2g sugars
- Cholesterol: 92mg cholesterol
- Protein: 13g protein.
- Total Fat: 8g fat (3g saturated fat)

648. Cranberry Turkey Salad

Serving: 12-15 servings. | Prep: 20mins | Cook: 0mins | Ready in:

Ingredients

- 1 package (3 ounces) lemon gelatin
- 2 cups boiling water, divided
- 2 cups cubed cooked turkey or chicken
- 4 celery ribs, chopped
- 8 ounces process cheese (Velveeta), cubed
- 1 cup chopped almonds
- 3 hard-boiled large eggs, chopped, optional
- 1 cup Miracle Whip
- 1 cup heavy whipping cream, whipped
- 1/2 teaspoon salt
- 1/2 teaspoon onion salt
- 1 package (3 ounces) raspberry gelatin
- 1 can (14 ounces) whole-berry cranberry sauce

Direction

- In 1 cup of boiling water in a bowl, dissolve lemon gelatin; keep it chilled in the refrigerator till lightly thickened for 60 minutes. Beat on high speed for 60 seconds. Mix in eggs if desired, onion salt, salt, cream, Miracle Whip, almonds, cheese, celery and turkey. Spread equally into a 13x9-in. dish. Keep it covered and chilled in the refrigerator till firm for about 2 hours.
- In the leftover boiling water, dissolve the raspberry gelatin; mix in cranberry sauce till blended and melted. Scoop on top of turkey mixture. Keep chilled in the refrigerator until set for 2 hours. Cut into squares.

Nutrition Information

- Calories: 379 calories
- Sodium: 460mg sodium
- Fiber: 2g fiber)
- Total Carbohydrate: 25g carbohydrate (19g sugars
- Cholesterol: 51mg cholesterol
- Protein: 12g protein.
- Total Fat: 27g fat (8g saturated fat)

649. Cranberry Chutney Turkey Salad

Serving: 6 servings. | Prep: 15mins | Cook: 0mins | Ready in:

Ingredients

- 3 cups diced cooked turkey breast
- 1/2 cup dried cranberries
- 1/3 cup chopped pecans
- 1/3 cup finely chopped onion
- 1/3 cup finely chopped green pepper
- 1/2 cup fat-free mayonnaise
- 1/2 cup reduced-fat sour cream
- 1 tablespoon lemon juice
- 1/2 teaspoon ground ginger
- 1/8 teaspoon cayenne pepper
- Leaf lettuce

Direction

- Mix green pepper, onion, pecans, cranberries, and turkey in a big bowl.
- Whisk cayenne, ginger, lemon juice, sour cream and mayonnaise in a small bowl.
- Put on top of turkey mixture; coat by mixing lightly. Keep it covered and let chill in the refrigerator till serving. Serve in a bowl lined with lettuce.

Nutrition Information

- Calories: 226 calories
- Cholesterol: 69mg cholesterol
- Protein: 23g protein. Diabetic Exchanges: 3 lean meat
- Total Fat: 8g fat (2g saturated fat)
- Sodium: 214mg sodium
- Fiber: 2g fiber)
- Total Carbohydrate: 15g carbohydrate (0 sugars

650. Cream Of Turkey And Wild Rice Soup

Serving: 6 servings. | Prep: 15mins | Cook: 20mins | Ready in:

Ingredients

- 1 medium onion, chopped
- 1 can (4 ounces) sliced mushrooms, drained
- 2 tablespoons butter
- 3 cups water
- 2 cups chicken broth
- 1 package (6 ounces) long grain and wild rice mix
- 2 cups diced cooked turkey
- 1 cup heavy whipping cream
- Minced fresh parsley

Direction

- Sauté mushrooms and onion with butter in a large saucepan until the onion becomes tender. Add rice mixed with seasoning, broth, and water, then boil. Decrease the heat and simmer until the rice becomes tender or for 20-25 minutes. Stir in cream and turkey, then heat through. Sprinkle with parsley.

Nutrition Information

- Calories: 364 calories
- Sodium: 857mg sodium
- Fiber: 1g fiber)

- Total Carbohydrate: 25g carbohydrate (3g sugars
- Cholesterol: 100mg cholesterol
- Protein: 19g protein.
- Total Fat: 21g fat (12g saturated fat)

651. Creamy Fruited Turkey Salad

Serving: 4 servings. | Prep: 25mins | Cook: 0mins |Ready in:

Ingredients

- 1 medium apple, diced
- 1-1/4 cups cubed cooked turkey
- 1 can (8 ounces) unsweetened pineapple chunks, drained
- 1 cup halved seedless grapes
- 1/4 cup fat-free cream cheese
- 2 tablespoons reduced-fat sour cream
- 1 tablespoon lemon juice
- 1 tablespoon reduced-fat mayonnaise

Direction

- Mix grapes, pineapple, turkey and apple in a serving bowl. Beat cream cheese till smooth in texture in another bowl. Put in mayonnaise, lemon juice and sour cream. Fold into the turkey mixture.

Nutrition Information

- Calories: 182 calories
- Sodium: 146mg sodium
- Fiber: 2g fiber)
- Total Carbohydrate: 20g carbohydrate (17g sugars
- Cholesterol: 38mg cholesterol
- Protein: 16g protein. Diabetic Exchanges: 2 lean meat
- Total Fat: 5g fat (1g saturated fat)

652. Creamy Turkey Noodle Soup

Serving: 8 servings (2 quarts). | Prep: 10mins | Cook: 20mins |Ready in:

Ingredients

- 1/3 cup butter, cubed
- 1 medium carrot, shredded
- 1 celery rib, finely chopped
- 1/3 cup all-purpose flour
- 1 carton (32 ounces) chicken broth
- 1/2 cup half-and-half cream
- 1/2 cup 2% milk
- 1 cup uncooked kluski or other egg noodles
- 2 cups cubed cooked turkey
- 1-1/2 cups shredded cheddar cheese
- 1/4 teaspoon salt
- 1/4 teaspoon pepper

Direction

- Use a big saucepan to heat butter on medium-high heat and sauté celery and carrot for 3 -5 minutes until tender. Stir in the flour until combined, then slowly add in milk, cream, and broth, allowing the mixture to boil while constantly stirring. Cook while stirring for 1 - 2 minutes until it thickens.
- Stir in the noodles and lower the heat. Simmer while uncovered for 7 - 10 minutes, occasionally stirring, until the noodles become al dente. Add in the other remaining ingredients and cook, stirring, until the cheese melts and the turkey heats through.

Nutrition Information

- Calories: 285 calories
- Fiber: 1g fiber)
- Total Carbohydrate: 11g carbohydrate (2g sugars
- Cholesterol: 92mg cholesterol
- Protein: 18g protein.

- Total Fat: 18g fat (11g saturated fat)
- Sodium: 823mg sodium

653. Creamy Turkey Soup

Serving: 8 | Prep: 30mins | Cook: | Ready in:

Ingredients

- 8 ounces red-skinned potatoes, cut in 1-inch pieces
- 8 ounces cremini mushrooms, sliced
- 1 cup coarsely chopped onion (1 large)
- 1 cup sliced celery (2 stalks)
- 2 turkey breast tenderloins (about 1½ pounds total)
- 3 (14.5 ounce) cans reduced-sodium chicken broth
- 1½ teaspoons dried thyme, crushed
- ½ teaspoon black pepper
- 1 (12 ounce) can (1½ cups) evaporated fat-free milk
- 3 tablespoons cornstarch
- ½ cup sliced green onions (4)
- 2 tablespoons lemon juice
- Toasted sliced almonds or chopped pecans and/or dried cranberries (see Tip) (optional)

Direction

- Combine the celery, onion, potatoes, and mushrooms in a 6-qt slow cooker. Top the mixture with turkey. Add the pepper, broth, and thyme.
- Cover the slow cooker and cook the mixture on low heat setting for 9-10 hours (or on high heat setting for 4 1/2-5 hours).
- Place the turkey in a cutting board. Shred the turkey using the two forks. Place it back into the cooker. Mix the cornstarch and evaporated milk in a small bowl and add it into the cooker. Set the setting into high heat if ever you're using the low heat.
- Cover the cooker and cook for 45-60 more minutes until the edges are bubbly. Mix in lemon juice and green onions.
- Top with nuts and/or cranberries if desired. Serve.

Nutrition Information

- Calories: 186 calories;
- Total Fat: 1
- Sodium: 480
- Cholesterol: 54
- Total Carbohydrate: 18
- Sugar: 8
- Saturated Fat: 0
- Fiber: 2
- Protein: 27

654. Creamy Turkey Vegetable Soup

Serving: 8 servings (2 quarts). | Prep: 25mins | Cook: 35mins | Ready in:

Ingredients

- 1 large onion, finely chopped
- 2 tablespoons butter
- 3 cups diced small red potatoes
- 2 cans (14-1/2 ounces each) chicken broth
- 2 cups cooked cubed turkey breast
- 2 cups frozen mixed vegetables, thawed
- 1/2 teaspoon salt
- 1/2 teaspoon white pepper
- 1/2 teaspoon poultry seasoning
- 2 cups heavy whipping cream

Direction

- Sauté onions in a big saucepan with butter until soft. Stir in broth and potatoes, bring the heat down, and let it boil with a cover for 20 minutes. Add turkey, vegetables, pepper, poultry seasoning powder, and salt. Cook for another 10-12 minutes or until the vegetables are cooked. Mix in cream, simmer, but do not let it boil.

Nutrition Information

- Calories: 235 calories
- Protein: 10g protein.
- Total Fat: 17g fat (10g saturated fat)
- Sodium: 292mg sodium
- Fiber: 2g fiber)
- Total Carbohydrate: 11g carbohydrate (3g sugars
- Cholesterol: 80mg cholesterol

655. Crispy Mashed Potato & Stuffing Patties

Serving: 12 patties. | Prep: 10mins | Cook: 20mins | Ready in:

Ingredients

- 2 large eggs, lightly beaten
- 2 tablespoons finely chopped onion
- 1/4 teaspoon pepper
- 2 cups leftover mashed potatoes
- 2 cups leftover chopped cooked turkey
- 2 cups leftover stuffing
- 2 tablespoons butter
- 2 tablespoons canola oil
- Unsweetened applesauce, optional

Direction

- Beat pepper, onion, and eggs together in a big bowl. Mix in stuffing, turkey, and potatoes.
- Heat oil and butter in a big frying pan over medium-high heat. Put in batches, drop 1/2 cupfuls of potato mixture in the frying pan; press to flatten slightly. Fry each side for 4-5 minutes until heated completely and golden brown. Put on paper towels to drain. Enjoy with applesauce if you want.

Nutrition Information

- Calories: 364 calories
- Total Carbohydrate: 28g carbohydrate (2g sugars
- Cholesterol: 118mg cholesterol
- Protein: 20g protein.
- Total Fat: 19g fat (6g saturated fat)
- Sodium: 628mg sodium
- Fiber: 2g fiber)

656. Crowd Pleasing Chicken Salad

Serving: 8 servings. | Prep: 15mins | Cook: 0mins | Ready in:

Ingredients

- 3 cups cubed cooked chicken or turkey
- 1 cup mayonnaise
- 1/4 cup sour cream
- 1/4 teaspoon salt
- Dash pepper
- 2 cups cooked rice
- 1 cup chopped celery
- 1/2 cup chopped green pepper
- 1/4 cup chopped onion
- 1 can (20 ounces) pineapple tidbits, drained
- 1 can (8 ounces) sliced water chestnuts, drained
- 1 cup shredded cheddar cheese
- 1/2 cup sliced almonds, toasted, optional
- Cantaloupe, optional

Direction

- Mix the initial 5 ingredients in a big bowl. Fold in cheese, water chestnuts, pineapple, onion, green pepper, celery and rice. Put in almonds just prior to serving if you want. Serve over wedges if desired or cantaloupe halves, or use as a sandwich spread.

Nutrition Information

- Calories: 463 calories
- Protein: 20g protein.
- Total Fat: 31g fat (8g saturated fat)
- Sodium: 377mg sodium
- Fiber: 2g fiber)
- Total Carbohydrate: 24g carbohydrate (8g sugars
- Cholesterol: 77mg cholesterol

657. Crunchy Turkey Salad

Serving: 6 | Prep: 15mins | Cook: | Ready in:

Ingredients

- 1 cup cooked, cubed turkey meat
- 2 stalks celery, chopped
- 2 tart apples, cored and cubed
- 1/2 cup chopped walnuts
- 1/4 cup sour cream
- 1/4 cup mayonnaise
- 2 tablespoons chopped fresh parsley
- 2 tablespoons lemon juice
- 1 tablespoon honey
- 1 tablespoon prepared Dijon-style mustard
- 1/4 teaspoon salt
- ground black pepper to taste

Direction

- Mix walnuts, apples, celery, and turkey in a big bowl.
- For dressing: Mix pepper, salt, mustard, honey, lemon juice, parsley, mayonnaise, and sour cream in a small bowl. Put on top of turkey mixture and coat evenly by tossing. Keep in the refrigerator till chilled.

Nutrition Information

- Calories: 237 calories;

- Sodium: 243
- Total Carbohydrate: 12.7
- Cholesterol: 25
- Protein: 8.8
- Total Fat: 17.7

658. Curried Turkey Salad

Serving: 6-8 servings. | Prep: 20mins | Cook: 0mins | Ready in:

Ingredients

- 3 cups cubed cooked turkey
- 1-1/2 cups seedless red grapes, halved
- 4 celery ribs, chopped
- 2/3 cup mayonnaise
- 2 tablespoons lemon juice
- 1 to 2 teaspoons curry powder
- 1/2 to 1 teaspoon salt
- 1 to 2 teaspoons sugar, optional
- 1/2 cup salted peanuts

Direction

- Combine celery, grapes and turkey in a large bowl. In a small bowl, combine curry powder, lemon juice, mayonnaise, and salt and sugar (these two are optional). Pour dressing over turkey mixture and toss until well coated. Cover and keep cold in refrigerator for 1 hour. Right before serving, stir in peanuts.

Nutrition Information

- Calories:
- Total Carbohydrate:
- Cholesterol:
- Protein:
- Total Fat:
- Sodium:
- Fiber:

659. Curried Turkey And Rice Salad

Serving: 8-10 servings. | Prep: 35mins | Cook: 0mins | Ready in:

Ingredients

- 4-1/2 cups chicken broth
- 2 cups uncooked long grain rice
- 1 to 2 teaspoons curry powder
- 1/2 teaspoon ground ginger
- 1/2 teaspoon ground turmeric
- 1/4 cup olive oil
- 1/4 cup lemon juice
- 2 cups cubed cooked turkey
- 1 cup golden raisins
- 1 can (8 ounces) water chestnuts, drained and chopped
- 1/2 cup chopped green pepper
- 1/2 cup chopped sweet red pepper
- 1/2 cup mayonnaise
- 1/2 cup sour cream
- 1/2 cup slivered almonds, toasted
- Salt and pepper to taste

Direction

- Boil broth in a saucepan; put in turmeric, ginger, curry and rice. Lower heat; keep it covered and let simmer till all of the broth is absorbed for 25 minutes. Take off the heat. Put in lemon juice and oil; stir well.
- Place in a big bowl; covered and chilled. Just prior to serving, pour in leftover ingredients and stir well.

Nutrition Information

- Calories: 434 calories
- Protein: 14g protein.
- Total Fat: 21g fat (4g saturated fat)
- Sodium: 510mg sodium
- Fiber: 3g fiber)
- Total Carbohydrate: 48g carbohydrate (12g sugars
- Cholesterol: 33mg cholesterol

660. Day After Thanksgiving Salad

Serving: 5 servings. | Prep: 30mins | Cook: 0mins | Ready in:

Ingredients

- 1 tablespoon butter
- 3/4 cup chopped walnuts
- 1 tablespoon sugar
- 1 package (8 ounces) ready-to-serve salad greens
- 3 cups cubed cooked turkey breast
- 1 small red onion, sliced
- 1 medium sweet yellow pepper, sliced
- 1 cup grape tomatoes, halved
- 1 cup chow mein noodles
- 3/4 cup jellied cranberry sauce
- 3 tablespoons seedless raspberry preserves
- 2 tablespoons balsamic vinegar
- 4-1/2 teaspoons vegetable oil
- 1 tablespoon water

Direction

- On medium heat, in a small skillet, melt butter. Put in walnuts; cook for about 4 minutes till toasted. Drizzle with sugar. Cook and stir for 2 to 4 minutes till melted sugar. Spread on foil to cool off.
- Mix sugared walnuts, noodles, tomatoes, and pepper, onion, turkey and salad greens in a big bowl. Mix the leftover ingredients in a blender; cover up and run the blender until smooth in consistency. Put on top of salad and coat by tossing.

Nutrition Information

- Calories: 464 calories
- Sodium: 136mg sodium
- Fiber: 4g fiber)
- Total Carbohydrate: 40g carbohydrate (23g sugars
- Cholesterol: 78mg cholesterol
- Protein: 32g protein.
- Total Fat: 21g fat (3g saturated fat)

661. Dressing For A Crowd

Serving: about 50 servings. | Prep: 20mins | Cook: 01hours30mins | Ready in:

Ingredients

- 5 loaves (1 pound each) day-old white bread, cubed
- 5 pounds Jones No Sugar Pork Sausage Roll, cooked and drained or 5 pounds giblets, cooked and chopped
- 2-1/2 cups chopped celery
- 1/2 cup finely chopped onion
- 2 pounds butter
- 3-3/4 to 4-1/2 cups chicken broth, divided
- 1 tablespoon salt
- 2 teaspoons rubbed sage
- 1-1/2 teaspoons pepper
- 1 teaspoon dried thyme
- 1 teaspoon celery salt
- 1 teaspoon poultry seasoning
- 1 teaspoon seasoned salt

Direction

- Mix sausage with bread cubes, put aside. Sauté onion and celery in butter in a big saucepan until soft. Take away from heat. Mix in seasonings and 3-3/4 cups broth; stir thoroughly. Put on the bread mixture and stir thoroughly. Add enough of the rest of the broth to reach the moistness you want.
- Move to 4 oiled 3-qt. baking dishes. Bake with a cover at 325° for 1-1/4 hours. Take away the cover and bake until thoroughly heated, about another 15 minutes.

Nutrition Information

- Calories: 249 calories
- Sodium: 662mg sodium
- Fiber: 0 fiber)
- Total Carbohydrate: 6g carbohydrate (1g sugars
- Cholesterol: 56mg cholesterol
- Protein: 4g protein.
- Total Fat: 23g fat (12g saturated fat)

662. Dutch Potato Poultry Stuffing

Serving: 10-12 servings. | Prep: 20mins | Cook: 04hours30mins | Ready in:

Ingredients

- 5 cups mashed potatoes (without added milk and butter or seasoning)
- 6 cups cubed crustless day-old white bread
- 2-1/2 cup chopped onion
- 1 cup chopped celery leaves
- 1 cup minced fresh parsley
- 3 tablespoons butter, melted
- 1 teaspoon salt
- 3/4 teaspoon pepper
- 1 tablespoon all-purpose flour
- 3/4 cup egg substitute
- 1 cup milk
- 1 turkey (12 to 14 pounds)

Direction

- Mix pepper, salt, butter, parsley, celery leaves, onion, bread cubes, and potatoes together in a big bowl. Whisk egg substitute and flour together in a small bowl. Mix in milk; put on the potato mixture and combine thoroughly. If the filling seems dry, add extra milk.

- Stuff the turkey right before baking. Skewer the openings, tie the drumsticks together. Put on a rack in a roasting pan.
- Bake for 4-1/2 to 5 hours at 325°, until a thermometer displays 165° for the stuffing and 180° for the turkey. Once the turkey starts to turn brown, use a tent of aluminum foil to lightly cover and baste if necessary. Take out all of the stuffing.

Nutrition Information

- Calories: 701 calories
- Sodium: 565mg sodium
- Fiber: 4g fiber)
- Total Carbohydrate: 27g carbohydrate (4g sugars
- Cholesterol: 256mg cholesterol
- Protein: 78g protein.
- Total Fat: 29g fat (9g saturated fat)

663. Easy Greek Pasta Salad

Serving: 4 servings. | Prep: 5mins | Cook: 15mins | Ready in:

Ingredients

- 1-1/2 cups uncooked penne pasta
- 1/2 cup cubed cooked turkey or chicken
- 1 can (3.8 ounces) sliced ripe olives, drained
- 1/4 cup chopped green pepper
- 1/4 cup chopped sweet red pepper
- 1/4 cup crumbled feta cheese
- 1/3 cup creamy Caesar salad dressing

Direction

- Cook pasta following package directions; drain and run pasta under cold water. Combine feta cheese, peppers, olives, turkey and pasta in a serving bowl. Add dressing on top of pasta mixture and toss until well coated. Cover and keep cold in refrigerator until serving.

Nutrition Information

- Calories:
- Fiber:
- Total Carbohydrate:
- Cholesterol:
- Protein:
- Total Fat:
- Sodium:

664. Easy Sausage Corn Chowder

Serving: 6-8 serving (2 quarts). | Prep: 10mins | Cook: 15mins | Ready in:

Ingredients

- 2 packages (7 ounces each) Jones No Sugar Pork Sausage Roll
- 2 cans (10-3/4 ounces each) condensed cream of chicken soup, undiluted
- 2-1/2 cups whole milk
- 2 cups fresh corn
- 2/3 cup sliced green onions
- 1/2 teaspoon hot pepper sauce
- 1 cup shredded Swiss cheese

Direction

- Crumble sausage in a big saucepan; brown on medium heat. Drain. Add hot pepper sauce, green onions, corn, milk and soup. Cook till corn is tender; lower to low heat. Add cheese. Heat till melted.

Nutrition Information

- Calories: 217 calories
- Total Carbohydrate: 15g carbohydrate (7g sugars
- Cholesterol: 35mg cholesterol
- Protein: 10g protein.

- Total Fat: 13g fat (6g saturated fat)
- Sodium: 472mg sodium
- Fiber: 2g fiber)

665. Easy Turkey Noodle Soup

Serving: 7 servings. | Prep: 10mins | Cook: 35mins | Ready in:

Ingredients

- 2 cans (14-1/2 ounces each) chicken broth
- 3 cups water
- 1-3/4 cups sliced carrots
- 1/2 cup chopped onion
- 2 celery ribs, sliced
- 1 package (12 ounces) frozen egg noodles
- 3 cups chopped cooked turkey
- 1 package (10 ounces) frozen peas
- 2 envelopes chicken gravy mix
- 1/2 cup cold water

Direction

- Boil onion, water, celery, and carrots in a large saucepan. Reduce the heat and cover the pan. Simmer the mixture for 4-6 minutes until the vegetables are crisp-tender. Add the noodles and simmer the mixture for 20 minutes, uncovered until the noodles are tender.
- Mix in peas and turkey. Mix cold water and gravy mixes until smooth, and then add it into the soup. Boil the mixture. Cook and stir for 2 minutes until thickened.

Nutrition Information

- Calories: 388 calories
- Sodium: 1106mg sodium
- Fiber: 5g fiber)
- Total Carbohydrate: 52g carbohydrate (6g sugars
- Cholesterol: 89mg cholesterol

- Protein: 28g protein.
- Total Fat: 7g fat (2g saturated fat)

666. Effortless Black Bean Chili

Serving: 6 servings. | Prep: 25mins | Cook: 06hours00mins | Ready in:

Ingredients

- 1 pound ground turkey
- 1 small onion, chopped
- 3 teaspoons chili powder
- 2 teaspoons minced fresh oregano or 3/4 teaspoon dried oregano
- 1 teaspoon chicken bouillon granules
- 1 jar (16 ounces) mild salsa
- 1 can (15-1/4 ounces) whole kernel corn, drained
- 1 can (15 ounces) black beans, rinsed and drained
- 1 can (14-1/2 ounces) diced tomatoes, undrained
- 1/2 cup water
- Optional toppings: sour cream, finely chopped red onion and corn chips

Direction

- Cook and crumble turkey with onion in a large skillet on medium-high heat for 5 - 7 minutes until the turkey meat is no longer pink, then transfer into a 4 quart slow cooker.
- Stir in all the other ingredients aside from the toppings. Cook while covered on a low setting for 6 - 8 hours until the flavors blend. Top the chili if you wish.

Nutrition Information

- Calories: 242 calories
- Protein: 20g protein.
- Total Fat: 6g fat (1g saturated fat)

- Sodium: 868mg sodium
- Fiber: 6g fiber)
- Total Carbohydrate: 26g carbohydrate (9g sugars
- Cholesterol: 50mg cholesterol

667. Fruit 'n' Spice Salad

Serving: 6-8 servings. | Prep: 20mins | Cook: 0mins | Ready in:

Ingredients

- 4 cups cooked long grain or wild rice
- 3 cups cubed fully cooked ham or turkey
- 1 small Granny Smith apple, cubed
- 1 small Red Delicious apple, cubed
- 1/2 cup sliced green onions
- 1/2 cup seedless green grapes, halved
- 1/2 cup seedless red grapes, halved
- 1/4 cup raisins
- 1/4 cup olive oil
- 1/4 cup white wine vinegar
- 1 teaspoon sugar
- 1/4 teaspoon curry powder
- 1/4 teaspoon ground cinnamon
- 1/4 teaspoon salt
- 1/4 cup slivered almonds

Direction

- Mix raisins, grapes, onions, apples, ham and rice in a big bowl. Mix salt, cinnamon, curry, sugar, vinegar and oil in a small bowl; put on top of rice mixture and coat by tossing. Keep chilled for no less than 2 hours. Just prior to serving, put in almonds and toss.

Nutrition Information

- Calories: 317 calories
- Protein: 13g protein.
- Total Fat: 13g fat (3g saturated fat)
- Sodium: 748mg sodium

- Fiber: 2g fiber)
- Total Carbohydrate: 37g carbohydrate (11g sugars
- Cholesterol: 28mg cholesterol

668. Fruited Tarragon Turkey Salad

Serving: 8 servings. | Prep: 10mins | Cook: 0mins | Ready in:

Ingredients

- 6 cups cubed cooked turkey
- 2 cups chopped celery
- 1 cup green grapes
- 3/4 cup sour cream
- 3/4 cup mayonnaise
- 1-1/2 teaspoons dried tarragon
- 1 teaspoon salt
- 1/8 teaspoon pepper
- 1/2 cup chopped walnuts, toasted
- Leaf lettuce

Direction

- Combine grapes, celery and turkey in a bowl. Combine salt, pepper, tarragon, mayonnaise and sour cream in a small bowl. Add dressing to turkey mixture and toss until well coated. Cover the salad and keep cold in refrigerator for 5 hours. Stir in walnuts right before serving. Serve in a lettuce-covered bowl.

Nutrition Information

- Calories: 442 calories
- Sodium: 520mg sodium
- Fiber: 1g fiber)
- Total Carbohydrate: 7g carbohydrate (5g sugars
- Cholesterol: 102mg cholesterol
- Protein: 34g protein.
- Total Fat: 30g fat (7g saturated fat)

669. Fruited Turkey Salad

Serving: 7 servings. | Prep: 15mins | Cook: 0mins | Ready in:

Ingredients

- 4 cups cubed cooked turkey
- 1 can (20 ounces) pineapple chunks, drained
- 1 cup seedless green grapes, halved
- 1 cup sliced celery
- 2 tablespoons vegetable oil
- 2 tablespoons orange juice
- 2 tablespoons lemon juice
- 1 tablespoon minced fresh parsley
- 1/2 teaspoon salt, optional
- 1/2 cup mayonnaise
- 1/2 cup salted sunflower kernels, optional

Direction

- Mix together celery, grapes, pineapple and turkey in a large bowl. In a small bowl, combine parsley, lemon juice, orange juice and oil, add salt if desired. Pour dressing over salad, toss until well coated. Allow salad to chill for 2 hours. Right before the salad is served, add sunflower kernels and mayonnaise if desired, mix properly.

Nutrition Information

- Calories: 184 calories
- Protein: 13g protein. Diabetic Exchanges: 2 very lean meat
- Total Fat: 6g fat (0 saturated fat)
- Sodium: 280mg sodium
- Fiber: 0 fiber)
- Total Carbohydrate: 18g carbohydrate (0 sugars
- Cholesterol: 49mg cholesterol

670. Garden Pasta Salad

Serving: 10 | Prep: 15mins | Cook: 15mins | Ready in:

Ingredients

- 1 (16 ounce) package uncooked tri-color spiral pasta
- 1/2 cup thinly sliced carrots
- 2 stalks celery, chopped
- 1/2 cup chopped green bell pepper
- 1/2 cup cucumber, peeled and thinly sliced
- 2 large tomatoes, diced
- 1/4 cup chopped onion
- 2 (16 ounce) bottles Italian-style salad dressing
- 1/2 cup grated Parmesan cheese

Direction

- In a big pot, cook pasta in boiling water until they're al dente. Rinse with cold water; drain.
- Combine onion, tomatoes, green pepper, cucumber, celery, and chopped carrots in a big bowl. Mix vegetables and cooled pasta in a big bowl. Pour Italian dressing on mixture, then put parmesan cheese and stir well.
- Chill for an hour before serving.

Nutrition Information

- Calories: 449 calories;
- Protein: 8.4
- Total Fat: 27.4
- Sodium: 1540
- Total Carbohydrate: 45.1
- Cholesterol: 4

671. Garden Fresh Chef Salad

Serving: 6 servings. | Prep: 25mins | Cook: 0mins | Ready in:

Ingredients

- 6 cups spring mix salad greens

- 2 medium tomatoes, coarsely chopped
- 6 hard-boiled large eggs, coarsely chopped
- 3 slices deli turkey, cut into thin strips
- 3 slices deli ham, cut into thin strips
- 1/2 cup shredded cabbage
- 4 green onions, sliced
- 4 fresh baby carrots, sliced
- 4 radishes, thinly sliced
- 1/4 teaspoon garlic powder
- 1/4 teaspoon pepper
- 1/2 cup reduced-fat Thousand Island salad dressing or dressing of your choice

Direction

- Mix the first 9 ingredients in a big bowl. Sprinkle pepper and garlic powder, toss until coated. Serve with the salad dressing.

Nutrition Information

- Calories: 171 calories
- Protein: 12g protein. Diabetic Exchanges: 2 lean meat
- Total Fat: 9g fat (2g saturated fat)
- Sodium: 508mg sodium
- Fiber: 2g fiber)
- Total Carbohydrate: 11g carbohydrate (6g sugars
- Cholesterol: 227mg cholesterol

672. Gizzard Soup

Serving: 12-14 servings (about 3-1/2 quarts). | Prep: 15mins | Cook: 02hours30mins | Ready in:

Ingredients

- 1/2 cup all-purpose flour
- 1 tablespoon seasoned salt
- 1-1/2 pounds chicken gizzards, trimmed and halved
- 1/4 cup vegetable oil
- 2 cans (49-1/2 ounces each) chicken broth
- 5 cups uncooked wide egg noodles

Direction

- In a big resealable plastic bag, mix together seasoned salt and flour. Add gizzards, shake to cover. Brown gizzards in oil in a Dutch oven or a soup kettle. Add chicken broth. Put a cover on and simmer until the gizzards are soft, about 2-3 hours. Add noodles; simmer without a cover for 30 minutes.

Nutrition Information

- Calories: 172 calories
- Cholesterol: 150mg cholesterol
- Protein: 13g protein.
- Total Fat: 7g fat (1g saturated fat)
- Sodium: 782mg sodium
- Fiber: 0 fiber)
- Total Carbohydrate: 15g carbohydrate (1g sugars

673. Greek Rice Salad

Serving: 8 | Prep: 20mins | Cook: 45mins | Ready in:

Ingredients

- 1 cup uncooked long grain brown rice
- 2 1/2 cups water
- 1 avocado - peeled, pitted, and diced
- 1/4 cup lemon juice
- 2 vine-ripened tomatoes, diced
- 1 1/2 cups diced English cucumbers
- 1/3 cup diced red onion
- 1/2 cup crumbled feta cheese
- 1/4 cup sliced Kalamata olives
- 1/4 cup chopped fresh mint
- 3 tablespoons olive oil
- 1 teaspoon lemon zest
- 1/2 teaspoon minced garlic
- 1/2 teaspoon kosher salt
- 1/2 teaspoon ground black pepper

Direction

- On high heat, boil water and brown rice in a saucepan. Lower the heat to medium-low, cover up, and let it simmer until the rice is soft and the liquid has been absorbed for 45 - 50 minutes; take off heat and allow to cool off, use a fork to fluff once in a while.
- In a big bowl, mix the lemon juice and avocado. Put the pepper, salt, garlic, lemon zest, olive oil, mint, olives, feta, onion, cucumber and tomatoes to the bowl; mixing gently till combined evenly. Fold the cooled rice lightly into the mixture. Serve instantly or keep chilled for the maximum of 1 hour; the salad cannot last well for more than a day as the cucumber and tomatoes start to release their juices and the salad becomes watery.

Nutrition Information

- Calories: 224 calories;
- Protein: 4.5
- Total Fat: 12.7
- Sodium: 304
- Total Carbohydrate: 24.6
- Cholesterol: 8

674. Grill Side Turkey Salad

Serving: 4 servings. | Prep: 15mins | Cook: 20mins | Ready in:

Ingredients

- 2 turkey breast tenderloins (1-1/2 pounds)
- 2 teaspoons dried tarragon, divided
- 1/2 cup thinly sliced celery
- 1/2 cup chopped green pepper
- 1/2 cup chopped red onion
- 2 tablespoons canola oil
- 1 tablespoon soy sauce
- 1 tablespoon lemon juice
- 1 tablespoon red wine vinegar
- 1/8 teaspoon pepper
- 1/4 teaspoon salt, optional
- Lettuce leaves
- Chopped salted peanuts, optional

Direction

- Season each of the tenderloins with 1/2 teaspoon of tarragon. Put the seasoned tenderloins on an open grill and let it grill for 8-10 minutes on every side over medium-hot heat until a thermometer inserted on the tenderloins indicate 170°F. Allow it to cool down.
- Cube the grilled tenderloins and put it in a big bowl. Put in the green pepper, onion and celery. Mix the remaining tarragon, pepper, salt if you want, vinegar, soy sauce, oil and lemon juice together in a small bowl. Drizzle the dressing mixture on top of the turkey mixture and mix well until coated. Keep in the fridge for a minimum of 3 hours.
- Place the salad mixture on lettuce leaves to serve then top it off with peanuts if you want.

Nutrition Information

- Calories: 258 calories
- Sodium: 261mg sodium
- Fiber: 0 fiber)
- Total Carbohydrate: 4g carbohydrate (0 sugars
- Cholesterol: 53mg cholesterol
- Protein: 41g protein. Diabetic Exchanges: 5 lean meat
- Total Fat: 9g fat (0 saturated fat)

675. Ham Salad

Serving: 10 servings. | Prep: 15mins | Cook: 0mins | Ready in:

Ingredients

- 3/4 cup mayonnaise
- 1/2 cup finely chopped celery

- 1/4 cup sliced green onions
- 2 tablespoons minced fresh chives
- 1 tablespoon honey
- 2 teaspoons spicy brown mustard
- 1/2 teaspoon Worcestershire sauce
- 1/2 teaspoon seasoned salt
- 5 cups diced fully cooked ham or turkey
- 1/3 cup chopped pecans and almonds, toasted
- Slider buns, split, optional

Direction

- Combine the initial 8 ingredients. Mix in ham. Keep chilled in the refrigerator, while covered, till serving.
- Mix in pecans prior to serving. If you want, serve this on buns.

Nutrition Information

- Calories: 254 calories
- Protein: 16g protein.
- Total Fat: 20g fat (3g saturated fat)
- Sodium: 1023mg sodium
- Fiber: 1g fiber)
- Total Carbohydrate: 4g carbohydrate (2g sugars
- Cholesterol: 43mg cholesterol

676. Ham And Turkey Pasta Salad

Serving: 10 servings. | Prep: 20mins | Cook: 0mins | Ready in:

Ingredients

- 3-3/4 cups uncooked bow tie pasta
- 1 cup chopped fully cooked lean ham
- 1 cup chopped cooked turkey breast
- 1 cup shredded reduced-fat cheddar cheese
- 1/4 cup chopped onion
- 1/4 cup chopped celery
- 1 hard-boiled large egg, chopped
- 1 cup fat-free mayonnaise
- 1/4 cup picante sauce
- 1 teaspoon salt
- 1/4 teaspoon pepper
- 1/4 teaspoon sugar

Direction

- Following the instruction on package to cook pasta; drain off and wash under cold water.
- At the same time, mix egg, celery, onion, cheese, turkey, ham and pasta in a big bowl. Mix the leftover ingredients in a small bowl. Put on top of salad; coat by lightly mixing. Keep it covered and let chilled in the refrigerator for 2 hours prior to serving.

Nutrition Information

- Calories: 0g sugar total.

677. Ham, Turkey And Wild Rice Salad

Serving: 8-10 servings. | Prep: 15mins | Cook: 0mins | Ready in:

Ingredients

- 5 cups cooked wild rice
- 1/2 cup Western salad dressing
- 1 cup cubed fully cooked ham
- 1 cup cubed cooked turkey
- 1 cup thinly sliced celery
- 1 cup frozen peas, thawed
- 2/3 cup thinly sliced radishes
- 1/2 cup finely chopped onion
- 1 cup mayonnaise
- 2 teaspoon prepared mustard
- 1/4 to 1/2 teaspoon curry powder
- 1/2 teaspoon salt
- 1/4 teaspoon pepper

Direction

- Combine dressing and rice in a large bowl; cover the mixture and allow it to chill overnight. Add onion, radishes, peas, celery, turkey and ham. Combine salt, pepper, curry, mustard and mayonnaise, mix thoroughly. Stir dressing into salad. Cover and keep cold in refrigerator for at least 2 hours.

Nutrition Information

- Calories: 360 calories
- Protein: 11g protein.
- Total Fat: 24g fat (4g saturated fat)
- Sodium: 573mg sodium
- Fiber: 3g fiber)
- Total Carbohydrate: 25g carbohydrate (5g sugars
- Cholesterol: 26mg cholesterol

678. Hamburger Soup

Serving: | Prep: 20 | Cook: mins | Ready in:

Ingredients

- 1 pound Ground Chicken
- 1 onion, chopped
- 3 stalks Celery, sliced
- 3 Carrots, sliced
- 1 Green pepper, chopped
- 1 Zucchini, diced
- 28 ounces Tomatoes, canned
- 14 ounces Chick peas or other beans, canned (rinsed and drained)
- 2 tablespoons Tomato paste
- 3 cups Chicken Stock
- 2 tablespoons Oregano and/or Basil (Herbs de Provence)
- 3 cloves Garlic
- 1/4 cup Rice or Barley
- 1 teaspoon Pepper, ground

Direction

- In a big pot, brown the meat with a bit olive oil. Add garlic and onions and cook until the onions are tender.
- Add carrots, green pepper, and celery and cook for 5 minutes. Add herbs.
- Add tomato paste, stock, tomatoes, and zucchini and mix. And then add beans if available.
- Boil the mixture, add rice and simmer for 20 minutes or more. Add pepper and salt to taste.

Nutrition Information

679. Harvest Turkey Soup

Serving: 22 servings (5-1/2 quarts). | Prep: 35mins | Cook: 02hours30mins | Ready in:

Ingredients

- 1 leftover turkey carcass (from a 12-pound turkey)
- 5 quarts water
- 2 large carrots, shredded
- 1 cup chopped celery
- 1 large onion, chopped
- 4 chicken bouillon cubes
- 1 can (28 ounces) stewed tomatoes
- 3/4 cup fresh or frozen peas
- 3/4 cup uncooked long grain rice
- 1 package (10 ounces) frozen chopped spinach
- 1 tablespoon salt, optional
- 3/4 teaspoon pepper
- 1/2 teaspoon dried marjoram
- 1/2 teaspoon dried thyme

Direction

- Place water and turkey carcass into a big soup kettle or Dutch oven, then boil. Lower the heat then simmer while covered for 1 1/2 hours. Remove the carcass and cool. Remove the

turkey meat from the bones and cut them into bite-sized pieces, then put aside.
- Strain the broth and add in bouillon, onion, celery, and carrots, then boil. Turn the heat down and simmer, covered, for 30 minutes. Add the reserved turkey, thyme, marjoram, pepper, salt (optional), spinach, rice, peas, and tomatoes, then bring back to a boil. Cook without a cover for 20 minutes or until the rice becomes tender.

Nutrition Information

- Calories: 0g saturated fat (0 sugars
- Sodium: 1 vegetable
- Total Carbohydrate: 1 fat.
- Cholesterol: 1 starch
- Total Fat: 0 fiber). Diabetic Exchanges: 4 very lean meat

680. Healthy Italian Market Salad

Serving: 9 servings. | Prep: 25mins | Cook: 0mins | Ready in:

Ingredients

- 2 cups cooked brown rice, cooled
- 2 cups shredded part-skim mozzarella cheese
- 4 plum tomatoes, seeded and chopped
- 1/2 medium green pepper, julienned
- 4 ounces sliced turkey pepperoni, quartered
- 1/2 cup cubed fully cooked ham
- 4 green onions, sliced
- 1 can (2-1/4 ounces) sliced ripe olives, drained
- 1/2 cup reduced-fat Italian salad dressing

Direction

- Mix the first 8 ingredients in a big bowl. Put the dressing on the salad, mix to coat. Put a cover on and chill for 2 hours until cold.

Nutrition Information

- Calories: 199 calories
- Total Fat: 9g fat (3g saturated fat)
- Sodium: 612mg sodium
- Fiber: 2g fiber)
- Total Carbohydrate: 15g carbohydrate (0 sugars
- Cholesterol: 36mg cholesterol
- Protein: 13g protein. Diabetic Exchanges: 2 lean meat

681. Hearty Alfredo Potatoes

Serving: 6-8 servings. | Prep: 20mins | Cook: 01hours15mins | Ready in:

Ingredients

- 1 jar (16 ounces) Alfredo sauce
- 1 cup whole milk
- 1 teaspoon garlic powder
- 3 pounds potatoes, peeled and thinly sliced
- 5 tablespoons grated Parmesan cheese, divided
- Salt and pepper to taste
- 2 to 3 cups cubed cooked turkey
- 3 cups frozen chopped broccoli, thawed
- 2 cups shredded Swiss cheese, divided

Direction

- Mix garlic powder, milk, and Alfredo sauce together in a big bowl. In an oil-coated 13x9-in. dish, put 1/4 of the mixture. Use 1/4 of the potatoes to layer, and scatter pepper, salt, and 1 tablespoon Parmesan cheese.
- Mix 1-1/2 cups Swiss cheese, broccoli, and turkey together in a big bowl. Put on the potatoes with 1/3 of the mixture. Do the layers 2 times more. Put the rest of the potatoes on top. Use the rest of the Parmesan and Swiss cheeses to sprinkle. Use the rest of the Alfredo sauce mixture to spread.

- Bake at 400° with a cover for 45 minutes. Lower the temperature to 350°. Bake without a cover until the potatoes are soft, about another 30 minutes. Let sit for 15 minutes prior to serving and enjoy.

Nutrition Information

- Calories: 420 calories
- Cholesterol: 74mg cholesterol
- Protein: 28g protein.
- Total Fat: 17g fat (11g saturated fat)
- Sodium: 412mg sodium
- Fiber: 4g fiber)
- Total Carbohydrate: 39g carbohydrate (7g sugars

682. Hearty Brunch Potatoes

Serving: 12 servings. | Prep: 25mins | Cook: 35mins | Ready in:

Ingredients

- 7 medium potatoes, peeled and cut into 1/2-inch cubes
- 1/2 cup chopped green pepper
- 1/2 cup chopped sweet red pepper
- 1/2 cup fresh or frozen corn
- 1 small onion, chopped
- 1 to 2 garlic cloves, minced
- 1/2 pound smoked turkey sausage links
- 2 tablespoons olive oil
- 1/4 teaspoon pepper

Direction

- In a saucepan, put potatoes and submerge in water. Boil it, lower the heat. Cook without a cover for 10 minutes until just soft.
- In the meantime, sauté garlic, onion, corn and peppers in a cooking spray-coated frying pan until soft. Slice sausage into small pieces, add to the vegetable mixture. Cook without a cover until fully heated, about 6-8 minutes.
- Drain the potatoes, add to the vegetable mixture. Add pepper and oil; stir thoroughly. Move to a non-oiled 13x9-in. baking dish. Bake without a cover at 350° until completely heated, about 35 minutes.

Nutrition Information

- Calories: 114 calories
- Fiber: 2g fiber)
- Total Carbohydrate: 18g carbohydrate (2g sugars
- Cholesterol: 7mg cholesterol
- Protein: 4g protein. Diabetic Exchanges: 1 starch
- Total Fat: 3g fat (1g saturated fat)
- Sodium: 164mg sodium

683. Hearty Meatball Soup

Serving: 22 servings (5-3/4 quarts). | Prep: 20mins | Cook: 45mins | Ready in:

Ingredients

- 2 large eggs
- 1 cup soft bread crumbs
- 1 teaspoon salt
- 1/2 teaspoon pepper
- 1 pound lean ground beef (90% lean)
- 1 pound ground pork
- 1/2 pound ground turkey
- 4 cups beef broth
- 1 can (46 ounces) tomato juice
- 2 cans (14-1/2 ounces each) stewed tomatoes
- 8 cups shredded cabbage
- 1 cup thinly sliced celery
- 1 cup thinly sliced carrots
- 8 green onions, sliced
- 3/4 cup uncooked long grain rice
- 2 teaspoons dried basil
- 3 tablespoons minced fresh parsley

- 2 tablespoons soy sauce

Direction

- Combine pepper, salt, breadcrumbs, and eggs in a big bowl. Crumble the meat over the mixture and blend well, then shape into 1 inch balls.
- Boil broth in a stockpot, then gently add in the meatballs. Add in basil, rice, vegetables, tomatoes, and tomato juice, then set to boil. Decrease the heat and simmer, covered, for 30 minutes.
- Add soy sauce and parsley, then simmer without a cover until the vegetables are tender and the meatballs no longer pink, about 10 minutes.

Nutrition Information

- Calories: 162 calories
- Sodium: 652mg sodium
- Fiber: 2g fiber)
- Total Carbohydrate: 13g carbohydrate (5g sugars
- Cholesterol: 50mg cholesterol
- Protein: 12g protein.
- Total Fat: 7g fat (2g saturated fat)

684. Hearty Pasta Salad

Serving: 4 servings. | Prep: 20mins | Cook: 0mins | Ready in:

Ingredients

- 2 cups uncooked spiral pasta
- 1 cup cubed pastrami, cooked turkey or roast beef
- 1/4 cup each chopped carrot, celery and onion
- 3/4 cup mayonnaise
- 1/4 cup grated Parmesan cheese
- 1/4 teaspoon salt
- 1/4 teaspoon pepper
- 1/4 teaspoon lemon juice

Direction

- Cook pasta based on package directions; drain and rinse the pasta in cold water.
- Combine onion, celery, carrot, pastrami and pasta in a large bowl. Mix together lemon juice, pepper, salt, Parmesan cheese and mayonnaise. Pour dressing over the pasta mixture; toss until well coated. Cover the salad and keep cold in refrigerator for 1 hour or until serving

Nutrition Information

- Calories: 535 calories
- Total Fat: 36g fat (6g saturated fat)
- Sodium: 483mg sodium
- Fiber: 2g fiber)
- Total Carbohydrate: 34g carbohydrate (2g sugars
- Cholesterol: 50mg cholesterol
- Protein: 18g protein.

685. Hearty Sausage Chicken Chili

Serving: 11 servings (2-3/4 quarts). | Prep: 20mins | Cook: 04hours00mins | Ready in:

Ingredients

- 1 pound Italian turkey sausage links, casings removed
- 1 medium onion, chopped
- 3/4 pound boneless skinless chicken thighs, cut into 3/4-inch pieces
- 2 cans (14-1/2 ounces each) diced tomatoes with mild green chilies, undrained
- 2 cans (8 ounces each) tomato sauce
- 1 can (16 ounces) kidney beans, rinsed and drained

- 1 can (15 ounces) white kidney or cannellini beans, rinsed and drained
- 1 can (15 ounces) pinto beans, rinsed and drained
- 1 can (15 ounces) black beans, rinsed and drained
- 1 teaspoon chili powder
- 1/2 teaspoon garlic powder
- 1/8 teaspoon pepper

Direction

- In a big nonstick skillet coated in cooking spray, crumble sausage. Put onion. Stir and cook on medium heat till meat isn't pink then drain.
- Put into 5-qt. slow cooker. Mix leftover ingredients in. Cook for 4-5 hours on low, covered, till chicken isn't pink.

Nutrition Information

- Calories: 272 calories
- Protein: 21g protein.
- Total Fat: 6g fat (1g saturated fat)
- Sodium: 826mg sodium
- Fiber: 8g fiber)
- Total Carbohydrate: 32g carbohydrate (7g sugars
- Cholesterol: 45mg cholesterol

686. Homemade Kielbasa Bean Soup

Serving: 8 servings (2 quarts). | Prep: 20mins | Cook: 20mins | Ready in:

Ingredients

- 1 small onion, chopped
- 2 garlic cloves, minced
- 2 teaspoons butter
- 2 cans (14-1/2 ounces each) reduced-sodium chicken broth
- 1 medium potato, peeled and cubed
- 1/2 pound smoked turkey kielbasa or turkey sausage, cut into 1/4-inch slices
- 3 cups shredded cabbage
- 1 can (15 ounces) garbanzo beans or chickpeas, rinsed and drained
- 1 cup sliced fresh carrots
- 2 tablespoons minced fresh parsley
- 1 tablespoon white wine vinegar
- 1/2 teaspoon pepper

Direction

- Sauté garlic and onion in butter in a big saucepan until soft. Mix in potato and broth. Boil it. Lower the heat, put a cover on and simmer for 10 minutes.
- Mix in the rest of the ingredients. Boil again. Lower the heat, put a cover on, and simmer for 10 minutes.

Nutrition Information

- Calories: 147 calories
- Cholesterol: 10mg cholesterol
- Protein: 9g protein. Diabetic Exchanges: 1 starch
- Total Fat: 2g fat (0 saturated fat)
- Sodium: 694mg sodium
- Fiber: 4g fiber)
- Total Carbohydrate: 23g carbohydrate (0 sugars

687. Hot Turkey Pecan Salad

Serving: 4 servings. | Prep: 10mins | Cook: 20mins | Ready in:

Ingredients

- 2 cups cubed cooked turkey or chicken
- 2 cups thinly sliced celery
- 1/2 cup sliced pimiento-stuffed olives
- 1/2 cup chopped pecans

- 1 tablespoon finely chopped onion
- 1 cup mayonnaise
- 2 tablespoons lemon juice
- 1/2 teaspoon salt
- 3/4 to 1 cup crushed potato chips
- 1/2 cup shredded cheddar cheese

Direction

- Mix onion, pecans, olives, celery and turkey in a big bowl. Mix salt, lemon juice and mayonnaise; put on top of turkey mixture and coat by tossing.
- Add into a greased square 8-inch baking dish. Use cheese and potato chips to drizzle. Bake it while uncovered, for 20-25 minutes till bubbly at 375 degrees.

Nutrition Information

- Calories: 773 calories
- Protein: 26g protein.
- Total Fat: 69g fat (12g saturated fat)
- Sodium: 1203mg sodium
- Fiber: 3g fiber)
- Total Carbohydrate: 13g carbohydrate (2g sugars
- Cholesterol: 88mg cholesterol

688. Hot Turkey Salad

Serving: 6 | Prep: 30mins | Cook: 10mins | Ready in:

Ingredients

- 2 cups cubed cooked turkey
- 2 cups chopped celery
- 2 teaspoons grated onion
- 1/2 cup pecans, chopped
- 1/2 teaspoon salt
- 1 cup mayonnaise
- 2 tablespoons fresh lemon juice
- 1/2 cup Cheddar cheese, grated
- 1 cup potato chips, crushed

Direction

- Set the oven to 450°F (230°C). Oil a 9x13 inch baking dish.
- In a mixing bowl, combine salt, pecans, onion, celery and turkey. Stir in lemon juice and mayonnaise until mixture is blended evenly. Place on prepared baking dish using a spoon. Add a sprinkle of cheddar cheese, then potato chips on top.
- Bake in preheated oven for 10 to 12 minutes, until cheese is evenly melted.

Nutrition Information

- Calories: 526 calories;
- Total Carbohydrate: 10.6
- Cholesterol: 59
- Protein: 18.4
- Total Fat: 46.4
- Sodium: 591

689. Italian Sausage Kale Soup

Serving: 8 servings (2 quarts). | Prep: 15mins | Cook: 20mins | Ready in:

Ingredients

- 1 package (19-1/2 ounces) Italian turkey sausage links, casings removed
- 1 medium onion, chopped
- 8 cups chopped fresh kale
- 2 garlic cloves, minced
- 1/4 teaspoon crushed red pepper flakes, optional
- 1/2 cup white wine or chicken stock
- 3-1/4 cups chicken stock (26 ounces)
- 1 can (15 ounces) white kidney or cannellini beans, rinsed and drained
- 1 can (14-1/2 ounces) no-salt-added diced tomatoes, undrained
- 1/2 cup sun-dried tomatoes (not packed in oil), chopped

- 1/4 teaspoon pepper

Direction

- Over medium heat, cook sausage and onion in a 6-qt. stockpot, while crumbling the sausage, for 6-8 minutes until sausage is not pink anymore. Move out using a slotted spoon.
- Mix in kale in the pot and cook and stir, about 2 minutes. Stir in garlic and, if you want, pepper flakes. Cook for about a minute. Pour in wine and cook for two minutes more.
- Mix in the remaining ingredients and the sausage mixture. Let it boil. Lower heat and simmer while covered until kale becomes tender, about 15-20 minutes.

Nutrition Information

- Calories: 217 calories
- Protein: 18g protein.
- Total Fat: 8g fat (2g saturated fat)
- Sodium: 868mg sodium
- Fiber: 4g fiber)
- Total Carbohydrate: 15g carbohydrate (5g sugars
- Cholesterol: 51mg cholesterol

690. Italian Sausage Pizza Soup

Serving: 12 servings (3 quarts) | Prep: 15mins | Cook: 06hours00mins | Ready in:

Ingredients

- 1 package (1 pound) Italian turkey sausage links
- 1 medium onion, chopped
- 1 medium green pepper, cut into strips
- 1 medium sweet red or yellow pepper, cut into strips
- 1 can (15 ounces) great northern or cannellini beans, rinsed and drained
- 1 can (14-1/2 ounces) diced tomatoes, undrained
- 1 jar (14 ounces) pizza sauce
- 2 teaspoons Italian seasoning
- 2 garlic cloves, minced
- 2 cans (14-1/2 ounces each) beef broth
- 1 package (5 ounces) Caesar salad croutons
- Shredded part-skim mozzarella cheese

Direction

- Take out the casings of the sausage. Over medium high heat, cook and crumble sausage in a big skillet until it is not pink anymore. Put in peppers and onion and cook until it becomes tender crisp. Drain out and move to a 6-qt. slow cooker.
- Put in the next five ingredients. Add the broth. Put the cover on and cook on low setting for 6-8 hours until veggies become tender. Serve with cheese and croutons.

Nutrition Information

- Calories: 158 calories
- Sodium: 828mg sodium
- Fiber: 4g fiber)
- Total Carbohydrate: 19g carbohydrate (4g sugars
- Cholesterol: 15mg cholesterol
- Protein: 9g protein.
- Total Fat: 5g fat (1g saturated fat)

691. Italian Sausage Tortellini Soup

Serving: 6 | Prep: 15mins | Cook: 55mins | Ready in:

Ingredients

- 1 (3.5 ounce) link sweet Italian sausage, casings removed
- 1 cup chopped onions
- 2 cloves garlic, minced

- 5 cups beef stock
- 1/3 cup water
- 1/2 cup red wine
- 4 tomatoes - peeled, seeded and chopped
- 1 cup chopped carrots
- 1/2 teaspoon dried basil
- 1/2 teaspoon dried oregano
- 1 cup tomato sauce
- 1 zucchini, chopped
- 8 ounces cheese tortellini
- 1 green bell pepper, chopped
- 1 tablespoon chopped fresh parsley
- 2 tablespoons grated Parmesan cheese for topping

Direction

- In a big pot, sauté sausage for 10 minutes over medium high heat until it is properly browned. Drain the grease but leave about 1 tablespoon and stir in garlic and onion. Sauté for about 5 minutes.
- Mix in tomato sauce, oregano, basil, carrots, tomatoes, wine, water, and beef stock. Let it boil and adjust heat to low. Let it simmer, while skimming any fat that may float, for 30 minutes.
- Mix in parsley, green bell pepper, tortellini and zucchini for added taste. Let it simmer until the tortellini is completely cooked, about 10 minutes. Put into individual bowls and top with cheese.

Nutrition Information

- Calories: 249 calories;
- Sodium: 542
- Total Carbohydrate: 27.7
- Cholesterol: 22
- Protein: 12.4
- Total Fat: 8.9

692. Kielbasa Summer Salad

Serving: 10 servings. | Prep: 15mins | Cook: 0mins | Ready in:

Ingredients

- 1 pound Johnsonville® Fully Cooked Polish Kielbasa Sausage Rope, halved and cut into 1/4-inch pieces
- 1 can (15-1/2 ounces) black-eyed peas, rinsed and drained
- 2 medium tart apples, cut into 1/2-inch chunks
- 1 medium green pepper, chopped
- 4 large green onions, thinly sliced
- DRESSING:
- 1/3 cup vegetable oil
- 3 tablespoons cider vinegar
- 1 tablespoon Dijon mustard
- 2 teaspoons sugar
- 1/2 to 1 teaspoon pepper

Direction

- Brown sausage in a nonstick skillet. Use paper towels to drain sausage. Put sausage, onions, green pepper, apples, and peas in a large bowl.
- In a small bowl, mix the dressing ingredients. Pour the dressing on top of the sausage mixture; toss to coat. Store in the fridge, while covered, for 4 hours or overnight.

Nutrition Information

- Calories: 192 calories
- Protein: 9g protein. Diabetic Exchanges: 1 starch
- Total Fat: 12g fat (0 saturated fat)
- Sodium: 561mg sodium
- Fiber: 0 fiber)
- Total Carbohydrate: 14g carbohydrate (0 sugars
- Cholesterol: 28mg cholesterol

693. Lemony Turkey Rice Soup

Serving: 8 servings (2 quarts). | Prep: 15mins | Cook: 15mins | Ready in:

Ingredients

- 2 cups diced cooked turkey
- 2 cups cooked long grain rice
- 1 can (10-3/4 ounces) condensed cream of chicken soup, undiluted
- 1/4 teaspoon pepper
- 6 cups chicken broth, divided
- 2 tablespoons cornstarch
- 1/4 to 1/3 cup lemon juice
- 1/4 to 1/2 cup minced fresh cilantro

Direction

- Combine the first 4 ingredients with 5 1/2 cups of broth into a large saucepan and boil, then cook for 3 minutes.
- Mix the remaining broth with cornstarch in a small bowl until smooth, then slowly stir into the soup. Allow the soup to boil, then cook while stirring for 1 - 2 minutes until it thickens. Take the pan off the heat then stir in the cilantro and lemon juice.

Nutrition Information

- Calories: 166 calories
- Total Fat: 4g fat (1g saturated fat)
- Sodium: 1047mg sodium
- Fiber: 1g fiber)
- Total Carbohydrate: 17g carbohydrate (1g sugars
- Cholesterol: 42mg cholesterol
- Protein: 13g protein.

694. Lentil Barley Soup

Serving: 8-10 servings (about 2-1/2 quarts). | Prep: 25mins | Cook: 40mins | Ready in:

Ingredients

- 1 medium onion, chopped
- 1/2 cup chopped green pepper
- 3 garlic cloves, minced
- 1 tablespoon butter
- 1 can (49-1/2 ounces) chicken broth
- 3 medium carrots, chopped
- 1/2 cup dried lentils
- 1-1/2 teaspoons Italian seasoning
- 1 teaspoon salt
- 1/4 teaspoon pepper
- 1 cup cubed cooked chicken or turkey
- 1/2 cup quick-cooking barley
- 2 medium fresh mushrooms, chopped
- 1 can (28 ounces) crushed tomatoes, undrained

Direction

- Sauté garlic, green pepper, and onion in butter in a soup kettle or a Dutch oven until soft. Add pepper, salt, Italian seasoning, lentils, carrots, and broth; boil it. Lower the heat, put a cover on and simmer for 25 minutes.
- Add mushrooms, barley, and chicken; boil again. Lower the heat, put a cover on and simmer until the carrots, barley, and lentils are soft, about 10-15 minutes. Add tomatoes, cook through.

Nutrition Information

- Calories: 155 calories
- Cholesterol: 16mg cholesterol
- Protein: 11g protein.
- Total Fat: 3g fat (1g saturated fat)
- Sodium: 949mg sodium
- Fiber: 7g fiber)
- Total Carbohydrate: 23g carbohydrate (4g sugars

695. Lentil Chili

Serving: 6 | Prep: | Cook: | Ready in:

Ingredients

- 2 tablespoons vegetable oil
- 1 onion, chopped
- 4 cloves garlic, minced
- 1 cup dry lentils
- 1 cup dry bulgur wheat
- 3 cups low fat, low sodium chicken broth
- 2 cups canned whole tomatoes, chopped
- 2 tablespoons chili powder
- 1 tablespoon ground cumin
- salt and pepper to taste

Direction

- Mix garlic, onion, and oil in a big pot over medium-high heat, and sauté for 5 minutes. Mix in bulgur wheat and lentils. Add pepper and salt to taste, cumin, chili powder, tomatoes, and broth. Boil it, lower the heat to low and simmer until the lentils are soft, about 30 minutes.

Nutrition Information

- Calories: 281 calories;
- Total Fat: 6.1
- Sodium: 376
- Total Carbohydrate: 45
- Cholesterol: 0
- Protein: 13.8

696. Lentil Sausage Soup

Serving: 13 servings. | Prep: 5mins | Cook: 30mins | Ready in:

Ingredients

- 1 package (19-1/2 ounces) turkey Italian sausage links, casings removed
- 13 cups water
- 1 cup chopped carrots
- 1/2 cup chopped celery
- 2 teaspoons onion powder
- 3/4 teaspoon dried oregano
- 1/2 teaspoon garlic powder
- 1/2 teaspoon dried basil
- 1/2 teaspoon seasoning salt
- 1/4 teaspoon pepper
- 2 cups dried lentils, rinsed
- 1/2 cup uncooked long grain rice
- 2 cans (one 15 ounces, one 8 ounces) tomato sauce
- 2-1/2 cups frozen cheese tortellini

Direction

- In nonstick skillet, crumble sausage. Cook till not pink anymore on medium heat; drain.
- Mix pepper, seasoning salt, basil, garlic powder, oregano, onion powder, celery, carrots and water in a big saucepan/Dutch oven; add rice and lentils. Boil; lower heat. Simmer, covered, till rice and lentils are tender, about 18-20 minutes.
- Mix tomato sauce in; boil. Add sausage and tortellini. Cook till tortellini are tender, about 3-4 minutes, mixing many times.

Nutrition Information

- Calories: 270 calories
- Sodium: 651mg sodium
- Fiber: 11g fiber)
- Total Carbohydrate: 36g carbohydrate (0 sugars
- Cholesterol: 27mg cholesterol
- Protein: 20g protein. Diabetic Exchanges: 2 starch
- Total Fat: 6g fat (2g saturated fat)

697. Lentil Spinach Soup

Serving: 5 servings. | Prep: 15mins | Cook: 30mins | Ready in:

Ingredients

- 1/2 pound bulk Italian turkey sausage
- 1 small onion, chopped
- 4 cups water
- 1/2 cup dried lentils, rinsed
- 2 teaspoons chicken bouillon granules
- 1/8 teaspoon crushed red pepper flakes
- 1 package (10 ounces) fresh spinach, coarsely chopped
- 2 tablespoons shredded Parmesan cheese

Direction

- Cook onion and sausage in a big saucepan until the meat is not pink anymore; drain. Mix in red pepper flakes, bouillon, lentils, and water. Boil it. Lower the heat, put a cover on and simmer until the lentils are soft, about 25-30 minutes. Mix in spinach, cook until the spinach is soft, about another 3-5 minutes. Use cheese to scatter.

Nutrition Information

- Calories: 136 calories
- Total Carbohydrate: 15g carbohydrate (1g sugars
- Cholesterol: 18mg cholesterol
- Protein: 11g protein. Diabetic Exchanges: 1 starch
- Total Fat: 4g fat (1g saturated fat)
- Sodium: 632mg sodium
- Fiber: 3g fiber)

698. Luncheon Spinach Salad

Serving: 10 servings. | Prep: 10mins | Cook: 0mins | Ready in:

Ingredients

- 3 packages (6 ounces each) fresh baby spinach, stems removed
- 2 medium tart apples, chopped
- 1 cup cubed cooked turkey
- 2/3 cup peanuts
- 1/2 cup raisins
- 1/4 cup thinly sliced green onions
- 2 tablespoons sesame seeds, toasted
- 2/3 cup vegetable oil
- 1/3 cup honey
- 1/4 cup vinegar
- 1 tablespoon grated orange zest
- 1 teaspoon salt
- 1 teaspoon curry powder
- 1 teaspoon ground mustard

Direction

- Mix sesame seeds, onions, raisins, peanuts, turkey, apples, and spinach in a salad bowl. Mix the leftover ingredients in a tight-fitting lidded jar; shake the mixture well. Sprinkle on top of salad and coat by tossing; serve right away.

Nutrition Information

- Calories: 297 calories
- Total Fat: 21g fat (3g saturated fat)
- Sodium: 312mg sodium
- Fiber: 3g fiber)
- Total Carbohydrate: 23g carbohydrate (17g sugars
- Cholesterol: 11mg cholesterol
- Protein: 8g protein.

699. Makeover Pizza Pasta Salad

Serving: 7 servings. | Prep: 20mins | Cook: 0mins | Ready in:

Ingredients

- 8 ounces uncooked spiral pasta
- 1/2 teaspoon cornstarch
- 1/3 cup water
- 1/4 cup Parmesan cheese
- 1/2 cup red wine vinegar
- 2 tablespoons olive oil
- 1 teaspoon dried oregano
- 1/2 teaspoon salt
- 1/2 teaspoon garlic powder
- 1/8 teaspoon pepper
- 1-1/2 cups halved cherry tomatoes
- 3/4 cup shredded reduced-fat cheddar cheese
- 3/4 cup shredded part-skim mozzarella cheese
- 1/2 cup sliced green onions
- 1/2 cup sliced turkey pepperoni (about 1-1/2 ounces)

Direction

- Follow the package directions to cook the pasta. Mix together the water and cornstarch in a small saucepan until smooth. Bring to a boil, then cook and stir until thickened or for 1 to 2 minutes. Take away from heat, then stir in pepper, garlic powder, salt, oregano, oil, vinegar and Parmesan cheese. Drain pasta and rinse under cold water. Mix the leftover ingredients in a big bowl, then put in pasta and dressing; toss to coat well. Cover and chill for a minimum of 1 hour before serving.

Nutrition Information

- Calories: 255 calories
- Cholesterol: 26mg cholesterol
- Protein: 14g protein. Diabetic Exchanges: 1-1/2 starch
- Total Fat: 11g fat (5g saturated fat)
- Sodium: 403mg sodium
- Fiber: 2g fiber)
- Total Carbohydrate: 25g carbohydrate (0 sugars

700. Makeover Sausage Pecan Stuffing

Serving: 12 servings. | Prep: 30mins | Cook: 30mins | Ready in:

Ingredients

- 1 pound lean ground turkey
- 2 cups sliced fresh mushrooms
- 2 celery ribs, chopped
- 1 medium onion, chopped
- 1 teaspoon fennel seed
- 1/4 teaspoon cayenne pepper
- 1/8 teaspoon ground nutmeg
- 3 garlic cloves, minced
- 1 loaf (16 ounces) day-old white bread, cubed
- 1 large tart apple, chopped
- 2 teaspoons rubbed sage
- 1-1/2 teaspoons salt
- 1-1/2 teaspoons poultry seasoning
- 1/2 teaspoon pepper
- 2 eggs
- 1 cup reduced-sodium chicken broth
- 1/2 cup chopped pecans

Direction

- Cook the nutmeg, cayenne, fennel seed, onion, celery, mushrooms and turkey in a Dutch oven on medium heat, until the turkey has no visible pink color. Add garlic and let it cook for an additional 1 minute, then drain.
- Move to a big bowl, then add the pepper, poultry seasoning, salt, sage, apple and bread. Whisk the broth and eggs, then pour it on top of the bread mixture and toss until coated. Move to a cooking spray coated 13x9-inch baking dish and sprinkle pecans on top.
- Let it bake for 30-35 minutes at 350 degrees without cover or until a thermometer registers 160 degrees and the top turns light brown.

Nutrition Information

- Calories: 226 calories
- Fiber: 2g fiber)

- Total Carbohydrate: 25g carbohydrate (5g sugars
- Cholesterol: 65mg cholesterol
- Protein: 12g protein. Diabetic Exchanges: 1-1/2 starch
- Total Fat: 9g fat (2g saturated fat)
- Sodium: 654mg sodium

- Calories: 298 calories
- Protein: 15g protein.
- Total Fat: 10g fat (5g saturated fat)
- Sodium: 717mg sodium
- Fiber: 3g fiber)
- Total Carbohydrate: 36g carbohydrate (0 sugars
- Cholesterol: 37mg cholesterol

701. Makeover Twice Baked Potatoes

Serving: 6 servings. | Prep: 01hours15mins | Cook: 30mins | Ready in:

Ingredients

- 6 large baking potatoes
- 2 tablespoons butter, softened
- 1 cup 1% milk
- 1/4 pound turkey bacon (about 9 slices), diced and cooked
- 1-1/2 cups shredded reduced-fat cheddar cheese, divided
- 2 tablespoons minced chives
- 1/2 teaspoon salt
- Dash pepper

Direction

- Let the potatoes bake for 1 hour at 375 degrees or until it becomes tender, then allow it to cool. Trim a thin slice off the top of every potato and get rid of it. Scoop out the pulp and leave a thin shell. Mash the pulp with butter in a big bowl, then stir in pepper, salt, chives, 1 cup of cheese, bacon and milk. Scoop it into the potato shells.
- Put it on ungreased baking tray and let it bake for 25 to 30 minutes at 375 degrees or until heated through. Sprinkle leftover cheese on top. Let it bake for 2 minutes more or until the cheese melts.

Nutrition Information

702. Mashed Potato Stuffing

Serving: 8-10 servings. | Prep: 20mins | Cook: 03hours00mins |Ready in:

Ingredients

- 8 cups riced cooked potatoes
- 4 cups fine soft bread crumbs
- 2 large onions, chopped
- 1 cup butter
- 1 cup egg substitute
- 1 to 2 tablespoons poultry seasoning
- 2 teaspoons salt
- 1/2 teaspoon pepper
- 1 turkey (10 to 12 pounds)

Direction

- Mix crumbs and potatoes together in a bowl; put aside. Sauté onions in butter in a frying pan until soft, add to the potato mixture. Mix in pepper, salt, poultry seasoning, and egg substitute.
- Stuff the turkey right before baking. Skewer and seal the openings. Tie the drumsticks together. Put the turkey on a rack in a roasting pan with the breast side turning up. Bake with a cover at 325° until a thermometer displays 165° for the stuffing and 180° for the turkey, about 3 to 3-3/4 hours.

Nutrition Information

- Calories: 735 calories

- Fiber: 6g fiber)
- Total Carbohydrate: 36g carbohydrate (3g sugars
- Cholesterol: 221mg cholesterol
- Protein: 73g protein.
- Total Fat: 30g fat (15g saturated fat)
- Sodium: 998mg sodium

703. Meatball Alphabet Soup

Serving: 9 servings. | Prep: 20mins | Cook: 35mins | Ready in:

Ingredients

- 1 large egg, lightly beaten
- 2 tablespoons quick-cooking oats
- 2 tablespoons grated Parmesan cheese
- 1/4 teaspoon garlic powder
- 1/4 teaspoon Italian seasoning
- 1/2 pound lean ground turkey
- 1 cup chopped onion
- 1 cup chopped celery
- 1 cup chopped carrots
- 1 cup diced peeled potatoes
- 1 tablespoon olive oil
- 2 garlic cloves, minced
- 4 cans (14-1/2 ounces each) reduced-sodium chicken broth
- 1 can (28 ounces) diced tomatoes, undrained
- 1 can (6 ounces) tomato paste
- 1/4 cup minced fresh parsley
- 1 teaspoon dried basil
- 1 teaspoon dried thyme
- 3/4 cup uncooked alphabet pasta

Direction

- Mix the first 5 ingredients together in a bowl. Break the turkey into small pieces over the mixture and combine thoroughly. Form into 1/2-in. balls. Working in small batches, put the meatballs in a nonstick frying pan to brown over medium heat until no pink anymore. Take away from heat, put aside.
- Sauté potatoes, carrots, celery, and onion in oil in a Dutch oven or a big saucepan until soft-crunchy, about 5 minutes. Add garlic, sauté for another 1 minute. Add thyme, basil, parsley, tomato paste, tomatoes, and broth; boil it. Add pasta, cook for 5-6 minutes. Lower the heat; add the meatballs. Simmer without a cover until the vegetables are soft, about 15-20 minutes.

Nutrition Information

- Calories: 192 calories
- Protein: 13g protein.
- Total Fat: 5g fat (1g saturated fat)
- Sodium: 742mg sodium
- Fiber: 4g fiber)
- Total Carbohydrate: 26g carbohydrate (8g sugars
- Cholesterol: 39mg cholesterol

704. Mediterranean Tortellini Salad

Serving: 6 servings. | Prep: 15mins | Cook: 15mins | Ready in:

Ingredients

- 1 package (19 ounces) frozen cheese tortellini
- 1 package (14 ounces) smoked turkey sausage, sliced
- 3/4 cup prepared pesto
- 2 cups fresh baby spinach, chopped
- 2 cups sliced baby portobello mushrooms
- 1 can (15 ounces) white kidney or cannellini beans, rinsed and drained
- 1 cup roasted sweet red peppers, chopped
- 1 cup (4 ounces) crumbled feta cheese
- 1/4 cup pitted Greek olives, sliced

Direction

- Cook tortellini following the directions on package.
- While cooking the pasta, put sausage into a large nonstick skillet with cooking spray and cook on medium heat until lightly browned or for 6-7 minutes. Place them in a large bowl.
- Drain the pasta and stir it into sausage. Add pesto and mix well. Toss in all other ingredients until well-combined. Serve when it is still warm or put it into the refrigerator until it chills.

Nutrition Information

- Calories: 334 calories
- Sodium: 981mg sodium
- Fiber: 4g fiber)
- Total Carbohydrate: 25g carbohydrate (2g sugars
- Cholesterol: 45mg cholesterol
- Protein: 19g protein.
- Total Fat: 17g fat (6g saturated fat)

705. Melon Turkey Salad

Serving: 7 servings. | Prep: 20mins | Cook: 0mins | Ready in:

Ingredients

- 4 medium cantaloupes, halved and seeded
- 4 cups cubed cooked turkey breast
- 1-1/2 cups seedless red grapes, halved
- 1 cup chopped celery
- 1/2 cup fat-free plain yogurt
- 1/4 cup reduced-fat mayonnaise
- 1 teaspoon lemon juice
- 1/2 teaspoon ground ginger
- 1/8 teaspoon salt
- 1/2 cup chopped unsalted dry roasted cashews

Direction

- Create melon balls from half of one cantaloupe; chill leftover cantaloupe halves. Mix the turkey, grapes, celery and reserved cantaloupe balls in a big bowl.
- In a small bowl, combine the salt, ginger, lemon juice, mayonnaise and yogurt. Put atop turkey mixture and mix slowly to coat. Cover and chill for an hour.
- Mix in cashews just prior to serving. Scoop a cup salad into every cantaloupe half.

Nutrition Information

- Calories: 342 calories
- Protein: 30g protein. Diabetic Exchanges: 3 lean meat
- Total Fat: 9g fat (2g saturated fat)
- Sodium: 209mg sodium
- Fiber: 3g fiber)
- Total Carbohydrate: 38g carbohydrate (32g sugars
- Cholesterol: 72mg cholesterol

706. Mexican White Chili

Serving: 8 servings (2 quarts). | Prep: 20mins | Cook: 06hours00mins | Ready in:

Ingredients

- 1 tablespoon olive oil
- 3 medium onions, chopped
- 2 garlic cloves, minced
- 4 cups cubed cooked chicken or turkey
- 2 cans (15 ounces each) white kidney or cannellini beans, rinsed and drained
- 1 can (15 ounces) garbanzo beans or chickpeas, rinsed and drained
- 2 cups chicken broth
- 1 can (4 ounces) chopped green chilies
- 2 teaspoons ground cumin
- 1/2 teaspoon dried oregano
- 1/4 teaspoon cayenne pepper
- 1/4 teaspoon salt

- 1/4 cup minced fresh cilantro
- Optional toppings: corn chips, shredded Monterey Jack cheese and sour cream

Direction

- Heat oil over medium-high heat in a big skillet. Put in onions; cook and mix till soft. Put garlic in; cook a minute more.
- Place in a 3-qt. slow cooker. Mix in dry seasonings, chilies, broth, beans and chicken.
- With cover, cook till heated through, about 6 to 8 hours on low. Mix in cilantro. If preferred, serve along with sour cream, cheese and corn chips.

Nutrition Information

- Calories: 271 calories
- Sodium: 561mg sodium
- Fiber: 6g fiber)
- Total Carbohydrate: 22g carbohydrate (5g sugars
- Cholesterol: 62mg cholesterol
- Protein: 26g protein. Diabetic Exchanges: 3 lean meat
- Total Fat: 8g fat (2g saturated fat)

707. Minute Minestrone

Serving: 10-12 servings. | Prep: 10mins | Cook: 15mins | Ready in:

Ingredients

- 4 cups water
- 1 package (1.7 ounces) vegetable soup mix
- 1 can (15-1/2 ounces) kidney beans, rinsed and drained
- 1 can (15-1/2 ounces) corn, drained
- 1 can (8 ounces) tomato sauce
- 2 cups cooked cubed beef, chicken or turkey
- 1 cup cooked leftover vegetables
- 1 cup sliced celery
- 1 cup chopped onion
- 3/4 teaspoon salt
- 1/8 teaspoon pepper
- 2 cups cooked elbow macaroni

Direction

- Combine soup mix and water in a big saucepan, then boil on medium heat. Add pepper, salt, onion, celery, vegetables, meat, tomato sauce, corn, and beans, then set to boil. Decrease heat and simmer, covered, for 10 minutes. Add the macaroni and heat thoroughly.

Nutrition Information

- Calories: 158 calories
- Total Fat: 2g fat (0 saturated fat)
- Sodium: 655mg sodium
- Fiber: 4g fiber)
- Total Carbohydrate: 21g carbohydrate (4g sugars
- Cholesterol: 21mg cholesterol
- Protein: 13g protein. Diabetic Exchanges: 1-1/2 starch

708. Mulligatawny Soup

Serving: Makes 8 first-course or 4 main-course servings | Prep: | Cook: | Ready in:

Ingredients

- 1/4 cup vegetable oil
- 3 cups chopped onions (about 1 pound)
- 5 garlic cloves, chopped
- 1 1/2 tablespoons garam masala
- 1 1/2 teaspoons ground coriander
- 1 teaspoon turmeric
- 1/2 teaspoon cayenne pepper
- 2 bay leaves
- 2 cups dried red lentils
- 8 cups low-salt chicken broth

- 2 cups diced cooked chicken
- 1 cup canned unsweetened coconut milk
- 3 tablespoons fresh lemon juice
- 2 cups cooked basmati rice
- Lemon wedges

Direction

- Put vegetable oil in a heavy large pot and heat it over medium-high heat. Add the onions and cook for 15 minutes, stirring constantly until golden brown. Add the garlic and cook for 2 minutes. Add the garam masala and the next 4 ingredients. Stir the mixture for 1 minute. Add the lentils and toss until well-coated. Add the chicken broth. Boil the soup. Adjust the heat to medium. Simmer the mixture for 20 minutes until the lentils are very tender. Discard the bay leaves.
- Puree the soup in the blender until smooth (do the blending by batches). Bring the pureed soup back into the pot. Whisk in coconut milk, lemon juice, and chicken. Season the mixture with salt and pepper to taste.
- Distribute the rice among bowls. Drizzle soup all over the rice and garnish each serving with lemon wedges.

Nutrition Information

- Calories: 465
- Protein: 28 g(56%)
- Total Fat: 18 g(27%)
- Saturated Fat: 7 g(35%)
- Sodium: 109 mg(5%)
- Fiber: 7 g(27%)
- Total Carbohydrate: 52 g(17%)
- Cholesterol: 26 mg(9%)

709. Okra Pilaf

Serving: 8 servings. | Prep: 15mins | Cook: 10mins | Ready in:

Ingredients

- 4 bacon strips, cut into 1/2-inch pieces
- 1 medium onion, chopped
- 1/2 cup chopped green pepper
- 1 cup sliced fresh or frozen okra, thawed
- 2 medium tomatoes, peeled, seeded and chopped
- 1/2 teaspoon salt, optional
- 1/4 teaspoon pepper
- 3 cups cooked rice

Direction

- Cook bacon in a big frying pan until crunchy, take out using a slotted spoon and put on paper towels to drain. In the drippings, sauté green pepper and onion for 6-8 minutes until soft.
- Mix in pepper, salt if wanted, tomatoes, and okra. Cook for 5 minutes over medium heat. Add rice, cook until the rice has absorbed the liquid and the okra is soft, about 10-15 minutes. Crumble the bacon, mix into the rice mixture.

Nutrition Information

- Calories: 134 calories
- Sodium: 97mg sodium
- Fiber: 0 fiber)
- Total Carbohydrate: 26g carbohydrate (0 sugars
- Cholesterol: 6mg cholesterol
- Protein: 4g protein. Diabetic Exchanges: 1-1/2 starch
- Total Fat: 2g fat (0 saturated fat)

710. Parsley Tortellini Toss

Serving: 12-15 servings. | Prep: 30mins | Cook: 0mins | Ready in:

Ingredients

- 1 package (16 ounces) frozen cheese tortellini
- 1-1/2 cups cubed provolone cheese
- 1-1/2 cups cubed part-skim mozzarella cheese
- 1 cup cubed fully cooked ham
- 1 cup cubed cooked turkey
- 1 cup frozen peas, thawed
- 2 medium carrots, shredded
- 1/2 medium sweet red pepper, diced
- 1/2 medium green pepper, diced
- 1 cup minced fresh parsley
- 1/2 cup olive oil
- 3 tablespoons cider vinegar
- 2 tablespoons grated Parmesan cheese
- 2 garlic cloves, minced

Direction

- Following the instructions on package, cook tortellini; wash under cold water and drain off water. Transfer into a big bowl; put in the following 8 ingredients.
- Mix the leftover ingredients in a tight-fitting lidded jar; shake the mixture well. Add on top of salad; coat by tossing. Keep it covered and let chill in the refrigerator till serving. Use a slotted spoon to serve.

Nutrition Information

- Calories: 257 calories
- Protein: 15g protein.
- Total Fat: 16g fat (6g saturated fat)
- Sodium: 417mg sodium
- Fiber: 1g fiber)
- Total Carbohydrate: 12g carbohydrate (2g sugars
- Cholesterol: 34mg cholesterol

711. Pear Harvest Salad

Serving: 6 servings. | Prep: 25mins | Cook: 0mins | Ready in:

Ingredients

- 6 tablespoons cider vinegar
- 1/4 cup olive oil
- 3 tablespoons honey
- 1 teaspoon Dijon mustard
- 1/2 teaspoon salt
- 1/4 teaspoon pepper
- 2 packages (5 ounces each) spring mix salad greens
- 4 cups cubed cooked turkey breast
- 2 medium pears, sliced
- 1 medium ripe avocado, peeled and cubed
- 1/2 cup pomegranate seeds
- 1/2 small red onion, thinly sliced
- 1/2 cup crumbled blue cheese
- 1/2 cup honey-roasted sliced almonds

Direction

- Mix the initial 6 ingredients in a big bowl. Put in the red onion, pomegranate seeds, avocado, pears, turkey and greens; coat by tossing. Drizzle with almonds and cheese. Serve right away.

Nutrition Information

- Calories: 438 calories
- Sodium: 549mg sodium
- Fiber: 5g fiber)
- Total Carbohydrate: 26g carbohydrate (18g sugars
- Cholesterol: 89mg cholesterol
- Protein: 34g protein.
- Total Fat: 23g fat (4g saturated fat)

712. Popover With Hot Turkey Salad

Serving: 10-12 servings. | Prep: 20mins | Cook: 35mins | Ready in:

Ingredients

- 1 cup all-purpose flour

- 1/2 teaspoon salt
- 2 large eggs
- 1 cup whole milk
- 4 cups diced cooked turkey
- 2 cups diced celery
- 2 cups shredded cheddar cheese
- 1 can (2-1/4 ounces) sliced ripe olives, drained
- 1 cup Miracle Whip
- 1/4 cup milk
- 1/8 teaspoon pepper
- Pinch onion powder
- 1-1/2 cups crushed potato chips
- Tomato wedges, optional

Direction

- Mix salt and flour in a big bowl. Mix milk and eggs then mix them into the dry ingredients till just blended. Add into a greased 10-inch glass pie dish. Bake till deep golden brown in color for 35-40 minutes at 400 degrees.
- Use a fork to prick right away in the middle to let steam escape. Mix the following 8 ingredients in a big saucepan, cook and stir on low heat till thoroughly heated.
- Mix in potato chips. Scoop into popover. Use tomato wedges to garnish if you want. Serve right away.

Nutrition Information

- Calories: 392 calories
- Protein: 21g protein.
- Total Fat: 27g fat (8g saturated fat)
- Sodium: 473mg sodium
- Fiber: 1g fiber)
- Total Carbohydrate: 15g carbohydrate (2g sugars
- Cholesterol: 101mg cholesterol

713. Potato Kale Sausage Soup

Serving: 7 servings. | Prep: 10mins | Cook: 25mins | Ready in:

Ingredients

- 3/4 cup chopped onion
- 1 tablespoon olive oil
- 2 garlic cloves, minced
- 4 cups reduced-sodium chicken broth
- 2 medium potatoes, peeled and cubed
- 1/4 teaspoon salt
- 1/4 teaspoon pepper
- 1 bunch kale, trimmed and chopped
- 1 can (15 ounces) white kidney or cannellini beans, rinsed and drained
- 1/2 pound reduced-fat fully cooked Polish sausage or turkey kielbasa, sliced

Direction

- Sauté onion in oil in a big saucepan/Dutch oven till tender. Add garlic; cook for a minute. Add pepper, salt, potatoes and broth; boil. Lower heat; cover. Simmer till potatoes are tender, about 10-15 minutes.
- Slightly mash potatoes with a potato masher. Add sausage, beans and kale; cook on medium-low heat till kale is tender.

Nutrition Information

- Calories: 194 calories
- Fiber: 50g fiber)
- Total Carbohydrate: 28g carbohydrate (50g sugars
- Cholesterol: 14mg cholesterol
- Protein: 11g protein. Diabetic Exchanges: 1-1/2 starch
- Total Fat: 4g fat (1g saturated fat)
- Sodium: 823mg sodium

714. Quick Pantry Salad

Serving: 16-18 servings. | Prep: 20mins | Cook: 0mins | Ready in:

Ingredients

- 4-1/2 cups cooked elbow macaroni
- 1 can (15 to 16 ounces) kidney beans, rinsed and drained
- 1 can (15-1/4 ounces) whole kernel corn, drained
- 2 cups cubed cooked turkey or chicken
- 1 small cucumber, seeded and chopped
- 2 celery ribs, thinly sliced
- 1 cup shredded carrots
- 1/2 cup chopped green pepper
- 1/2 cup chopped onion
- 1/2 cup frozen peas, thawed
- 6 hard-boiled large eggs, chopped
- 1 cup mayonnaise
- 1/4 cup milk
- 1/2 teaspoon salt
- 1/4 to 1/2 teaspoon poultry seasoning
- 1/4 to 1/2 teaspoon ground cumin
- 1/4 teaspoon pepper

Direction

- Mix in a big bowl the first 11 ingredients. In a small bowl, mix seasonings, milk and mayonnaise. Put on salad and toss. Serve right away or keep in the refrigerator until serving time.

Nutrition Information

- Calories: 232 calories
- Sodium: 280mg sodium
- Fiber: 3g fiber)
- Total Carbohydrate: 17g carbohydrate (3g sugars
- Cholesterol: 87mg cholesterol
- Protein: 10g protein.
- Total Fat: 13g fat (2g saturated fat)

715. Quick Pasta Sausage Soup

Serving: 10 servings (2-1/2 quarts). | Prep: 10mins | Cook: 30mins | Ready in:

Ingredients

- 1-1/2 pounds turkey Italian sausage links
- 1 medium green pepper, cut into 1-inch strips
- 1/2 cup chopped onion
- 1 garlic clove, minced
- 6 cups water
- 1 can (28 ounces) diced tomatoes, undrained
- 1 tablespoon sugar
- 1 tablespoon Worcestershire sauce
- 2 teaspoons chicken bouillon granules
- 1 teaspoon salt
- 1 teaspoon dried basil
- 1 teaspoon dried thyme
- 2-1/2 cups uncooked bow tie pasta

Direction

- Take out the casings of the sausage. Slice links into half inch portions. Over medium heat, cook sausage in a soup kettle or Dutch oven until it is not pink anymore, about 5-7 minutes. Take it out using a slotted spoon. Let it drain and keep 2 tablespoons drippings.
- Sauté garlic, onion, and green pepper in the drippings until they become tender, about 4-5 minutes.
- Put in sausage, thyme, basil, salt, bouillon, Worcestershire sauce, sugar, tomatoes, and water. Let it boil and put in the pasta. Lower the heat. Without cover, let it simmer until the pasta becomes tender, about 18-22 minutes.

Nutrition Information

- Calories: 0g sugar total.

716. Quick Turkey Salad

Serving: 2 servings. | Prep: 20mins | Cook: 0mins | Ready in:

Ingredients

- 1 cup cubed cooked turkey breast
- 1/4 cup seedless red grapes, halved
- 3 tablespoons chopped celery
- 4 teaspoons chopped pecans
- 4 teaspoons chopped water chestnuts
- DRESSING:
- 3 tablespoons mayonnaise
- 1-1/2 teaspoons dried minced onion
- 1 teaspoon red wine vinegar
- 1/2 teaspoon reduced-sodium soy sauce
- 1/4 teaspoon ground ginger
- Dash curry powder

Direction

- Combine water chestnuts, pecans, celery, grapes and turkey in a small bowl. Combine the dressing ingredients in another small bowl. Pour dressing on top of turkey mixture; toss until well coated. Chill till serving.

Nutrition Information

- Calories: 232 calories
- Cholesterol: 68mg cholesterol
- Protein: 22g protein.
- Total Fat: 12g fat (2g saturated fat)
- Sodium: 280mg sodium
- Fiber: 1g fiber)
- Total Carbohydrate: 8g carbohydrate (5g sugars

717. Quick Turkey Bean Soup

Serving: 14-16 servings (4 quarts). | Prep: 30mins | Cook: 0mins | Ready in:

Ingredients

- 1 pound ground turkey
- 2 garlic cloves, minced
- 1 medium onion, chopped
- 1 tablespoon canola oil
- 1-1/2 cups chopped celery
- 1 medium green pepper, chopped
- 1 medium sweet red pepper, chopped
- 2 cans (14-1/2 ounces each) beef broth
- 1 can (28 ounces) stewed tomatoes
- 3 tablespoons tomato paste
- 1/2 teaspoon cayenne pepper
- 1/4 teaspoon dried basil
- 1/4 teaspoon dried oregano
- 2 cans (16 ounces each) kidney beans, rinsed and drained
- 1 can (15 ounces) black beans, rinsed and drained
- 1 can (15 ounces) pinto beans, rinsed and drained
- 1 can (15-1/4 ounces) whole kernel corn, drained

Direction

- In a Dutch oven or soup kettle, brown onion, garlic, and turkey in oil on medium heat, then drain. Add peppers and celery, then cook, stirring, for 2 minutes.
- Add oregano, basil, cayenne, tomato paste, tomatoes, and broth, mixing well. Set to boil, then add corn and beans. Decrease heat and simmer, covered, for 15 minutes.

Nutrition Information

- Calories: 182 calories
- Sodium: 426mg sodium
- Fiber: 5g fiber)
- Total Carbohydrate: 23g carbohydrate (6g sugars
- Cholesterol: 19mg cholesterol
- Protein: 10g protein.
- Total Fat: 6g fat (1g saturated fat)

718. Rainy Day Soup

Serving: 12 servings (3 quarts). | Prep: 20mins | Cook: 60mins | Ready in:

Ingredients

- 1 pound ground turkey
- 1 can (46 ounces) V8 juice
- 1 jar (16 ounces) thick and chunky salsa
- 1 can (14-1/2 ounces) chicken broth
- 1 can (16 ounces) kidney beans, rinsed and drained
- 1 package (10 ounces) frozen mixed vegetables
- 4 cups shredded cabbage
- 1 cup chopped onion
- 1/2 cup cubed peeled potatoes
- 1/3 cup medium pearl barley

Direction

- Coat a Dutch oven with cooking spray and use to cook turkey on medium heat until it is no longer pink, then drain. Add in the remainder of the ingredients and set to boil. Turn the heat down and simmer, covered, until the barley and vegetables are tender, or for about 60 - 70 minutes.

Nutrition Information

- Calories: 196 calories
- Total Carbohydrate: 23g carbohydrate (8g sugars
- Cholesterol: 26mg cholesterol
- Protein: 11g protein. Diabetic Exchanges: 2 vegetable
- Total Fat: 6g fat (2g saturated fat)
- Sodium: 703mg sodium
- Fiber: 6g fiber)

719. Red Bean 'N' Sausage Soup

Serving: 8 servings (2 quarts). | Prep: 10mins | Cook: 55mins | Ready in:

Ingredients

- 1 pound turkey Italian sausage links, casings removed
- 1 medium onion, diced
- 3 cups chicken broth
- 3 medium tart apples, peeled and chopped
- 1 can (14-1/2 ounces) crushed tomatoes, undrained
- 2 tablespoons cider vinegar
- 2 tablespoons chopped green pepper
- 2 tablespoons chopped sweet red pepper
- 2 tablespoons brown sugar
- 1/2 teaspoon seasoned salt
- 1/2 teaspoon ground mustard
- 1/4 teaspoon rubbed sage
- 1/4 teaspoon chili powder
- 1/4 teaspoon pepper
- 1 can (16 ounces) kidney beans, rinsed and drained

Direction

- Cook onion and sausage in soup kettle/big saucepan till meat is not pink anymore; drain. Add the following 12 ingredients; boil. Lower heat; cover. Simmer, occasionally mixing, for 45 minutes. Add beans and heat through.

Nutrition Information

- Calories: 232 calories
- Cholesterol: 47mg cholesterol
- Protein: 14g protein. Diabetic Exchanges: 2 lean meat
- Total Fat: 8g fat (2g saturated fat)
- Sodium: 1132mg sodium
- Fiber: 5g fiber)
- Total Carbohydrate: 29g carbohydrate (0 sugars

720. Refreshing Turkey Salad

Serving: 8 servings. | Prep: 20mins | Cook: 0mins | Ready in:

Ingredients

- 3 cups cooked wild rice
- 2 cups cubed cooked turkey
- 2 cups thinly sliced celery
- 1/2 cup seedless green grapes, halved
- 1/2 cup seedless red grapes, halved
- 1/4 cup chopped green pepper
- 1/4 cup chopped sweet red pepper
- 1 jar (2 ounces) chopped pimientos, drained
- 1/2 cup mayonnaise
- 1/2 cup sour cream
- 1 tablespoon honey
- 1 teaspoon Dijon mustard
- 1 teaspoon celery seed
- 1/2 teaspoon poppy seeds
- 1/2 teaspoon salt, optional
- 1/4 teaspoon pepper
- 1 tablespoon slivered almonds, toasted, optional

Direction

- Mix pimientos, peppers, grapes, celery, turkey and rice in a bowl; put aside. Mix poppy seeds, celery seed, mustard, honey, sour cream, mayonnaise, salt if desired and pepper in a small bowl; combine well. Put on top of rice mixture; coat by tossing. Keep it covered and chilled for no less than 60 minutes. If you want, use almonds to garnish just prior to serving.

Nutrition Information

- Calories: 160 calories
- Protein: 9g protein. Diabetic Exchanges: 1 starch
- Total Fat: 1g fat (0 saturated fat)
- Sodium: 340mg sodium
- Fiber: 0 fiber)
- Total Carbohydrate: 27g carbohydrate (0 sugars
- Cholesterol: 13mg cholesterol

721. Rosemary Split Pea Soup

Serving: 5 servings. | Prep: 25mins | Cook: 01hours30mins | Ready in:

Ingredients

- 3 celery ribs, finely chopped
- 1 cup finely chopped onion
- 1 garlic clove, minced
- 1 tablespoon minced fresh rosemary or 1 teaspoon dried rosemary, crushed
- 3 tablespoons butter
- 6 cups chicken broth
- 1-1/4 cups dried split peas, rinsed
- 1 teaspoon salt, optional
- MEATBALLS
- 1/2 pound ground pork or turkey
- 1-1/2 teaspoons minced fresh rosemary or 1/2 teaspoon dried rosemary, crushed
- 1/4 teaspoon pepper

Direction

- In a Dutch oven or big kettle, sauté rosemary, garlic, onions, and celery with butter until they are tender. Add in salt (if desired), peas, and broth, then boil. Decrease heat and simmer, covered, for 1 1/2 hour until the peas are soft. Take off the heat and cool.
- To make the meatballs, combine pepper, rosemary, and pork, then shape into 1/2 inch balls. In a big pan, brown the meatballs for 5 minutes until no longer pink.
- In a food processor or blender, ladle in half of the soup and puree. Return to the soup with the meatballs to the kettle and heat thoroughly.

Nutrition Information

- Calories: 359 calories
- Fiber: 0 fiber)
- Total Carbohydrate: 37g carbohydrate (0 sugars
- Cholesterol: 24mg cholesterol
- Protein: 26g protein. Diabetic Exchanges: 2 starch
- Total Fat: 13g fat (0 saturated fat)
- Sodium: 1mg sodium

722. Sausage & Cannellini Bean Soup

Serving: 4 servings. | Prep: 15mins | Cook: 15mins | Ready in:

Ingredients

- 3 Italian turkey sausage links (4 ounces each), casings removed
- 1 medium onion, chopped
- 2 garlic cloves, minced
- 1 can (15 ounces) cannellini or white kidney beans, rinsed and drained
- 1 can (14-1/2 ounces) reduced-sodium chicken broth
- 1 cup water
- 1/4 cup white wine or additional reduced-sodium chicken broth
- 1/4 teaspoon pepper
- 1 bunch escarole or spinach, chopped
- 4 teaspoons shredded Parmesan cheese

Direction

- Over medium heat, cook onion and sausage in a big saucepan until the sausage is not pink anymore. Let it drain. Put in garlic and cook for one more minute.
- Mix in the pepper, wine, water, broth, and beans and let it boil. Put in escarole and heat it through. Drizzle with cheese.

Nutrition Information

- Calories: 232 calories
- Sodium: 837mg sodium
- Fiber: 9g fiber)
- Total Carbohydrate: 24g carbohydrate (3g sugars
- Cholesterol: 33mg cholesterol
- Protein: 17g protein.
- Total Fat: 6g fat (2g saturated fat)

723. Sausage Potato Salad

Serving: 5 servings. | Prep: 20mins | Cook: 15mins | Ready in:

Ingredients

- 1 pound small red potatoes
- 2 tablespoons olive oil
- 2 tablespoons honey mustard
- 1 tablespoon white vinegar
- 1 tablespoon minced fresh parsley
- 1 teaspoon minced fresh tarragon or 1/4 teaspoon dried tarragon
- 1/4 teaspoon salt
- 1/4 teaspoon pepper
- 1/4 pound smoked turkey sausage, halved and sliced
- 1 small onion, chopped

Direction

- Clean potatoes; put into a small saucepan then pour water over. Heat up the saucepan until the water is boiling, lower the heat and cook covered until tender or for 15 to 20 minutes.
- To make the dressing, mix seasonings with vinegar, honey mustard, and oil in a small bowl, then set aside. Coat a small nonstick skillet with cooking spray, add sausage until thoroughly heated.
- Take potatoes out for draining, leave them to cool slightly for a while. Slice into 1/4 inch portion then put into a bowl. Drizzle dressing

and put sausage and onion in; coat by tossing. Serve right away or chilled.

Nutrition Information

- Calories: 162 calories
- Protein: 6g protein. Diabetic Exchanges: 1-1/2 fat
- Total Fat: 7g fat (1g saturated fat)
- Sodium: 398mg sodium
- Fiber: 2g fiber)
- Total Carbohydrate: 19g carbohydrate (4g sugars
- Cholesterol: 14mg cholesterol

724. Sausage Tomato Soup

Serving: 6 servings. | Prep: 25mins | Cook: 10mins | Ready in:

Ingredients

- 1/2 pound Johnsonville® Ground Mild Italian sausage
- 1 medium onion, chopped
- 1 small green pepper, chopped
- 1 can (28 ounces) diced tomatoes, undrained
- 1 can (14-1/2 ounces) beef broth
- 1 can (8 ounces) tomato sauce
- 1/2 cup picante sauce
- 1-1/2 teaspoons sugar
- 1 teaspoon dried basil
- 1/2 teaspoon dried oregano
- 1/2 to 3/4 cup shredded part-skim mozzarella cheese

Direction

- Over medium heat, cook green pepper, onion and sausage in a saucepan until sausage is not pink anymore. Let it drain. Mix in the oregano, basil, sugar, picante sauce, tomato sauce, broth and tomatoes. Let it boil. Lower the heat and simmer for 10 minutes with the cover on. Drizzle with cheese.

Nutrition Information

- Calories: 161 calories
- Protein: 12g protein. Diabetic Exchanges: 3 vegetable
- Total Fat: 6g fat (2g saturated fat)
- Sodium: 870mg sodium
- Fiber: 4g fiber)
- Total Carbohydrate: 16g carbohydrate (0 sugars
- Cholesterol: 26mg cholesterol

725. Sausage And Corn Bread Dressing

Serving: 12 servings. | Prep: 30mins | Cook: 40mins | Ready in:

Ingredients

- 1 package (19-1/2 ounces) Italian turkey sausage links, casings removed
- 4 medium onions, chopped (about 3 cups)
- 1/2 cup chopped celery
- 6 cups cubed day-old white or French bread
- 6 cups coarsely crumbled corn bread
- 2 large eggs
- 2 tablespoons steak sauce
- 2 teaspoons onion salt
- 2 teaspoons poultry seasoning
- 2 teaspoons dried parsley flakes
- 1 teaspoon garlic powder
- 1 teaspoon baking powder
- 2-1/2 to 3 cups reduced-sodium chicken broth

Direction

- Preheat the oven to 350°. Cook sausage for 6 to 8 minutes in a 6-quart stockpot over medium heat or till not pink anymore, breaking up into

crumbles. Take off using a slotted spoon, setting aside drippings in pot.
- Put celery and onions to the drippings; let cook and mix for 6 to 8 minutes till soft. Take off from heat; mix in sausage. Put corn bread and cubed bread; combine by tossing.
- Beat baking powder, seasonings, steak sauce and eggs in a small bowl till incorporated; mix into the bread mixture. Mix in sufficient broth to attain preferred moistness.
- Put to an oiled 3-quart or 13x9-inch baking dish. Let bake for 40 to 50 minutes till browned lightly.

Nutrition Information

- Calories: 240 calories
- Protein: 11g protein.
- Total Fat: 6g fat (1g saturated fat)
- Sodium: 1112mg sodium
- Fiber: 3g fiber)
- Total Carbohydrate: 35g carbohydrate (4g sugars
- Cholesterol: 48mg cholesterol

726. Sausage Pecan Turkey Stuffing

Serving: 12-14 servings. | Prep: 25mins | Cook: 05hours00mins | Ready in:

Ingredients

- 9 cups soft bread crumbs
- 1 pound Jones No Sugar Pork Sausage Roll sausage
- 2 cups chopped onion
- 1/4 cup butter, cubed
- 3 unpeeled tart apples, coarsely chopped
- 1 cup chopped pecans
- 1/2 cup minced fresh parsley
- 1-1/2 teaspoons dried thyme
- 1 teaspoon rubbed sage
- 1/4 teaspoon salt
- 1/4 teaspoon pepper
- 1/4 cup apple juice
- Chicken broth
- 1 turkey (14 to 16 pounds)

Direction

- In a big bowl, put bread crumbs and put aside. Cook onion and sausage in butter in a big frying pan until the onion is soft and the sausage is not pink anymore; avoid draining. Add to the bread crumbs. Mix in pepper, salt, sage, thyme, parsley, pecans, and apples; mix in enough broth to moisten and apple juice.
- Stuff the turkey right before baking. Skewer the openings; tie the drumsticks together. Put on a rack in a roasting pan. Bake at 325° until a thermometer displays 185°, about 5 to 5-1/2 hours. Once the turkey starts to turn brown, use an aluminum foil tents to cover and baste if necessary. Take out all of the stuff.

Nutrition Information

- Calories: 849 calories
- Sodium: 558mg sodium
- Fiber: 3g fiber)
- Total Carbohydrate: 23g carbohydrate (8g sugars
- Cholesterol: 294mg cholesterol
- Protein: 86g protein.
- Total Fat: 44g fat (13g saturated fat)

727. Savory Meatball Minestrone

Serving: 12 servings. | Prep: 45mins | Cook: 40mins | Ready in:

Ingredients

- 1 egg white
- 2 tablespoons quick-cooking oats
- 2 tablespoons nonfat Parmesan cheese topping

- 1/8 teaspoon Italian seasoning
- 1/8 teaspoon garlic powder
- 1/2 pound lean ground turkey
- 1 cup chopped onion
- 1 cup chopped celery
- 2 garlic cloves, minced
- 3 cans (14-1/2 ounces each) reduced-sodium chicken broth
- 1 can (28 ounces) no-salt-added diced tomatoes, undrained
- 1 can (6 ounces) tomato paste
- 1 cup chopped carrots
- 1 cup diced peeled potatoes
- 1/2 cup minced fresh parsley
- 1 teaspoon dried basil
- 1 teaspoon dried thyme
- 1 cup uncooked spiral pasta

Direction

- Mix the first 5 ingredients together in a bowl. Break the turkey into small pieces over the mixture; mix thoroughly. Form into 3/4-in. balls. On a cooking spray-coated rack in a shallow baking pan, put the meatballs. Bake without a cover at 350° until the meat is not pink anymore, about 20 minutes; drain.
- Sauté garlic, celery, and onion in a big cooking spray-coated saucepan until soft-crunchy. Add seasonings, vegetables, tomato paste, tomatoes, and broth. Boil it. Lower the heat, put a cover on and simmer for 30 minutes.
- Mix in meatballs and pasta. Cook without a cover over medium heat until the pasta and vegetables are soft, about 10-12 minutes.

Nutrition Information

- Calories: 118 calories
- Protein: 9g protein. Diabetic Exchanges: 1 starch
- Total Fat: 1g fat (0 saturated fat)
- Sodium: 128mg sodium
- Fiber: 0 fiber)
- Total Carbohydrate: 19g carbohydrate (0 sugars
- Cholesterol: 11mg cholesterol

728. Shortcut Sausage Minestrone

Serving: 6 servings (2 quarts). | Prep: 5mins | Cook: 20mins | Ready in:

Ingredients

- 3/4 pound Italian turkey sausage links, casings removed
- 1 small green pepper, chopped
- 1 small onion, chopped
- 2 cups cut fresh green beans or frozen cut green beans
- 2 cups water
- 1 can (16 ounces) kidney beans, rinsed and drained
- 1 can (14-1/2 ounces) diced tomatoes with basil, oregano and garlic, undrained
- 1 can (14-1/2 ounces) reduced-sodium chicken broth
- 3/4 cup uncooked ditalini or other small pasta

Direction

- Over medium heat, cook onion, pepper, sausage in a 6-qt. stockpot, while crumbling the sausage, until the meat is not pink anymore, about 5-7 minutes. Let it drain.
- Put in broth, tomatoes, kidney beans, water, and green beans and boil. Mix in ditalini. Without cover, cook and stir from time to time until pasta becomes tender, about 10-11 minutes.

Nutrition Information

- Calories: 232 calories
- Sodium: 773mg sodium
- Fiber: 7g fiber)
- Total Carbohydrate: 34g carbohydrate (6g sugars

- Cholesterol: 21mg cholesterol
- Protein: 16g protein.
- Total Fat: 4g fat (1g saturated fat)

729. Skinny Cobb Salad

Serving: 4 servings. | Prep: 25mins | Cook: 0mins | Ready in:

Ingredients

- 1/4 cup fat-free plain Greek yogurt
- 2 tablespoons reduced-fat ranch salad dressing
- 1 to 2 teaspoons cold water
- SALAD:
- 3 cups coleslaw mix
- 3 cups chopped lettuce
- 1 large apple, chopped
- 1/2 cup crumbled reduced-fat feta or blue cheese
- 1 cup cubed cooked chicken breast
- 2 green onions, chopped
- 4 turkey bacon strips, chopped and cooked
- 1 can (15 ounces) garbanzo beans or chickpeas, rinsed and drained
- 1 small ripe avocado, peeled and cubed

Direction

- Combine dressing and yogurt, use water to thin if you want. Mix lettuce with coleslaw and split into 4 dishes.
- Transfer the rest of the ingredients on top in rows. Use the yogurt mixture to sprinkle on.

Nutrition Information

- Calories: 324 calories
- Sodium: 646mg sodium
- Fiber: 9g fiber)
- Total Carbohydrate: 31g carbohydrate (11g sugars
- Cholesterol: 48mg cholesterol

- Protein: 23g protein. Diabetic Exchanges: 2 lean meat
- Total Fat: 13g fat (3g saturated fat)

730. Slow Cooker Turkey Chili

Serving: 6 | Prep: 10mins | Cook: 6hours | Ready in:

Ingredients

- 1 1/4 pounds lean ground turkey
- 1 (28 ounce) can crushed tomatoes
- 1 (16 ounce) can kidney beans, rinsed and drained
- 1 (16 ounce) can pinto beans, rinsed and drained
- 1 cup chicken stock
- 1 small onion, chopped
- 1 tablespoon hot sauce (such as Frank's® Redhot®), or more to taste (optional)
- 1 tablespoon chili powder
- 2 teaspoons salt
- 1 teaspoon minced garlic
- 1/2 teaspoon paprika
- 1/2 teaspoon dried oregano
- 1/2 teaspoon cayenne pepper, or more to taste
- 1/2 teaspoon ground cumin
- 1/2 teaspoon ground black pepper

Direction

- In a slow cooker, combine black pepper, cumin, cayenne pepper, oregano, paprika, minced garlic, salt, chili powder, hot sauce, onion, chicken stock, pinto beans, kidney beans, tomatoes, and ground turkey. Mix to crumble the turkey into small pieces.
- Cook for 6-8 hours on Low (or for 4 hours on High).

Nutrition Information

- Calories: 323 calories;
- Sodium: 1575

- Total Carbohydrate: 35.2
- Cholesterol: 70
- Protein: 29.1
- Total Fat: 8.8

731. Slow Cooked Turkey White Bean Soup

Serving: 8 servings (3 quarts). | Prep: 35mins | Cook: 05hours00mins | Ready in:

Ingredients

- 1 pound Jones No Sugar Pork Sausage Roll sausage
- 4 cups cubed cooked turkey
- 2 cans (14-1/2 ounces each) beef broth
- 1 can (15 ounces) white kidney or cannellini beans, rinsed and drained
- 1 can (14-1/2 ounces) diced tomatoes, undrained
- 4 medium carrots, chopped
- 1 medium onion, chopped
- 1 medium green pepper, chopped
- 1 celery rib, chopped
- 2 teaspoons Italian seasoning
- 1/4 teaspoon cayenne pepper

Direction

- In a large pan, crumble the sausage and cook, stirring, until the meat is no longer pink, then drain. Move to a 5 - 6-quart slow cooker. Stir in all the remaining ingredients and cook, covered, on a low setting until the vegetables become tender, about 5 - 6 hours.

Nutrition Information

- Calories: 318 calories
- Sodium: 902mg sodium
- Fiber: 5g fiber)
- Total Carbohydrate: 16g carbohydrate (5g sugars

- Cholesterol: 74mg cholesterol
- Protein: 29g protein.
- Total Fat: 15g fat (5g saturated fat)

732. Smoked Turkey And Apple Salad

Serving: 4 servings. | Prep: 20mins | Cook: 0mins | Ready in:

Ingredients

- 5 tablespoons olive oil
- 2 tablespoons cider vinegar
- 1 tablespoon Dijon mustard
- 1/2 teaspoon lemon-pepper seasoning
- SALAD:
- 6 to 8 cups watercress or torn romaine
- 1 medium carrot, julienned
- 10 cherry tomatoes, halved
- 8 ounces sliced deli smoked turkey, cut into strips
- 4 medium apples, sliced
- 1/3 cup chopped walnuts, toasted

Direction

- Mix the first four ingredients.
- On a dish, put watercress, put apples, turkey, tomatoes, and carrots on top. Use the dressing to sprinkle, put walnuts on top. Eat immediately.

Nutrition Information

- Calories:
- Protein:
- Total Fat:
- Sodium:
- Fiber:
- Total Carbohydrate:
- Cholesterol:

733. Southern Cornbread Dressing

Serving: 18 | Prep: 1hours15mins | Cook: 30mins | Ready in:

Ingredients

- 4 skinless, boneless chicken breast halves
- 1 (16 ounce) package dry corn bread mix
- 1 (1 pound) loaf day-old white bread, torn into small pieces
- 4 tablespoons margarine
- 1/2 cup chopped onions
- 1/2 cup chopped celery
- 1 (10.75 ounce) can condensed cream of chicken soup
- 1/8 teaspoon garlic powder
- 2 teaspoons poultry seasoning
- 1/2 teaspoon ground black pepper
- 6 eggs

Direction

- In a big saucepan with sufficient water to submerge, put chicken breast halves. Boil. Allow to cook for an hour till meat is soft and easily shredded. Shred the chicken and reserve. Set aside 4 to 6 cups of leftover broth.
- Prepare an 8x8 inch pan of cornbread following packaging instructions. Into a big bowl, crumble corn bread. Add in white bread.
- Preheat the oven to 175 °C or 350 °F.
- Liquefy margarine and mix in celery and onions in a medium saucepan over medium heat. Gradually cook, mixing from time to time till soft.
- Mix celery and onions into bread mixture. Add in eggs, pepper, poultry seasoning, garlic powder, cream of chicken soup, 4 cups of reserved broth and chicken. Combine using a potato masher till mixture is the consistency of gelatin. Put additional leftover broth as needed to reach preferred consistency. Put to a baking dish, 9x13 inch in size.
- In the prepared oven, bake for half hour till golden brown.

Nutrition Information

- Calories: 284 calories;
- Total Fat: 8.9
- Sodium: 772
- Total Carbohydrate: 31.4
- Cholesterol: 94
- Protein: 18.6

734. Southwestern Turkey Dumpling Soup

Serving: 8 servings (2-1/2 quarts). | Prep: 15mins | Cook: 30mins | Ready in:

Ingredients

- 1 can (15 ounces) tomato sauce
- 1 can (14-1/2 ounces) diced tomatoes, undrained
- 1-3/4 cups water
- 1 envelope chili seasoning
- 3 cups diced cooked turkey or chicken
- 1 can (16 ounces) kidney beans, rinsed and drained
- 1 can (15 ounces) black beans, rinsed and drained
- 1 can (15-1/4 ounces) whole kernel corn, drained
- DUMPLINGS:
- 1-1/2 cups biscuit/baking mix
- 1/2 cup cornmeal
- 3/4 cup shredded cheddar cheese, divided
- 2/3 cup milk

Direction

- Use a Dutch oven to combine the first 5 of the ingredients, then boil. Decrease heat, cover, and simmer for 10 minutes, occasionally stirring. Add in the corn and beans.

- In a big bowl, combine 1/2 cup cheese, cornmeal, and biscuit mix, then stir in milk. Drop heaping tablespoonfuls of the mixture into the simmering soup. Cook while covered until the dumplings are firm, about 12 - 15 minutes. Sprinkle the remaining cheese and cook, covered, for another 1 minute until cheese melts.

Nutrition Information

- Calories: 424 calories
- Cholesterol: 54mg cholesterol
- Protein: 29g protein.
- Total Fat: 11g fat (4g saturated fat)
- Sodium: 1358mg sodium
- Fiber: 8g fiber)
- Total Carbohydrate: 51g carbohydrate (8g sugars

735. Spice It Up Soup

Serving: 8 servings (2-1/2 quarts). | Prep: 10mins | Cook: 40mins | Ready in:

Ingredients

- 1 pound uncooked hot turkey Italian sausage links, sliced
- 1/2 pound lean ground beef (90% lean)
- 1 large onion, chopped
- 1 medium green pepper, chopped
- 3 garlic cloves, minced
- 2 cans (14-1/2 ounces each) beef broth
- 2 cups water
- 2 cups fresh or frozen corn
- 1 can (14-1/2 ounces) diced tomatoes with green chilies, undrained
- 1 cup diced carrots
- 1/3 cup minced fresh cilantro
- 2 jalapeno peppers, seeded and chopped
- 1/2 teaspoon salt
- 1/2 teaspoon ground cumin

Direction

- Cook green pepper, onion, beef, and sausage over medium heat in a Dutch oven until the meat is not pink anymore. Add garlic, cook for another 1 minute. Drain.
- Mix in the rest of the ingredients. Boil it. Lower the heat, put a cover on and simmer so that the flavors combine, about 30-40 minutes.

Nutrition Information

- Calories: 222 calories
- Fiber: 2g fiber)
- Total Carbohydrate: 18g carbohydrate (0 sugars
- Cholesterol: 41mg cholesterol
- Protein: 18g protein. Diabetic Exchanges: 2 lean meat
- Total Fat: 9g fat (3g saturated fat)
- Sodium: 1153mg sodium

736. Spicy Kielbasa Soup

Serving: 5 servings. | Prep: 15mins | Cook: 08hours00mins | Ready in:

Ingredients

- 1/2 pound reduced-fat smoked turkey kielbasa, sliced
- 1 medium onion, chopped
- 1 medium green pepper, chopped
- 1 celery rib with leaves, thinly sliced
- 4 garlic cloves, minced
- 2 cans (14-1/2 ounces each) reduced-sodium chicken broth
- 1 can (15-1/2 ounces) great northern beans, rinsed and drained
- 1 can (14-1/2 ounces) stewed tomatoes, cut up
- 1 small zucchini, sliced
- 1 medium carrot, shredded
- 1 tablespoon dried parsley flakes
- 1/4 teaspoon crushed red pepper flakes

- 1/4 teaspoon pepper

Direction

- Cook kielbasa in a nonstick frying pan over medium heat until brown lightly. Add celery, green pepper, and onion, stir and cook for 3 minutes. Add garlic, cook for another 1 minute.
- Move to a 5-qt. slow cooker. Mix in the rest of the ingredients. Put a cover on and cook on low until the vegetables are soft, about 8-9 hours.

Nutrition Information

- Calories: 194 calories
- Protein: 14g protein.
- Total Fat: 2g fat (0 saturated fat)
- Sodium: 1187mg sodium
- Fiber: 7g fiber)
- Total Carbohydrate: 32g carbohydrate (0 sugars
- Cholesterol: 16mg cholesterol

737. Spicy Turkey Bean Soup

Serving: 4 servings. | Prep: 20mins | Cook: 05hours00mins | Ready in:

Ingredients

- 2 cans (15 ounces each) white kidney or cannellini beans, rinsed and drained
- 2 cups cubed cooked turkey
- 1 can (14-1/2 ounces) chicken broth
- 1 can (10 ounces) diced tomatoes and green chilies, undrained
- 1 cup salsa
- 1/2 teaspoon ground cumin
- 1/4 teaspoon curry powder
- 1/4 teaspoon ground ginger
- 1/4 teaspoon paprika

Direction

- Combine all of the ingredients into a 3 quart slow cooker, then cook while covered on a low setting until it heats through, or about 5 - 6 hours.

Nutrition Information

- Calories: 322 calories
- Total Fat: 5g fat (1g saturated fat)
- Sodium: 1283mg sodium
- Fiber: 9g fiber)
- Total Carbohydrate: 37g carbohydrate (2g sugars
- Cholesterol: 55mg cholesterol
- Protein: 30g protein.

738. Spicy Turkey Chili

Serving: 8 | Prep: 10mins | Cook: 3hours | Ready in:

Ingredients

- 2 (5 ounce) cans turkey meat, drained
- 2 (15 ounce) cans kidney beans
- 2 (14.5 ounce) cans Italian-style stewed tomatoes
- 2 (1.25 ounce) packages chili seasoning mix
- 1 (4 ounce) can green chile peppers
- 1 (8 ounce) can tomato sauce
- 1 onion, diced
- 1 cup water

Direction

- Mix turkey, tomato sauce, water, onion, chili peppers, beans, chili seasoning, and tomatoes in a slow cooker. Let it cook on Low setting for 3-4 hours. Serve it warm.

Nutrition Information

- Calories: 213 calories;
- Sodium: 1751
- Total Carbohydrate: 30.8

- Cholesterol: 23
- Protein: 17
- Total Fat: 3.7

739. Submarine Sandwich Salad

Serving: 6 servings. | Prep: 15mins | Cook: 0mins | Ready in:

Ingredients

- 5 to 6 cups torn lettuce
- 1 to 2 hard rolls, cubed
- 1 medium tomato, chopped
- 1/2 cup thinly sliced red onion
- 1/2 cup shredded Swiss cheese
- 2 ounces each ham, turkey and salami, julienned
- 1/2 cup sliced pepperoni
- DRESSING:
- 1/3 cup canola oil
- 2 tablespoons tarragon vinegar
- 1/4 to 1/2 teaspoon dried oregano
- 1/4 teaspoon salt
- 1/8 teaspoon garlic powder
- Dash pepper

Direction

- Mix pepperoni, salami, turkey, ham, cheese, onion, tomato, rolls, and lettuce in a big salad bowl. Mix the dressing ingredients in a tight-fitting lidded jar; shake the mixture well. Sprinkle on top of salad; coat by tossing.

Nutrition Information

- Calories:
- Total Fat:
- Sodium:
- Fiber:
- Total Carbohydrate:
- Cholesterol:

- Protein:

740. Summer Spiral Salad

Serving: 8 servings. | Prep: 15mins | Cook: 0mins | Ready in:

Ingredients

- 4 cups cooked spiral pasta
- 1 can (15 ounces) garbanzo beans or chickpeas, rinsed and drained
- 1 cup cherry tomatoes, halved
- 4 ounces part-skim mozzarella cheese, cut into thin strips
- 2 ounces turkey salami, cut into thin strips
- 1/2 cup pitted ripe olives
- 3 tablespoons canola oil
- 1/4 cup tarragon vinegar
- 1-1/2 teaspoons salt
- 4-1/2 teaspoons minced fresh oregano or 1-1/2 teaspoons dried oregano
- 4-1/2 teaspoons minced fresh basil or 1-1/2 teaspoons dried basil
- 1/8 teaspoon pepper

Direction

- Mix the first six ingredients in a big bowl. Mix seasonings, vinegar and oil in a jar with a tight-fitting lid, then shake well. Drizzle over pasta mixture and toss to coat well. Cover and chill for a couple of hours or overnight.

Nutrition Information

- Calories: 269 calories
- Protein: 11g protein. Diabetic Exchanges: 2 fat
- Total Fat: 10g fat (2g saturated fat)
- Sodium: 801mg sodium
- Fiber: 4g fiber)
- Total Carbohydrate: 34g carbohydrate (0 sugars
- Cholesterol: 13mg cholesterol

741. Summer Squash And Bell Pepper Saute With Bacon

Serving: 2 servings. | Prep: 10mins | Cook: 5mins | Ready in:

Ingredients

- 1 bacon strip, diced
- 1 tablespoon finely chopped onion
- 1 tablespoon each finely chopped green, sweet red and yellow pepper
- 1 garlic clove, minced
- 1 medium yellow summer squash, cut into 1/2-inch cubes

Direction

- Cook bacon in a frying pan until crunchy. Mix in garlic, peppers, and onion; cook until the vegetables are tender, about 2 minutes. Add squash, put a cover on and cook for 3-4 minutes over medium heat until soft.

Nutrition Information

- Calories: 83 calories
- Cholesterol: 9mg cholesterol
- Protein: 3g protein. Diabetic Exchanges: 1 vegetable
- Total Fat: 6g fat (2g saturated fat)
- Sodium: 101mg sodium
- Fiber: 1g fiber)
- Total Carbohydrate: 5g carbohydrate (3g sugars

742. Sweet And Savory Turkey Salad

Serving: 6-8 servings. | Prep: 25mins | Cook: 0mins | Ready in:

Ingredients

- 1/3 cup vegetable oil
- 3 tablespoons lemon juice
- 3 tablespoons white wine vinegar
- 2 to 3 tablespoons Dijon mustard
- 3 tablespoons minced red onion
- 3 tablespoons poppy seeds
- 1 tablespoon honey
- 1/4 teaspoon salt
- 1 to 2 teaspoons grated orange zest
- 1/2 cup finely chopped dried apricots
- 1/2 cup finely chopped dried figs
- 5 cups shredded cooked turkey or cubed fully cooked ham
- 4 celery ribs, sliced
- 4 ounces cheddar cheese, julienned
- 3/4 cup coarsely chopped pecans, toasted

Direction

- In a small bowl, whisk salt, honey, poppy seeds, onion, mustard, vinegar, lemon juice and oil. Stir in figs, apricots and orange peel; cover the mixture and allow it to stand at room temperature for 1 hour. In a large bowl, combine dressing, cheese, celery and turkey. Keep cold in refrigerator for several hours. Stir in pecans right before serving.

Nutrition Information

- Calories:
- Total Fat:
- Sodium:
- Fiber:
- Total Carbohydrate:
- Cholesterol:
- Protein:

743. Tangy Turkey Salad

Serving: 4 servings. | Prep: 20mins | Cook: 0mins | Ready in:

Ingredients

- DRESSING:
- 1/2 cup Miracle Whip Light
- 1/4 cup sour cream
- 1 tablespoon sugar
- 1 tablespoon lemon juice
- 1 tablespoon minced chives
- 1 teaspoon ground ginger
- 1/2 teaspoon grated lemon zest
- 1/4 teaspoon salt
- SALAD:
- 2 to 3 cups cubed cooked turkey breast
- 1 cup seedless green grapes, halved if desired
- 1 cup sliced celery
- 1 cup pineapple chunks, drained and halved if desired
- Leaf lettuce
- 4 cantaloupe rings, peeled and seeded (about 3/4 inch thick)
- 1/2 cup pecans, toasted

Direction

- Mix dressing ingredients in a small bowl. Keep in the refrigerator.
- Prepare salad ingredients then mix them gently with dressing. Use the base of lettuce to cover separate luncheon dishes and fill the middle with salad. Use pecans to garnish.

Nutrition Information

- Calories: 403 calories
- Cholesterol: 86mg cholesterol
- Protein: 34g protein. Diabetic Exchanges: 2 fat.
- Total Fat: 17g fat (0 saturated fat)
- Sodium: 389mg sodium
- Fiber: 0 fiber)
- Total Carbohydrate: 29g carbohydrate (0 sugars

744. Tarragon Turkey Salad

Serving: 8 servings. | Prep: 20mins | Cook: 0mins | Ready in:

Ingredients

- 4 cups uncooked bow tie pasta
- 2 cups cubed cooked turkey breast
- 3/4 cup sliced celery
- 1 can (11 ounces) mandarin oranges, drained
- 1/2 cup reduced-fat mayonnaise
- 1 tablespoon orange juice
- 1 tablespoon Dijon mustard
- 2 teaspoons minced fresh tarragon or 3/4 teaspoon dried tarragon
- 1 teaspoon grated orange zest
- 3/4 teaspoon salt
- 1/8 teaspoon white pepper
- Lettuce leaves

Direction

- Following the instruction on the package, cook pasta; wash under cold water and drain off. Transfer into a big bowl; put in oranges, celery and turkey. Mix pepper, salt, orange zest, tarragon, mustard, orange juice and mayonnaise in a small bowl. Put on top of pasta mixture and coat by tossing. Keep it covered and let chill in the refrigerator for 60 minutes. Serve on top of lettuce.

Nutrition Information

- Calories: 0g sugar total.

745. Tasty Reuben Soup

Serving: 10 servings (2-1/2 quarts). | Prep: 10mins | Cook: 15mins | Ready in:

Ingredients

- 4 cans (14-1/2 ounces each) chicken broth

- 4 cups shredded cabbage
- 2 cups uncooked medium egg noodles
- 1 pound Johnsonville® Fully Cooked Polish Kielbasa Sausage Rope, halved and cut into 1-inch slices
- 1/2 cup chopped onion
- 1 teaspoon caraway seeds
- 1/4 teaspoon garlic powder
- 1 cup shredded Swiss cheese

Direction

- Mix the first 7 ingredients together in a big saucepan; boil it. Lower the heat, put a cover on and simmer until the noodles and cabbage are soft, about 15 minutes. Use cheese to sprinkle.

Nutrition Information

- Calories: 125 calories
- Cholesterol: 41mg cholesterol
- Protein: 12g protein. Diabetic Exchanges: 1 meat
- Total Fat: 5g fat (0 saturated fat)
- Sodium: 455mg sodium
- Fiber: 0 fiber)
- Total Carbohydrate: 9g carbohydrate (0 sugars

746. Tasty Turkey Soup

Serving: 4 servings. | Prep: 10mins | Cook: 0mins | Ready in:

Ingredients

- 2 tablespoons chopped celery
- 2 tablespoons chopped onion
- 1 tablespoon butter
- 1 package (3 ounces) chicken-flavored ramen noodles
- 1-1/2 cups water
- 1 can (10-3/4 ounces) condensed turkey noodle soup, undiluted
- 1 cup chicken broth
- 1 cup cubed cooked turkey
- Pepper to taste

Direction

- Sauté onion and celery with butter in a large saucepan until tender. Discard or save the packet from the ramen noodles.
- Stir in pepper, turkey, broth, soup, water, and noodles, then cook until the noodles become tender and heated completely, about 3 minutes.

Nutrition Information

- Calories: 166 calories
- Total Carbohydrate: 22g carbohydrate (0 sugars
- Cholesterol: 18mg cholesterol
- Protein: 10g protein. Diabetic Exchanges: 1-1/2 starch
- Total Fat: 4g fat (0 saturated fat)
- Sodium: 1042mg sodium
- Fiber: 1g fiber)

747. Texas Turkey Soup

Serving: 10-12 servings (3 quarts). | Prep: 20mins | Cook: 35mins | Ready in:

Ingredients

- 8 cups chicken broth
- 4 cups cubed cooked turkey
- 2 large white onions, halved
- 2 celery ribs, sliced
- 3 medium carrots, sliced
- 1 cup each frozen corn, cut green beans and peas
- 2 bay leaves
- 1/2 to 1 teaspoon dried tarragon
- 3/4 teaspoon garlic powder
- 1/4 to 1/2 teaspoon hot pepper sauce

- Salt and pepper to taste
- 1-1/2 cups uncooked noodles
- 1 tablespoon cornstarch
- 1 tablespoon water

Direction

- In a soup kettle or Dutch oven, combine seasonings, vegetables, turkey, and broth, then boil. Decrease the heat, cover, and simmer until the vegetables become tender, about 20 - 30 minutes.
- Bring the soup back to a boil and add in the noodles. Lower heat and simmer, covered, until the noodles are soft, about 15 - 20 minutes.
- Combine water and cornstarch until blended and add to the soup, then boil. Boil, continually stirring, for 2 minutes, then remove the bay leaves.

Nutrition Information

- Calories: 152 calories
- Total Fat: 3g fat (1g saturated fat)
- Sodium: 692mg sodium
- Fiber: 2g fiber)
- Total Carbohydrate: 14g carbohydrate (5g sugars
- Cholesterol: 40mg cholesterol
- Protein: 17g protein.

748. Texican Chili

Serving: 16-18 servings. | Prep: 25mins | Cook: 09hours00mins | Ready in:

Ingredients

- 8 bacon strips, diced
- 2-1/2 pounds beef stew meat, cut into 1/2-inch cubes
- 2 cans (one 28 ounces, one 14-1/2 ounces) stewed tomatoes, undrained
- 2 cans (8 ounces each) tomato sauce
- 1 can (16 ounces) kidney beans, rinsed and drained
- 2 cups sliced carrots
- 1 cup chopped celery
- 3/4 cup chopped onion
- 1/2 cup chopped green pepper
- 1/4 cup minced fresh parsley
- 1 tablespoon chili powder
- 1 teaspoon salt, optional
- 1/2 teaspoon ground cumin
- 1/4 teaspoon pepper

Direction

- Cook bacon in a big frying pan until crunchy. Transfer onto paper towels to strain. In the drippings, brown beef over medium heat, drain.
- Move to a 5-qt. slow cooker; add the rest of the ingredients and bacon. Put a cover on and cook on low until the meat is soft, about 8-10 hours; tossing from time to time.

Nutrition Information

- Calories: 163 calories
- Fiber: 0 fiber)
- Total Carbohydrate: 12g carbohydrate (0 sugars
- Cholesterol: 44mg cholesterol
- Protein: 16g protein. Diabetic Exchanges: 2 lean meat
- Total Fat: 6g fat (0 saturated fat)
- Sodium: 242mg sodium

749. Thick Turkey Bean Chili

Serving: 8-10 servings. | Prep: 5mins | Cook: 30mins | Ready in:

Ingredients

- 1 pound ground turkey

- 2 cans (16 ounces each) baked beans, undrained
- 1 can (16 ounces) kidney beans, rinsed and drained
- 1 can (15-1/2 ounces) sloppy joe sauce
- 1 can (14-1/2 ounces) diced tomatoes, undrained
- 1 tablespoon brown sugar
- 1/4 teaspoon each garlic powder, salt and pepper
- Shredded cheddar cheese, sour cream and tortilla chips, optional

Direction

- Brown turkey in a big saucepan until the meat is not pink anymore; drain. Mix in seasonings, brown sugar, tomatoes, sloppy joe sauce, and beans. Simmer without a cover until heated completely, about 30 minutes. Enjoy with tortilla chips, sour cream, and cheese if you want.

Nutrition Information

- Calories: 213 calories
- Protein: 13g protein.
- Total Fat: 7g fat (2g saturated fat)
- Sodium: 680mg sodium
- Fiber: 6g fiber)
- Total Carbohydrate: 24g carbohydrate (9g sugars
- Cholesterol: 34mg cholesterol

750. Thrive On Five Soup

Serving: 7 servings. | Prep: 25mins | Cook: 01hours10mins | Ready in:

Ingredients

- 1 cup chopped onion
- 1/2 cup chopped celery
- 1/2 cup chopped green pepper
- 1/2 cup chopped peeled turnip
- 1/3 cup sliced fresh carrot
- 1 tablespoon olive oil
- 3 cups reduced-sodium chicken broth
- 1 can (14-1/2 ounces) stewed tomatoes, cut up
- 1-1/2 teaspoons dried thyme
- 1 bay leaf
- 1 cup coarsely chopped green cabbage
- 1 cup cut fresh green beans (2-inch pieces)
- 1-1/2 cups cubed cooked turkey breast
- 1 tablespoon cider vinegar
- 1/2 teaspoon salt
- 1/8 teaspoon pepper

Direction

- Use a large saucepan to sauté carrot, turnip, green pepper, celery, and onion with oil for 7 minutes. Stir in the bay leaf, thyme, tomatoes, and broth, then allow to boil. Lower heat, cover, and let it simmer for 30 minutes.
- Stir in beans and cabbage, then bring back to a boil. Decrease heat and simmer, covered, for 10 minutes. Stir in the turkey and allow to simmer for 5 minutes longer. Stir in pepper, salt, and vinegar, heating the soup through. Throw away the bay leaf.

Nutrition Information

- Calories: 112 calories
- Sodium: 550mg sodium
- Fiber: 3g fiber)
- Total Carbohydrate: 9g carbohydrate (6g sugars
- Cholesterol: 26mg cholesterol
- Protein: 12g protein. Diabetic Exchanges: 2 vegetable
- Total Fat: 3g fat (1g saturated fat)

751. Tomato Turkey Soup

Serving: 14 servings. | Prep: 10mins | Cook: 01hours45mins | Ready in:

Ingredients

- 6 cups chicken or turkey broth
- 2 cans (14-1/2 ounces each) diced tomatoes, undrained
- 1/3 cup quick-cooking barley
- 1 tablespoon dried parsley flakes
- 1 teaspoon salt
- 1/2 teaspoon garlic powder
- 1/2 teaspoon dried oregano
- 1/2 teaspoon dried basil
- 1/4 teaspoon pepper
- 2 cups cubed cooked turkey
- 1-1/2 cups sliced carrots
- 1-1/2 cups sliced celery
- 1 medium onion, chopped
- 1 cup chopped green pepper
- 1 package (10 ounces) frozen chopped okra

Direction

- Combine first 9 of the ingredients in a big saucepan, then boil. Decrease heat and simmer, covered, for 50 minutes. Add in the vegetables and turkey, then simmer while covered for another 50 minutes until the vegetables become tender.

Nutrition Information

- Calories: 85 calories
- Protein: 5g protein. Diabetic Exchanges: 1 vegetable
- Total Fat: 2g fat (0 saturated fat)
- Sodium: 714mg sodium
- Fiber: 3g fiber)
- Total Carbohydrate: 11g carbohydrate (0 sugars
- Cholesterol: 14mg cholesterol

752. Tropical Turkey Salad

Serving: 12 | Prep: 20mins | Cook: | Ready in:

Ingredients

- 1/3 cup low-fat sour cream
- 2 tablespoons mango chutney
- 1 tablespoon fresh lemon juice
- 1 tablespoon honey
- 1/4 teaspoon curry powder
- 4 cups chopped cooked turkey
- 1 cup diced red bell pepper
- 1 cup diced celery
- 1 cup pineapple chunks
- 1 cup chopped orange segments
- 1/2 cup chopped green onion

Direction

- To make the dressing, mix curry powder, honey, lemon juice, chutney and sour cream in a small bowl and mix well until well combined, keep cold in refrigerator until ready to use.
- Mix together green onion, orange segments, pineapple, celery, red pepper and turkey in a large bowl. Pour dressing and toss until well coated. Keep cold in refrigerator for 1 hour before serving.

Nutrition Information

- Calories: 126 calories;
- Total Fat: 3.2
- Sodium: 46
- Total Carbohydrate: 9.6
- Cholesterol: 38
- Protein: 14.4

753. Turkey Almond Salad

Serving: 6 servings. | Prep: 20mins | Cook: 0mins | Ready in:

Ingredients

- 2/3 cup Miracle Whip
- 1 tablespoon milk

- 2 teaspoons prepared mustard
- 1-1/2 teaspoons sugar
- 1/2 teaspoon salt
- 1/4 teaspoon pepper
- 3 cups cubed cooked turkey
- 2 cups shredded cabbage
- 3/4 cup diced celery
- 1/2 cup sliced green onion
- 1-1/2 cups chow mein noodles
- 1/2 cup slivered almonds, toasted
- 2 tablespoons sesame seeds, toasted

Direction

- Combine the first six ingredients in a large bowl. Add green onions, celery, cabbage and turkey; toss until well combined. Cover the salad and allow to chill for several hours. Right before serving, add sesame seeds, almonds and chow mein noodles; toss to mix.

Nutrition Information

- Calories: 388 calories
- Protein: 25g protein.
- Total Fat: 25g fat (4g saturated fat)
- Sodium: 518mg sodium
- Fiber: 3g fiber)
- Total Carbohydrate: 16g carbohydrate (5g sugars
- Cholesterol: 62mg cholesterol

754. Turkey Barley Soup

Serving: 10 | Prep: 20mins | Cook: 3hours15mins | Ready in:

Ingredients

- Stock:
- 2 tablespoons vegetable oil
- 3 pounds turkey bones
- 1 onion, quartered
- 1 stalk celery, coarsely chopped
- 1 carrot, coarsely chopped
- 16 cups water
- 2 sprigs fresh thyme
- Soup:
- 2 1/2 cups water
- 1 cup barley
- 2 tablespoons olive oil
- 1 onion, diced
- 2 carrots, sliced
- 2 stalks celery, sliced
- 2 cloves garlic, minced
- 2 cups chopped cooked turkey
- 1/4 cup chopped fresh parsley
- 2 sprigs fresh thyme, leaves stripped
- 1/4 teaspoon salt
- 1/4 teaspoon ground black pepper
- 1/8 teaspoon cayenne pepper
- 1/2 lemon, juiced

Direction

- In a large stockpot, heat vegetable oil on medium-high heat and add the turkey bones, then cook, occasionally turning, for 10 minutes until it browns. Transfer the bones into a bowl.
- Use the same stockpot to cook, stirring, coarsely chopped carrots, coarsely chopped celery, and quartered onion with hot oil for 2 minutes until fragrant. Place the turkey bones into the stockpot and add sprigs of thyme and 16 cups of water. Allow to boil and skim off the foam. Turn the heat to medium - low and simmer for 2 hours until the liquid reduces to 10 cups. Strain the stock into a big bowl and allow to stand for 15 minutes. Spoon the fat off the top of the stock.
- In a saucepan, boil barley with 2 1/2 cup of water. Cover, turn heat to low, and simmer for 30 - 40 minutes until the barley becomes tender.
- In a large stockpot, heat olive oil on medium-high heat and cook while stirring garlic, sliced celery, sliced carrots, and diced onion for 5 minutes until they are slightly soft. Add in the turkey stock and set to boil.
- Mix cayenne pepper, black pepper, salt, thyme leaves, parsley, barley, and turkey meat into

the soup. Turn the heat to medium-low and allow to simmer for 20 minutes. Stir in the lemon juice.

Nutrition Information

- Calories: 262 calories;
- Protein: 13.7
- Total Fat: 14.1
- Sodium: 126
- Total Carbohydrate: 21
- Cholesterol: 38

755. Turkey Barley Tomato Soup

Serving: 6 servings. | Prep: 15mins | Cook: 40mins | Ready in:

Ingredients

- 1 pound lean ground turkey
- 3/4 cup sliced or baby carrots
- 1 medium onion, chopped
- 1 celery rib, chopped
- 1 garlic clove, minced
- 1 envelope reduced-sodium taco seasoning, divided
- 3-1/2 cups water
- 1 can (28 ounces) Italian diced tomatoes, undrained
- 3/4 cup quick-cooking barley
- 1/2 teaspoon minced fresh oregano or 1/8 teaspoon dried oregano

Direction

- Cook 1 tablespoon taco seasoning, garlic, celery, onion, carrots, and turkey in a Dutch oven on medium heat until the turkey meat is no longer pink. Stir in the remaining taco seasoning, tomatoes, and water, then boil. Lower heat, cover, and simmer for 20 minutes. Add the barley and simmer, covered, until the barley becomes tender, or for 15 - 20 minutes longer. Stir in the oregano.

Nutrition Information

- Calories: 275 calories
- Sodium: 923mg sodium
- Fiber: 6g fiber)
- Total Carbohydrate: 36g carbohydrate (0 sugars
- Cholesterol: 60mg cholesterol
- Protein: 18g protein.
- Total Fat: 7g fat (2g saturated fat)

756. Turkey Bean Chili

Serving: 6 servings. | Prep: 10mins | Cook: 20mins | Ready in:

Ingredients

- 2 cups cubed cooked turkey breast
- 2 cans (14-1/2 ounces each) diced tomatoes, undrained
- 1 can (15 ounces) black beans, rinsed and drained
- 1 can (15 ounces) great norther beans, rinsed and drained
- 1 cup barbecue sauce
- 1 medium onion, chopped
- 1 teaspoon chili powder
- 1 teaspoon ground cumin

Direction

- Mix all the ingredients together in a big saucepan. Boil it. Lower the heat; simmer without a cover until the flavors combine, about 15-20 minutes.

Nutrition Information

- Calories: 236 calories
- Sodium: 757mg sodium

- Fiber: 9g fiber)
- Total Carbohydrate: 32g carbohydrate (9g sugars
- Cholesterol: 40mg cholesterol
- Protein: 23g protein.
- Total Fat: 2g fat (0 saturated fat)

- Protein: 16g protein.
- Total Fat: 11g fat (3g saturated fat)
- Sodium: 1052mg sodium
- Fiber: 6g fiber)
- Total Carbohydrate: 25g carbohydrate (4g sugars
- Cholesterol: 39mg cholesterol

757. Turkey Bean Soup

Serving: 8 servings. | Prep: 10mins | Cook: 40mins | Ready in:

Ingredients

- 1 pound ground turkey
- 1 cup chopped onion
- 1 cup chopped celery
- 1 tablespoon olive oil
- 1 can (49-1/2 ounces) chicken broth
- 2 cups frozen corn
- 1 can (15 ounces) white kidney or cannellini beans, rinsed and drained
- 1 cup frozen lima beans
- 1 can (4 ounces) chopped green chilies
- 1 teaspoon dried oregano
- 1 teaspoon ground cumin
- 1 teaspoon chili powder
- 1/2 teaspoon salt
- Shredded cheddar cheese, optional

Direction

- Use a Dutch oven to cook celery, onion, and turkey with oil on medium heat until the turkey is no longer pink. Add in salt, chili powder, cumin, oregano, chilies, beans, corn, and broth, then allow to boil. Lower the heat and simmer, covered, until it heats through, about 30 minutes. If desired, you can serve with cheese.

Nutrition Information

- Calories: 259 calories

758. Turkey Cabbage Soup

Serving: 10 servings (about 3-1/2 quarts). | Prep: 15mins | Cook: 20mins | Ready in:

Ingredients

- 1 pound lean ground turkey
- 2 medium onions, chopped
- 1 tablespoon canola oil
- 3 pounds potatoes, peeled and cut into 1-inch pieces
- 3 medium carrots, sliced
- 1 small head cabbage, chopped
- 1 can (49-1/2 ounces) reduced-sodium chicken broth
- 1 tablespoon prepared Dijon mustard
- 1-1/2 teaspoons prepared horseradish
- 3/4 teaspoon salt
- 1/2 teaspoon pepper
- 2 teaspoons cornstarch
- 1 tablespoon cold water

Direction

- In a big soup kettle, cook onions and turkey with oil on medium heat until the turkey meat is no longer pink, then drain. Add in pepper, salt, horseradish, mustard, broth, cabbage, carrots, and potatoes, then boil. Lower the heat and simmer, covered, occasionally stirring, for 15 - 20 minutes until potatoes become tender.
- Mix cold water and cornstarch together until smooth, then stir into the soup slowly. Bring to a boil, then cook and stir until thickened a little, about 2 minutes.

Nutrition Information

- Calories: 242 calories
- Protein: 14g protein. Diabetic Exchanges: 2 vegetable
- Total Fat: 6g fat (1g saturated fat)
- Sodium: 661mg sodium
- Fiber: 6g fiber)
- Total Carbohydrate: 36g carbohydrate (0 sugars
- Cholesterol: 36mg cholesterol

759. Turkey Cashew Salad

Serving: 8 servings. | Prep: 30mins | Cook: 0mins | Ready in:

Ingredients

- 1 cup small ring pasta
- 4 cups cubed cooked turkey or chicken
- 1 cup thinly sliced celery
- 1 cup seedless green grapes, halved
- 1 cup mayonnaise
- 2 tablespoons orange juice
- 2 tablespoons vinegar
- 1 tablespoon olive oil
- 1-1/2 teaspoons grated orange zest
- 3/4 teaspoon salt
- 1/4 teaspoon ground ginger
- 3/4 cup salted cashews

Direction

- Cook pasta following packaging instruction; drain. Wash in cold water; put in a big bowl. Put in the grapes, celery and turkey. Mix together ginger, salt, orange zest, oil, vinegar, orange juice and mayonnaise in a small bowl. Put atop salad; coat by tossing. Refrigerate for a minimum of 1 hour. Mix in cashews just prior to serve.

Nutrition Information

- Calories: 477 calories
- Total Fat: 35g fat (6g saturated fat)
- Sodium: 529mg sodium
- Fiber: 1g fiber)
- Total Carbohydrate: 15g carbohydrate (5g sugars
- Cholesterol: 63mg cholesterol
- Protein: 25g protein.

760. Turkey Chili

Serving: Makes 6 to 8 servings | Prep: 20mins | Cook: 45mins | Ready in:

Ingredients

- 1 large white onion, coarsely chopped
- 2 bell peppers (any color), cut into 1-inch pieces
- 3 tablespoons vegetable oil
- 1 tablespoon chili powder
- 1 teaspoon chipotle chile powder
- 2 teaspoon packed brown sugar
- 1 (28-ounce) can whole tomatoes in juice
- 1 (19-ounce) can black beans, rinsed and drained
- 1/2 cup water
- 2 cups cooked turkey, cut into 1-inch pieces
- Accompaniments: sour cream; sliced avocado; chopped white onion; lime wedges

Direction

- In a heavy medium-sized pot, cook peppers and onion in oil over medium heat, tossing from time to time for 12-15 minutes till golden. Add brown sugar and spices, and cook, mixing for 1 minute until aromatic. Add tomatoes with juice; use the back of a spoon to crumble, and then add 1 teaspoon of salt, water, and beans. Simmer with a cover for 15 minutes.
- Mix in turkey and let sit with a cover for 5 minutes until heated completely.

Nutrition Information

- Calories: 272
- Cholesterol: 47 mg(16%)
- Protein: 21 g(42%)
- Total Fat: 10 g(15%)
- Saturated Fat: 1 g(6%)
- Sodium: 378 mg(16%)
- Fiber: 11 g(42%)
- Total Carbohydrate: 27 g(9%)

761. Turkey Chutney Salad

Serving: 10-12 servings. | Prep: 15mins | Cook: 0mins | Ready in:

Ingredients

- 1-1/2 cups mayonnaise
- 1/2 cup prepared chutney
- 1 to 2 teaspoons curry powder
- 1/4 teaspoon salt
- 4 cups diced cooked turkey
- 1 cup sliced celery
- 1 can (8 ounces) pineapple chunks, drained
- 1/2 cup golden raisins
- 2 firm red apples, cubed
- 2 medium bananas, sliced
- 1/2 cup chopped pecans, toasted
- 1/2 cup sweetened shredded coconut, toasted, optional

Direction

- Mix salt, curry, chutney and mayonnaise in a big bowl. Mix in raisins, pineapple, celery, and turkey. Keep chilled for no less than 2 hours. Just prior to serving, mix in pecans, bananas, and apples and coconut if you want.

Nutrition Information

- Calories: 390 calories
- Protein: 15g protein.
- Total Fat: 28g fat (4g saturated fat)
- Sodium: 244mg sodium
- Fiber: 2g fiber)
- Total Carbohydrate: 20g carbohydrate (16g sugars
- Cholesterol: 45mg cholesterol

762. Turkey Curry Salad

Serving: 4-6 servings. | Prep: 10mins | Cook: 0mins | Ready in:

Ingredients

- 3/4 cup mayonnaise
- 3/4 cup sour cream or plain yogurt
- 1 to 2 teaspoons curry powder
- 4 cups diced cooked turkey
- 2 cups chopped apples
- 1 cup chopped celery
- 1 cup chopped peeled cucumber
- 2 tablespoons chopped onion

Direction

- Mix yogurt or sour cream and mayonnaise together in a big bowl; mix in curry powder. Tuck in the rest of the ingredients. Refrigerate for a minimum of 2 hours before eating.

Nutrition Information

- Calories: 451 calories
- Fiber: 2g fiber)
- Total Carbohydrate: 9g carbohydrate (6g sugars
- Cholesterol: 101mg cholesterol
- Protein: 29g protein.
- Total Fat: 32g fat (8g saturated fat)
- Sodium: 248mg sodium

763. Turkey Dumpling Soup

Serving: 16 servings (4 quarts). | Prep: 20mins | Cook: 20mins | Ready in:

Ingredients

- 1 meaty leftover turkey carcass (from an 11-pound turkey)
- 6 cups chicken broth
- 6 cups water
- 2 celery ribs, cut into 1-inch slices
- 1 medium carrot, cut into 1-inch slices
- 1 tablespoon poultry seasoning
- 1 bay leaf
- 1/2 teaspoon salt
- 1/2 teaspoon pepper
- SOUP INGREDIENTS:
- 1 medium onion, chopped
- 2 celery ribs, chopped
- 2 medium carrots, sliced
- 1 cup fresh or frozen cut green beans
- 1 package (10 ounces) frozen corn
- 1 package (10 ounces) frozen peas
- 2 cups biscuit/baking mix
- 2/3 cup milk

Direction

- Mix the first 9 ingredients in a stockpot. Boil the mixture before reducing the heat. Cover the pot and simmer the mixture for 3 hours.
- Remove the carcass and allow the mixture to cool. Remove the meat and reserve 4 cups of it for the soup. Refrigerate the remaining meat for another use, discarding the bones. Cut the meat into bite-size pieces. Strain the broth and discard the bay leaf and vegetables.
- Pour the broth back into the pan. Add the carrots, beans, celery, and onion. Boil the mixture before reducing the heat. Cover the pan and simmer the mixture for 10 minutes until the vegetables are tender. Add the reserved turkey, corn, and peas. Bring the mixture to a boil; reduce heat.
- Combine the milk and biscuit mix. Drop teaspoonfuls of the mixture into the simmering broth. Cover the pan and simmer the mixture for 10 minutes until an inserted toothpick inside the dumpling comes out clean. Take note not to lift the cover while the mixture is still simmering.

Nutrition Information

- Calories: 185 calories
- Total Carbohydrate: 19g carbohydrate (4g sugars
- Cholesterol: 30mg cholesterol
- Protein: 14g protein.
- Total Fat: 5g fat (1g saturated fat)
- Sodium: 724mg sodium
- Fiber: 2g fiber)

764. Turkey Fried Rice

Serving: 4 servings. | Prep: 50mins | Cook: 10mins | Ready in:

Ingredients

- 2 cups reduced-sodium chicken broth
- 1 cup uncooked brown rice
- 2 cups cubed cooked turkey breast
- 3 tablespoons reduced-sodium soy sauce
- 1 egg, lightly beaten
- 1 small onion, chopped
- 1/4 cup chopped green pepper
- 1/4 cup chopped celery
- 1 tablespoon canola oil
- 1 cup shredded romaine

Direction

- Boil broth in a big saucepan. Mix in rice. Lower the heat, put a cover on, and simmer until the rice is soft and has absorbed all the liquid, about 45-50 minutes. Take away from heat, let cool. Chill overnight with a cover on.
- Mix soy sauce and turkey together in a small bowl. Put a cover on and chill. Stir and cook

the egg in a big nonstick frying pan over medium heat until fully set. Take out and put aside.
- Sauté celery, green pepper, and onion in oil in the same frying pan until soft. Add turkey and rice; stir and cook for 6-8 minutes over medium heat. Add the saved egg and lettuce, stir and cook for 1-2 minutes. Enjoy immediately.

Nutrition Information

- Calories: 367 calories
- Protein: 28g protein. Diabetic Exchanges: 3 lean meat
- Total Fat: 10g fat (2g saturated fat)
- Sodium: 994mg sodium
- Fiber: 2g fiber)
- Total Carbohydrate: 40g carbohydrate (0 sugars
- Cholesterol: 106mg cholesterol

765. Turkey Fruit Salad

Serving: 8 servings. | Prep: 10mins | Cook: 0mins | Ready in:

Ingredients

- 1/2 cup mayonnaise
- 2 tablespoons honey
- 1/8 teaspoon ground ginger
- 2 cups cubed cooked turkey
- 1 can (11 ounces) mandarin oranges, drained
- 1 cup chopped unpeeled apple
- 1 cup grape halves
- 1 can (8-1/4 ounces) pineapple chunks, drained
- 1/2 cup pecan halves, toasted

Direction

- Combine ginger, honey and mayonnaise in a large bowl. Stir in pineapple, grapes, apple, oranges and turkey. Cover the mixture and keep in refrigerator for 1 hour. Sprinkle with pecans right before serving.

Nutrition Information

- Calories: 280 calories
- Sodium: 104mg sodium
- Fiber: 2g fiber)
- Total Carbohydrate: 20g carbohydrate (18g sugars
- Cholesterol: 32mg cholesterol
- Protein: 11g protein.
- Total Fat: 18g fat (3g saturated fat)

766. Turkey Ginger Noodle Soup

Serving: 8 servings (about 3 quarts). | Prep: 20mins | Cook: 04hours15mins | Ready in:

Ingredients

- 2 medium carrots, sliced
- 2 cans (8 ounces each) sliced water chestnuts, drained
- 3 to 4 tablespoons minced fresh gingerroot
- 2 tablespoons minced fresh parsley
- 2 teaspoons chili powder
- 1 carton (32 ounces) chicken stock
- 1 can (11.8 ounces) coconut water
- 3 tablespoons lemon juice
- 2 pounds uncooked skinless turkey breast, cut into 1-inch cubes
- 2 teaspoons pepper
- 1/2 teaspoon salt
- 2 tablespoons canola oil
- 1 cup frozen corn (about 5 ounces), thawed
- 1 cup frozen peas (about 4 ounces), thawed
- 8 ounces rice noodles or thin spaghetti

Direction

- In a 4 or 5 quart slow cooker, place in the first 8 of the ingredients.

- Toss salt and pepper with the turkey. In a big skillet, heat oil on medium-high heat and brown the turkey in batches, then add into the slow cooker.
- Cover and cook on a low heat for 4 - 5 hours until the turkey and carrots become tender. Stir in peas and corn, then heat thoroughly.
- Cook noodles according to the package instructions, then drain. Before serving, add the noodles into the soup.

Nutrition Information

- Calories: 351 calories
- Total Carbohydrate: 41g carbohydrate (5g sugars
- Cholesterol: 65mg cholesterol
- Protein: 33g protein. Diabetic Exchanges: 3 starch
- Total Fat: 6g fat (1g saturated fat)
- Sodium: 672mg sodium
- Fiber: 4g fiber)

767. Turkey Mandarin Salad

Serving: 6-8 servings. | Prep: 15mins | Cook: 0mins | Ready in:

Ingredients

- 2 cups cubed cooked turkey
- 1 tablespoon finely chopped onion
- 1/2 teaspoon salt
- 1 cup halved seedless red grapes
- 1 cup diced celery
- 1 can (15 ounces) mandarin oranges, drained
- 1 cup cooked macaroni
- 3/4 cup heavy whipping cream, whipped
- 3/4 cup mayonnaise
- 1/3 cup slivered almonds
- Toasted almonds, optional

Direction

- Combine salt, onion and turkey in a large bowl; mix properly. Add macaroni, oranges, celery and grapes; lightly toss until well mixed. Cover the mixture and keep cold in refrigerator.
- Right before serving, fold whipped cream into mayonnaise; fold almonds and mayonnaise mixture into salad. Put toasted almonds on top if desired.

Nutrition Information

- Calories: 382 calories
- Cholesterol: 65mg cholesterol
- Protein: 13g protein.
- Total Fat: 29g fat (8g saturated fat)
- Sodium: 310mg sodium
- Fiber: 2g fiber)
- Total Carbohydrate: 18g carbohydrate (13g sugars

768. Turkey Meatball Salad

Serving: 4 servings. | Prep: 20mins | Cook: 10mins | Ready in:

Ingredients

- 1 egg
- 6 teaspoons soy sauce, divided
- 1 can (8 ounces) water chestnuts, drained and chopped
- 1/3 cup thinly sliced green onions
- 1/4 cup dry bread crumbs
- 1 pound ground turkey
- 1 tablespoon cornstarch
- 1 teaspoon sugar
- 1-1/2 cups chicken broth
- 1/2 teaspoon vinegar
- 1 medium head iceberg lettuce, finely shredded
- Additional green onions
- 1 medium lemon, cut into wedges

Direction

- Beat 4 teaspoons of soy sauce and egg in a big bowl; put in bread crumbs, green onions and water chestnuts. Put in turkey and stir them well. Form into 1-inch balls. Put meatballs on a greased shallow rack in a shallow baking pan. Bake, while uncovered, for 10-12 minutes at 400 degrees until meat is not pink anymore.
- At the same time, to make dressing, in a saucepan, mix sugar and cornstarch. Combine leftover soy sauce, vinegar, and broth until smooth in texture. Boil; cook and stir till thickened for 2 minutes. To serve, arrange meatballs on top of lettuce; use lemon and onions to decorate. Serve alongside the dressing.

Nutrition Information

- Calories: 346 calories
- Cholesterol: 130mg cholesterol
- Protein: 24g protein.
- Total Fat: 19g fat (6g saturated fat)
- Sodium: 1019mg sodium
- Fiber: 4g fiber)
- Total Carbohydrate: 21g carbohydrate (5g sugars

769. Turkey Meatball Soup

Serving: 12 servings (3 quarts). | Prep: 30mins | Cook: 10mins | Ready in:

Ingredients

- MEATBALLS:
- 1/4 cup cooked rice
- 1/4 cup finely chopped onion
- 1/4 cup finely chopped celery
- 2 tablespoons all-purpose flour
- 2 tablespoons water
- 1/2 teaspoon ground cumin
- 1/2 teaspoon salt, optional
- 1/8 teaspoon pepper
- 3/4 pound ground turkey breast
- SOUP:
- 6 cup chicken broth
- 1 cup uncooked fine egg noodles
- 1/2 teaspoon pepper
- 1/4 teaspoon garlic salt, optional
- 1/8 teaspoon dill weed
- 1 tablespoon minced fresh parsley

Direction

- Combine the first 8 of the ingredients into a bowl. Add the turkey and mix properly, then shape the mixture into 1 inch balls. Place the meatballs onto 2 racks coated with cooking spray in shallow baking pans. Bake in the oven, uncovered, at 450 degrees for 15 minutes or until the turkey meatballs are no longer pink, then drain. Boil the broth using a large soup kettle or Dutch oven. Add dill, pepper, noodles, and meatballs (You can also add garlic salt if you want), then set to boil; lower the heat and simmer without a cover for 5 minutes or until the noodles become tender. Stir in the parsley.

Nutrition Information

- Calories: 65 calories
- Cholesterol: 19mg cholesterol
- Protein: 9g protein. Diabetic Exchanges: 1 lean meat
- Total Fat: 2g fat (0 saturated fat)
- Sodium: 77mg sodium
- Fiber: 0 fiber)
- Total Carbohydrate: 5g carbohydrate (0 sugars

770. Turkey Meatballs Soup

Serving: 6 servings. | Prep: 10mins | Cook: 20mins | Ready in:

Ingredients

- 1 package (12 ounces) refrigerated fully cooked Italian turkey meatballs
- 1 can (49-1/2 ounces) chicken broth
- 2 cups uncooked egg noodles
- 2 cups cut fresh green beans
- 1 cup sliced fresh carrots
- 1 cup chopped celery
- 1 cup chopped onion
- 1 tablespoon dried parsley flakes
- 1 teaspoon garlic powder
- 1 teaspoon dried oregano
- 1 teaspoon dried basil
- 1/4 teaspoon pepper

Direction

- Combine all the ingredients into Dutch oven and set to boil. Decrease the heat and simmer without a cover until the noodles become tender, about 20 - 25 minutes.

Nutrition Information

- Calories: 227 calories
- Protein: 17g protein.
- Total Fat: 8g fat (2g saturated fat)
- Sodium: 1357mg sodium
- Fiber: 4g fiber)
- Total Carbohydrate: 22g carbohydrate (6g sugars
- Cholesterol: 55mg cholesterol

771. Turkey Minestrone

Serving: 16 servings (4 quarts). | Prep: 30mins | Cook: 0mins | Ready in:

Ingredients

- 2/3 cup chopped onion
- 2 tablespoons canola oil
- 1/2 pound lean ground turkey
- 1/2 pound hot Italian turkey sausage links, casings removed
- 1/2 cup minced fresh parsley
- 2 garlic cloves, minced
- 1 teaspoon dried oregano
- 1 teaspoon dried basil
- 2 cans (14-1/2 ounces each) Italian stewed tomatoes
- 6 cups chicken broth
- 1 medium zucchini, sliced
- 1 package (10 ounces) frozen mixed vegetables
- 1 can (16 ounces) kidney beans, rinsed and drained
- 1-1/2 cups cooked elbow macaroni
- 2 tablespoons cider vinegar
- 1/2 teaspoon salt, optional
- Pinch pepper

Direction

- Sauté onion in oil in a stockpot that is set over medium heat for 4 minutes until tender. Add the next six ingredients. Cook the mixture until the meat is no longer pink.
- Add the broth, mixed vegetables, zucchini, and tomatoes. Cover the pot and cook the mixture on low heat for 5 minutes. Mix on vinegar, beans, macaroni, and salt and pepper if desired. Simmer the mixture for 3-4 minutes until heated through.

Nutrition Information

- Calories: 132 calories
- Fiber: 3g fiber)
- Total Carbohydrate: 15g carbohydrate (4g sugars
- Cholesterol: 20mg cholesterol
- Protein: 9g protein. Diabetic Exchanges: 1 starch
- Total Fat: 4g fat (1g saturated fat)
- Sodium: 538mg sodium

772. Turkey Noodle Soup

Serving: 6 servings (3 quarts). | Prep: 20mins | Cook: 01hours15mins | Ready in:

Ingredients

- 9 cups homemade turkey or chicken broth
- 4 medium carrots, shredded
- 3 celery ribs, sliced
- 1 medium onion, chopped
- 1 teaspoon rubbed sage
- 1/2 teaspoon pepper
- 3 whole cloves
- 1 bay leaf
- 2 cups diced cooked turkey
- 1 cup uncooked macaroni
- 1/4 cup chopped fresh parsley

Direction

- Mix the first six ingredients in a Dutch oven or large kettle. Knot bay leaf and cloves in a cheesecloth bag and put to kettle; make it boil. Lower heat; cover and gently boil for 1 hour. Stir in parsley, macaroni and turkey; cover and gently boil for 15-20 minutes or until macaroni is soft and the soup is heated through. Get rid of spice bag.

Nutrition Information

- Calories: 179 calories
- Sodium: 1462mg sodium
- Fiber: 3g fiber)
- Total Carbohydrate: 18g carbohydrate (6g sugars
- Cholesterol: 35mg cholesterol
- Protein: 19g protein.
- Total Fat: 4g fat (1g saturated fat)

773. Turkey Pasta Salad

Serving: 8 servings | Prep: 30mins | Cook: | Ready in:

Ingredients

- 1 pkg. (13.25 oz.) whole wheat medium pasta shell, uncooked
- 1 small zucchini, cut lengthwise in half, then crosswise into 1/4-inch-thick slices
- 1 env. (0.75 oz.) GOOD SEASONS Garlic & Herb Dressing Mix
- 1/4 cup olive oil, divided
- 1 pkg. (7.5 oz.) OSCAR MAYER CARVING BOARD Oven Roasted Turkey Breast, cut into bite-size pieces
- 1 cup cherry tomatoes, halved
- 1/4 cup KRAFT Grated Parmesan Cheese
- 2 Tbsp. chopped assorted pitted olives
- 1 Tbsp. chopped fresh chives

Direction

- 1. Based on package directions, cook pasta, omitting salt.
- 2. At the same time, combine dressing mix with zucchini. Over medium high heat, heat 1tbsp. of oil in a large skillet. Put in zucchini; cook and stir for two minutes. Put in turkey; cook and stir for 1 - 2 minutes or turkey is heated through and zucchini is tender-crisp. Take off the heat.
- 3. Drain pasta; Add into a big bowl. Put in all the leftover ingredients and turkey mixture, including leftover oil; gently stir.

Nutrition Information

- Calories: 280
- Saturated Fat: 2 g
- Sodium: 690 mg
- Total Carbohydrate: 39 g
- Fiber: 5 g
- Sugar: 4 g
- Cholesterol: 15 mg
- Protein: 14 g
- Total Fat: 9 g

774. Turkey Pasta Soup

Serving: 10 servings. | Prep: 10mins | Cook: 20mins | Ready in:

Ingredients

- 1 cup uncooked small pasta shells
- 1 pound lean ground turkey
- 2 medium onions, chopped
- 2 garlic cloves, minced
- 3 cans (14-1/2 ounces each) reduced-sodium chicken broth
- 2 cans (15 ounces each) white kidney or cannellini beans, rinsed and drained
- 2 cans (14-1/2 ounces each) Italian stewed tomatoes
- 2 teaspoons dried oregano
- 2 teaspoons dried basil
- 1 teaspoon fennel seed, crushed
- 1 teaspoon pepper
- 1/2 teaspoon salt
- 1/4 teaspoon crushed red pepper flakes

Direction

- Cook pasta according to package instructions. At the same time, cook onions and turkey in a big stockpot on medium heat until turkey is no longer pink. Add in the garlic; cook for a minute longer, then drain. Stir in seasonings, tomatoes, beans, and broth, then boil. Lower the heat and simmer while uncovered for 10 minutes.
- Drain the pasta and add into the soup, then cook for 5 minutes longer or until it heats through.

Nutrition Information

- Calories: 211 calories
- Sodium: 868mg sodium
- Fiber: 6g fiber)
- Total Carbohydrate: 28g carbohydrate (7g sugars
- Cholesterol: 36mg cholesterol
- Protein: 15g protein. Diabetic Exchanges: 2 lean meat
- Total Fat: 4g fat (1g saturated fat)

775. Turkey Ramen Noodle Salad

Serving: 6 servings. | Prep: 20mins | Cook: 0mins | Ready in:

Ingredients

- 1/3 cup white wine vinegar
- 1/4 cup canola oil
- 3 tablespoons sugar
- 1/2 teaspoon pepper
- 2 packages (3 ounces each) Oriental ramen noodles
- 1 package (14 ounces) coleslaw mix
- 1 pound sliced deli turkey, chopped
- 1/2 cup sliced almonds, toasted
- 1/4 cup sesame seeds
- Thinly sliced green onions, optional

Direction

- Mix contents of ramen noodle seasoning packets, pepper, sugar, oil, and vinegar in a small bowl until blended.
- Chop noodles into small pieces and put in a big bowl. Add in turkey and coleslaw mix. Use the dressing to sprinkle on, mix to coat. Use sesame seeds and almonds to drizzle. If you want, you can put green onions on top. Serve immediately.

Nutrition Information

- Calories: 406 calories
- Cholesterol: 27mg cholesterol
- Protein: 21g protein.
- Total Fat: 22g fat (4g saturated fat)
- Sodium: 1222mg sodium
- Fiber: 4g fiber)

- Total Carbohydrate: 32g carbohydrate (10g sugars
- Sodium: 299mg sodium
- Fiber: 3g fiber)

776. Turkey Ranch Salad

Serving: 9 servings. | Prep: 20mins | Cook: 0mins | Ready in:

Ingredients

- 1 can (20 ounces) pineapple tidbits
- 3 cups cubed cooked turkey
- 1 can (8 ounces) sliced water chestnuts, drained and halved
- 1 cup thinly sliced fresh mushrooms
- 1 cup thinly sliced celery
- 1/2 cup thinly sliced green onions
- 3/4 cup ranch salad dressing
- 1/8 teaspoon garlic powder
- 1/8 teaspoon onion powder
- 7 cups torn mixed greens, divided
- 2 tablespoons slivered almonds, toasted, optional

Direction

- Drain the pineapple, put aside 3 tbsps. of juice. Mix onions, celery, mushrooms, water chestnuts, turkey and pineapple together in a big bowl. Mix onion powder, garlic powder, dressing and reserved juice together in a small bowl. Put into turkey mixture; coat by tossing. Separate greens into 9 dishes; put on top of each with one cup of turkey mixture. If you want, drizzle with almonds.

Nutrition Information

- Calories: 168 calories
- Total Carbohydrate: 20g carbohydrate (10g sugars
- Cholesterol: 36mg cholesterol
- Protein: 15g protein. Diabetic Exchanges: 2 lean meat
- Total Fat: 3g fat (1g saturated fat)

777. Turkey Rice Salad

Serving: 2 servings. | Prep: 20mins | Cook: 0mins | Ready in:

Ingredients

- 2/3 cup frozen peas
- 1-1/4 cups cubed cooked turkey
- 1/4 cup long grain rice, cooked
- 1/4 cup finely chopped carrot
- 2 tablespoons chopped onion
- 1/3 cup sour cream
- 1 tablespoon lemon juice
- 1 tablespoon chutney
- 1 tablespoon canola oil
- 1/4 to 1/2 teaspoon curry powder
- 1/4 teaspoon salt
- 1/8 teaspoon pepper
- Lettuce leaves and tomato wedges

Direction

- In a saucepan, pour 1 in. of water; boil. Put in peas. Lower heat; keep it covered and let it simmer till soft for 4 to 6 minutes. Drain off.
- Mix onion, carrot, rice, turkey and peas in a big bowl. Combine pepper, salt, curry powder, oil, chutney, lemon juice and sour cream in a small bowl. Pour to turkey mixture and coat by tossing. Keep chilled in the refrigerator for no less than 2 hours. Serve on top of lettuce; Put tomato wedges on top.

Nutrition Information

- Calories: 436 calories
- Protein: 32g protein.
- Total Fat: 18g fat (7g saturated fat)
- Sodium: 496mg sodium
- Fiber: 4g fiber)

- Total Carbohydrate: 33g carbohydrate (9g sugars
- Cholesterol: 93mg cholesterol

778. Turkey Rice Soup

Serving: 6 | Prep: 10mins | Cook: 15mins | Ready in:

Ingredients

- 4 cups chicken broth
- 1 cup water
- 1/4 teaspoon rosemary (optional)
- 1/4 teaspoon black pepper
- 1 (10 ounce) package frozen mixed vegetables
- 1 (6 ounce) box long grain white rice and wild rice, fast cooking
- 2 cups cooked turkey, chopped
- 2 (14.5 ounce) cans RED GOLD® Petite Diced Tomatoes

Direction

- In a big soup kettle, combine black pepper, rosemary, water, and broth, then set to boil. Stir in seasoning packet, a box of rice, and mixed vegetables.
- Bring back to a boil, then lower the heat. Simmer, covered, until the rice and vegetables become tender, or for 10 - 15 minutes. Stir in tomatoes and turkey, then heat thoroughly. Stir in the black pepper.

Nutrition Information

- Calories: 269 calories;
- Sodium: 1368
- Total Carbohydrate: 35.2
- Cholesterol: 42
- Protein: 19.2
- Total Fat: 5.4

779. Turkey Rice And Barley Soup

Serving: 12 servings. | Prep: 20mins | Cook: 03hours00mins | Ready in:

Ingredients

- 1 leftover turkey breast carcass (from an 8-pound turkey breast)
- 3 quarts water
- 4 teaspoons chicken bouillon granules
- 2 bay leaves
- 1/2 cup uncooked instant rice
- 1/2 cup uncooked quick-cooking barley
- 1-1/2 cups sliced carrots
- 1 cup chopped onion
- 1 cup sliced celery
- 1 garlic clove, minced
- 1 teaspoon salt
- 1/4 teaspoon pepper
- 1 cup cubed cooked turkey
- 2 tablespoons minced fresh parsley or 2 teaspoons dried parsley flakes

Direction

- In a Dutch oven, place in bay leaves, bouillon, water, and carcass, then boil. Decrease heat, then simmer, covered, for 1 1/2 hour. Take out the carcass and cool.
- Remove the turkey meat from the bones and cut into bite-sized pieces, then set aside, discarding the bones. Strain broth and skim off the fat, then throw away the bay leaves. Add in barley and rice, then bring the mixture to a boil. Decrease heat and simmer, covered, for 30 minutes.
- Stir in pepper, salt, garlic, celery, onion, and carrots, then simmer, covered, until the vegetables become tender, another 20 - 25 minutes. Add the reserved turkey meat, cubed turkey and parsley, then heat thoroughly.

Nutrition Information

- Calories:

- Protein:
- Total Fat:
- Sodium:
- Fiber:
- Total Carbohydrate:
- Cholesterol:

780. Turkey Salad

Serving: 24 | Prep: 20mins | Cook: |Ready in:

Ingredients

- 3/4 pound cooked turkey meat
- 2 stalks celery
- 2 green onions
- 1/2 red bell pepper
- 3 tablespoons mayonnaise
- 2 tablespoons prepared Dijon-style mustard
- 1 tablespoon cider vinegar
- 1 teaspoon white sugar
- 1/4 teaspoon salt

Direction

- In a blender or food processor, place red bell pepper, green onions, celery and cooked turkey meat. Finely chop ingredients using the pulse setting.
- Move turkey mixture to a medium bowl. Mix in salt, white sugar, cider vinegar, prepared Dijon-style mustard and mayonnaise. Cover the salad and keep cold in refrigerator for 8 hours or overnight before serving.

Nutrition Information

- Calories: 40 calories;
- Total Carbohydrate: 0.8
- Cholesterol: 11
- Protein: 4.2
- Total Fat: 2.1
- Sodium: 78

781. Turkey Salad Sundaes

Serving: 6 servings. | Prep: 30mins | Cook: 0mins |Ready in:

Ingredients

- 12 slices whole wheat bread, crusts removed
- Refrigerated butter-flavored spray
- 2 tablespoons grated Parmesan cheese
- 1/8 teaspoon onion powder
- SALAD:
- 3 cups cubed cooked turkey
- 1/4 cup finely chopped celery
- 1/4 cup finely chopped onion
- 1/2 cup fat-free mayonnaise
- 1/2 teaspoon seasoned salt
- 1 cup shredded lettuce
- 6 tablespoons salsa
- 1 cup (8 ounces) fat-free cottage cheese
- 2 tablespoons crumbled blue cheese
- 3 tablespoons minced fresh parsley
- 6 pitted ripe olives

Direction

- Put on a bread slice halfway atop another for every toast cup; roll to flatten. Push into jumbo muffin cups that have been coated by cooking spray. Use butter spray to spritz bread cups. Mix onion powder and Parmesan cheese; drizzle on top of cups. Bake for 13-15 minutes till the bread is toasted at 350 degrees. Let it cool down for 5 minutes prior to taking off from pan to a wire rack to totally cool off.
- To make salad, in a bowl, mix onion, celery and turkey. Mix in salt and mayonnaise; scoop into toast cups. Use lettuce and salsa to put on top. Mix cheese in; dollop on top of every serving. Use olives and parsley to garnish.

Nutrition Information

- Calories: 334 calories
- Sodium: 945mg sodium

- Fiber: 5g fiber)
- Total Carbohydrate: 32g carbohydrate (6g sugars
- Cholesterol: 60mg cholesterol
- Protein: 32g protein. Diabetic Exchanges: 3-1/2 lean meat
- Total Fat: 8g fat (3g saturated fat)

782. Turkey Salad For 50

Serving: 50 servings. | Prep: 30mins | Cook: 0mins | Ready in:

Ingredients

- 18 cups diced cooked turkey (about one 14-pound turkey)
- 8 cups thinly sliced celery
- 8 cups seedless grapes
- 18 hard-boiled large eggs, chopped
- 2 cups slivered almonds, toasted
- DRESSING:
- 1 quart Miracle Whip
- 1 pint heavy whipping cream, whipped
- 1/4 cup lemon juice
- 1/4 cup sugar
- 1 teaspoon salt
- 1/2 teaspoon pepper

Direction

- Mix almonds, eggs, grapes, celery and turkey in several small bowls or a big bowl. Mix dressing ingredients until smooth in consistency. Put on top of salad and lightly mixing. Keep chilled till serving.

Nutrition Information

- Calories: 286 calories
- Protein: 18g protein.
- Total Fat: 19g fat (5g saturated fat)
- Sodium: 247mg sodium
- Fiber: 1g fiber)

- Total Carbohydrate: 10g carbohydrate (7g sugars
- Cholesterol: 134mg cholesterol

783. Turkey Salad For 60

Serving: 60 servings. | Prep: 30mins | Cook: 05hours00mins | Ready in:

Ingredients

- 1 turkey (20 to 22 pounds)
- 4 packages (7 ounces each) uncooked ring macaroni, cooked and drained
- 3 bunches celery, thinly sliced
- 3 cans (8 ounces each) sliced water chestnuts, drained
- 2 packages (16 ounces each) frozen tiny sweet peas, thawed
- 1 large onion, finely chopped
- 2 quarts mayonnaise
- 2 tablespoons seasoned salt
- 4 cups slivered almonds, toasted

Direction

- Roast the turkey. Once cool enough to touch, take the turkey from its bones; get rid of the bones. Slice turkey meat into bite-size portions.
- Mix onion, peas, water chestnuts, celery, macaroni and turkey in several big bowls. Stir seasoned salt and mayonnaise together then mix into the salad. Let it chill for a couple of hours. Put almonds just prior to serving.

Nutrition Information

- Calories: 409 calories
- Protein: 25g protein.
- Total Fat: 31g fat (5g saturated fat)
- Sodium: 406mg sodium
- Fiber: 2g fiber)

- Total Carbohydrate: 7g carbohydrate (2g sugars
- Cholesterol: 68mg cholesterol

784. Turkey Salad With Grapes & Cashews

Serving: 4 servings. | Prep: 20mins | Cook: 0mins | Ready in:

Ingredients

- 1/4 cup mayonnaise
- 1/4 cup plain yogurt
- 1 tablespoon honey Dijon mustard
- 3 cups cubed cooked turkey
- 1 cup halved green grapes
- 2 celery ribs, chopped
- 1/2 cup chopped cashews
- 2 green onions, thinly sliced
- Lettuce leaves

Direction

- Combine mustard, yogurt and mayonnaise in a bowl. Put in green onions, cashews, celery, grapes and turkey; coat by tossing. Serve over lettuce.

Nutrition Information

- Calories: 415 calories
- Protein: 34g protein.
- Total Fat: 24g fat (5g saturated fat)
- Sodium: 348mg sodium
- Fiber: 1g fiber)
- Total Carbohydrate: 16g carbohydrate (9g sugars
- Cholesterol: 113mg cholesterol

785. Turkey Salad With Pear Dressing

Serving: 4 servings. | Prep: 25mins | Cook: 0mins | Ready in:

Ingredients

- 3 tablespoons olive oil
- 2 tablespoons lemon juice
- 1 tablespoon honey
- 1/4 teaspoon salt
- 1/4 teaspoon ground ginger
- 2 medium ripe pears, divided
- SALAD:
- 8 cups fresh arugula or baby spinach
- 2 cups cubed cooked turkey
- 1/2 cup pomegranate seeds
- 1/4 cup chopped pecans, toasted
- 1/4 cup dried cranberries
- 2 green onions, sliced
- Coarsely ground pepper

Direction

- To make dressing, in a blender, add initial 5 ingredients. Peel, cut into 2 halves and core one pear; add into blender. Cover up and run the blender until smooth in consistency.
- Peel off the skin, core and cut thinly the leftover pear. Separate arugula between four dishes; put green onions, cranberries, pecans, pomegranate seeds, sliced pear and turkey on top. Sprinkle with dressing; drizzle with pepper. Serve right away.

Nutrition Information

- Calories: 364 calories
- Fiber: 5g fiber)
- Total Carbohydrate: 31g carbohydrate (22g sugars
- Cholesterol: 71mg cholesterol
- Protein: 23g protein. Diabetic exchanges: 3 lean meat
- Total Fat: 18g fat (3g saturated fat)
- Sodium: 232mg sodium

786. Turkey Salad With Raspberries

Serving: 6 servings. | Prep: 20mins | Cook: 0mins | Ready in:

Ingredients

- 6 cups torn romaine
- 6 cups torn Bibb or Boston lettuce
- 1 can (15 ounces) mandarin oranges, drained
- 1 can (8 ounces) sliced water chestnuts, drained
- 1 cup fresh raspberries
- 1/3 cup salted sunflower kernels
- 2 tablespoons chopped chives
- 3/4 pound turkey breast tenderloin, cooked and sliced
- DRESSING:
- 1/2 cup raspberry or red wine vinegar
- 1/2 cup honey
- 2 tablespoons soy sauce
- 2 teaspoons Dijon mustard

Direction

- Toss chives, sunflower kernels, raspberries, water chestnuts, oranges and lettuces together in a large bowl.
- Distribute the salad among 6 salad plates; put turkey on top of each salad. In a jar that comes with a tight-fitting lid, combine dressing ingredients; shake properly. Drizzle dressing over salad and serve.

Nutrition Information

- Calories: 291 calories
- Fiber: 5g fiber)
- Total Carbohydrate: 47g carbohydrate (36g sugars
- Cholesterol: 28mg cholesterol
- Protein: 18g protein.
- Total Fat: 6g fat (1g saturated fat)
- Sodium: 440mg sodium

787. Turkey Sausage Bean Soup

Serving: 8 servings (2 quarts). | Prep: 15mins | Cook: 25mins | Ready in:

Ingredients

- 4 Italian turkey sausage links, casings removed
- 1 large onion, chopped
- 1 cup chopped fennel bulb
- 1 cup chopped peeled celery root or turnip
- 1 can (14-1/2 ounces) no-salt-added diced tomatoes, undrained
- 3 cups water
- 4 bay leaves
- 1 tablespoon reduced-sodium beef base
- 2 teaspoons Italian seasoning
- 1/2 teaspoon pepper
- 2 cans (15 ounces each) white kidney or cannellini beans, rinsed and drained
- Shaved Parmesan cheese, optional

Direction

- Cook celery root, fennel, onion and sausage in Dutch oven on medium heat till sausage is not pink anymore, about 4-5 minutes, breaking into crumbles; drain. Mix pepper, Italian seasoning, beef base, bay leaves, water and tomatoes in.
- Boil; lower heat. Simmer till veggies are tender, covered, about 20 minutes. Mix beans in; heat through. Discard bay leaves. Top servings with cheese if desired. For freezing: In freezer containers, freeze soup without cheese. To use, thaw partially in the fridge overnight. In a saucepan, heat through, occasionally mixing. Top with cheese if desired.

Nutrition Information

- Calories: 168 calories
- Fiber: 6g fiber)
- Total Carbohydrate: 22g carbohydrate (3g sugars
- Cholesterol: 20mg cholesterol
- Protein: 11g protein. Diabetic Exchanges: 1-1/2 starch
- Total Fat: 4g fat (1g saturated fat)
- Sodium: 585mg sodium

788. Turkey Sausage Potato Salad

Serving: 7 servings. | Prep: 30mins | Cook: 0mins | Ready in:

Ingredients

- 6 medium red potatoes, cubed
- 3 turkey Italian sausage links, casings removed
- 1/2 cup reduced-fat mayonnaise
- 1/2 cup reduced-fat sour cream
- 1 tablespoon red wine vinegar
- 1 tablespoon Dijon mustard
- 1 teaspoon dried oregano
- 3/4 teaspoon salt
- 1/8 teaspoon white pepper
- 6 green onions, sliced
- Leaf lettuce, optional

Direction

- In a large sauce pan, place potatoes and cover with water; bring to a boil. Lower the heat; cover and simmer for 15 to 20 minutes or until potatoes becomes soft. Drain and run potatoes under cold water; set aside.
- Cut sausage into bite-size pieces; put in a nonstick skillet and cook over medium heat until sausages are no longer pink. Drain and allow them to cool.
- Combine salt, pepper, oregano, mustard, vinegar, sour cream and mayonnaise in a small bowl. In a large bowl, combine onions, sausage and potatoes; pour dressing over potato mixture and toss until well coated. Cover and keep cold in refrigerator for a minimum of 2 hours. Serve in a lettuce-covered bowl if desired.

Nutrition Information

- Calories: 233 calories
- Total Carbohydrate: 27g carbohydrate (0 sugars
- Cholesterol: 31mg cholesterol
- Protein: 11g protein. Diabetic Exchanges: 1-1/2 starch
- Total Fat: 11g fat (3g saturated fat)
- Sodium: 682mg sodium
- Fiber: 3g fiber)

789. Turkey Sausage And Lentil Soup

Serving: 12 servings (3-3/4 quarts). | Prep: 25mins | Cook: 45mins | Ready in:

Ingredients

- 1 package (19-1/2 ounces) Italian turkey sausage links, casings removed
- 1 large onion, chopped
- 2 celery ribs, chopped
- 1 medium carrot, chopped
- 2 garlic cloves, minced
- 1 bay leaf
- 1/2 teaspoon fennel seed
- 1/2 teaspoon dried oregano
- 1/2 teaspoon dried thyme
- 1/2 teaspoon pepper
- 1/8 teaspoon crushed red pepper flakes, optional
- 2 cups dried brown lentils, rinsed

- 2 cans (14-1/2 ounces each) no-salt-added diced tomatoes, undrained
- 2 cartons (32 ounces each) reduced-sodium chicken broth
- Fat-free plain Greek yogurt and minced fresh parsley, optional

Direction

- Over medium high heat, cook and crumble sausage for 5-7 minutes in a 6-qt. stockpot until it is not pink anymore. Take out the sausage using a slotted spoon.
- Sauté carrot, celery and onion for 4-6 minutes in the same pot until tender. Mix in seasonings and garlic. Cook and stir for about a minute. Mix in broth, tomatoes, lentils, and sausage and let it boil. Lower the heat. Let it simmer with cover, while stirring regularly, for 30-40 minutes until lentils becomes tender. Discard the bay leaf.
- In a blender, put in 5 cups of soup. Let it slightly cool. Put on cover and process in the blender until it becomes smooth. Transfer to the pot again and heat it through. Put parsley and yogurt on top of servings if you want. You also have the option to freeze the soup. Freeze it in freezer containers and slightly thaw overnight in the refrigerator to use. In a saucepan, heat it through while stirring from time to time. If necessary, add a small amount of broth.

Nutrition Information

- Calories: 187 calories
- Protein: 15g protein. Diabetic Exchanges: 1-1/2 starch
- Total Fat: 3g fat (1g saturated fat)
- Sodium: 639mg sodium
- Fiber: 5g fiber)
- Total Carbohydrate: 25g carbohydrate (4g sugars
- Cholesterol: 17mg cholesterol

790. Turkey Shrimp Salad

Serving: 20-22 servings. | Prep: 15mins | Cook: 0mins | Ready in:

Ingredients

- 12 cups cooked elbow macaroni
- 6 cups cubed cooked turkey
- 2 cups cooked deveined salad shrimp
- 1 cup thinly sliced celery
- 1/2 cup thinly sliced green onions
- 1 can (20 ounces) pineapple chunks, drained
- 1 can (15 ounces) sliced peaches, drained and diced
- 1 can (14 ounces) sweetened condensed milk
- 1/2 cup lemon juice
- 1/2 cup vegetable oil
- 1/4 cup Dijon mustard
- 1/2 teaspoon salt
- 1/8 teaspoon lemon-pepper seasoning
- hard-boiled large eggs, sliced, optional
- Orange slices, optional

Direction

- Mix the first 7 ingredients in a big bowl. Mix in a small bowl the lemon-pepper, salt, mustard, oil, lemon juice, and milk; stir well. Place on salad; then toss to coat. Let it chill for a minimum of 2 hours, covered. Decorate with oranges and eggs if wished.

Nutrition Information

- Calories:
- Sodium:
- Fiber:
- Total Carbohydrate:
- Cholesterol:
- Protein:
- Total Fat:

791. Turkey Soup

Serving: | Prep: | Cook: | Ready in:

Ingredients

- 2 Turkey Drumsticks, cooked
- 2 Turkey Wings, cooked
- 8 quarts Chicken Stock
- 2 Onions, chopped
- 1 Bay Leaf
- 1 tablespoon Salt
- 1 teaspoon Pepper
- 4 sprigs Parsley
- 1/2 teaspoon Thyme
- 2 cloves Garlic, chopped
- 4 Carrots, thinly sliced
- 1 bunch Celery, thinly sliced
- 28 ounces Canned Chopped Tomatoes
- 2 tablespoons Fresh Dill
- 1 cup Rice

Direction

- In a large soup kettle, combine the turkey pieces and broth. Simmer the mixture for 1 hour.
- Get the turkey bones and remove the meat from its bones; reserve.
- Add the pepper, thyme, garlic, salt, bay leaf, onions, and parsley. Let the mixture boil and simmer it for 1 more hour.
- Add the remaining ingredients except for the turkey meat. Simmer the mixture for 35-45 more minutes. Add the turkey meat and heat the mixture through.

Nutrition Information

792. Turkey Soup With Slickers

Serving: 8-10 servings (2-1/2 quarts). | Prep: 20mins | Cook: 02hours30mins | Ready in:

Ingredients

- 1 leftover turkey carcass (from a 14-pound turkey)
- 5 quarts water
- 1/2 cup chopped onion
- 1/2 cup chopped carrot
- 1/2 cup chopped celery
- 3 tablespoons dried parsley flakes
- 2 teaspoons salt
- 1/2 teaspoon pepper
- 2 bay leaves
- 1 egg
- 2-1/2 to 3 cups all-purpose flour
- 1/2 teaspoon dill weed
- 1/2 teaspoon poultry seasoning
- 1 cup frozen peas

Direction

- Add the first 9 of the ingredients into a soup kettle or Dutch oven and slowly boil, then skim off the foam. Lower heat, cover, and allow to simmer for 2 hours, then discard the bay leaves. Remove the carcass and put aside until cool enough to handle, then, remove the meat from the bones. Throw away the bones and cut the meat into bite-sized pieces, then put aside.
- Beat together egg and 1 cup broth in a big bowl, then stir enough flour to make a stiff dough. Turn out onto a floured surface and knead until smooth, or 8 - 10 times. Divide the dough into half and roll each piece 1/8 inches thick, then cut into 2x1/4-inch strips.
- Add poultry seasoning and dill to the remaining broth and allow to gently boil. Drop the slickers into the broth and cook, covered, until tender, or for 30 - 35 minutes. Add the reserved turkey and peas, then heat through.

Nutrition Information

- Calories:
- Protein:
- Total Fat:
- Sodium:
- Fiber:
- Total Carbohydrate:
- Cholesterol:

793. Turkey Vegetable Barley Soup

Serving: 10 servings (3 quarts). | Prep: 15mins | Cook: 55mins | Ready in:

Ingredients

- 2 cans (one 49-1/2 ounces, one 14-1/2 ounces) chicken broth
- 4 cups cubed cooked turkey
- 2 medium carrots, halved and thinly sliced
- 1 large potato, peeled and cubed
- 2 cups frozen cut green beans
- 1 medium green pepper, chopped
- 1 celery rib, chopped
- 3 garlic cloves, minced
- 1/2 cup uncooked medium pearl barley
- 2 bay leaves
- 1 teaspoon dried thyme
- 1 teaspoon rubbed sage
- 1/2 teaspoon salt

Direction

- Combine all of the ingredients in a Dutch oven, and boil. Decrease heat and simmer without a cover until vegetables and barley become tender, about 45 - 55 minutes, then discard the bay leaves.
- This soup can freeze up to 3 months.

Nutrition Information

- Calories:
- Total Carbohydrate:
- Cholesterol:
- Protein:
- Total Fat:
- Sodium:
- Fiber:

794. Turkey Vegetable Pasta Salad

Serving: 12-14 servings. | Prep: 25mins | Cook: 0mins | Ready in:

Ingredients

- DRESSING:
- 1 cup vegetable oil
- 1/2 cup red wine or cider vinegar
- 1/4 cup honey
- 1/4 cup Dijon mustard
- SALAD:
- 1 package (12 ounces) tri-colored spiral pasta
- 3 cups broccoli florets
- 3 cups cubed cooked turkey breast
- 1/2 cup thinly sliced green onions
- 1/2 cup chopped sweet red pepper

Direction

- In a small bowl, mix all dressing; put aside. Based on the instruction on package, cook pasta; drain off. Transfer into a big bowl. While pasta is warm, mix in half cup dressing. Keep covered and chilled. Put in leftover dressing, red pepper, onions, turkey and broccoli; coat by tossing. Keep it covered and chilled 3-4 hours or overnight.

Nutrition Information

- Calories: 302 calories
- Cholesterol: 26mg cholesterol
- Protein: 13g protein.

- Total Fat: 17g fat (2g saturated fat)
- Sodium: 132mg sodium
- Fiber: 1g fiber)
- Total Carbohydrate: 26g carbohydrate (6g sugars

795. Turkey White Chili

Serving: 6 servings (6 cups). | Prep: 15mins | Cook: 01hours10mins | Ready in:

Ingredients

- 2 tablespoons canola oil
- 1/2 cup chopped onion
- 3 garlic cloves, minced
- 2-1/2 teaspoons ground cumin
- 1 pound boneless skinless turkey breast, cut into 1-inch cubes
- 1/2 pound ground turkey
- 3 cups chicken broth
- 1 can (15 ounces) garbanzo beans or chickpeas, rinsed and drained
- 1 tablespoon minced jalapeno pepper
- 1/2 teaspoon dried marjoram
- 1/4 teaspoon dried savory
- 2 teaspoons cornstarch
- 1 tablespoon water
- Shredded Monterey Jack cheese and sliced red onion, optional

Direction

- Use a Dutch oven or a big saucepan to heat canola oil in medium heat and add the onion, then sauté for about 5 minutes until tender. Add in the garlic to cook for a minute more. Stir in the cumin and cook for 5 minutes. Add the turkey, then cook and crumble the ground turkey until it is no longer pink. Add savory, marjoram, jalapeno, beans, and broth, then allow to boil. Lower the heat. Simmer while covered for 45 minutes, occasionally stirring.
- Cook, uncovered, for 15 more minutes. Dissolve the cornstarch in water and stir into the chili, then boil. Cook while stirring for 2 minutes. If you want, you can serve this with red onion slices and cheese.

Nutrition Information

- Calories: 288 calories
- Protein: 29g protein. Diabetic Exchanges: 3 lean meat
- Total Fat: 12g fat (2g saturated fat)
- Sodium: 635mg sodium
- Fiber: 3g fiber)
- Total Carbohydrate: 15g carbohydrate (3g sugars
- Cholesterol: 73mg cholesterol

796. Turkey Wild Rice Soup

Serving: 9 | Prep: 15mins | Cook: 1hours | Ready in:

Ingredients

- 3 (10.5 ounce) cans condensed chicken broth
- 2 cups water
- 1/2 cup finely chopped green onions
- 1/2 cup uncooked wild rice
- 8 slices bacon
- 1/2 cup margarine
- 3/4 cup all-purpose flour
- 1/2 teaspoon salt
- 1/4 teaspoon poultry seasoning
- 1/8 teaspoon ground black pepper
- 2 cups half-and-half cream
- 1 1/2 cups cooked, diced turkey meat
- 2 tablespoons dry sherry

Direction

- Combine wild rice, green onions, water, and chicken broth in a large pot over medium heat. Bring to a boil then lower heat and simmer for 35 to 40 minutes until rice is tender.
- In the meantime, cook bacon in a big skillet

over medium heat until it is crisp. Let it cool then crumble. Put aside.
- When the rice is soft, melt margarine in a medium-sized saucepan over medium-low heat. Mix in pepper, poultry seasoning, salt and flour all at once. Cook and mix until it is bubbly and smooth. Mix in half-and-half and cook for 2 minutes until thick. Mix in half-and-half mixture into rice mixture. Mix in sherry, turkey and bacon. Heat through and serve.

Nutrition Information

- Calories: 409 calories;
- Total Fat: 29.8
- Sodium: 1137
- Total Carbohydrate: 17
- Cholesterol: 56
- Protein: 17.9

797. Turkey And Dumpling Soup

Serving: 8 servings. | Prep: 10mins | Cook: 20mins | Ready in:

Ingredients

- 1 tablespoon olive oil
- 2 celery ribs, chopped
- 1/2 cup chopped onion
- 1-1/2 pounds red potatoes (about 5 medium), cut into 1/2-inch cubes
- 3-1/2 cups frozen mixed vegetables (about 16 ounces)
- 1/2 teaspoon pepper
- 1/2 teaspoon dried thyme
- 2 cartons (32 ounces each) reduced-sodium chicken broth
- 2-1/2 cups coarsely shredded cooked turkey or chicken
- 2 cups biscuit/baking mix
- 2/3 cup 2% milk

Direction

- Put oil in a 6-qt stockpot and heat it over medium heat. Sauté onion and celery for 3-4 minutes until tender. Mix in mixed vegetables, broth, seasonings, and potatoes. Bring the mixture to a boil. Reduce the heat and cook the mixture for 8-10 minutes, covered until the potatoes are almost tender. Add the turkey and simmer the mixture.
- In the meantime, mix milk and baking mix until it forms a soft dough. Drop the mixture by tablespoonfuls on top of the simmering soup. Cook the mixture over low heat, covered, for about 8-10 minutes until the inserted toothpick inside the dumpling comes out clean.

Nutrition Information

- Calories: 350 calories
- Cholesterol: 46mg cholesterol
- Protein: 23g protein.
- Total Fat: 8g fat (2g saturated fat)
- Sodium: 1036mg sodium
- Fiber: 6g fiber)
- Total Carbohydrate: 47g carbohydrate (7g sugars

798. Turkey And Fruit Salad

Serving: 5 servings. | Prep: 25mins | Cook: 0mins | Ready in:

Ingredients

- 1/4 cup fat-free plain yogurt
- 1/4 cup reduced-fat mayonnaise
- 1 tablespoon honey
- 1 tablespoon spicy brown mustard
- 1/2 teaspoon dried marjoram
- 1/8 teaspoon ground ginger
- 3 cups cubed cooked turkey breast
- 1 large red apple, finely chopped

- 2 celery ribs, thinly sliced
- 1/2 cup dried cranberries
- 1/4 cup chopped walnuts, toasted

Direction

- Combine initial 6 ingredients. Mix the leftover ingredients in a big bowl. Mix in yogurt mixture. Keep chilled in the refrigerator, while covered, till serving.

Nutrition Information

- Calories: 278 calories
- Sodium: 208mg sodium
- Fiber: 2g fiber)
- Total Carbohydrate: 23g carbohydrate (17g sugars
- Cholesterol: 77mg cholesterol
- Protein: 28g protein. Diabetic Exchanges: 3 lean meat
- Total Fat: 9g fat (1g saturated fat)

799. Turkey And Ham Salad With Greens

Serving: 4-6 servings. | Prep: 15mins | Cook: 0mins | Ready in:

Ingredients

- 1/4 cup vegetable oil
- 2 tablespoons white wine vinegar, divided
- 1/4 teaspoon salt, divided
- 1/4 teaspoon pepper, divided
- 4 cups thinly sliced salad greens
- 1/3 cup mayonnaise
- 4 teaspoons spicy brown mustard
- 1/4 teaspoon dried thyme
- 2-1/2 cups cubed cooked turkey
- 2 cups julienned fully cooked ham
- 1 cup halved seedless green grapes
- 1/4 cup thinly sliced green onions
- 1/4 cup slivered almonds, toasted

Direction

- Mix 1/8 tsp. of pepper, 1/8 tsp. of salt and 1 tbsp. of vinegar; toss with greens. Arrange on an individual plates or a platter. Mix pepper, salt, leftover vinegar, thyme, mustard and mayonnaise in a bowl. Put in onions, grapes, ham and turkey; coat by tossing. Scoop on top of greens. Use almonds to garnish.

Nutrition Information

- Calories: 401 calories
- Protein: 27g protein.
- Total Fat: 28g fat (5g saturated fat)
- Sodium: 856mg sodium
- Fiber: 2g fiber)
- Total Carbohydrate: 9g carbohydrate (5g sugars
- Cholesterol: 74mg cholesterol

800. Turkey And Vegetable Barley Soup

Serving: 6 servings. | Prep: 10mins | Cook: 20mins | Ready in:

Ingredients

- 1 tablespoon canola oil
- 5 medium carrots, chopped
- 1 medium onion, chopped
- 2/3 cup quick-cooking barley
- 6 cups reduced-sodium chicken broth
- 2 cups cubed cooked turkey breast
- 2 cups fresh baby spinach
- 1/2 teaspoon pepper

Direction

- Use a large saucepan to heat oil on medium-high heat and add onion and carrots, then cook, stirring, for 4 - 5 minutes or until the carrots become tender-crisp.

- Stir in broth and barley, then boil. Turn down the heat and simmer while covered for 10 - 15 minutes or until the barley and carrots become tender. Stir in pepper, spinach, and turkey, heating the soup through.

Nutrition Information

- Calories: 208 calories
- Sodium: 662mg sodium
- Fiber: 6g fiber)
- Total Carbohydrate: 23g carbohydrate (4g sugars
- Cholesterol: 37mg cholesterol
- Protein: 21g protein. Diabetic Exchanges: 2 lean meat
- Total Fat: 4g fat (1g saturated fat)

801. Turkey And Wild Rice Soup

Serving: 8 servings (2-1/2 quarts). | Prep: 20mins | Cook: 01hours05mins | Ready in:

Ingredients

- 1/2 cup uncooked wild rice
- 4 cups water
- 1/2 cup butter, cubed
- 8 ounces red potatoes (about 2 medium), chopped
- 1 medium onion, chopped
- 1 celery rib, chopped
- 1 medium carrot, chopped
- 2 garlic cloves, minced
- 1/2 cup all-purpose flour
- 3 cups chicken broth
- 2 cups half-and-half cream
- 1 teaspoon salt
- 1/2 teaspoon dried rosemary, crushed
- 2 cups cubed cooked turkey or chicken

Direction

- Mix water and rice in a saucepan. Bring the mixture to a boil over high heat before reducing the heat. Cover and simmer the mixture for 30 minutes.
- Put butter in a Dutch oven and heat it over medium heat. Add the carrot, onion, celery, and potatoes. Cook and stir the mixture for 6-8 minutes until almost tender. Add the garlic and cook the mixture for 1 minute.
- Mix in flour and cook for 2 minutes until well-blended. Stir in undrained rice and broth gradually. Bring the mixture to a boil over medium-high heat. Cook and stir the mixture for 1-2 minutes until slightly thickened.
- Add the rosemary, cream, and salt. Bring the mixture to a boil. Simmer for 15-20 minutes, uncovered and stirring occasionally until the rice is tender. Mix in turkey until heated through.

Nutrition Information

- Calories: 338 calories
- Sodium: 832mg sodium
- Fiber: 2g fiber)
- Total Carbohydrate: 23g carbohydrate (4g sugars
- Cholesterol: 98mg cholesterol
- Protein: 16g protein.
- Total Fat: 19g fat (12g saturated fat)

802. Turkey Berry Stuffing Balls

Serving: 4-6 servings. | Prep: 20mins | Cook: 35mins | Ready in:

Ingredients

- 1 pound ground turkey
- 1 celery rib, finely chopped
- 1/4 cup finely chopped onion
- 2 eggs, beaten
- 1-1/4 cups chicken broth

- 4 cups seasoned stuffing croutons
- 3/4 cup fresh or frozen cranberries, halved

Direction

- Cook onion, celery, and turkey in a big frying pan over medium heat until the meat is not pink anymore; drain. Mix stuffing, broth, and eggs together in a big bowl. Let sit for 5 minutes. Mix in cranberries and the turkey mixture.
- Form into 12 balls and put on an oiled 11x7-in. baking dish. Bake without a cover at 325° until heated completely, about 35-40 minutes.

Nutrition Information

- Calories: 314 calories
- Total Carbohydrate: 28g carbohydrate (4g sugars
- Cholesterol: 122mg cholesterol
- Protein: 18g protein.
- Total Fat: 14g fat (4g saturated fat)
- Sodium: 770mg sodium
- Fiber: 3g fiber)

803. Turkey Blue Cheese Pasta Salad

Serving: 12 servings. | Prep: 15mins | Cook: 0mins | Ready in:

Ingredients

- 1 package (16 ounces) pasta shells, cooked, drained and cooled
- 3 cups cubed cooked turkey or chicken
- 1 cup diced green pepper
- 1/4 cup chopped onion
- 1 cup blue cheese salad dressing
- 1/4 cup sour cream
- 2 teaspoons celery seed
- 1/4 teaspoon pepper
- 1/2 teaspoon salt, optional

Direction

- In a large bowl, mix onion, green pepper, turkey and pasta. Mix pepper, celery seed, sour cream, and dressing and salt if you want in a small bowl; put on top of salad and toss. Serve right away.

Nutrition Information

- Calories: 213 calories
- Protein: 11g protein. Diabetic Exchanges: 2 starch
- Total Fat: 2g fat (0 saturated fat)
- Sodium: 240mg sodium
- Fiber: 0 fiber)
- Total Carbohydrate: 38g carbohydrate (0 sugars
- Cholesterol: 22mg cholesterol

804. Turkey Melon Pasta Salad

Serving: 4 servings. | Prep: 10mins | Cook: 15mins | Ready in:

Ingredients

- 2 cups uncooked bow tie pasta
- 1-1/2 cups cubed cooked turkey breast
- 1-1/2 cups diced seedless watermelon
- 1/2 cup sliced celery
- 2 tablespoons chopped green onion
- 1/4 cup fat-free plain yogurt
- 2 tablespoons reduced-fat mayonnaise
- 2 tablespoons lime juice
- 1-3/4 teaspoons sugar

Direction

- Follow the package directions to cook the pasta. At the same time, mix together the onion, celery, watermelon and turkey in a big bowl, then set aside.

- Whisk together the sugar, lime juice, mayonnaise and yogurt in a small bowl until smooth. Drain pasta and rinse under cold water, then stir into turkey mixture. Drizzle the yogurt mixture over and toss to coat well. Chill until serving.

Nutrition Information

- Calories:
- Fiber:
- Total Carbohydrate:
- Cholesterol:
- Protein:
- Total Fat:
- Sodium:

805. Turkey White Bean Soup

Serving: 6 servings (2 quarts). | Prep: 20mins | Cook: 40mins | Ready in:

Ingredients

- 2 garlic cloves, minced
- 2 teaspoons olive oil
- 1/2 teaspoon dried rosemary, crushed
- 1/4 teaspoon crushed red pepper flakes
- 1 can (28 ounces) whole tomatoes in puree, cut up
- 1 can (14-1/2 ounces) reduced-sodium chicken broth
- 2 cups shredded carrots
- 2 cans (15 ounces each) white kidney or cannellini beans, rinsed and drained
- 1 package (6 ounces) fresh baby spinach, chopped
- 1-1/2 cups cubed cooked turkey breast
- Shredded Parmesan cheese, optional

Direction

- Cook garlic with oil in a big saucepan on medium heat for 1 minute. Add pepper flakes and rosemary and cook for 1 minute longer.
- Stir in carrots, broth, and tomatoes, then set to boil. Decrease heat and simmer, covered, for 15 minutes. Stir in turkey, spinach, and beans, then bring back to a boil. Decrease the heat and simmer while covered for 10 minutes longer. You can serve the soup with cheese.

Nutrition Information

- Calories: 233 calories
- Sodium: 893mg sodium
- Fiber: 9g fiber)
- Total Carbohydrate: 32g carbohydrate (6g sugars
- Cholesterol: 30mg cholesterol
- Protein: 20g protein.
- Total Fat: 3g fat (0 saturated fat)

806. Two Bean Turkey Salad

Serving: 8-10 servings. | Prep: 20mins | Cook: 0mins | Ready in:

Ingredients

- 12 cups torn fresh spinach
- 2 cups cubed cooked turkey
- 2 cups fresh broccoli florets
- 1 can (15-1/2 ounces) black-eyed peas or navy beans, rinsed and drained
- 1 can (15 ounces) garbanzo beans or chickpeas, rinsed and drained
- 1 large unpeeled red apple, cubed
- 1/2 cup coarsely chopped walnuts
- 1/3 cup dried cranberries
- 3/4 cup ranch salad dressing
- 1/2 cup apricot preserves
- 1 teaspoon Dijon mustard
- 3/4 teaspoon ground ginger

Direction

- Toss the first eight ingredients in a large salad bowl. In a small bowl, put ginger, mustard, preserves, and salad dressing, mix until well blended. Pour dressing over salad and toss until well coated.

Nutrition Information

- Calories: 323 calories
- Total Carbohydrate: 33g carbohydrate (17g sugars
- Cholesterol: 24mg cholesterol
- Protein: 15g protein.
- Total Fat: 16g fat (2g saturated fat)
- Sodium: 357mg sodium
- Fiber: 5g fiber)

807. White Bean Bisque

Serving: 2 servings. | Prep: 15mins | Cook: 20mins | Ready in:

Ingredients

- 1/4 cup shredded Parmesan cheese
- Cayenne pepper
- 1/4 pound Johnsonville® Ground Mild Italian sausage
- 2 tablespoons chopped onion
- 1 teaspoon olive oil
- 1 garlic clove, minced
- 1 can (15 ounces) white kidney or cannellini beans, rinsed and drained
- 1 cup chicken broth
- 1/4 cup heavy whipping cream
- 2 teaspoons sherry, optional
- 1 teaspoon minced fresh parsley
- 1/8 teaspoon salt
- 1/8 teaspoon dried thyme

Direction

- On a cookie sheet lined with a parchment paper, put 6 mounds of Parmesan cheese 3 in. apart. Spread the mounds into 1-1/2-in. circles. Use a dash of cayenne to scatter over the mounds. Bake for 5-6 minutes at 400°, until the mounds turn pale golden brown. Let cool.
- Cook onion and sausage in oil in a saucepan over medium heat until the meat is not pink anymore; drain. Take out and keep warm.
- Sauté garlic in the same pan until soft, about 1-2 minutes. Mix in a dash of cayenne, thyme, salt, parsley, sherry if desired, cream, broth, and beans. Boil it. Lower the heat, simmer without a cover until completely heated, about 12-15 minutes. Let cool slightly.
- Move to a blender. Put the lid on and blend on high until nearly blended. Put in the soup bowls, use Parmesan crisps and the sausage mixture to scatter over.

Nutrition Information

- Calories: 440 calories
- Total Fat: 22g fat (11g saturated fat)
- Sodium: 1256mg sodium
- Fiber: 8g fiber)
- Total Carbohydrate: 34g carbohydrate (2g sugars
- Cholesterol: 78mg cholesterol
- Protein: 24g protein.

808. White Bean Sausage Soup

Serving: 2 servings. | Prep: 15mins | Cook: 20mins | Ready in:

Ingredients

- 1/4 cup shredded Parmesan cheese
- Cayenne pepper
- 1 Italian turkey sausage link, casing removed
- 2 tablespoons chopped onion
- 1 teaspoon olive oil
- 1 garlic clove, minced
- 1 can (15 ounces) white kidney or cannellini beans, rinsed and drained

- 1 cup reduced-sodium chicken broth
- 1/4 cup heavy whipping cream
- 2 teaspoons sherry, optional
- 1 teaspoon minced fresh parsley
- 1/8 teaspoon salt
- 1/8 teaspoon dried thyme

Direction

- On a parchment paper-lined baking sheet, scoop cheese into six mounds and set them 3 inches apart. Form into circles measuring 1 and a half inch. Season with a dash of cayenne. Bake at 400° F until it becomes light golden brown in color, about 5-6 minutes. Let it cool.
- Over medium heat in a big saucepan, cook onion and sausage in oil until the meat is not pink anymore. Drain the sausage and remove from the pan to keep warm.
- Sauté garlic in the same saucepan until it becomes tender, about a minute. Mix in a dash of cayenne, thyme, salt, parsley, sherry if you want, cream, broth and beans. Let it boil. Lower the heat. Without cover, simmer until it is heated through, about 12 to 15 minutes. Let it slightly cool.
- Move it to a blender. Process on high heat while covered until it is nearly blended. Put into soup bowls. Drizzle with Parmesan crisps and sausage mixture.

Nutrition Information

- Calories: 425 calories
- Protein: 23g protein.
- Total Fat: 22g fat (10g saturated fat)
- Sodium: 1218mg sodium
- Fiber: 8g fiber)
- Total Carbohydrate: 33g carbohydrate (1g sugars
- Cholesterol: 82mg cholesterol

809. White Bean Turkey Chili

Serving: 12 servings. | Prep: 10mins | Cook: 01hours05mins | Ready in:

Ingredients

- 1-1/2 pounds lean ground turkey
- 2 medium onions, chopped
- 1-1/2 teaspoons dried oregano
- 1-1/2 teaspoons ground cumin
- 1 can (28 ounces) diced tomatoes, undrained
- 3 cups beef broth
- 1 can (8 ounces) tomato sauce
- 1 tablespoon chili powder
- 1 tablespoon baking cocoa
- 2 bay leaves
- 1 teaspoon salt
- 1/4 teaspoon ground cinnamon
- 3 cans (15 ounces each) white kidney beans or 15 ounces cannellini beans, rinsed and drained

Direction

- Cook onions and turkey in a big soup kettle or a Dutch oven over medium heat until the meat is not pink anymore; drain. Add cumin and oregano; stir and cook for another 1 minute. Mix in cinnamon, salt, bay leaves, cocoa, chili powder, tomato sauce, broth, and tomatoes. Boil it. Lower the heat, put a cover on and simmer for 45 minutes. Add beans, cook through. Dispose the bay leaves.

Nutrition Information

- Calories: 276 calories
- Fiber: 13g fiber)
- Total Carbohydrate: 34g carbohydrate (0 sugars
- Cholesterol: 45mg cholesterol
- Protein: 22g protein. Diabetic Exchanges: 2 starch
- Total Fat: 6g fat (1g saturated fat)
- Sodium: 948mg sodium

810. White Bean And Chicken Chili

Serving: 6 servings. | Prep: 10mins | Cook: 10mins | Ready in:

Ingredients

- 3 cans (15 ounces each) cannellini beans, undrained
- 1 can (4 ounces) chopped green chilies
- 3 teaspoons chicken bouillon granules
- 3 teaspoons ground cumin
- 2 cups water
- 3 cups cubed cooked chicken or turkey
- Minced fresh cilantro, optional

Direction

- Mix the initial 5 ingredients, in a big saucepan; boil. Lower heat; without cover, allow to simmer for 2 to 3 minutes to let flavors to incorporate, mixing from time to time.
- Mix in chicken; heat through. Put cilantro over, if wished. Freeze choice: in freezer containers, freeze cooled chili. Thaw in refrigerator in part overnight to use. In a saucepan, heat through, mixing from time to time and putting a bit water if needed.

Nutrition Information

- Calories: 323 calories
- Protein: 34g protein.
- Total Fat: 6g fat (1g saturated fat)
- Sodium: 1113mg sodium
- Fiber: 10g fiber)
- Total Carbohydrate: 34g carbohydrate (3g sugars
- Cholesterol: 63mg cholesterol

811. White Christmas Chili

Serving: 12-14 servings (3 quarts). | Prep: 20mins | Cook: 01hours45mins | Ready in:

Ingredients

- 1 pound dried navy beans
- 6 cups turkey or chicken broth
- 1 cup chopped onion
- 4 garlic cloves, minced
- 1 teaspoon white pepper
- 1/2 teaspoon crushed red pepper flakes
- 1/4 to 1/2 teaspoon curry powder
- 1/4 teaspoon ground cumin
- 2 pounds turkey or chicken breast, cooked and cubed
- 1 can (15-1/4 ounces) white sweet corn
- 1 cup heavy whipping cream
- Chopped green and sweet red peppers, optional

Direction

- In a Dutch oven or big saucepan, put beans; submerge in water. Allow to boil for 2 minutes. Take off heat and immerse till beans are softened for 1 to 4 hours. Drain and wash beans; put back to the pan. Put seasonings, garlic, onion and broth.
- Cover and let simmer till beans are tender for 1-1/2 hours. Put corn and turkey; allow to simmer for 15 minutes. Just prior serving put cream; heat through. Top each serving with peppers if wished.

Nutrition Information

- Calories:
- Cholesterol:
- Protein:
- Total Fat:
- Sodium:
- Fiber:
- Total Carbohydrate:

812. White Turkey Chili

Serving: 6 | Prep: 20mins | Cook: 30mins | Ready in:

Ingredients

- 1 tablespoon olive oil
- 1 1/2 cups chopped onion
- 3 cloves garlic, minced
- 2 teaspoons dried oregano
- 1 1/2 teaspoons ground cumin
- 1/2 teaspoon ground ginger
- 1/2 cup low-sodium chicken broth
- 1/2 cup dry white wine
- 1 bay leaf
- 2 cups shredded cooked turkey
- 2 cups white kidney beans (cannellini), undrained
- 2 fresh jalapeno peppers, chopped
- 1 1/2 cups shredded Monterey Jack cheese
- 1/2 teaspoon salt
- 1/2 teaspoon coarsely ground black pepper
- 2 tablespoons lime juice

Direction

- In a skillet, heat olive oil on medium heat. Cook onion in the oil for 5 minutes till onion is translucent and soft. Mix ginger, cumin, oregano and garlic in. cook for 1 more minute. Put white wine and chicken broth in. Add bay leaf. Cook till slightly reduced for 5-8 minutes, uncovered.
- Mix jalapeno, beans and turkey in. Simmer, occasionally mixing, for 10 minutes, uncovered.
- To thicken sauce, mash 1/4 beans with a back of spoon. Lower heat to low. 1/2 cup at a time, start mixing cheese in. Mix till cheese is melted completely. Season with pepper and salt. Take off heat. Mix lime juice in. Serve while hot.

Nutrition Information

- Calories: 315 calories;
- Protein: 25
- Total Fat: 13.8
- Sodium: 571
- Total Carbohydrate: 18.5
- Cholesterol: 61

813. Wild Rice Stuffing

Serving: 8-10 servings. | Prep: 02hours15mins | Cook: 25mins | Ready in:

Ingredients

- Turkey giblets
- 4 cups water
- 1 package (6 ounces) long grain and wild rice mix
- 1 celery rib, chopped
- 1 small onion, chopped
- 1/2 cup butter
- 2-1/2 cups crushed seasoned stuffing
- 1-1/2 cups chicken broth

Direction

- You can remove the liver from giblets if you want. In a saucepan, put water and giblets. Put a cover on and simmer until soft, about 2 hours.
- In the meantime, cook the rice as the package directs. Sauté onion and celery in butter in a small skillet; add to the rice. Strain and dice the giblets. Mix giblets, broth, and stuffing into the rice.
- Put into a non-oiled 1-1/2-qt. baking plate. Bake without a cover at 350° until heated completely, about 25-30 minutes.

Nutrition Information

- Calories: 231 calories
- Protein: 9g protein.
- Total Fat: 11g fat (6g saturated fat)
- Sodium: 685mg sodium

- Fiber: 1g fiber)
- Total Carbohydrate: 25g carbohydrate (2g sugars
- Cholesterol: 93mg cholesterol

814. Wild Rice Turkey Salad

Serving: 6-7 servings. | Prep: 10mins | Cook: 0mins | Ready in:

Ingredients

- 3 cups cooked wild rice
- 3 cups cubed cooked turkey
- 1/3 cup chopped green onions
- 1/3 cup chopped celery
- 1 can (8 ounces) sliced water chestnuts, drained and halved
- 2/3 cup mayonnaise
- 2/3 cup sour cream
- 1 teaspoon salt
- 1/2 teaspoon white pepper
- 1/2 teaspoon dill weed
- 1 cup cashews, divided
- 1 cup halved seedless red grapes

Direction

- Mix water chestnuts, celery, onions, turkey and rice in a big bowl. Mix the dill, pepper, salt, sour cream and mayonnaise; put on top of salad and coat by lightly mixing. Keep it covered and let chill in the refrigerator for no less than 2 hours.
- Chop coarsely three quarters cup cashews. Just prior to serving, mix chopped cashews and grapes into salad. Use the leftover cashews to garnish.

Nutrition Information

- Calories: 544 calories
- Protein: 26g protein.
- Total Fat: 35g fat (8g saturated fat)
- Sodium: 661mg sodium
- Fiber: 3g fiber)
- Total Carbohydrate: 30g carbohydrate (8g sugars
- Cholesterol: 68mg cholesterol

815. Wild Rice And Turkey Salad

Serving: 9 servings. | Prep: 15mins | Cook: 0mins | Ready in:

Ingredients

- 4 cups torn fresh spinach
- 2 cups cubed cooked turkey breast
- 2 cups cooked wild rice
- 1 medium onion, chopped
- 1 cup sliced fresh mushrooms
- 2 medium tomatoes, chopped
- 1 jar (2 ounces) chopped pimientos, drained
- 1 bottle (8 ounces) Italian salad dressing

Direction

- Mix the initial 7 ingredients in a big bowl. Put in dressing just prior to serving; coat by tossing.

Nutrition Information

- Calories: 157 calories
- Cholesterol: 10mg cholesterol
- Protein: 14g protein. Diabetic Exchanges: 1 starch
- Total Fat: 2g fat (0 saturated fat)
- Sodium: 71mg sodium
- Fiber: 0 fiber)
- Total Carbohydrate: 21g carbohydrate (0 sugars

816. Williamsburg Inn Turkey Soup

Serving: 4 to 4-1/2 quarts. | Prep: 15mins | Cook: 30mins | Ready in:

Ingredients

- 1 turkey carcass (from a 12- to 14-pound turkey)
- 4 quarts water
- 3 large onions, finely chopped
- 3 celery ribs, finely chopped
- 2 large carrots, finely chopped
- 1/4 cup uncooked long grain rice
- 1 cup butter, cubed
- 1-1/2 cups all-purpose flour
- 1 pint half-and-half cream
- 3 cups diced cooked turkey
- 1/2 teaspoon poultry seasoning, optional
- Salt and pepper to taste

Direction

- Cook the turkey carcass with water in a big kettle enough to make 3 quarts of stock. Remove the bones and set aside the turkey meat for the soup. Strain the stock and reserve. Combine 1-quart stock, rice, carrots, celery, and onions in a big saucepan. Cook for 20 minutes and put aside.
- Melt butter in a big soup kettle and stir in flour until it becomes smooth. Add in the remaining 2 quarts of stock and cream, then set to boil. Cook, stirring, for 2 minutes or until the soup thickens. Stir in vegetable mixture and the reserved turkey, then season with pepper and salt. Heat the soup thoroughly.

Nutrition Information

- Calories:
- Cholesterol:
- Protein:
- Total Fat:
- Sodium:
- Fiber:
- Total Carbohydrate:

817. Wilted Green Salad

Serving: 8 servings. | Prep: 10mins | Cook: 0mins | Ready in:

Ingredients

- 10 cups torn leaf lettuce
- 6 cups torn fresh spinach
- 2 green onions, sliced
- 1/4 cup cider vinegar
- 2 tablespoons water
- 2 tablespoons canola oil
- Sugar substitute equivalent to 2 teaspoons sugar
- 4 turkey bacon strips, cooked and crumbled

Direction

- Combine onions, spinach, and lettuce in a big salad bowl; put aside. Add sugar substitute, oil, water, and vinegar to a small saucepan and boil it. Put on the lettuce and mix, use bacon to sprinkle.

Nutrition Information

- Calories: 71 calories
- Sodium: 132mg sodium
- Fiber: 1g fiber)
- Total Carbohydrate: 5g carbohydrate (0 sugars
- Cholesterol: 6mg cholesterol
- Protein: 3g protein. Diabetic Exchanges: 1 vegetable
- Total Fat: 5g fat (1g saturated fat)

818. Zesty Turkey Chili

Serving: 8 servings. | Prep: 15mins | Cook: 15mins | Ready in:

Ingredients

- 1 large onion, chopped
- 3 garlic cloves, minced
- 1 teaspoon canola oil
- 1 can (4 ounces) green chilies
- 2 teaspoons ground cumin
- 1-1/2 teaspoons dried oregano
- 1/4 teaspoon ground cloves
- 1/8 teaspoon hot pepper sauce
- 1/8 teaspoon cayenne pepper
- 2 cans (15-1/2 ounces each) great northern beans, drained
- 3 cups reduced-sodium chicken broth
- 3 cups cubed cooked turkey breast

Direction

- Sauté garlic and onion in oil for 5 minutes. Add seasonings and chilies, stir and cook for 3 minutes. Mix in turkey, broth, beans; simmer for 15 minutes.

Nutrition Information

- Calories: 219 calories
- Total Fat: 3g fat (0 saturated fat)
- Sodium: 554mg sodium
- Fiber: 0 fiber)
- Total Carbohydrate: 31g carbohydrate (0 sugars
- Cholesterol: 32mg cholesterol
- Protein: 17g protein. Diabetic Exchanges: 2 starch

Chapter 6: Whole Turkey Recipes

***

819. Apple Stuffed Turkey

Serving: 15 | Prep: 30mins | Cook: 2hours30mins | Ready in:

Ingredients

- 1 (12 pound) whole turkey - thawed, neck and giblets removed
- 1/4 cup vegetable oil, or as needed
- 5 apples, cored and quartered
- 5 pounds whole unpeeled apples

Direction

- Preheat the oven to 190°C or 375°F.
- If needed, untie legs of turkey. Wash and use paper towels to dry the turkey. Into the roasting pan with a lid, put the turkey, and massage the entire turkey with oil, inside and out. With apple quarters, fill the neck and body cavities of turkey; in roasting pan, place whole apples surrounding turkey. Into the pan, scatter any excess apple quarters. Put cover on roasting pan.
- In the prepped oven, roast for 2 1/2 to 3 hours till meat is starting to part from legs and skin turns browned. Uncover during the final 20 minutes of roasting in case needed to brown the skin. Use the pan drippings for the gravy, if wished.

Nutrition Information

- Calories: 671 calories;
- Total Fat: 29.1
- Sodium: 177
- Total Carbohydrate: 27.3
- Cholesterol: 212
- Protein: 73

820. Awesome Tangerine Glazed Turkey

Serving: 13 | Prep: 45mins | Cook: 3hours30mins | Ready in:

Ingredients

- 3/4 cup unsalted butter, divided
- 3/4 cup canola oil
- 1 1/2 cups tangerine juice
- 1 (10 pound) whole turkey, neck and giblets reserved
- 2 1/4 cups sausage stuffing
- salt and pepper to taste
- 2 1/4 cups turkey stock
- 3 tablespoons all-purpose flour

Direction

- In a saucepan over moderate heat, liquify 6 tablespoons of butter with tangerine juice and canola oil. Take off heat, and let cool for 5 minutes. Submerge a cheesecloth piece in mixture, big enough to drape on turkey.
- Preheat the oven to 220°C or 425°F. Rinse the turkey, and put pepper and salt to season body cavity. Fill the body cavity and neck cavity loosely with stuffing. Bind the drumsticks together, scatter 6 tablespoons of butter on turkey, and add pepper and salt to season. In a shallow roasting pan, put the turkey.
- In the prepped oven, allow the turkey to roast for 25 minutes, and then place the submerged cheesecloth on top of the turkey. Lower the oven heat to 110°C or 325°F. Keep roasting for an hour. Retaining cheesecloth draped on top of turkey, baste with tangerine juice mixture. Keep roasting for 2 hours, basting from time to time, till the inner temperature of the chunkiest part of thigh reads 80°C or 180°F and the filling inside the body cavity reads 70°C or 165°F. Get rid of the cheesecloth, and put the turkey on serving platter. Let turkey cool for 25 minutes prior to carving.
- Remove fat from pan juices, and setting a quarter cup fat and skimmed pan juices aside. Combine 1 cup turkey stock and pan juices in the baking pan; allow to cook over high heat, mixing to scratch the base of pan.
- Mix together flour and the reserved quarter cup of fat in a saucepan for 3 minutes over low heat till thickened. Mix in the rest of turkey stock and the pan juices, and put giblets and neck. Allow to simmer for 10 minutes, mixing continuously, till giblets are cooked completely. Filter through sieve, and serve along with stuffing and turkey.

Nutrition Information

- Calories: 807 calories;
- Sodium: 316
- Total Carbohydrate: 8.9
- Cholesterol: 256
- Protein: 74
- Total Fat: 51.1

821. BBQ Turkey

Serving: 12 | Prep: 45mins | Cook: 5hours | Ready in:

Ingredients

- 2 cups butter, divided
- 1 (15 pound) whole turkey, neck and giblets removed
- 1/4 cup chicken soup base
- 3 sweet onions, peeled and cut into wedges
- 5 apples, cored and cut into wedges
- 2 tablespoons minced garlic, or to taste
- 1 (750 milliliter) bottle dry white wine

Direction

- Prepare a gas grill by preheating over low heat.
- Brush some butter on the turkey, all over it, inside and out; for the chicken base, rub all

over the turkey with it as well. Cube the remaining butter and mix with onions, garlic, and apples in a large bowl, tossing them together. Stuff the mixture inside the bird and put the turkey in an aluminum roasting pan.
- Cover the hole by folding the skin of the turkey around the neck area then turn it over and add wine by pouring it into the opening on the other end until the bottle is empty or the turkey is full.
- Place the turkey with the breast side up.
- Cover the pan loosely using an aluminum foil and put the roasting pan on the grill. Use a heat safe meat thermometer or a pop-up timer if you have one and insert it into the turkey breast then close the lid.
- Roast the turkey for about 4 hours depending on the temperature of your grill, until the temperature inserted in the breast reads 170° F (75° C) and the temperature on the thigh's thickest part shows 180° F (80° C). When you see the temperature getting close, take off the aluminum foil cover from the turkey and allow the turkey to brown until it has reached the last minutes of cooking. If the turkey begins to brown too much, put the aluminum cover back. Leave the turkey for 20 minutes to rest before carving it.

Nutrition Information

- Calories: 1294 calories;
- Protein: 117.7
- Total Fat: 76.7
- Sodium: 1310
- Total Carbohydrate: 16.2
- Cholesterol: 468

822. Best Greek Stuffed Turkey

Serving: 18 | Prep: 30mins | Cook: 4hours | Ready in:

Ingredients

- 1 (12 pound) whole turkey, thawed
- 3 lemons, juiced
- 1/4 cup butter
- 4 medium onions, chopped
- 2 turkey livers, finely chopped
- 1 pound ground lamb
- 2 1/2 cups long grain white rice
- 1 tablespoon ground cinnamon
- 1/4 cup chopped fresh mint leaves
- 2 tablespoons tomato paste
- 3 cups water
- salt and pepper to taste
- 1/2 cup butter, melted

Direction

- Preheat an oven to 230°C or 450°F. Wash turkey inside and out, and pat it dry using paper towels. Massage lemon juice on the entire outer part of turkey and inside the cavity. Reserve.
- In a big skillet, liquify a quarter cup of butter over moderate heat. Put in onion, and cook for 5 minutes, till soft. Put in ground lamb and chopped livers. Cook, mixing to break up, till equally browned. Mix in tomato paste, mint, cinnamon and rice. Stir in 1 cup water, and add pepper and salt to season. Allow to cook for 10 minutes over low heat, mixing continuously.
- Stuff the turkey with filling mixture, and truss. In shallow roasting pan, put on a rack, and add the leftover 2 cups water into pan. Combine together the melted butter and the rest of the lemon juice. It will be the basting sauce.
- In the prepped oven, bake for an hour, then lower oven temperature to 175°C or 350°F and keep roasting for 2 hours longer, or till the inner temperature of chunkiest part of the thigh reads 80°C or 180°F. Baste from time to time with lemon juice and liquified butter.

Nutrition Information

- Calories: 703 calories;
- Total Fat: 33.7
- Sodium: 240
- Total Carbohydrate: 26.7
- Cholesterol: 246
- Protein: 69.8

823. Brined Thanksgiving Turkey

Serving: 12 | Prep: 30mins | Cook: 6hours30mins | Ready in:

Ingredients

- 4 (32 ounce) containers chicken broth
- 1 cup apple juice (optional)
- 1 cup light brown sugar
- 1 cup kosher salt
- 2 tablespoons dried sage
- 4 peppercorns
- 4 red apples, halved
- 5 cloves garlic, crushed
- 10 pounds ice cubes, or as needed
- 1 (20 pound) turkey whole turkey - thawed, neck and giblets removed
- 3 apples, cored and quartered
- 1 onion, cut into 8 wedges
- 3 cloves garlic
- 6 fresh sage leaves
- 3 tablespoons olive oil, or as needed

Direction

- In large stock pot, stir together peppercorns, dried sage, salt, brown sugar, apple juice and chicken broth. Put in crushed garlic cloves and apple halves. Boil the mixture, stirring to dissolve salt and sugar. Immediately discard from the heat.
- In the large food-safe container, fill enough ice to be about 1/2 full. Add the chicken broth mixture over ice. Let cool the liquid evenly and completely by stirring.
- Lower turkey gently into liquid, the breast side down.
- Brine the turkey 24-36 hours; if needed, adding ice to keep turkey and brine cold.
- Start preheating the oven to 500°F (260°C).
- Discard the turkey from brine. Then rinse well under the cold water. Using paper towels, pat the turkey dry.
- In a bowl, mix fresh sage leaves, whole garlic cloves, onion wedges and apple quarters. Loosely fill into the turkey cavity. Transfer turkey to the shallow roasting pan. Coat the skin of turkey lightly with olive oil.
- Bake turkey in prepared oven for half an hour or until skin on the turkey breast turns golden brown.
- Lower the heat to 350°F (175°C), wrap turkey in aluminum foil. Keep roasting turkey for 6 hours or until juices run clear and bone is no longer pink. An instant-read thermometer should register 180°F (85°C) when inserted into the thigh's thickest part. Discard turkey from oven, wrap in doubled sheet of the aluminum foil. Let rest 10-15 mins in a warm place. Then slice.

Nutrition Information

- Calories: 1320 calories;
- Total Carbohydrate: 35.9
- Cholesterol: 455
- Protein: 155.4
- Total Fat: 57.4
- Sodium: 9411

824. Brined Turkey

Serving: 16 | Prep: 20mins | Cook: | Ready in:

Ingredients

- 2 quarts water
- 2 cups kosher salt
- 1 cup white sugar

- 2 gallons cold water
- 3 sprigs fresh rosemary, or more to taste
- 3 sprigs fresh thyme, or more to taste
- 1 tablespoon crushed garlic
- 1 teaspoon ground allspice
- 1 teaspoon ground black pepper
- 1 (16 pound) whole turkey, neck and giblets removed

Direction

- Bring 2 quarts of water in a large pot to a boil; stir in white sugar and kosher salt until completely dissolved. Turn off the heat and allow to cool slightly before pouring into large food-safe container that is big enough to hold a turkey and brine, but still small enough to fit in the fridge. Add 2 gallons of cold water to the container; put in black pepper, allspice, garlic, thyme sprigs, and rosemary sprigs.
- Carefully immerse turkey into the brine until completely covered; chill for 12-36 hours in the fridge.
- Take turkey out of the brine and wash both outside and inside carefully. Pour off brine.

Nutrition Information

- Calories: 730 calories;
- Total Carbohydrate: 12.9
- Cholesterol: 268
- Protein: 92
- Total Fat: 31.9
- Sodium: 11627

825. Brined And Roasted Whole Turkey

Serving: 10 | Prep: | Cook: | Ready in:

Ingredients

- 1 cup Morton® Coarse Kosher Salt
- 1 cup sugar
- 2 gallons cool water
- 1 (12 pound) fresh, whole, bone-in skin-on turkey, rinsed and patted dry
- 5 tablespoons unsalted butter, softened
- 1/2 teaspoon ground black pepper
- 3 tablespoons unsalted butter, melted
- 1 cup white wine, chicken broth or water

Direction

- Overnight Brine: In a big, clean stockpot, mix sugar and Morton(R) Kosher Salt in cool water till fully melted. Put the whole turkey in brine till entirely soaked. Place cover on and chill overnight, up to 14 hours. Take turkey out of the brine, wash the inner and outer sides in cool running water for a few minutes to get rid of every trace of salt; using paper towel, pat it dry.
- For 4 to 5 hours Brine: To brine turkey in less time, for 4 to 5 hours, use 2 cups sugar and two cups of Morton(R)Coarse Kosher Salt. Place cover on and chill for 4 to 5 hours.
- To Roast: Combine pepper and softened butter. In roasting pan, put the turkey on rack. Massage seasoned butter beneath the skin. Brush skin with liquified butter. Add 1 cup liquid either water, broth or wine on pan bottom to keep drippings from burning. Let the turkey roast for 25 minutes at 450°F, baste and then rotate the roasting pan. Keep roasting for 25 minutes longer till skin becomes golden brown; baste once more. Lower the oven temperature to 325°F; keep roasting, basting and rotating pan one time approximately midway through cooking, till the inner heat registers a minimum of 165°F. Take turkey out of the oven. Allow to sit for 20 minutes prior to carving.

Nutrition Information

- Calories: 985 calories;
- Sodium: 9504
- Total Carbohydrate: 20.7
- Cholesterol: 342
- Protein: 108.9

- Total Fat: 46.9

826. Brining And Cooking The Perfect Turkey With Delicious Gravy

Serving: 24 | Prep: 30mins | Cook: 3hours5mins | Ready in:

Ingredients

- Brine:
- 4 (32 ounce) cartons low-sodium chicken broth
- 1 cup kosher salt
- 2 tablespoons dried savory
- 2 tablespoons dried thyme
- 2 tablespoons dried sage
- 2 tablespoons dried rosemary
- 1 gallon apple juice
- 1 gallon water, or as needed to cover
- Roast Turkey:
- 1 (22 pound) whole turkey
- 4 large onions, chopped
- 8 stalks celery, chopped
- 8 carrots, chopped
- 1/4 cup butter, melted
- 2 cups white cooking wine
- 2 (32 ounce) cartons chicken broth
- 1/4 cup butter, melted
- Gravy:
- 2 cups water
- 1 (32 ounce) carton turkey broth
- 1/4 cup cornstarch

Direction

- Into a big stock pot, put 4 cartons of 32-ounce low-sodium chicken broth and mix in rosemary, sage, thyme, savory and kosher salt. Boil, lower the heat to moderate, and let the brine cook for 7 minutes to incorporate the flavors. Allow to cool. Into a big brining bag, big cooler or 5-gallon food-grade bucket, put the mixture. Into the mixture, mix 1 gallon of water and apple juice. Into the brine, put the turkey, breast side facing down, and add additional water if necessary to cover. Refrigerate and brine for a minimum of 36 hours.
- Preheat an oven to 175°C or 350°F.
- Take turkey out and throw away used brine. Wash turkey and pat it dry using paper towels. On roasting rack placed into a roasting pan, set turkey with breast side facing down. Fill the turkey with 4 carrots, 4 stalks of celery and 2 onions; into the roasting pan, put the leftover 4 carrots, 4 stalks of celery and 2 onions around the turkey. Brush the outer side of turkey with a quarter cup liquified butter and into the pan, add two 32-ounce cartons of chicken broth and white cooking wine.
- In the prepped oven, roast for half an hour; baste using pan juices. Put an aluminum foil tent on turkey in case skin starts to darken very fast. Keep roasting for 1 1/2 hours longer, basting every half an hour. Flip turkey over to make it breast side up; brush with the leftover a quarter cup liquified butter. Keep roasting, basting every half an hour, till an inserted instant-read meat thermometer into the chunkiest part of thigh without touching the bone registers 80°C or 180°F, 1 hour longer (in a total of 3 hours roasting time).
- Take turkey out and put aside while preparing gravy. Into a big saucepan, filter all pan drippings through a mesh strainer. Boil, turn heat to moderately low, and allow to simmer. In a bowl, mix cornstarch, one 32-ounce carton turkey broth, and 2 cups water together till smooth. Into the hot pan drippings, mix cornstarch mixture and cook till thickened, mixing continuously for 5 minutes. Allow the gravy to cool to slightly thicken. To get rid of extra fat, use a gravy separator if wished. Serve the turkey along with gravy.

Nutrition Information

- Calories: 796 calories;
- Total Carbohydrate: 29.1

- Cholesterol: 261
- Protein: 87.5
- Total Fat: 33.9
- Sodium: 4792

827. Cajun Deep Fried Turkey

Serving: 12 | Prep: 30mins | Cook: 45mins | Ready in:

Ingredients

- 2 cups butter
- 1/4 cup onion juice
- 1/4 cup garlic juice
- 1/4 cup Louisiana-style hot sauce
- 1/4 cup Worcestershire sauce
- 2 tablespoons ground black pepper
- 1 teaspoon cayenne pepper
- 7 fluid ounces beer
- 3 gallons peanut oil for frying, or as needed
- 1 (12 pound) whole turkey, neck and giblets removed

Direction

- Melt butter in big saucepan on medium heat then add beer, cayenne pepper, black pepper, hot sauce, Worcestershire sauce, garlic juice and onion juice; mix till blended well.
- Inject marinade with turkey baster with injector tip/marinade injecting syringe all over turkey including breasts, thighs, wings, back and legs. Put in big plastic bag; marinate in the fridge overnight. Don't use kitchen trash bag. Use oven bag if your turkey is big.
- Lower turkey into fryer to measure amount of oil needed when it's time to fry; fill with sufficient oil to cover turkey. Remove turkey; put aside.
- Heat oil to 185°C/365°F. Slowly lower turkey into hot oil using hanging device from turkey deep fryers when oil reaches the temperature; turkey must be fully submerged in oil. Cook for 3 minutes per turkey pound or for 36 minutes. When temperature in thickest portion of thigh reads 80°C/180°F, turkey is done. Turn flame off; remove from oil slowly, draining all oil from cavity. Rest for 20 minutes on serving platter then carve.

Nutrition Information

- Calories: 1036 calories;
- Total Fat: 70.9
- Sodium: 682
- Total Carbohydrate: 2.8
- Cholesterol: 346
- Protein: 91.2

828. Carl's Turkey Stuffing

Serving: 20 | Prep: 15mins | Cook: 6hours10mins | Ready in:

Ingredients

- 1 (18 pound) whole turkey, neck and giblets removed
- 1 (16 ounce) package sage pork sausage (such as Bob Evans®)
- 2 (14 ounce) packages dry herb-flavored stuffing mix (such as Pepperidge Farm Herb Seasoned Stuffing®)
- 2 bunches green onion, chopped (green part only)
- 1 cup dried parsley flakes
- 1/2 cup butter, softened
- 1 1/2 tablespoons dry rubbed sage
- 1 teaspoon salt
- 1 teaspoon ground black pepper
- 2 (32 ounce) cans chicken broth
- 1/4 cup water, or as needed (optional)
- 1/4 cup butter, softened, or as needed
- salt to taste

Direction

- Preheat an oven to 220°C or 425°F. For durability, nest 2 big aluminum turkey-roasting pans together. Wash and use paper towels to pat turkey dry, and put turkey into doubled pans.

- Into a big skillet, put the sausage over moderate heat, and cook till crumbly and browned, crumbling it into pieces as it cooks. Into a big mixing bowl, put sausage together with pan drippings.
- Stir in black pepper, salt, sage, 1/2 cup of softened butter, parsley flakes, green onion and dry stuffing mix till well incorporated, then with chicken broth, dampen stuffing. In case stuffing looks dry, stir in water, approximately a tablespoon at a time, till stuffing reaches preferred consistency.
- With the stuffing, slightly fill the main and neck cavities; into baking dish, put any excess stuffing, and cover using foil. Chill the stuffing pan. Liberally massage the outer side of turkey with a quarter cup of the softened butter, or as necessary; scatter salt on turkey. Using foil, cover the turkey.
- In the prepped oven, roast for 4 hours till juices run clear and drumstick of the turkey twists effortlessly in the socket. Check the pan drippings level, and remove extra drippings if necessary. Allow the turkey to roast for an hour longer and recheck and pour off drippings if needed. Bake for half an hour longer and remove cover of turkey.
- Heat an oven's broiler. Let the turkey broil for 15 minutes longer, basting frequently, till golden brown. An instant-read meat thermometer pricked into the chunkiest portion of a thigh should register 80°C or 180°F. Approximately 2 hours prior to serving, bake the pan of dressing if wished.

Nutrition Information

- Calories: 895 calories;
- Total Fat: 41.9
- Sodium: 1731
- Total Carbohydrate: 31.6
- Cholesterol: 275
- Protein: 92.1

829. Chef John's Boneless Whole Turkey

Serving: 20 | Prep: 20mins | Cook: 1hours50mins | Ready in:

Ingredients

- 1 (15 pound) whole turkey, boned
- kosher salt and ground black pepper to taste
- 3 cups prepared stuffing, or more to taste
- 2 tablespoons heavy whipping cream, or more to taste

Direction

- Preheat the oven to 230°C or 450°F.
- On a work area, put turkey, skin-side facing down, and use hands to set the meat into an even, flat surface. Add black pepper and salt to season. Push the stuffing on the entire surface of meat.
- Fold the lengthy turkey edges surrounding the stuffing into the middle of turkey and cautiously flip turkey seam-side facing down. To cinch turkey together, bind leg-end of turkey using kitchen twine. Redo binds at 2-inch spaces throughout the length of turkey, finishing with a single tie along the length of turkey. Add salt to season and put in a big roasting pan.
- In the prepped oven, let the turkey roast for 15 minutes. Lower the heat to 165°C or 325°F and roast for 1 1/2 hours till an inserted instant-read thermometer into the chunkiest part of turkey registers 68°C or 155°F. Turn turkey onto platter; take off and throw away twine. Allow to sit for 20 minutes till inner heat raises to 74°C or 165°F.
- Over moderately high heat, set the roasting pan and into pan drippings, mix the cream. Cook and mix for 3 to 7 minutes till sauce cooks down and thickens. Into a gravy boat or bowl, put through a fine mesh sieve. Cut

turkey crosswise and put gravy on top of slices.

Nutrition Information

- Calories: 567 calories;
- Sodium: 350
- Total Carbohydrate: 6.6
- Cholesterol: 203
- Protein: 69.8
- Total Fat: 26.9

830. Chef John's Roast Turkey And Gravy

Serving: 16 | Prep: 1hours | Cook: 3hours45mins | Ready in:

Ingredients

- 2 tablespoons kosher salt
- 1 tablespoon ground black pepper
- 1 tablespoon poultry seasoning
- 1 (12 pound) whole turkey, neck and giblets reserved
- 2 onions, coarsely chopped
- 3 ribs celery, coarsely chopped
- 2 carrots, coarsely chopped
- 3 sprigs fresh rosemary
- 1/2 bunch fresh sage
- 1/2 cup butter
- 1 bay leaf
- 6 cups water
- 2 tablespoons turkey fat
- 1 tablespoon butter
- 1/4 cup all-purpose flour
- 3 cups turkey pan drippings
- 1/4 teaspoon balsamic vinegar (optional)
- 1 tablespoon chopped fresh sage
- salt and ground black pepper to taste

Direction

- Set the oven to 325°F (165°C) for preheating.
- In a small bowl, mix the poultry seasoning, 2 tbsp. of salt, and 1 tbsp. of pepper. Tuck the wings of the turkey under the bird and season the cavity with 1 tbsp. of the poultry seasoning mixture. Set the remaining poultry seasoning mix aside.
- In a bowl, toss the celery, carrots, and onion. Stuff the cavity of the turkey with rosemary sprigs, 1/2 bunch of sage, and a 1/2 cup of the vegetable mixture. Use a kitchen string to tie the legs together. You can use a small spatula or your fingers to loosen the skin on top of the breast of turkey. Fill 2 tbsp. of butter under its skin and spread it evenly. Coat the outside of the skin all over with the remaining butter, about 2 tbsp. of it. Sprinkle the remaining poultry seasoning mix all over the outside of the turkey.
- In a large roasting pan, spread the celery, carrots, and the remaining onion. Top the vegetables with turkey. Pour water into the pan, filling it about 1/2-inch. Place a sheet of aluminum foil over the turkey's breast.
- Roast the turkey inside the preheated oven for 3 1/2 hours until its juices run clear, the bone is no longer pink, and an inserted instant-read thermometer into the thigh's thickest part (near the bone) reads 165°F (75°C). During the last hour of roasting, remove the foil and baste the pan juices all over the turkey.
- While waiting for the turkey to cook, prepare for the stock. In a saucepan, mix the heart, gizzards, neck, water and bay leaf. Simmer the mixture for 2 hours over medium heat. Strain the turkey giblets from the stock and discard it. The stock should measure at least 4 cups in total.
- Remove the turkey from the oven and cover it with a doubled sheet of aluminum foil. Let the turkey rest in a warm area for 10-15 minutes before slicing it. Pour 3 cups of pan juices into the saucepan; put aside. Skim off any fat from the pan juices, reserving about 2 tbsp. of it.
- Pour 2 tbsp. of the turkey fat and 1 tbsp. of butter in a saucepan and heat it over medium heat. Get the onion from the roasting pan and transfer it into the skillet. Cook and stir the

onion for 5 minutes until browned. Stir in flour and cook for 5 more minutes. Mix in the reserved pan juices and 4 cups of skimmed turkey stock until smooth, skimming off any formed foam. Mix in balsamic vinegar. Simmer the mixture for 10 minutes, stirring often until the gravy is thick. Mix in 1 tbsp. of chopped sage. Season the mixture with salt and black pepper to taste.

Nutrition Information

- Calories: 942 calories;
- Total Fat: 70.1
- Sodium: 950
- Total Carbohydrate: 4.6
- Cholesterol: 256
- Protein: 68.7

831. Classic Turkey And Rice Soup

Serving: 8 | Prep: 20mins | Cook: 1hours25mins | Ready in:

Ingredients

- Stock:
- 1 turkey carcass
- 1 large onion, halved and skin left on
- 1 large carrot, roughly chopped
- 1 stalk celery, roughly chopped
- 1 head garlic, halved
- 1 teaspoon dried rosemary
- 1 teaspoon dried thyme
- 2 bay leaves
- salt and ground black pepper to taste
- water to cover
- Soup:
- 2 large onions, diced
- 2 carrots, diced
- 2 stalks celery, diced
- 2 cloves garlic, minced
- 1 teaspoon poultry seasoning
- 1 teaspoon dried rosemary
- 1 teaspoon onion powder
- 2 cups cooked rice

Direction

- In a stockpot, combine pepper, salt, bay leaves, thyme, 1 teaspoon of rosemary, garlic head and onion (halved), and celery and carrot (roughly chopped), and turkey carcass. Cover with enough water. Allow the mixture to boil, cover, lower heat, and simmer for about 1 hour until the flavors blend.
- Remove the turkey carcass and pull out any remaining meat from the bones, then discard carcass and put meat aside. Use a slotted spoon to remove the bay leaves and vegetables, then discard.
- Into the stock, stir in onion powder, 1 teaspoon of rosemary, poultry seasoning, minced garlic, diced celery, diced carrots, and diced onions, then set to boil. Reduce heat and simmer, covered, for 20 - 30 minutes until the vegetables become very tender. Add the turkey meat and cooked rice into the soup, then season with pepper and salt. Cook for about 5 minutes until turkey meat and rice are warm.

Nutrition Information

- Calories: 115 calories;
- Total Fat: 1.7
- Sodium: 37
- Total Carbohydrate: 22.4
- Cholesterol: 4
- Protein: 3.2

832. Cola Roast Turkey

Serving: 12 | Prep: 10mins | Cook: 4hours | Ready in:

Ingredients

- 1 (16 pound) whole turkey - thawed, neck and giblets removed
- 1/2 cup butter, softened
- 2 cups cola-flavored carbonated beverage (such as Coke®)
- salt and ground black pepper to taste

Direction

- Start preheating oven to 165°C (or 325°F).
- Rinse turkey well, then use paper towels to pat dry. Lather butter on the entire turkey, front and back, using your hands. Make sure both leg ends and wing tips are buttered. Set turkey on a roasting pan and pour cola onto the turkey. Add black pepper and salt to season the whole turkey.
- Roast for 4-5 hours, checking turkey's doneness after 4 hours of roasting. Use turkey drippings to baste turkey every 30 minutes. Wrap turkey's breast with aluminum foil in case it browns too fast. The instant-read thermometer that is inserted into the thickest thigh part (near the bone) should register 82°C (180°F). Take turkey out of the oven, wrap the top with a doubled sheet of aluminum foil, and rest for 10-15 minutes in a warm place prior to slicing.

Nutrition Information

- Calories: 993 calories;
- Total Fat: 50.1
- Sodium: 353
- Total Carbohydrate: 4.6
- Cholesterol: 378
- Protein: 122.6

833. Deep Fried Turkey

Serving: 16 | Prep: 30mins | Cook: 45mins | Ready in:

Ingredients

- 3 gallons peanut oil for frying, or as needed
- 1 (12 pound) whole turkey, neck and giblets removed
- 1/4 cup Creole seasoning
- 1 white onion

Direction

- Preheat oil to 400 degrees F (200 degrees C) in a big turkey fryer or a stockpot. Make sure not to fill the pot with too much oil or it will spill. Prepare a big platter and line it with paper towels or food-safe paper bags. Pat the rinsed turkey with paper towels until thoroughly dry. Massage the outside and cavity of the bird with Creole seasoning. See to it that the neck hole has a two-inch opening to ensure that the oil will reach the inside of the turkey. Put the turkey and whole onions in the drain basket, positioning the turkey neck end first. Carefully submerge the basket into the hot oil, completely submerging the turkey. Fry the turkey for 45 minutes or 3 1/2 minutes per pound, make sure that the oil stays at 350 degrees F (175 degrees C) throughout the cooking process. Slowly and carefully lift the basket from oil and drain the turkey. Thermometer inserted inside thickest area of thigh should read 180 degrees F (80 degrees C). Drain excess oil on prepared platter.

Nutrition Information

- Calories: 603 calories;
- Total Fat: 33.6
- Sodium: 571
- Total Carbohydrate: 1.5
- Cholesterol: 228
- Protein: 68.8

834. Dry Brine Turkey

Serving: 15 | Prep: 15mins | Cook: 2hours30mins | Ready in:

Ingredients

- 1 (15 pound) whole turkey, neck and giblets removed
- 3 tablespoons kosher salt
- black pepper to taste
- 1 onion, cut into wedges
- 4 stalks celery, halved

Direction

- Using paper towels, pat turkey dry. Add kosher salt to season inside and out of turkey, especially on thighs and breast. In roasting pan, put turkey, breast-side facing up, and cover using plastic wrap. Chill turkey for 2 days.
- Turn turkey over, breast-side facing down, cover with plastic wrap, and chill for a day longer.
- Unwrap and night prior to roasting, put the turkey on rack over a baking sheet. Let turkey to air-dry in refrigerator for a minimum of 8 hours.
- Let turkey come to room temperature, about an hour or two; using paper towels, pat dry. Add black pepper to season the turkey and insert celery and onion in cavity.
- Preheat the oven to 220°C or 425°F. In a roasting pan, put the turkey, breast-side facing down.
- In the prepped oven, roast for 30 minutes till skin turns golden. Take turkey out of oven and turn to breast-side facing up. Lower the oven heat to 165°C or 325°F; keep roasting for 2 hours till an inserted instant-read thermometer into the chunkiest part of thigh registers 74°C or 165°F.
- Turn the turkey onto a big platter and tent loosely with aluminum foil; let the turkey sit for half an hour prior to carving.

Nutrition Information

- Calories: 684 calories;
- Sodium: 1383
- Total Carbohydrate: 1
- Cholesterol: 268
- Protein: 91.9
- Total Fat: 31.8

835. Easy Beginner's Turkey With Stuffing

Serving: 12 | Prep: 30mins | Cook: 4hours | Ready in:

Ingredients

- 12 pounds whole turkey
- 1 (6 ounce) package dry bread stuffing mix
- 1 cup water
- 1 tablespoon butter
- 1 cup chopped celery
- 1/4 cup chopped onion
- 4 slices toasted white bread, torn into small pieces
- salt and pepper to taste
- 2 tablespoons vegetable oil

Direction

- Set the oven to 350°F (175°C) for preheating. Wash the turkey and remove all the giblets. Place it in a shallow roasting pan.
- Follow the package directions on how to prepare the stuffing; stir in water.
- In a medium saucepan, melt the butter over medium heat. Cook and stir onion and celery slowly until tender.
- Mix the onion, celery, and toasted bread pieces into the stuffing. Season the mixture with salt and pepper. Spoon the stuffing loosely into the body and neck cavity of the turkey. Rub vegetable oil into the exterior part of the turkey.
- Cover the turkey loosely with an aluminum foil. Roast the turkey into the preheated oven for 3 1/2-4 hours until the thickest part of the thigh has a temperature of 180°F (85°C) and the stuffing inside has a temperature of 165°F (70°C). During the last half hour of cooking

time, remove the foil to allow the bird to brown.

Nutrition Information

- Calories: 835 calories;
- Protein: 95
- Total Fat: 40.4
- Sodium: 593
- Total Carbohydrate: 15.6
- Cholesterol: 311

836. Easy Herb Roasted Turkey

Serving: 16 | Prep: 15mins | Cook: 3hours30mins | Ready in:

Ingredients

- 1 (12 pound) whole turkey
- 3/4 cup olive oil
- 2 tablespoons garlic powder
- 2 teaspoons dried basil
- 1 teaspoon ground sage
- 1 teaspoon salt
- 1/2 teaspoon black pepper
- 2 cups water

Direction

- Preheat the oven to 165°C or 325°F. Rinse the turkey, throw away the organs and giblets, and put in a roasting pan with a lid.
- Mix black pepper, salt, ground sage, dried basil, garlic powder and olive oil in a small bowl. Apply the mixture to outer of uncooked turkey with a basting brush. Into the base of roasting pan, add water, and place the cover.
- Allow to bake for 3 to 3 1/2 hours, or till inner temperature of the chunkiest portion of thigh reads 82°C or 180°F. Take turkey out of oven, and let sit for half an hour prior to carving.

Nutrition Information

- Calories: 597 calories;
- Total Fat: 33.7
- Sodium: 311
- Total Carbohydrate: 0.9
- Cholesterol: 198
- Protein: 68.2

837. Easy Smoked Turkey

Serving: 12 | Prep: 20mins | Cook: 4hours | Ready in:

Ingredients

- 1 (12 pound) thawed whole turkey, neck and giblets removed
- 1 tablespoon chopped fresh savory
- 1 tablespoon chopped fresh sage
- 1 tablespoon salt (optional)
- 1 tablespoon ground black pepper
- 1/8 cup olive oil
- 1/2 cup water

Direction

- Wash turkey and using paper towels, pat it dry. In a bowl, mix black pepper, salt, sage and savory; massage 1/2 of herb mix on the inside of turkey's cavity and neck cavity. Loosen turkey skin on legs and breast; massage the leftover 1/2 of herb mixture beneath the loosened skin. Massage the olive oil all over the turkey.
- Light 20 charcoal briquettes and on lower grate of kettle charcoal grill, put 1/2 of them on every side. Put a disposable aluminum baking pan or drip pan in the center of lower grate and add water. Once coals turn gray with ash, put a 2-inch square piece of hickory or different hardwood onto every coals' bank.
- Over cooking grate, put the turkey and place cover on grill. Using grill thermometer, check the temperature to keep heat between 65 to 120°C or 150 and 250°F; put in about 3 to 5

coals to every side approximately every 1 1/2 hours. Once hardwood pieces burn away, put in additional to maintain a consistent stream of smoke rising from wood. In case open flames erupt once you open the lid, extinguish them with a drizzle of beer or water.
- Let the turkey smoke for approximately 4 hours total, 20 minutes each pound; allow the temperature to raise to 120°C or 250°F on the final hour of smoking. An inserted instant-read meat thermometer into the chunkiest part of a thigh without touching bone should register 75°C or 165°F.

Nutrition Information

- Calories: 692 calories;
- Protein: 90.7
- Total Fat: 33.7
- Sodium: 801
- Total Carbohydrate: 0.4
- Cholesterol: 264

838. English Honey Roasted Turkey

Serving: 10 | Prep: 45mins | Cook: 2hours30mins | Ready in:

Ingredients

- 1 (10 pound) whole turkey - thawed, neck and giblets removed
- 1 lemon, cut in half
- salt and black pepper to taste
- 1 small apple, peeled
- 1 small onion, peeled
- 1 small potato, peeled
- 3 ounces butter
- 6 ounces honey
- 1 cup chicken stock (optional)

Direction

- Using paper towels, pat dry the turkey in and out. Lightly stroke the cut side of lemon halves on turkey skin. Season to taste the inner and outer with pepper and salt. Into turkey cavity, put potato, onion, apple and lemon halves. Put into a tight-fitting roasting pan.
- In a small saucepan over moderately-low heat, mix honey and butter together till butter has liquified the mixture is equally incorporated. Scoop honey mixture on turkey, covering the whole outer surface. Let sit for half an hour, reapplying honey mixture a few times.
- Preheat the oven to 200°C or 400°F.
- In the prepped oven, let the turkey bake for half an hour, basting twice or thrice with honey mixture and drippings. Lower heat to 175°C or 350°F, and let cook for half an hour longer, basting often. In case necessary, add a cup of chicken stock to prevent pan juices from drying out.
- Cover aluminum foil on turkey, and keep roasting for an additional of 1 1/2 to 2 hours till juices run clear and not pink anymore at the bone. An inserted instant-read thermometer into the chunkiest portion of thigh, close to the bone should register 82°C or 180°F. Take off foil on the final 15 minutes and baste once more. Take turkey out of the oven, cover using a double thickness of aluminum foil, and let sit in a warm place for 15 minutes prior to cutting.

Nutrition Information

- Calories: 816 calories;
- Sodium: 342
- Total Carbohydrate: 20.2
- Cholesterol: 286
- Protein: 92.7
- Total Fat: 38.8

839. Erick's Deep Fried Rosemary Turkey

Serving: 16 | Prep: 30mins | Cook: 55mins | Ready in:

Ingredients

- 1 (12 pound) whole turkey, neck and giblets removed
- 1/2 cup minced garlic
- salt and ground black pepper to taste
- 3 gallons peanut oil for frying
- 3 sprigs fresh rosemary
- 12 cloves garlic, peeled
- 1/2 cup chopped fresh ginger root

Direction

- Pour peanut oil on an outdoor deep-fryer and fill it up then heat the oil for 30 minutes at 325° F (160° C).
- Rub minced garlic, pepper, and salt on the inside and the outside of the turkey. Fill the inside or the cavity of the turkey with rosemary, ginger, and garlic cloves then leave it to marinate, refrigerating it for 30 minutes.
- Take out the garlic and herbs from the turkey's cavity and throw them away. The gash on the turkey's neck should be at least 2 inches wide. Snip the skin back if needed to avoid the pressure from building inside the turkey. Remove the turkey ahead of time if it has a pop-up doneness indicator.
- Put the turkey to the fryer basket or on a hanging device, then carefully lower it down into the hot oil. The temperature of the oil should be maintained while the turkey is frying. Cook until the internal temperature is at 180° F (82° C) when you test the thickest part of the thigh, about 3 1/2 minutes per pound.
- Slowly lift the turkey out from the hot oil and turn the deep-fryer off. Leave the turkey for 5 minutes to cool then dry by patting it.

Nutrition Information

- Calories: 573 calories;
- Protein: 68.4
- Total Fat: 30.2
- Sodium: 166
- Total Carbohydrate: 2.7
- Cholesterol: 198

840. Evil Turkey

Serving: 30 | Prep: 20mins | Cook: 3hours30mins | Ready in:

Ingredients

- 1 onion, chopped
- 1 (12 ounce) jar roasted red peppers, drained and chopped
- 1 cup whiskey
- 1/2 cup minced garlic
- 1 (22 pound) whole turkey, neck and giblets removed
- 1 (7 ounce) can chipotle chilies in adobo sauce
- roasting bag for a large turkey

Direction

- Preheat the oven to 165 °C or 325 °F.
- Mix together the garlic, whiskey, roasted red peppers and onion and put the mixture in the turkey cavity of the bird. In a food processor, mince chipotle peppers till almost the consistency of spaghetti sauce. Massage the outer part turkey with half of chipotles, and put the remaining inside the cavity of turkey. In a roasting bag, put the turkey; seal bag following bag instruction, and put onto roasting pan.
- In the prepped oven, let the turkey bake for 3 1/2 hours till juices run clear and not pink anymore at the bone. An instant-read thermometer pricked into the chunkiest part of thigh, close the bone should register 82 ° C or 180 °F. Take turkey off the oven, and let rest in warm place for 10 to 15 minutes prior cutting.

Nutrition Information

- Calories: 529 calories;
- Cholesterol: 196
- Protein: 67.6
- Total Fat: 23.5
- Sodium: 234
- Total Carbohydrate: 2.1

841. Fruity Tutti Turkey Brine

Serving: 15 | Prep: | Cook: 5hours | Ready in:

Ingredients

- 9 (14 ounce) cans vegetable broth
- 1 1/2 cups chopped candied ginger
- 1 1/2 cups dried cherries
- 4 ounces dried pears
- 4 ounces dried apples
- 2 1/2 cups brown sugar
- 1 cup kosher salt
- 2 tablespoons whole peppercorns
- 1 teaspoon whole allspice berries
- 3 cinnamon sticks
- 5 leaves fresh sage
- 1 gallon ice water
- 1 (15 pound) frozen whole turkey, unthawed
- 1 white onion, quartered
- 1 red apple, cored and quartered
- 1 sprig fresh rosemary, or to taste
- 2 cinnamon sticks
- 1 leaf fresh sage, or to taste
- 3 cups water, or amount to cover
- 1 tablespoon vegetable oil, or as needed

Direction

- In large stockpot, stir together 5 sage leaves, 3 sticks of cinnamon, allspice berries, black peppercorns, kosher salt, brown sugar, dried apples, dried pears, dried cherries, candied ginger and vegetable broth until salt and brown sugar are completely dissolved. Boil. Lower the heat to medium-low; cook, stirring occasionally, for 60 mins.
- Discard brine from the heat. Put in ice water. Melt ice by stirring. Let chill brine. Place in the refrigerator at least 120 mins, until cold. Put still-frozen turkey into brine and place in the refrigerator for 3 days. On the second day of brining, flip the turkey in brine.
- After 3 days of brining (the serving day), start preheating the oven to 350°F (175°C). Discard turkey from brine. Put into the roasting pan. Remove brine.
- In a 5-cup microwave-safe measuring cup, put one sage leaf, 2 more sticks of cinnamon, 1 sprig of rosemary, red apple and onion, add enough water to cup to cover. Place into microwave oven and cook on high power until hot, about 5 mins. Add the cup contents to the turkey cavity. Rub vegetable oil over the turkey skin.
- Roast in prepared oven for 4-4 1/2 hours or until juices run clear and turkey turns golden brown. An instant-read meat thermometer should register 165°F (75°C) when inserted into thickest part of the thigh.

Nutrition Information

- Calories: 985 calories;
- Sodium: 6881
- Total Carbohydrate: 60.4
- Cholesterol: 308
- Protein: 94.9
- Total Fat: 38

842. Garbage Can Turkey

Serving: 12 | Prep: 30mins | Cook: 2hours | Ready in:

Ingredients

- aluminum foil
- 15 inch wooden stake

- 1 (12 pound) whole turkey, neck and giblets removed
- new 15 gallon metal garbage can with lid

Direction

- Make a square of about 3x3 feet on the grass by laying 3 long sheets of aluminum foil that's heavy duty. In the center of the aluminum foil, strike the wooden stake into the ground.
- Fill up the garbage can's lid with a large pile of charcoal and light it up. Position the thawed turkey onto the stake with the legs down. Reverse the garbage can, turning it upside down and put it over the turkey. Put loads of the lighted coals around the sides and on the top of the can.
- Cook the turkey for at least 1 1/2 hours and continue until the coals have gone out. Do not take off the can while cooking. Remove the charcoals off and lift the can carefully for the heat not to rush out when you lift. Check the internal temperature of the turkey which should read at least 180° F (83° C) when taken in the thigh's thickest part.

Nutrition Information

- Calories: 671 calories;
- Cholesterol: 264
- Protein: 90.6
- Total Fat: 31.4
- Sodium: 219
- Total Carbohydrate: 0

843. General Tso's Whole Turkey

Serving: 15 | Prep: 1hours | Cook: 3hours30mins | Ready in:

Ingredients

- Marinade/Glaze:
- 3 tablespoons vegetable oil
- 3 small dried red chiles, or more to taste
- 1 teaspoon ground black pepper
- 2 green onions, chopped
- 1/4 cup light sesame oil
- 1 small shallot, chopped
- 1/2 (16 ounce) can whole berry cranberry sauce
- 1 cup turkey broth
- 1/2 cup soy sauce
- 1/4 cup orange juice
- 1/4 cup white vinegar
- 1/4 cup plum wine
- 1/4 cup white sugar
- 2 tablespoons chopped fresh ginger root
- 2 tablespoons chopped garlic
- 2 teaspoons grated orange zest
- 1 (12 pound) whole turkey, neck and giblets removed
- 3 tablespoons cornstarch
- Dressing:
- 2 cups cooked white rice
- 1/2 cup cooked wild rice
- 1/3 cup dried cranberries
- 1/4 cup chopped walnuts
- 2 small green onions, chopped
- 1 small shallot, chopped
- 1 tablespoon sesame oil
- Basting Oil:
- 1/3 cup vegetable oil
- 1/3 cup sesame oil

Direction

- In a small skillet, put in 3 tablespoons of vegetable oil and let it heat up over medium heat setting. Put in the dried red chiles and let it toast in the hot oil for about 2 minutes until it is dark red in color. Add in the light sesame oil, black pepper, 1 small chopped shallot and 2 chopped green onions and mix everything together in the hot oil; remove the skillet away from the heat.
- Use a blender to mix the orange juice, garlic, cranberry sauce, plum wine, soy sauce, orange zest, ginger, white vinegar and turkey broth together until it is smooth in consistency. Put

the mixture in a bowl. Add in the toasted red chile mixture and mix everything together. Divide the glaze mixture to 2 equal portions.

- Put the turkey inside a big basting bag then put in 1/2 of the prepared glaze mixture all over the turkey and inside the cavity. Seal the basting bag and keep it in the fridge throughout the night.
- Mix the cornstarch with the remaining 1/2 of the prepared glaze mixture until the cornstarch has dissolved; put it in a covered container and keep it in the fridge as well.
- Preheat the oven to 325°F (165°C).
- Take the marinated turkey and throw away the marinade mixture. Put the marinated turkey on top of the wire rack placed inside a roasting pan.
- In a bowl, combine the dried cranberries, 1 chopped shallot, white rice, walnuts, 1 tablespoon of sesame oil, wild rice and 2 small chopped green onions together. Stuff the prepared rice mixture lightly inside the cavity of the marinated turkey. In a bowl, mix 1/3 cup of sesame oil and 1/3 cup of vegetable oil together and put it aside.
- Put it in the preheated oven and let it roast for about 2 hours while basting the turkey with the prepared oil mixture in 15-minute intervals until the turkey skin turns brown in color and is already crispy. Give the reserved chilled glaze-cornstarch mixture a thorough mix and baste the turkey with this mixture in 15-minute intervals for 1 1/2 to 2 more hours until the glaze has seeped through the baked turkey and a poked instant-read meat thermometer in the thickest part of the turkey's thigh indicates 165°F (75°C).

Nutrition Information

- Calories: 802 calories;
- Total Fat: 43.6
- Sodium: 685
- Total Carbohydrate: 23.1
- Cholesterol: 212
- Protein: 74.5

844. Greek Traditional Turkey With Chestnut And Pine Nut Stuffing

Serving: 12 | Prep: 30mins | Cook: 4hours15mins | Ready in:

Ingredients

- 1 cup chestnuts
- 2/3 cup butter
- 1/4 cup orange juice
- 1/4 cup tangerine juice
- 2/3 cup lemon juice
- 1 (10 pound) whole turkey
- salt and ground black pepper to taste
- 1/2 pound ground beef
- 1/2 pound ground pork
- 1/4 cup chopped onion
- 1/2 cup uncooked instant rice
- 1/4 cup pine nuts
- 1/4 cup raisins (optional)
- 1/3 cup butter
- 1/2 cup chicken broth
- 2 tablespoons brandy
- 1 teaspoon salt
- 1/2 teaspoon ground black pepper

Direction

- Preheat the oven to 165°C or 325°F.
- Create a small cut on sides of every chestnut, and put in a skillet over moderate heat. Cook till toasted, mixing frequently. Take off heat, skin, and cut.
- In a saucepan, liquify 2/3 cup of butter, and stir in lemon juice, tangerine juice and orange juice. Massage the mixture on the inside and outside of turkey, setting aside some for basting. Put pepper and salt to season the turkey.
- Cook onion, ground pork, and ground beef in a big skillet over moderate heat till pork and

beef are equally brown and onion is soft. Drain oil. Stir in rice. Mix in brandy, broth, 1/3 cup butter, raisins, pine nuts and chestnuts. Add 1/2 teaspoon pepper and 1 teaspoon salt to season. Keep cooking till all liquid has been soaked up. Fill every turkey cavity with the mixture, and use kitchen twine to tie in place.
- On a rack in roasting pan, put the turkey, and cover thighs and breast loosely using aluminum foil. Into the base of pan, add approximately a quarter inch of water. Keep this water level throughout the cook time. In the prepped oven, let turkey roast for 3 to 4 hours, brushing from time to time with the rest of the juice and butter mixture. Raise the oven temperature to 200°C or 400°F on the last hour of roasting, and take off foil. Let the turkey cook to a minimum internal temperature of 82°C or 180°F.

Nutrition Information

- Calories: 930 calories;
- Total Carbohydrate: 22.3
- Cholesterol: 322
- Protein: 86.1
- Total Fat: 52.2
- Sodium: 572

845.   Grilled Turkey

Serving: 24 | Prep: 30mins | Cook: 3hours | Ready in:

Ingredients

- 1 large onion, diced
- 1 (750 milliliter) bottle red wine
- salt and pepper to taste
- 12 pounds whole turkey

Direction

- Fill the bottom of the pot style grill with a 5-pound bag of charcoals. Light the charcoal and spread it to cover the bottom of the grill.
- Rinse the turkey thoroughly and stuff it with onion. Rub its exterior down with salt and pepper.
- Lay the turkey in a deep aluminum roasting pan and place it on the grill's grate. Pour wine over the turkey. Cover the turkey's top with foil.
- Using the grill's lid, cover the grill and open its vents. Grill the turkey for 60-90 minutes, basting it constantly until the meat reached its desired doneness. Add more water if the wine evaporates.

Nutrition Information

- Calories: 369 calories;
- Total Fat: 15.9
- Sodium: 113
- Total Carbohydrate: 1.4
- Cholesterol: 134
- Protein: 46

846.   Grilled Whole Turkey

Serving: 18 | Prep: 15mins | Cook: 4hours | Ready in:

Ingredients

- 12 pounds whole turkey
- 2 cups water
- 3 tablespoons chicken bouillon powder
- 2 teaspoons garlic powder
- 2 teaspoons onion powder
- 1 teaspoon poultry seasoning
- 1/2 teaspoon chopped parsley
- 1 teaspoon paprika

Direction

- Wash turkey in cold water, dry well with paper towels. Preheat your outdoor grill on medium, and brush grate lightly with oil. Breast side down, position the turkey on the grill, searing both sides of the turkey until golden brown. Combine water, garlic powder, onion powder, bouillon powder, parsley, poultry seasoning and paprika in a big roasting pan. Position the turkey on the roasting pan breast side down, bathe the turkey with the mixture. Cover properly with aluminum foil and place the pan on the grill. Cook on the grill until thermometer inserted in the thigh hits 180 degrees F (85 degrees C) about 3 to 4 hours. Take out turkey from grill and roasting pan, let rest for 15 minutes before slicing.

Nutrition Information

- Calories: 461 calories;
- Sodium: 508
- Total Carbohydrate: 1
- Cholesterol: 179
- Protein: 61.7
- Total Fat: 21.4

847. Herb Glazed Roasted Turkey

Serving: 16 | Prep: 30mins | Cook: 4hours | Ready in:

Ingredients

- 1 (16 pound) whole turkey, neck and giblets removed
- 1/4 cup extra-virgin olive oil
- 1 teaspoon salt
- 1/2 teaspoon ground black pepper
- 1 teaspoon ground thyme
- 1 cup honey
- 1/2 cup melted butter
- 2 teaspoons dried sage leaves
- 1 tablespoon minced fresh parsley
- 1 teaspoon dried basil
- 1 teaspoon salt
- 1 teaspoon ground black pepper

Direction

- Preheat an oven to 165°C or 325°F. Wash turkey, and using paper towels, pat dry well. Brush inside and out of the turkey with olive oil.
- In a small bowl, combine thyme, 1/2 teaspoon of pepper and 1 teaspoon of salt, and scatter the mixture on turkey.
- On a rack positioned in a roasting pan, put the turkey, and in the prepped oven, allow to roast for 2 hours.
- Mix together the 1 teaspoon pepper, 1 teaspoon salt, basil, parsley, sage, melted butter and honey in a bowl till mixture is well incorporated and smooth. Brush the honey glaze on turkey, and put back to oven.
- Allow the turkey roast for 2 hours longer till juices run clear and not pink anymore at the bone. An inserted instant-read thermometer into the chunkiest portion of thigh, close to the bone should register 82°C or 180°F. Keep brushing honey glaze on turkey often as it roasts. Take the turkey out from oven, cover using a double thickness of aluminum foil, and let sit in a warm place for 10 to 15 minutes prior to cutting.

Nutrition Information

- Calories: 828 calories;
- Total Carbohydrate: 17.7
- Cholesterol: 283
- Protein: 92.1
- Total Fat: 41.1
- Sodium: 555

848. Holiday Turkey With Honey Orange Glaze

Serving: 20 | Prep: 20mins | Cook: 6hours15mins | Ready in:

Ingredients

- 2 teaspoons rubbed sage

- 2 teaspoons salt
- 1 pinch dried thyme
- 1 (16 pound) whole turkey, neck and giblets removed
- 1/4 cup butter
- 1/3 cup orange juice
- 1/3 cup orange marmalade
- 1 1/2 teaspoons honey
- 1 orange, peeled, sectioned, and cut into bite-size pieces

Direction

- Preheat the oven to 165°C or 325°F.
- In a small bowl, mix thyme, salt and sage. Massage 1/2 of sage mixture on the entire turkey, then put turkey in a big roasting pan. Reserve the rest of sage mixture. In a saucepan, boil orange sections, honey, orange marmalade, orange juice and butter over moderately high heat. Lower the heat and allow to simmer without a cover for 15 to 20 minutes till thickened, mixing from time to time. Mix in the rest of the sage mixture. Brush glaze over turkey.
- In the prepped oven, let the turkey bake for 5 and a half hours, basting every half an hour. Using foil, lightly cover the turkey and keep baking for half an hour to 1 hour till juices run clear and not pink anymore at the bone, brushing with glaze from time to time. An inserted instant-read thermometer into the chunkiest portion of thigh close to the bone should register 82°C or 180°F. Take turkey out of the oven, cover using doubled aluminum foil sheet, and let sit in warm place for 10 to 15 minutes prior to cutting.

Nutrition Information

- Calories: 582 calories;
- Protein: 73.6
- Total Fat: 27.8
- Sodium: 430
- Total Carbohydrate: 4.5
- Cholesterol: 221

849. Homestyle Turkey, The Michigander Way

Serving: 16 | Prep: 10mins | Cook: 5hours | Ready in:

Ingredients

- 1 (12 pound) whole turkey
- 6 tablespoons butter, divided
- 4 cups warm water
- 3 tablespoons chicken bouillon
- 2 tablespoons dried parsley
- 2 tablespoons dried minced onion
- 2 tablespoons seasoning salt

Direction

- Set the oven to 350°F (175°C) for preheating. Rinse and wash the turkey well, discarding the giblets or put into pan if someone likes them.
- Place the turkey in a roasting pan or Dutch oven. Separate the skin over the breast so that it would look like little pockets. Pour 3 tbsp. of butter on both sides between the breast meat and skin to make juicier breast meat.
- Mix the bouillon and water in a medium bowl. Sprinkle the mixture with minced onion and parsley. Pour the mixture on top of the turkey. Season the turkey with seasoning salt.
- Use a foil to cover the pan. Let it bake inside the preheated oven for 3 1/2-4 hours until the meat's internal temperature registers 180°F or 80°C. Make sure that in the last 45 minutes of the baking time, you already removed the foil so that the turkey turns brown nicely.

Nutrition Information

- Calories: 545 calories;
- Cholesterol: 210
- Protein: 68.1
- Total Fat: 27.9
- Sodium: 560
- Total Carbohydrate: 0.9

850. Honey Brined Smoked Turkey

Serving: 12 | Prep: 10mins | Cook: 4hours | Ready in:

Ingredients

- 1 gallon hot water
- 1 pound kosher salt
- 2 quarts vegetable broth
- 1 pound honey
- 1 (7 pound) bag of ice cubes
- 1 (15 to 20) pound turkey, giblets removed
- 1/4 cup vegetable oil, or as needed
- 1 cup wood chips

Direction

- In a 54 quarts cooler, mix salt and hot water; mix till salt dissolves. Into the water, mix honey and vegetable broth. Put ice and mix. With breast side facing up, put turkey in brine; cover using the cooler lid. Allow to brine overnight to 12 hours.
- From brine, take off turkey and pat it dry using paper towel; coat turkey with vegetable oil by massaging it over. Get rid of the brine.
- In the middle of every of the 2 big aluminum foil sheets, place a cup wood chips. Wrap the edges around wood chips to create little pouches, retaining small gaps on surface.
- Preheat the outdoor grill to 200°C or 400°F and grease grate lightly. Put a wood chip pouch right on top of flame under the grate.
- Place turkey on indirect heat, into the chunkiest portion of breast, prick a probe thermometer, and set the alarm for 70°C or 160°F. Seal the lid and allow to cook for an hour till skin of turkey turn golden brown. Take off and get rid of the initial wood chips pouch; put a new one from the rest of the pouch.
- Using aluminum foil, cover the turkey, put cover back to grill and keep cooking for 3 hours longer till juices run clear and turkey is not pink anymore at the bone. An inserted instant-read thermometer into the chunkiest portion of thigh, close the bone should register 82°C or 180°F.
- Take turkey out of the grill, cover using aluminum foil, and let sit in warm place for an hour prior to carving to serve.

Nutrition Information

- Calories: 1308 calories;
- Total Fat: 57.9
- Sodium: 15829
- Total Carbohydrate: 34.5
- Cholesterol: 447
- Protein: 153.9

851. Honey Smoked Turkey

Serving: 16 | Prep: 30mins | Cook: 3hours15mins | Ready in:

Ingredients

- 1 (12 pound) whole turkey
- 2 tablespoons chopped fresh sage
- 2 tablespoons ground black pepper
- 2 tablespoons celery salt
- 2 tablespoons chopped fresh basil
- 2 tablespoons vegetable oil
- 1 (12 ounce) jar honey
- 1/2 pound mesquite wood chips

Direction

- Prepare the grill, set on high heat. Use twice the normal amount of charcoal if using charcoal grill. Put wood chips in a pile of water, let it soak near grill. Prepare the turkey by removing neck and the giblets and gravy packet. Rinse well over cold water and pat dry with paper towels. Put turkey in a big disposable roasting pan. Combine vegetable oil, sage, ground black pepper, basil and celery salt in a bowl. Rub the mixture evenly all over turkey. With the bird facing breast side down in the pan, tent the pan loosely with aluminum foil. Put a handful of soaked wooden chips into the coals, place the roasting pan on the prepared grill. Cook for one hour with the grill lid closed. Add 2 extra handfuls of wood chips to the coals. Pour half of the honey on the turkey and replace the aluminum foil. Keep cooking with the lid closed for 1 1/2 to 2 hours, or until thickest area of thigh's inner temperature is 180 degrees F (80 degrees C). Remove aluminum foil and gently turn over the turkey breast side up. Brush the surface with remaining half of the honey and cook uncovered for another 15 minutes. The cooked turkey will be very dark because of the cooked honey.

Nutrition Information

- Calories: 647 calories;
- Sodium: 776
- Total Carbohydrate: 25.3
- Cholesterol: 228
- Protein: 68.9
- Total Fat: 28.8

852. How To Cook A Turkey

Serving: 24 | Prep: 30mins | Cook: 3hours | Ready in:

Ingredients

- 1 onion, coarsely chopped
- 1 stalk celery, coarsely chopped
- 1 carrot, coarsely chopped
- 1 (12 pound) whole turkey, neck and giblets reserved
- 2 tablespoons kosher salt
- 1 tablespoon ground black pepper
- 1 teaspoon cayenne pepper
- 3 tablespoons butter
- 4 sprigs fresh rosemary
- 1/2 bunch chopped fresh sage

Direction

- Preheat the oven to 165°C or 325°F.
- In a big, shallow roasting pan, put the carrot, celery and onion.
- In roasting pan, set the turkey, breast side facing up, over the vegetables. Using paper towels, pat in and outside of turkey dry.
- In a small bowl, mix cayenne pepper, black pepper and salt. Season the inner of turkey with approximately a third of salt mixture. Tuck wing tips beneath the turkey.
- In small saucepan, liquify the butter for 2 minutes over moderate heat till edges start to become golden. Cook and mix sage and rosemary for a minute.
- Put sage and rosemary inside the turkey cavity; set liquified butter aside. Tie legs together using twine.
- With the melted butter, brush the entire outer side of turkey. Add leftover 2/3 of salt mixture to season.
- In the prepped oven, let the turkey bake without a cover for 3 hours till juices run clear and not pink anymore at the bone. An inserted instant-read thermometer into the thickest part of thigh, close to the bone should register 82°C or 180°F. Take the turkey out of the oven and let sit in a warm place for 10 to 15 minutes prior to cutting.

Nutrition Information

- Calories: 355 calories;
- Sodium: 604
- Total Carbohydrate: 1.5
- Cholesterol: 136
- Protein: 45.5
- Total Fat: 17.2

853. Juicy Thanksgiving Turkey

Serving: 20 | Prep: 20mins | Cook: 3hours | Ready in:

Ingredients

- 2 tablespoons dried parsley
- 2 tablespoons ground dried rosemary
- 2 tablespoons rubbed dried sage
- 2 tablespoons dried thyme leaves
- 1 tablespoon lemon pepper
- 1 tablespoon salt
- 1 (15 pound) whole turkey, neck and giblets removed
- 2 stalks celery, chopped
- 1 orange, cut into wedges
- 1 onion, chopped
- 1 carrot, chopped
- 1 (14.5 ounce) can chicken broth
- 1 (750 milliliter) bottle champagne

Direction

- Preheat the oven to 175°C or 350°F. Line lengthy sheets of aluminum foil on a turkey roaster, it should be long enough to wrap on turkey.
- In a small bowl, mix together the salt, lemon pepper, thyme, sage, rosemary and parsley. Into the turkey cavity, massage the herb mixture, then fill with the carrot, onion, orange and celery. Truss if wished, and put turkey into roasting pan. Add champagne and chicken broth on turkey, ensuring to place some champagne in cavity. Over the top of turkey place the aluminum foil, and enclose. Try to prevent foil from touching skin of turkey legs or breast.
- In the prepped oven, let the turkey bake for 2 1/2 to 3 hours till juices run clear and not pink anymore at the bone. Remove turkey cover, and keep baking for an additional of 30 minutes to 1 hour till skin becomes golden brown. An inserted instant-read thermometer into the chunkiest portion of thigh, close to the bone should register 82°C or 180°F. Take turkey out of the oven, cover using a double thickness of aluminum foil, and let sit in a warm place for 10 to 15 minutes prior to cutting.

Nutrition Information

- Calories: 556 calories;
- Sodium: 680
- Total Carbohydrate: 4.3
- Cholesterol: 201
- Protein: 69.3
- Total Fat: 24

854. Lauren's Apple Cider Roast Turkey

Serving: 15 | Prep: | Cook: |Ready in:

Ingredients

- 1 (16 pound) whole turkey, neck and giblets removed
- 1 1/2 gallons water
- 1 gallon apple cider
- 1 1/2 cups kosher salt
- 1 cup white sugar
- 1/4 cup extra-virgin olive oil
- 1/4 teaspoon dried thyme
- 1/4 teaspoon poultry seasoning

Direction

- Wash in and out of turkey using cold water; pat it dry using paper towels.
- In a big pot or 5 gallons food-grade bucket, combine sugar, kosher salt, apple cider and water, mixing to dissolve sugar and salt. Soak turkey in brine, put a cover on the container, and refrigerate for 8 hours or overnight.
- Preheat the oven to 165°C or 325°F.
- Take turkey off brine and get rid of used brine. Into a roasting pan, put the turkey, breast side facing up; using paper towels pat dry turkey and cavity. Using your fingers, loosen the skin of turkey over thighs and breast.
- In a small bowl, combine poultry seasoning, thyme and olive oil. Massage the entire turkey and beneath the loosened skin with seasoned

oil. Loosely cover the turkey using aluminum foil.

- In the prepped oven, let roast for 4 to 4 1/2 hours till an inserted instant-read meat thermometer into the chunkiest portion of a thigh, without touching bone, registers 75 to 80°C or 165 to 175°F. Take foil tent off on the final 45 minutes of roasting time to allow the skin to brown. Allow the turkey to sit for 30 to 45 minutes prior to carving.

Nutrition Information

- Calories: 952 calories;
- Total Fat: 37.7
- Sodium: 9387
- Total Carbohydrate: 48.6
- Cholesterol: 286
- Protein: 98.1

855. Lemon Herb Turkey

Serving: 12 | Prep: 30mins | Cook: 2hours | Ready in:

Ingredients

- 3 tablespoons chopped fresh marjoram
- 3 tablespoons chopped fresh rosemary
- 3 tablespoons chopped fresh thyme
- 3 tablespoons chopped fresh basil
- 3 tablespoons garlic, minced
- 1 pinch ground black pepper to taste
- 1 (12 pound) whole turkey, neck and giblets removed
- 1/4 cup olive oil
- 2 large lemons, juiced, lemon halves reserved
- 1 tablespoon all-purpose flour
- 1 turkey-size oven roasting bag

Direction

- Set the oven to 350°F (175°c) for preheating. In a small dish, mix the basil, black pepper, rosemary, marjoram, garlic, and thyme; put the mixture aside.
- Lift the skin of the turkey away from the meat gently. Brush the meat with olive oil lightly. Sprinkle it with lemon juice, and then with 2/3 of the mixed herbs. Slowly pat the skin of the turkey into the meat. Sprinkle the turkey cavity with the remaining herbs. Add the squeezed lemon halves. Fill the turkey roasting bag with the flour. Shake the bag well to coat evenly. Place the turkey inside the bag. Use a nylon tie to seal the end of the bag. Place the bag into the deep roasting pan and cut its top into six 1/2-inch slits.
- Bake the turkey inside the preheated oven for 2-2 1/2 hours until the juices run clear and the bone is no longer pink. The inserted instant-read thermometer into the thigh's thickest part, the one that is near on the bone, should read 180°F or 82°C. Remove the turkey from the oven. Use a doubled sheet of aluminum foil to cover the turkey. Let the turkey rest in a warm area for 10-15 minutes before slicing it.

Nutrition Information

- Calories: 722 calories;
- Sodium: 221
- Total Carbohydrate: 3.6
- Cholesterol: 264
- Protein: 91.2
- Total Fat: 36

856. Ma Lipo's Apricot Glazed Turkey With Roasted Onion And Shallot Gravy

Serving: 30 | Prep: 30mins | Cook: 4hours30mins | Ready in:

Ingredients

- 1 cup apricot nectar
- 1 cup apricot preserves

- 2 tablespoons minced fresh ginger root
- 1 tablespoon honey
- 3/4 cup unsalted butter, softened
- 3 tablespoons chopped fresh sage
- 1 1/2 teaspoons salt
- 1 teaspoon ground black pepper
- 2 tablespoons unsalted butter
- 3 onions, thinly sliced
- 6 ounces thinly sliced shallots
- 22 pounds whole turkey
- 2 cups low-sodium chicken broth
- 1 teaspoon chopped fresh thyme
- 1/2 teaspoon dried sage
- 2 cups low-sodium chicken broth
- salt and pepper to taste

Direction

- In a small saucepan, mix honey, ginger, preserves and apricot nectar, and boil. Turn the heat to moderately low, and allow to simmer for 15 minutes till thickened and cooked down to 1-1/4 cups.
- In small bowl, mix pepper, salt, 3 tablespoons chopped fresh sage and 3/4 cup unsalted butter at room temperature. Reserve.
- In a big heavy skillet, liquify 2 tablespoons of unsalted butter over moderate heat. Put on the shallots and onions; sauté for 20 minutes till light brown and really tender.
- In the lowest third of the oven, place the rack. Preheat to 200°C or 400°F.
- Put pepper and salt on the turkey cavity to season. On a rack in a big roasting pan, put the turkey, breast side facing up. To loosen skin, slip hand beneath the turkey breast skin. Scatter 1/2 of herb butter on breast beneath the skin. Massage the rest of the herb butter on the outer part of the turkey.
- Scoop the stuffing loosely into the primary cavity if stuffing the turkey; as it cooks, it will expand. Loosely bind legs together to keep the form of turkey.
- In the prepped oven, let the turkey roast for half an hour. Lower the oven heat to 165°C or 325°F, and keep roasting for an hour and 30 minutes, basting from time to time with pan drippings. Using an aluminum foil, tent the turkey; roast for an additional of 45 minutes.
- Into the roasting pan, put 1/2 teaspoon chopped fresh sage, thyme, 1 cup broth and onion mixture. Roast for 15 minutes longer prior to brushing half a cup of apricot glaze on turkey. Keep roasting the turkey without a cover, brushing from time to time with glaze. Into pan, put additional broth if needed. For unstuffed turkey, bake for an additional of 40 minutes, and an hour and 10 minutes more for stuffed turkey, or till an inserted meat thermometer into the chunkiest part of thigh reads 75°C or 165°F. Put the turkey on platter, and tent using foil. Allow to sit for half an hour. For gravy, set mixture aside in pan.
- Into a strainer placed on top of a big bowl, put the contents of roasting pan. Remove fat from the pan juices with a big spoon. Into blender, put the onion mixture. Put in a cup of pan juices, and process till smooth, putting in additional chicken broth and pan juices if needed to thin the sauce to preferred consistency. Turn the sauce into a big saucepan, and boil. Let cook for 5 minutes till color darkens, removing any froth. Add pepper and salt to season.

Nutrition Information

- Calories: 591 calories;
- Total Carbohydrate: 10.9
- Cholesterol: 211
- Protein: 68.2
- Total Fat: 28.8
- Sodium: 301

857. Maple Basted Roast Turkey With Cranberry Pan Gravy

Serving: 12 | Prep: 15mins | Cook: 3hours50mins | Ready in:

Ingredients

- 1 (12 pound) Butterball® Turkey, thawed if frozen
- 8 fresh sage leaves
- 1/4 cup fresh lemon juice
- 2/3 cup pure maple syrup
- 2 1/2 cups chicken broth
- 2 cups cranberry juice
- 2 tablespoons cornstarch
- 3/4 cup sweetened dried cranberries

Direction

- Preheat the oven to 325 °F.
- Cut off giblets and neck from neck and body cavities of the turkey. Chill for another use or throw. Let juices form turkey drain. Using paper towels, pat it dry. Turn the wings backward to keep skin of neck on back of turkey. On a flat roasting rack in the shallow roasting pan, put the turkey, breast side facing up. Put 4 sage leaves beneath the skin on each breast side. On shallow rack in pan, put the turkey. Brush the entire skin with lemon juice.
- Allow to bake for about 3-1/2 hours, or till meat thermometer inserted in deepest part of thigh reads 180°F. Using aluminum foil, cover breast and surface of drumsticks 2 hours later to avoid overcooking of the breast.
- With maple syrup, baste turkey every 15 minutes on the final half hour of baking.
- Take turkey off roasting pan and allow to sit while making gravy.
- Over moderate heat, put the roasting pan on burners. Put half cup of broth. Boil, while scratching dripping from base of pan. Take pan off heat. Into a big saucepan, filter the mixture.
- Into saucepan, mix cranberry juice and 1-1/2 cups of broth. Boil on moderate heat, mixing often; turn the heat to moderately-low.
- Into the leftover half-cup of broth, mix the cornstarch. Slowly mix into the simmering mixture. Mix in the cranberries. Allow to simmer for 5 minutes, mixing often.
- Carve the turkey and serve together with gravy.

Nutrition Information

- Calories: 783 calories;
- Total Carbohydrate: 25.6
- Cholesterol: 269
- Protein: 92.2
- Total Fat: 32
- Sodium: 425

858. Maple Roast Turkey

Serving: 12 | Prep: 1hours | Cook: 3hours30mins | Ready in:

Ingredients

- 2 cups apple cider
- 1/3 cup real maple syrup
- 2 1/2 tablespoons chopped fresh thyme
- 2 tablespoons chopped fresh marjoram
- 1 1/2 teaspoons grated lemon zest
- 3/4 cup butter, softened
- salt and pepper to taste
- 1 (12 pound) whole turkey, neck and giblets reserved
- 2 cups chopped onion
- 1 1/2 cups chopped celery
- 1 1/2 cups chopped carrots
- 3 cups chicken broth
- 1/4 cup all-purpose flour
- 1 bay leaf
- 1/2 cup apple brandy

Direction

- In a saucepan, mix maple syrup and apple cider, and let come to a boil over moderately high heat. Keep cooking till reduced to half a cup, then take pan off heat. Mix in lemon zest, 1 tablespoon marjoram and 1 tablespoon thyme. Mix in butter till liquified, and add

pepper and salt to season. Place cover on, and chill till cold.
- Preheat an oven to 190°C or 375°F. In the lower third of the oven, position the rack.
- On a rack placed in roasting pan, put the turkey. Set 1/4 cup of maple butter aside for gravy, and massage the rest of the maple butter beneath the breast skin and on the outer side of turkey. Set giblets, turkey neck, carrots, celery and onion surrounding the turkey. Scatter a tablespoon of thyme and a tablespoon of marjoram on top of vegetables. Into pan, add 2 cups broth.
- In the prepped oven, let the turkey roast for half an hour. Lower temperature of oven to 175°C or 350°F. Loosely cover the whole turkey in foil. Keep roasting for 2 1/2 hours, or till an inserted meat thermometer into chunkiest part of thigh reads 85°C or 180°F. Turn turkey onto platter, and allow to sit for 30 minutes.
- Into a big measuring cup, strain pan juices, and get rid of any extra fat. Into pan juices, put sufficient chicken broth to get 3 cups. Turn liquid into saucepan, and boil. Combine 1/3 cup flour and 1/4 cup maple butter in a small bowl till smooth. Into the broth mixture, mix butter mixture and flour. Mix in the bay leaf and the rest of the thyme. Boil till cooked down to sauce consistency, mixing from time to time for 10 minutes. Stir in apple brandy, if wished. Season to taste with pepper and salt.

Nutrition Information

- Calories: 872 calories;
- Cholesterol: 295
- Protein: 91.6
- Total Fat: 43.1
- Sodium: 331
- Total Carbohydrate: 21.2

859. Maple Roast Turkey And Gravy

Serving: 20 | Prep: 30mins | Cook: 4hours | Ready in:

Ingredients

- 2 cups apple cider
- 1/3 cup real maple syrup
- 2 tablespoons chopped fresh thyme
- 2 tablespoons chopped fresh marjoram
- 2 1/2 teaspoons grated lemon zest
- 3/4 cup butter
- salt and ground black pepper to taste
- 14 pounds whole turkey, neck and giblets reserved
- 2 cups chopped onion
- 1 cup chopped celery
- 1 cup coarsely chopped carrots
- 2 cups chicken stock
- 3 tablespoons all-purpose flour
- 1 teaspoon chopped fresh thyme
- 1 bay leaf
- 2 tablespoons apple brandy (optional)

Direction

- In a heavy saucepan set on medium-high heat, put the maple syrup and apple cider the simmer for approximately 20 minutes, until lessened to 1/2 cup. Separate from heat and stir in marjoram and 1/2 of the thyme and all of the lemon zest. Stir in the butter until dissolved. Add ground pepper and salt to taste. Keep in the refrigerator, covered, until cold (syrup can be prepared up to 2 days in advance.)
- Prepare the oven by preheating to 375°F (190°C). Set the oven rack at the lowest third of the oven.
- Rinse and dry the turkey, then put in a big roasting pan. Under the skin of the breast, slide your hand to loosen. Then rub 1/2 cup of the maple butter mix under the breast skin. If you are planning on stuffing the turkey, do it now. Use 1/4 cup of the maple butter mixture

to rub the outside of turkey. Tie legs of turkey loosely using a kitchen string.

- Then place the chopped carrot, chopped celery, and chopped onion to surround turkey in the roasting pan. You may add also the giblets and neck to the vegetables if wished. Dust the rest of the marjoram and thyme on the vegetables, then add the chicken stock in the pan.
- Place turkey in the preheated oven and roast for 30 minutes. Minimize oven temperature to 350°F (175°C), then use a foil to loosely cover the turkey. Keep on roasting for approximately 3-4 hours unstuffed or 4-5 hours stuffed, until the internal temperature of the stuffing achieves 165°F (75°C) and thigh achieves 180°F (80°C). Place the turkey on a platter and use foil to cover. Set aside the pan mixture for gravy. Let the turkey sit for approximately 25 minutes prior to taking off the carving and stuffing.
- For Gravy: Drain pan juices to a measuring cup. Scoop fat from the juices. Put enough chicken stock to create 3 cups. Place liquid in a heavy saucepan and make it boil. Combine flour and leftover maple butter to make a paste, then stir in the broth. Mix in apple brandy, bay leaf, and thyme. Boil until it reduces and gets slightly thick. Add pepper and salt to season.

Nutrition Information

- Calories: 584 calories;
- Total Fat: 29.3
- Sodium: 314
- Total Carbohydrate: 10.5
- Cholesterol: 206
- Protein: 65

860. McCormick® Savory Herb Rub Roasted Turkey

Serving: 12 | Prep: 20mins | Cook: 3hours30mins | Ready in:

Ingredients

- 2 tablespoons McCormick® Rubbed Sage or McCormick® Poultry Seasoning
- 1 tablespoon McCormick® Paprika
- 1 tablespoon seasoned salt
- 2 teaspoons McCormick® Garlic Powder
- 1 teaspoon McCormick® Black Pepper, Ground
- 3/4 teaspoon McCormick® Ground Nutmeg
- 1 turkey (12 to 14 pounds), fresh or frozen, thawed
- 1 large onion, cut into wedges
- 6 McCormick® Bay Leaves
- 1 tablespoon vegetable oil

Direction

- Position the oven rack in the lowest part of the oven. Set it to 325°F for preheating. Place the roasting rack in the shallow roasting pan. In a small bowl, mix the garlic powder, nutmeg, seasoned salt, poultry seasoning or sage, pepper, and paprika.
- Wash the turkey well and pat it to dry. Position the turkey into the prepared pan, breast-side up. Inside the turkey, sprinkle half of the seasoning mixture and stuff it with bay leaves and onion. Coat the turkey breast with the oil. Spread the remaining seasoning mixture all over the turkey's surface and the skin under the turkey. Pour 1/2 cup of water into the pan. Use a heavy-duty foil to cover the turkey loosely.
- Roast the turkey for 1 hour. Remove the foil and roast the turkey for 2-2 1/2 more hours, basting it with the pan juices occasionally or until the internal temperature reaches 165°F and the thigh's temperature is 175°F. Remove the turkey from the oven and allow it to stand for 20 minutes. Slice the turkey in a carving

board or platter. Reserve the remaining pan juices for the gravy or you can also serve it immediately together with the turkey.

Nutrition Information

- Calories: 815 calories;
- Sodium: 490
- Total Carbohydrate: 2.5
- Cholesterol: 313
- Protein: 107.5
- Total Fat: 38.5

861. Megaturkey

Serving: 12 | Prep: 25mins | Cook: 4hours | Ready in:

Ingredients

- 1 (12 pound) whole turkey, neck and giblets removed
- 1/2 cup butter, cubed
- 1 cup chopped celery
- 1 1/2 cups toasted bread cubes
- 1/4 cup chopped onion
- 1 tablespoon garlic powder
- salt and pepper to taste
- 2 apples, cored and halved
- 2 cups apple juice

Direction

- Set the oven to 350°F (175°C) for preheating.
- Slide your hand between the breast of the bird and the skin to loosen it. Stuff butter pieces between the breast and the skin.
- Toss the bread cubes, onion, and celery in a medium bowl. Season the mixture with salt, pepper, and garlic powder. Stuff the turkey cavity with the mixture together with the apple halves. Place the turkey inside the roasting bag. Pour apple juice all over the inner and outer parts of the turkey. Seal the bag and place it in a large roasting pan, positioning the turkey breast side up.
- Bake the turkey for 3-3 1/2 hours inside the preheated oven or until the thigh's meatiest part has an internal temperature of 180°F or 85°C. Open the bag. Transfer the turkey into the serving platter. Allow it to stand for 20 minutes before carving it.

Nutrition Information

- Calories: 787 calories;
- Cholesterol: 285
- Protein: 91.3
- Total Fat: 39.3
- Sodium: 314
- Total Carbohydrate: 11.4

862. Orange And Maple Glazed Turkey

Serving: 25 | Prep: 20mins | Cook: 3hours10mins | Ready in:

Ingredients

- 1 teaspoon salt
- 1/4 teaspoon ground black pepper
- 1/4 cup butter, softened
- 3 tablespoons chopped fresh thyme
- 3 tablespoons chopped fresh sage
- 1 (20 pound) whole turkey, neck and giblets removed
- 3 tablespoons olive oil
- 1/4 cup orange juice
- 1/2 cup maple syrup
- 1 cup chicken broth, divided
- 1/2 cup dry vermouth

Direction

- Preheat the oven to 230 °C or 450 °F. Oil a roasting pan. In a small bowl, combine pepper and salt together, and put aside.

- In a small bowl, mix sage, thyme and butter together. In the preheated roasting pan, put the turkey, and separate skin from breast along neck cavity. On the breast, scatter the butter mixture equally, then force skin back down over butter. With olive oil, brush the outer of turkey, then scatter pepper and salt mixture over. Mix together the 1/2 the chicken broth, maple syrup and orange juice, and put aside.
- In preheated oven, let the turkey bake for 3 hours, or till juices run clear and no sign of pink remains at bone. Baste with maple syrup mixture every half an hour. An instant-read thermometer inserted into the thickest portion of thigh, close to the bone should register 82 °C or 180 °F. Take turkey out of oven, cover in a double layer of aluminum foil, and let sit in warm place for 10 to 15 minutes prior to cutting.
- After turkey has sat, take it out of roasting pan, and put it on serving platter. On the stove, put the roasting pan, and mix in the rest of chicken broth together with the vermouth. Simmer over medium -high heat. Scratch the base of roasting pan thoroughly to melt the browned bits, then let simmer over medium-low heat till gravy is thick, about 10 minutes in all. Drain prior to serving with turkey.

Nutrition Information

- Calories: 601 calories;
- Protein: 73.7
- Total Fat: 29
- Sodium: 324
- Total Carbohydrate: 5.3
- Cholesterol: 220

863. Perfect Turkey

Serving: 24 | Prep: 30mins | Cook: 4hours | Ready in:

Ingredients

- 1 (18 pound) whole turkey, neck and giblets removed
- 2 cups kosher salt
- 1/2 cup butter, melted
- 2 large onions, peeled and chopped
- 4 carrots, peeled and chopped
- 4 stalks celery, chopped
- 2 sprigs fresh thyme
- 1 bay leaf
- 1 cup dry white wine

Direction

- Rub kosher salt inside and out the turkey. In large stock pot, place bird, add cold water to cover. Place in fridge, let turkey soak in water and salt mixture for half a day or overnight.
- Start preheating the oven to 350°F (175°C). Rinse turkey thoroughly. Remove brine mixture.
- Brush half melted butter over turkey. In a shallow roasting pan, arrange the breast side down on the roasting rack. Stuff bay leaf, one thyme sprig, 1/2 celery, 1/2 carrots and one onion into turkey cavity. Scatter around the roasting pan bottom with remaining thyme and vegetables. Add white wine to cover.
- Roast uncovered in prepared oven, until temperature reaches 180°F (85°C) internal of the thigh, about 3 1/2 to 4 hours. About 2/3 through roasting time, flip turkey carefully, the breast side facing up. Then brush remaining butter over. Let bird stand for half an hour before carving.

Nutrition Information

864. Roast Peruvian Turkey

Serving: 12 | Prep: 30mins | Cook: 3hours25mins | Ready in:

Ingredients

- 1 (12 pound) whole turkey, neck and giblets removed
- Spice rub:
- 1/2 cup ground cumin
- 1/2 cup soy sauce
- 1/2 cup white vinegar
- 1/3 cup vegetable oil
- 12 cloves garlic, peeled
- 3 tablespoons paprika
- 2 tablespoons freshly ground black pepper
- 1 tablespoon smoked paprika
- 1 tablespoon dried oregano
- 2 teaspoons kosher salt, or as needed
- 1 tablespoon vegetable oil
- 2 teaspoons water, or as needed
- Sauce:
- 1 (8 ounce) container creme fraiche
- 1 cup chicken broth
- 1 lime, juiced
- 2 jalapeno peppers, stemmed
- 1/2 cup chopped fresh cilantro
- salt and freshly ground black pepper to taste
- 1 pinch cayenne pepper, or to taste
- 1 pinch cayenne pepper, or to taste

Direction

- Use paper towels to tap dry turkey. Insert a spatula underneath the skin of each side of the breastbone to loosen skin.
- In a blender, put oregano, smoked paprika, black pepper, paprika, garlic, vegetable oil, vinegar, soy sauce, and cumin. Blend the spice rub for 1 minute until it forms a thick paste. Put aside 1/2 cup of the rub in a bowl to use later; put the rest of the rub on the turkey and put approximately 2 tablespoons of the mixture under the loosened skin on each side of the breast using a spatula. Rub the mixture on every part of the turkey. Let the turkey sit at room temperature for 1 hour.
- Start preheating the oven to 325°F (165°C). Fold an aluminum foil sheet into a round piece approximately the size of the turkey breast, put the foil aside.
- Set a rack in a big roasting pan and put the turkey on it. Use a string of kitchen twine to tie the legs together at the bottom. Spread into the cavity of the turkey the 1/4 cup of the saved wet rub, save the leftover 1/4 cup for later. Sprinkle kosher salt over the whole sides and top of the turkey.
- Put the turkey in the preheated oven and roast for 1 1/2 hours; put the foil tent on the turkey breast. Put back to the oven and keep roasting for another 75 minutes. In a small bowl, mix together water, 1 tablespoon vegetable oil, and the leftover 1/4 cup spice rub. Brush the turkey's sides, legs, and top with the mixture. Roast for another 30 minutes until an instant-read meat thermometer displays 170 to 175°F (75 to 80°C) when you insert it in the thickest part of a thigh without touching the bone. Move the turkey to a serving dish and let sit for a minimum of 20 minutes, saving the drippings in the roasting pan.
- In a blender, put cilantro, jalapeno peppers, lime juice, chicken broth, and creme fraiche and process until smooth. Remove the extra grease from the turkey roasting pan, add the creme fraiche mixture, and put the roasting pan on a burner over medium-high heat. Transfer the browned pan drippings to the sauce mixture, boil it, and cook for 10 minutes until the gravy thickens and decreases by half. Stir frequently to avoid lumps. Use cayenne pepper, black pepper, and salt to season the gravy. Carve and enjoy the turkey with the pan gravy.

Nutrition Information

- Calories: 840 calories;
- Total Carbohydrate: 7
- Cholesterol: 292
- Protein: 93.5
- Total Fat: 47.3
- Sodium: 1237

865. Roast Spatchcock Turkey

Serving: 10 | Prep: 15mins | Cook: 1hours45mins | Ready in:

Ingredients

- 1 (10 pound) whole turkey
- 1/2 cup olive oil
- 1 tablespoon salt
- 1 tablespoon chopped fresh sage
- 1 tablespoon fresh thyme leaves
- 1 tablespoon finely chopped fresh rosemary
- 1 teaspoon crushed black pepper

Direction

- Preheat the oven 175°C or 350°F. Put a roasting rack over a baking sheet.
- Upturn the turkey with the breast-side down. Slice along one side of the backbone with a pair of sharp heavy-duty kitchen shears. Repeat with the backbone's other side. Save the backbone to make the turkey stock for the gravy. Flatten the turkey by firmly pushing down on both sides.
- Tuck the tips of the wing beneath the turkey then arrange on a roasting rack. Pat the skin dry then brush olive oil all over the turkey; sprinkle black pepper, salt, rosemary, thyme, and sage to season.
- Bake for 1 hour 30 minutes in the preheated oven, rotate the baking sheet every half hour. Turn the heat to 200°C or 400°F; roast for another 15 minutes until the skin is crisp. An inserted instant-read thermometer in the thickest thigh part should register 74°C or 165°F. Take the turkey out of the oven then tent with two sheets of aluminum foil. Let it sit for 10-15 minutes before carving.

Nutrition Information

- Calories: 777 calories;
- Total Fat: 42.7
- Sodium: 920
- Total Carbohydrate: 0.3
- Cholesterol: 268
- Protein: 92

866. Roast Turkey With Tasty Chestnut Stuffing

Serving: 16 | Prep: 45mins | Cook: 4hours30mins | Ready in:

Ingredients

- 2 pounds chestnuts
- 2 cups butter
- 2 cups minced onion
- 2 cups minced celery
- 10 cups dried bread crumbs
- 1 teaspoon dried thyme
- 1 teaspoon dried marjoram
- 1 teaspoon dried savory
- 1 teaspoon dried rosemary
- 12 pounds whole turkey, neck and giblets removed
- salt and freshly ground black pepper to taste

Direction

- On flat side of every chestnut, cut a cross using a sharp knife. In a saucepan, simmer for 5 minutes, covered in water. Let drain. Take off shells and inner brown skins while hot. Use fresh water to cover. Allow to boil for 20 minutes to half an hour till soft. Allow to drain. Chop roughly.
- To make stuffing, in a medium saucepan, liquify the butter over moderate heat. Mix in celery and onions, and cook till soft. Combine in chestnuts and bread crumbs well. Add rosemary, savory, marjoram and thyme to season.
- Preheat the oven to 175°C or 350°F.
- Rinse turkey in cold water, and pat it dry. Massage pepper and salt into body cavities. Scoop stuffing loosely into cavities. Seal the skin using kitchen twine or skewers, and bind

drumsticks together. On a rack in medium roasting pan, put the turkey.
- In the prepped oven, let turkey roast for 3 1/2 to 4 1/2 hours till inner temperature of thigh reads 80°C or 180°F and stuffing attains 75°C or 165°F. A tent of foil may be put on turkey during the final half of the roasting time to prevent overbrowning. Take out of oven, put on platter, and let turkey sit for 20 minutes prior to carving.

Nutrition Information

- Calories: 1103 calories;
- Total Fat: 51.2
- Sodium: 838
- Total Carbohydrate: 76.3
- Cholesterol: 262
- Protein: 79.4

867. Roast Turkey With Cranberry And Pomegranate Glaze

Serving: 8 | Prep: 20mins | Cook: 4hours | Ready in:

Ingredients

- Glaze:
- 3/4 cup honey
- 1/2 cup white wine
- 1/2 cup unsalted butter
- 1/2 cup cranberry juice
- 1/2 cup pomegranate juice
- Turkey:
- 1 (10 pound) whole turkey, neck and giblets removed
- 1/2 cup unsalted butter, melted
- 1/2 cup extra virgin olive oil
- 1 tablespoon dried crushed rosemary leaves
- 1 teaspoon kosher salt
- 1 teaspoon dried thyme leaves
- 1/4 teaspoon black pepper
- 2 cups fresh whole cranberries
- 1 diced sweet onion
- 4 cups turkey or chicken stock
- 8 sprigs chopped fresh rosemary
- 3 bay leaves
- Reynolds Wrap® Aluminum Foil

Direction

- Boil the pomegranate juice, cranberry juice, butter, white wine and honey in a medium pot over medium-high heat. Turn heat to low and let the mixture simmer for 10 minutes. Take off from heat and reserve to cool down.
- Preheat an oven to 450 °F. Wash turkey and pat it dry. Forcefully mix together black pepper, thyme, salt, rosemary, olive oil and melted butter till smooth. Massage mixture around the whole outer and inner of turkey, including beneath the breast skin of the bird, careful not to tear the skin.
- Scatter evenly the onion and cranberries on the base of roasting pan. Put turkey in the roasting pan, breast side up. Stuff if wished, and tie turkey's legs together using cooking twine. Mix together the turkey stock with 2/3 cup of glaze and put mixture into roasting pan, on surrounding of turkey but not over it. Set 4 sprigs of rosemary surrounding the bird in the stock and put bay leaves in the pan.
- Loosely cover the entire top of roasting pan with Reynolds Wrap® Aluminum Foil, keeping an inch between foil and skin. Leave a small opening to allow for basting bird as it cooks.
- Roast for half hour then reduce heat to 350 °F, keep cooking for 15 to 20 minutes per pound of turkey. Baste after every 20 minutes with pan drippings and baste with glaze once every hour. Rotate the roasting pan once after every hour to aid in even cooking.
- Once skin starts to turn lightly golden, check temperature, when it attains 165 °F in the breast, stuffing cavity and thigh, it is done. In case you desire to brown a little more, take off the foil and roast for 10 to 15 minutes longer.

- Ensure to keep an eye for browning will be very fast due to glaze's sugar content.
- Once taken off, garnish with the leftover 4 sprigs of fresh rosemary surrounding the turkey. Let it rest for half hour prior carving and serving.

Nutrition Information

- Calories: 1338 calories;
- Sodium: 1096
- Total Carbohydrate: 37.1
- Cholesterol: 399
- Protein: 116.2
- Total Fat: 77.3

868. Roast Turkeys With Rich Pan Gravy

Serving: 24 | Prep: | Cook: | Ready in:

Ingredients

- 2 turkeys (10 to 12 pounds each), neck and giblets discarded
- 3 cups kosher salt (do not use regular table salt)
- 2 cups granulated sugar
- 2 unpeeled medium onions, coarsely chopped
- 2 unpeeled medium carrots, coarsely chopped
- 2 stalks celery stalks, coarsely chopped
- 2 tablespoons melted butter
- 1 cup dry white wine or vermouth
- 4 cups low-sodium chicken broth
- 1/4 cup cornstarch

Direction

- In a big clean ice chest or any alike container, dissolve sugar and salt in three gallons of cold water then place in a cold area like an unheated garage or basement the night before roasting. If you live in a warm area, put ice packs to cool turkeys. Place the turkeys in the container with the breast-side down then cover; let it sit for 12hrs. The brine will season the turkey to the bone and prevents it from drying. Drain the turkey, rinse, then pat dry.
- Place the oven rack in the lower middle part of the oven then set it to 425°Fahrenheit about 5hrs before serving. Put one turkey with the breast-side down then use kitchen shears to cut open the back. Then flip the turkey breast-side up, and flatten it down with your palms. Put the turkey with skin-side up on a lipped cookie sheet over a layer of 1/2 of the chopped veggies. Brush the butter all over the turkey.
- Roast for 1 - 1 1/2hrs until an inserted meat thermometer in the thigh reads 175°Fahrenheit. Watch the pan drippings and veggies while roasting, they must be dry enough to brown and make a rich brown mixture to brush the second turkey with and to produce a rich gravy, but also just moist enough to avoid burning. If needed, add water throughout the roasting process.
- Take the pan out of the oven then move the turkey on a cutting board; set aside the juices and veggies in the pan for the second turkey. Let the turkey sit for half to a full hour before slicing to firm the meat up. Crave some turkey slices then move them to a baking pan or ovenproof serving platter, use aluminum foil to cover. Chill in the refrigerator or place in a cool area just under 40°F until serving. Reheat gently while covered on a baking pan or platter.
- Once you remove the first turkey, turn the oven to 400°Fahrenheit right away then place the rack in the bottom position. Scrape the first turkey's pan drippings and veggies to a roasting pan. Then place a V-rack in the pan. Put the rest of the raw veggies in the second turkey's cavity then tie the legs together using kitchen twine for presentation. Place the turkey on a rack with the breast-side down. Slather with the collected pan drippings from the first turkey.
- Roast for an hour then take it out of the oven; use the pan drippings to baste the sides and back. Carefully flip the turkey breast-side up

using tow paper towel wads then baste. Roast for another 1- 1 1/2hr until an inserted thermometer in the leg reads 175°Fahrenheit. Watch the drippings and veggies while roasting, adding water if necessary. Move to a platter for display or leftovers and seconds.
- Prepare the gravy. On medium-high heat, place the roasting pan over two burners. Pour in wine then stir to loosen any brown bits with a wooden spoon. Use a big strainer to strain the contents in the pan to a pot; pour in broth then boil. Dissolve cornstarch in a half cup of water; stir into the pan juices gradually then boil. Turn to low heat; let it simmer until thick. Serve right away.

Nutrition Information

- Calories: 845 calories;
- Total Fat: 36.1
- Sodium: 11664
- Total Carbohydrate: 19.7
- Cholesterol: 298
- Protein: 101.9

869. Roasted Turkey, Navy Style

Serving: 15 | Prep: 30mins | Cook: 7hours30mins | Ready in:

Ingredients

- 1 (18 pound) whole turkey, thawed
- 1 1/4 cups chilled butter, diced
- 1 pound baby carrots
- 2 large onions, roughly chopped
- 3 stalks celery, roughly chopped
- 1 whole head garlic, cut in half crosswise
- 3 tablespoons chopped fresh thyme
- 3 tablespoons chopped fresh sage
- 2 bay leaves
- 1 (750 milliliter) bottle chilled Chardonnay wine
- salt and ground black pepper to taste

Direction

- Preheat the oven to 150°C or 300°F. In roasting pan, place a turkey roasting rack.
- Take giblet package and neck off the inner of turkey, in case there is any, and wash the turkey well, in and out. Using paper towels, pat turkey dry. Onto roasting rack, put the turkey. Using fingers, aim beneath the skin over the breast, and loosen the skin. Put butter cubes beneath breast skin, dividing them as equally as can be on the entire breast. To support the skin as it cooks, prick 4 or 5 wooden toothpicks all the way from skin into meat.
- Combine black pepper, salt, bay leaves, sage, thyme, the two garlic head halves, celery, onions and carrots in a bowl. Fill the turkey cavity with as much seasonings and vegetables will accommodate; scatter the remaining, in case there is any, into the base of roasting pan. Raise turkey upright to make cavity opening is topmost, and into the turkey, put the entire Chardonnay bottle to make wine stream into the pan. Onto the rack, set the turkey back facing down, and truss if preferred. Using aluminum foil, cover the turkey.
- In the prepped, oven, let roast for 7 hours till juices run clear and not pink anymore at the bone. Take turkey out of the oven, take off foil, and let roast for 25 to 30 minutes longer till skin becomes crisp and brown. An inserted instant-read thermometer into the chunkiest portion of thigh, close to the bone should register 82°C or 180°F. Take off from oven and allow to sit for 10 minutes prior to carving. Serve turkey with cooked celery, onion, and carrots on the side, if wished.

Nutrition Information

- Calories: 1019 calories;
- Total Fat: 53.7
- Sodium: 410

- Total Carbohydrate: 7.3
- Cholesterol: 363
- Protein: 111.3

870. Rosemary Roasted Turkey

Serving: 16 | Prep: 25mins | Cook: 4hours | Ready in:

Ingredients

- 3/4 cup olive oil
- 3 tablespoons minced garlic
- 2 tablespoons chopped fresh rosemary
- 1 tablespoon chopped fresh basil
- 1 tablespoon Italian seasoning
- 1 teaspoon ground black pepper
- salt to taste
- 1 (12 pound) whole turkey

Direction

- Preheat the oven to 165°C or 325°F.
- Combine the salt, black pepper, Italian seasoning, basil, rosemary, garlic and olive oil in a small bowl. Reserve.
- Rinse turkey inside and out; pat it dry. Get rid any big fat deposits. Loosen the breast skin by gently working fingers between breast and skin. Loosen it to the end of drumstick, ensuring not to tear the skin.
- Apply a liberal amount of rosemary mixture beneath the breast skin and down the thigh and leg with your hand. Massage the rest of the rosemary mixture on the outer part of breast. Secure the skin over any exposed breast meat with toothpicks.
- In roasting pan, put turkey on rack. Into the base of pan, put approximately a quarter inch of water. In the prepped oven, roast for 3 to 4 hours, or till the inner temperature of turkey reads 80°C or 180°F.

Nutrition Information

- Calories: 596 calories;
- Sodium: 165
- Total Carbohydrate: 0.8
- Cholesterol: 198
- Protein: 68.1
- Total Fat: 33.7

871. Salvadorian Roasted Turkey

Serving: 12 | Prep: 25mins | Cook: 3hours20mins | Ready in:

Ingredients

- 10 large Roma (plum) tomatoes, halved and seeded
- 1 large green bell pepper, halved and seeded
- 2 tablespoons vegetable oil
- 1 (10 pound) whole turkey, neck and giblets removed
- 1 Granny Smith apple - peeled, quartered, and cored
- 1 (5 ounce) jar pitted green olives, drained
- 2 dried ancho chiles, stemmed and seeded
- 1/2 cup raw pumpkin seeds
- 2 bay leaves
- 1 onion, cut into chunks
- salt and pepper to taste

Direction

- In the topmost place, position the oven rack and preheat the oven on broil setting. Line aluminum foil on a baking sheet.
- Onto the baking sheet, put the bell pepper and tomatoes, cut-side facing down. Broil on top rack of prepped oven for 5 minutes till skins start to blacken. Into a bowl, put the charred vegetables and enclose in plastic wrap to steam till skins loosen. Bring oven rack lower to fit a roasting pan, and set oven to 165°C or 325°F.
- In the meantime, into a roasting pan or skillet big enough to accommodate the turkey, put

the vegetable oil, and set over moderately high heat. Once hot, put in the turkey and sear on every side for 10 minutes till browned. When turkey has browned, into roasting pan, set breast side facing up, and fill with olives and quartered apples. Reserve.
- Over moderately high heat, heat a skillet. Put in bay leaves, pumpkin seeds and ancho chilies. Cook and mix for 5 minutes till pumpkin seeds start to smell toasted, then into the blender, put the mixture.
- When peppers and tomatoes have steamed enough to loosen the skins, peel and throw away the skins. Into the blender with pumpkin seeds, put the onion, green peppers and tomatoes. Process till it turns into smooth, thick sauce. Season to taste with pepper and salt, putting in a small amount of olive liquid if wished.
- Brush the turkey with sauce, and put into prepped oven. Allow to cook for 3 hours till an inserted meat thermometer in meaty portion of thigh registers 80°C or 180°F, basting from time to time.

Nutrition Information

- Calories: 662 calories;
- Protein: 79.3
- Total Fat: 33.3
- Sodium: 472
- Total Carbohydrate: 7.9
- Cholesterol: 224

872. Sherry's German Turkey

Serving: 18 | Prep: 25mins | Cook: 4hours | Ready in:

Ingredients

- 1 (18 pound) whole turkey, neck and giblets removed
- 1 medium onion, peeled
- 1 large carrot, peeled
- 1 stalk celery
- 1 apple, stem removed
- 1 orange
- 1/4 cup vegetable oil
- 1 teaspoon salt
- 1 tablespoon coarsely ground black pepper
- 1 teaspoon soul food seasoning
- 1 pound sliced smoked bacon
- 1 turkey sized oven bag

Direction

- Preheat an oven to 175°C or 350°F.
- Wash turkey, pat it dry and put in big roasting pan. Stuff turkey cavity with celery, carrot, and onion. Poke holes in the orange and apple to release their juices, and insert them inside the turkey. You may need to halve some things to make everything all inside. Scatter oil on the entire outside of turkey, and put soul food seasoning, pepper and salt to season.
- Into an oven bag, put the turkey, and return to the pan with breast-side up. Arrange bacon strips on the whole surface. Seal the bag.
- Let the turkey roast for approximately 4 hours, or till the inserted thermometer in the thickest part of the thigh reads 82°C or 180°F. Allow the turkey to sit for 10 or 15 minutes prior to carving, and use drippings in your preferred gravy recipe.

Nutrition Information

- Calories: 883 calories;
- Total Fat: 50.9
- Sodium: 666
- Total Carbohydrate: 3.6
- Cholesterol: 326
- Protein: 96

873. Simple Classic Roasted Turkey

Serving: 12 | Prep: 10mins | Cook: 6hours | Ready in:

Ingredients

- 1 (10 pound) whole turkey, neck and giblets optional
- salt and ground black pepper to taste
- 1/3 cup water, or as needed

Direction

- Preheat the oven to 135°C or 275°Fahrenheit.
- Sprinkle pepper and salt on the turkey then place in a roaster with the breast-side down; put in giblets and neck then add water in the pan.
- Bake for 6 hours in the preheated oven until the juices run clear and not pink at the bone, baste as necessary. An inserted instant-read thermometer in the thigh's thickest part should register 74°C or 165°Fahrenheit. If desired, roast until the meat falls off the bone.

Nutrition Information

- Calories: 567 calories;
- Sodium: 186
- Total Carbohydrate: 0
- Cholesterol: 224
- Protein: 76.6
- Total Fat: 26.5

874. Simple Deep Fried Turkey

Serving: 12 | Prep: 10mins | Cook: 35mins | Ready in:

Ingredients

- 3 1/2 gallons peanut oil for frying
- 1 (10 pound) whole turkey, neck and giblets removed
- 1 tablespoon salt, or to taste
- 1 tablespoon ground black pepper, or to taste

Direction

- Pour oil on a turkey fryer or a big stockpot and heat it to 350 degrees F (175 degrees C). For safety purposes, please make sure that the fryer is in a safe area outdoors, away from buildings and other objects that could catch fire. For extra measures, have a fire extinguisher nearby. The turkey must be thawed completely. All extra skin trimmed, and neck hole is at least one inch wide. Using paper towels, pat the turkey completely dry. Rub pepper and salt generously outside and inside the bird. Position the turkey neck-side first on a drain basket. Very carefully and slowly, lower the drain basket into the oil until the turkey is completely submerged. Cook the turkey for approximately 35 minutes or 3 1/2 minutes per pound. Keep the oil temperature at 350 degrees (175 degrees C) so the bird will be cooked evenly.
- After carefully removing the drain basket from the oil, check inner temperature of the bird by inserting a meat thermometer into the thick area of thigh; it should be 180 degrees F (80 degrees C). Remove turkey from basket and drain excess oil with paper towels. Let rest for 15 minutes before carving.

Nutrition Information

- Calories: 9644 calories;
- Total Fat: 1053.2
- Sodium: 768
- Total Carbohydrate: 0.3
- Cholesterol: 224
- Protein: 76.7

875. Smoked Turkey

Serving: 18 | Prep: 30mins | Cook: 6hours | Ready in:

Ingredients

- 1 (12 pound) whole turkey, neck and giblets removed

- 1 (20 pound) bag high quality charcoal briquettes
- hickory chips or chunks

Direction

- Brush the grate lightly with oil. Light the coals on the bottom pan of the smoker. Wait till the temperature to reach 240 degrees F (115 degrees C).
- Under cold water, rinse the turkey thoroughly, then pat dry with paper towels. Soak hickory chips in a pan with water.
- Put the turkey on the oiled grate. Toss 2 handfuls of soaked hickory chips before cooking and add a handful every 2 hours throughout the cooking process. DO NOT let the heat out by checking the turkey every now and then. You can cook the turkey till the coals die out or check the internal temperature of the turkey. It should be 165 degrees F (74 degrees C).

Nutrition Information

- Calories: 447 calories;
- Sodium: 146
- Total Carbohydrate: 0
- Cholesterol: 176
- Protein: 60.4
- Total Fat: 20.9

876. Sugar Free Citrus Turkey Brine

Serving: 12 | Prep: 30mins | Cook: 3hours30mins | Ready in:

Ingredients

- 1 (10 pound) whole turkey, neck and giblets removed
- 1 large, sturdy food-grade plastic bag
- 1 large cooler
- 2 gallons water
- 2 cups kosher salt
- 2 unpeeled navel oranges, cut into chunks
- 2 unpeeled lemons, cut into chunks
- 2 unpeeled clementines (Mandarin oranges), cut into chunks
- 1 bunch fresh rosemary sprigs
- 1 bunch fresh thyme
- 2 tablespoons butter, softened
- 1 tablespoon olive oil (optional)
- 1 teaspoon poultry seasoning, or to taste (optional)
- 1 teaspoon ground black pepper, or to taste (optional)

Direction

- Rinse both inside and outside of the turkey; put to one side. Put a plastic bag into the cooler; open the bag.
- Add water into the plastic bag, put in salt; smush the bag around with your fingers a few times until salt is dissolved. Add juices squeezed from clementine chunks, lemon, and orange into the salty water; put the chunks into the bag. Add thyme and rosemary and mix well. Lay turkey, breast side down, into the brine. Close the bag, squeeze to remove any excess air, and seal carefully; put the lid onto the cooler, and put into the fridge for 1 day.
- Turn oven to 350°F (175°C) to preheat.
- Take turkey out of the brine, saving 4 to 5 chunks each of lemon and navel oranges and sprigs of thyme and rosemary from the brine. Pour off the remaining used brine. Rinse turkey thoroughly both inside and outside, and remove to a roasting pan.
- Put herb sprigs and pieces of fruit inside the turkey. Use your fingers to loosen the skin over the breast, spread butter over the breast under the skin. Rub olive oil all over the turkey, and season with black pepper and poultry seasoning. Cover the turkey breast with aluminum foil, if desired.
- Roast turkey for 3.5 to 4 hours in the preheated oven until juices run clear and golden brown.

Take off the foil for the last 30 to 45 minutes of roasting. Cook until internal temperature of the thickest part of a thigh of the turkey reaches at least 165°F (75°C).

Nutrition Information

- Calories: 624 calories;
- Total Fat: 29.9
- Sodium: 15402
- Total Carbohydrate: 8.2
- Cholesterol: 229
- Protein: 77.4

877. Super Easy Smoked Turkey

Serving: 12 | Prep: 10mins | Cook: 6hours | Ready in:

Ingredients

- 1 (12 pound) whole turkey, thawed if frozen, neck and giblets removed
- 3/4 cup kosher salt
- 3/4 cup unsalted butter, melted

Direction

- Massage salt outside and inside the turkey, place in a roasting pan and set aside for an hour. Fill water pan of the smoker with water, preheat to 250 degrees F (120 degrees C). Rinse the turkey to remove the salt and dry thoroughly with paper towels. Put it back to the roasting pan and brush with melted butter. Cover top of the pan with aluminum foil and place it in the smoker. Remove the foil after 3 hours of cooking, cook uncovered for another 3 1/2 hours or until thermometer inserted into thickest area of thigh says 165 degrees F (74 degrees C). Take the turkey out of smoker then tent it using aluminum foil. Let the bird rest for 45 to 60 minutes in a warm place before slicing.

Nutrition Information

- Calories: 773 calories;
- Total Fat: 42.9
- Sodium: 5914
- Total Carbohydrate: 0
- Cholesterol: 295
- Protein: 90.7

878. Thanksgiving Turkey Brine

Serving: 20 | Prep: | Cook: 5hours | Ready in:

Ingredients

- 1 gallon water
- 4 quarts chicken broth
- 1 1/2 cups kosher salt
- 2 tablespoons minced garlic
- 2 tablespoons dried rosemary
- 2 tablespoons dried minced onion
- 2 tablespoons dried basil
- 2 tablespoons dried savory
- 2 tablespoons dried marjoram
- 2 tablespoons dried thyme
- 2 tablespoons dried tarragon
- 1 tablespoon dried oregano
- 1 tablespoon ground black pepper
- 1 tablespoon coriander seeds
- 2 gallons ice, divided, or more as needed
- 1 (20 pound) whole turkey, neck and giblets removed

Direction

- In a 5-gallon bucket with lid, combine salt, chicken broth, and water until salt is dissolved. Mix in coriander, pepper, oregano, tarragon, thyme, marjoram, savory, basil, onion, rosemary, and garlic until well combined. Whisk 2 cups ice into brine.

- Put turkey into the brine, filling brine into the cavity. Put enough ice into bucket to cover the turkey. Set lid on the bucket. Swiss the bucket from side-to-side to make water chilled. Chill bucket and turkey, refilling with ice after each 2 hours if necessary, 12 hours to 1 day.
- Set oven to 350°F (175°C) to preheat.
- Take turkey out of the brine; pat turkey dry. Pour off used brine. Arrange turkey on a rack inside a roasting pan.
- Bake turkey at 350°F (175°C) for 5 to 6.5 hours, basting after each 30 to 40 minutes, until no pink remains at the bone and turkey juices run clear. An instant-read thermometer pierced into the thickest area of the thigh should register 165°F (74°C). Take turkey out of the oven, tent with a double sheet of aluminum foil, and let stand for 5 to 10 minutes before carving.

Nutrition Information

- Calories: 704 calories;
- Total Fat: 32.5
- Sodium: 7841
- Total Carbohydrate: 3.2
- Cholesterol: 272
- Protein: 93.2

879. The Attention Hungry Turkey Of Moistness

Serving: 18 | Prep: 20mins | Cook: 4hours | Ready in:

Ingredients

- 1 (18 pound) whole turkey, neck and giblets removed
- 8 cups prepared stuffing
- 1/2 cup softened butter
- salt and pepper to taste

Direction

- Preheat an oven to 165°C or 325°F. Position oven rack to lowest position so the turkey can fit.
- Wash the turkey and pat it dry. Put in a big roasting pan and stuff the cavity loosely with filling. Massage butter on the entire outside, and add pepper and salt to season. Create a tent on top of the turkey using a big aluminum foil sheet.
- Put in prepped oven. Baste all over after every 5 to 10 minutes. Baste constantly. After 2 hours, take off the foil tent. Continue roasting till inner temperature in the chunkiest part of thigh reads 82°C or 180°F. It will take approximately 4 hours in total.

Nutrition Information

- Calories: 883 calories;
- Total Carbohydrate: 19.3
- Cholesterol: 282
- Protein: 94.8
- Total Fat: 44.6
- Sodium: 871

880. The Best Ugly Turkey

Serving: 12 | Prep: 30mins | Cook: 3hours | Ready in:

Ingredients

- 1 (12 pound) whole turkey, neck and giblets removed
- 1/2 cup extra virgin olive oil
- 2 tablespoons salt
- 1 apple - peeled, cored and cubed

Direction

- Preheat an oven to 175°C or 350°F. Wash turkey inside and out and use paper towels to pat it dry. Massage the entire turkey with salt and olive oil. Put apple pieces inside of the cavity. In a big roasting pan, set the turkey breast side facing down.

- In the prepped oven, let roast for 3 hours. Take out of the oven and cautiously flip the turkey, making breast side face up. Put back to oven and cook till the inner temperature of the thickest part of thigh has read 82°C or 180°F. Let the turkey sit for approximately 30 minutes prior to carving.

Nutrition Information

- Calories: 807 calories;
- Protein: 91.5
- Total Fat: 45.3
- Sodium: 1454
- Total Carbohydrate: 1.6
- Cholesterol: 305

881. The Greatest Grilled Turkey

Serving: 18 | Prep: 30mins | Cook: 3hours | Ready in:

Ingredients

- 12 pounds whole turkey
- 1 tablespoon vegetable oil
- 1 teaspoon Italian seasoning
- salt and pepper to taste

Direction

- Preheat your outdoor grill to indirect medium to high heat. Wash turkey with cold water then pat dry. Tuck the legs and turn the wings back to keep the neck skin stable. Brush the skin using oil and rub thoroughly using Italian seasoning, salt and the pepper outside and inside the cavity.
- Place a metal grate on the bottom of a big roasting pan and position the bird with the breast side up. Put the pan on preheated grill. Cook for 2-3 hours or until meat thermometer inserted on the thickest area of thigh reads 180 degrees F (85 degrees C). Take out the turkey and allow to rest for 15 minutes before cutting.

Nutrition Information

- Calories: 460 calories;
- Sodium: 148
- Total Carbohydrate: 0.1
- Cholesterol: 179
- Protein: 61.2
- Total Fat: 22

882. The World's Best Turkey

Serving: 16 | Prep: 20mins | Cook: 3hours30mins | Ready in:

Ingredients

- 1 (12 pound) whole turkey, neck and giblets removed
- 1/2 cup butter, cubed
- 2 apples, cored and halved
- 1 tablespoon garlic powder
- salt and pepper to taste
- 2/3 (750 milliliter) bottle Champagne

Direction

- Set the oven to 350°F (175°C) for preheating.
- Wash the turkey and pat it to dry. Loosen the turkey breast skin gently. Stuff the pieces of butter between breast and skin. Stuff the apples inside the cavity of the turkey. Sprinkle it with pepper, garlic powder, and salt. Position the turkey in the roasting bag. Pour Champagne all over the inner and outer parts of the bird. Seal the bag and place it into the roasting pan.
- Bake the turkey in the preheated oven for 3-3 1/2 hours or until the internal temperature of the meatiest part of the thigh reaches 180°F (85°C). Get the turkey from the bag. Before carving, allow it to stand for at least 20 minutes.

Nutrition Information

- Calories: 591 calories;
- Sodium: 207
- Total Carbohydrate: 3.6
- Cholesterol: 214
- Protein: 68.2
- Total Fat: 29.3

883. Thyme Roasted Turkey

Serving: 14 | Prep: 20mins | Cook: 3hours30mins | Ready in:

Ingredients

- 2 teaspoons McCormick® Garlic Powder
- 2 teaspoons McCormick® Paprika
- 1 teaspoon McCormick® Thyme Leaves
- 1 teaspoon McCormick® Black Pepper, Ground
- 1 teaspoon salt
- 1 tablespoon oil
- 1 (14 pound) whole turkey, fresh or frozen, thawed

Direction

- Position oven rack in the lowest level of the oven. Turn oven to 325°F to preheat. Set roasting rack in a shallow roasting pan. In a small bowl, combine salt, pepper, thyme, paprika, and garlic powder.
- Place turkey in the prepared baking pan, breast-side up. Brush oil over the turkey. Scatter evenly seasoning mixture all over the turkey. Tent chicken loosely with heavy duty foil.
- Roast chicken in the preheated oven for 2 hours, adding an additional 15 minutes per pound for bigger turkeys. Take off the foil. Keep roasting until a thermometer inserted in chick thigh reads 165°F (or 175°F in thigh), basting with pan juices occasionally, about 1 hour longer. Take turkey out of the oven. Allow to cool for 20 minutes before placing on a cutting board or platter. Save the pan juice for making gravy or serving with turkey.

Nutrition Information

- Calories: 691 calories;
- Total Fat: 32.8
- Sodium: 389
- Total Carbohydrate: 0.6
- Cholesterol: 268
- Protein: 91.9

884. Tiffany's Herb Roasted Turkey

Serving: 8 | Prep: | Cook: | Ready in:

Ingredients

- Reynolds® Oven Bag, turkey size
- 1 tablespoon all-purpose flour
- 2 stalks celery
- 1 medium onion
- 1 (8 pound) turkey, fresh or thawed*
- 2 tablespoons vegetable oil
- 1 teaspoon ground thyme
- 1 teaspoon dried basil
- 1 teaspoon dried rosemary
- 1 teaspoon paprika
- 1 teaspoon seasoned salt
- 1 tablespoon dried sage
- 1/2 teaspoon ground black pepper

Direction

- Prepare the oven by preheating to 350°F.
- In Reynolds® Oven bag, add flour and shake; transfer to a large roasting pan at least 2-inch deep. Use nonstick cooking spray to coat inside of the bag, if wished to lessen sticking with large turkeys.

- Put vegetables to the bag. Take off giblets and neck from the turkey. Wash the turkey, pat dry and use oil to brush it. In a small bowl mix the seasonings; dust and rub evenly over the turkey.
- Put the turkey in the oven bag on top of vegetables.
- Use a nylon tie to seal the oven bag; slice six slits (1/2-inch) at the top. Tuck the meat thermometer through the slit in the bag into the thickest part of the inner thigh without touching the bone. Insert ends of the bag in the pan.
- Bake based on the times below or until the meat thermometer registers 180°F.
- Allow it to stand for 15 minutes in the oven bag. Slice open the top of the bag. With the two carving forks, tuck one in each end, to get the turkey from the bag.
- Roasting times:
- For 8 to 12 lb. turkeys, bake for 1 1/2-2 hours.
- For 12 to 16 lb. turkeys, bake for 2-2 1/2 hours.
- For 16 to 20 lb. turkeys, bake for 2 1/2-3 hours.
- For 20 to 24 lb. turkeys, bake for 3-3 1/2 hours.

Nutrition Information

- Calories: 723 calories;
- Total Fat: 35.3
- Sodium: 345
- Total Carbohydrate: 3.1
- Cholesterol: 267
- Protein: 92.1

885. Turducken

Serving: 24 | Prep: 1hours | Cook: 4hours | Ready in:

Ingredients

- 1 (3 pound) whole chicken, boned
- salt and pepper to taste
- Creole seasoning to taste
- 1 (4 pound) duck, boned
- 1 (16 pound) turkey, boned
- 3 cups prepared sausage and oyster dressing

Direction

- Start preheating oven to 375 degrees F or 190 degrees C. With the skin-side down, put the boned chicken on a plate and generously season with Creole seasoning, pepper, and salt. With the skin-side down, put the boned duck on top the chicken and generously season with Creole seasoning, pepper, and salt. Cover; place in refrigerator.
- Skin-side down, put the boned turkey on a flat surface. Add a layer of chilled Sausage and Oyster Dressing, make sure to push it into the wing and leg cavities so it looks like the bones are still there.
- Put the duck, skin-side down on top the turkey and add a layer of the chilled dressing. Put the chicken, skin-side down on top the duck and add a layer of the chilled dressing.
- With someone's help, wrap the turkey skin around and use toothpicks to secure them. Take kitchen string and lace it between the toothpicks to help hold everything in. Gently put the turducken in a big roasting pan breast side up.
- With the cover on, roast until turducken is golden brown, 4 hours. Remove cover and roast until thermometer poked into thigh reads 180 degrees F and when poked in stuffing says 165 degrees F, 1 hour. Check every few hours to baste and remove any extra liquid. There should be enough cooking juices to make one gallon of gravy. Carve the turducken and enjoy.

Nutrition Information

- Calories: 836 calories;
- Total Fat: 52.8
- Sodium: 360
- Total Carbohydrate: 5.3
- Cholesterol: 262
- Protein: 78.7

886. Turkey Mercedes

Serving: 20 | Prep: 40mins | Cook: 5hours | Ready in:

Ingredients

- 3 heads garlic, peeled
- 1 tablespoon black pepper
- 1 tablespoon ground cumin
- 1 tablespoon dried oregano
- 2 tablespoons salt (or to taste)
- 2 cups fresh lemon juice
- 1 cup dry white wine
- 1/2 (12 fluid ounce) can frozen orange juice concentrate, thawed
- 1 (16 pound) turkey

Direction

- Mash peeled garlic cloves and put into big bowl. Add salt, oregano, cumin and pepper to season. Add orange juice concentrate, wine and lemon juice; mix together till thoroughly combined.
- Prick turkey legs, thighs, and breast with a sharp paring knife, making holes to penetrate the marinade. Add marinade on top of turkey, and into holes. Lastly, fill holes with garlic pieces. Cover turkey thoroughly, and marinate by chilling overnight.
- Preheat the oven to 165°C or 325°F.
- In the prepped oven, let the turkey roast for 5 hours till inner temperature of the chunkiest part of thigh reads 80°C or 180°F. Baste turkey every 30 to 45 minutes. When breast turns brown, loosely cover with aluminum foil to keep from becoming burnt.

Nutrition Information

- Calories: 589 calories;
- Total Fat: 25.6
- Sodium: 879
- Total Carbohydrate: 8.9
- Cholesterol: 215
- Protein: 74.5

887. Turkey And Stuffing

Serving: 18 | Prep: 30mins | Cook: 3hours30mins | Ready in:

Ingredients

- 1 (12 ounce) package dry bread stuffing mix
- 5 cups water
- 1 large onion, chopped
- 4 celery, chopped
- 4 tablespoons dried sage
- 12 pounds whole turkey, neck and giblets removed

Direction

- Follow the package instructions on how to prepare the stuffing. Place it in a large bowl and put aside.
- Set the oven to 350°F (175°C) for preheating.
- Boil the water in a medium saucepan over medium heat. Stir in celery, sage, and onion. Boil the mixture for 10 minutes or until the onion is soft. Mix the mixture into the prepared stuffing.
- Wash the turkey and pat it to dry. Fill the neck and body cavities loosely with the stuffing mixture.
- Position the turkey in a large roasting pan. Cook the turkey inside the preheated oven for 3-3 1/2 hours or until the thigh meat's internal temperature reaches 180°F or 80°C and the stuffing's temperature reaches at least 165°F or 75°C.

Nutrition Information

- Calories: 533 calories;
- Sodium: 460
- Total Carbohydrate: 15.8
- Cholesterol: 179
- Protein: 63.5

- Total Fat: 21.9

888. Turkey In A Bag

Serving: 12 | Prep: 20mins | Cook: 3hours | Ready in:

Ingredients

- 12 pounds whole turkey
- salt and pepper to taste
- 2 tablespoons all-purpose flour
- 5 stalks celery
- 2 large onions, quartered

Direction

- Set the oven to 350°F (175°C) for preheating.
- Wash the turkey well and remove the giblets. Season it with salt and pepper to taste.
- Sprinkle flour into the bottom of an oven bag with a size of a turkey. Arrange the onions, celery, and turkey into the bag. Seal the bag. Use a fork to poke several holes all over the bag.
- Let it bake inside the oven for 3-3 1/2 hours or until the thigh meat's internal temperature reaches 180°F or 85°C.

Nutrition Information

- Calories: 744 calories;
- Sodium: 309
- Total Carbohydrate: 3.8
- Cholesterol: 309
- Protein: 93.2
- Total Fat: 36.5

889. Turkey In A Smoker

Serving: 13 | Prep: 20mins | Cook: 10hours | Ready in:

Ingredients

- 1 (10 pound) whole turkey, neck and giblets removed
- 4 cloves garlic, crushed
- 2 tablespoons seasoned salt
- 1/2 cup butter
- 2 (12 fluid ounce) cans cola-flavored carbonated beverage
- 1 apple, quartered
- 1 onion, quartered
- 1 tablespoon garlic powder
- 1 tablespoon salt
- 1 tablespoon ground black pepper

Direction

- Prepare smoker, preheat to 225 to 250 degrees R (110 to 120 degrees C).
- Under cold running water, wash the turkey thoroughly and dry with paper towels. Rub salt and crushed garlic on the outside until every surface is seasoned. Put in a disposable roasting pan and fill the cavity with a mixture of butter, apple, onions, cola, ground black pepper and salt. Cover loosely using aluminum foil. Transfer the roasting pan into the smoker and cook for 10 hours at 225 to 250 degrees F (110 to 120 degrees C), basting every 1-2 hours with drippings from the bottom of the pan. Inner temperature of the thickest area of thigh should be 180 degrees F (80 degrees C) to know if the bird is cooked through.

Nutrition Information

- Calories: 625 calories;
- Total Carbohydrate: 9.8
- Cholesterol: 225
- Protein: 71.2
- Total Fat: 31.7
- Sodium: 1185

890. Turkey With Cornbread Stuffing

Serving: 12 | Prep: 1hours | Cook: 4hours | Ready in:

Ingredients

- 3/4 cup cornmeal
- 1 1/4 cups water
- 1 cup whole wheat flour
- 1/3 cup white sugar
- 1 tablespoon baking powder
- 1/2 teaspoon salt
- 1 egg
- 1/4 cup vegetable oil
- 1/4 pound bacon, or more to taste
- 1 large onion, chopped
- 2 cloves garlic, minced
- 6 celery stalk, chopped
- 1 red bell pepper, diced (optional)
- 4 teaspoons poultry seasoning
- 4 teaspoons dried rubbed sage
- 4 teaspoons dried oregano
- 1 (1 pound) loaf rye bread, cubed
- 2 cups low-sodium chicken broth
- 1 whole turkey, neck and giblets removed

Direction

- Set the oven at 200° C (400° F) to preheat. Coat a pie pan with cooking spray.
- Mix water and cornmeal in a bowl and let it sit for 10 minutes. Meanwhile, in a big bowl, whip salt, baking powder, sugar and whole wheat flour together. Whip vegetable oil and eggs into wet cornmeal; stir this wet mixture into the flour mixture until just blended and transfer to the prepared pie pan.
- In the preheated oven, bake the cornbread until it is lightly browned and a knife inserted into the middle of the cornbread comes out clean, about 20-30 minutes. Take it out of the oven and put aside to cool.
- Reduce the heat to 165° C (325° F).
- In a big skillet, cook the bacon over medium-high heat until it is crispy and browned, approximately 6 minutes on each side; place on a paper towel-lined plate to drain. When the bacon is cool, crumble it. Stir oregano, sage, poultry seasoning, red bell pepper, celery, garlic and onion into the bacon drippings left in the skillet; cook while stirring until the onion becomes translucent, approximately 10 minutes.
- Take the cooled cornbread out of the pie pan and chop into small cubes; put them in a big bowl and blend in rye bread cubes. Stir cooked vegetables and bacon into the filling until well mixed, pour chicken broth into the dressing, stirring so the bread cubes are moistened evenly.
- Rinse both the inside and outside of the turkey and use paper towels to pat dry. Transfer turkey to a big roasting pan with a lid. Loosely stuff the body and neck cavities with the filling, folding neck's skin over the filling and use toothpicks to secure. Put all remaining stuffing onto a big square aluminum foil, fold and seal edges to enclose the stuffing. Put stuffing packet in the fridge until 45 minutes before serving.
- Put the turkey in the oven, roast until a thermometer inserted in the thickest part of the thigh indicates 80° C (180° F), about 3 1/2 to 4 hours. After 2 1/2 hours, remove the lid to brown the skin. Baste with pan drippings occasionally. Bake the additional stuffing 45 minutes before serving, if necessary.

Nutrition Information

- Calories: 1324 calories;
- Protein: 158.7
- Total Fat: 60.1
- Sodium: 809
- Total Carbohydrate: 27.3
- Cholesterol: 466

891. Upside Down Turkey

Serving: 18 | Prep: 30mins | Cook: 3hours | Ready in:

Ingredients

- 13 pounds whole turkey
- 1/2 cup butter
- 1 cup water

Direction

- Preheat the oven to 175°C or 350°F.
- Wash the turkey and get rid of giblets. In a roasting pan, set the turkey upside, the breast facing down. Stuff quarter cup of butter into the turkey. Arrange leftover butter in few pieces around the turkey. Add water into pan.
- In the prepped oven, allow to cook with a cover for 3 to 3 1/2 hours till inner temperature of thigh reads 80°C or 180°F.

Nutrition Information

- Calories: 536 calories;
- Total Fat: 28.1
- Sodium: 197
- Total Carbohydrate: 0
- Cholesterol: 207
- Protein: 66.4

892. Very Moist And Flavorful Roast Turkey

Serving: 12 | Prep: 20mins | Cook: 3hours30mins | Ready in:

Ingredients

- 1/2 cup cold butter
- 1 (12 pound) whole turkey, neck and giblets removed
- 1 tablespoon vegetable oil
- 2 Granny Smith apples - cored, peeled, and cut into 8 wedges each
- 1 large onion, cut into 8 wedges
- 1/2 whole head garlic, separated into cloves and peeled
- 1 pound celery, cut into 2-inch lengths
- 1 tablespoon poultry seasoning

Direction

- Set the oven to 165°Celcious or 325°Fahrenheit.
- Cut the butter into 1tbsp portions then cut them again into quarters then chill in the refrigerator until ready to use.
- Loosen the skin on the thighs and breast of the turkey with your fingers. On the part of skin between the body and tail, slit a hole to affix the legs latter. Slit a hole under each turkey wing to affix the wings. Rub or brush vegetable oil on the entire surface of the turkey skin.
- In a big bowl, toss together celery, apple, garlic cloves, and onion wedges; toss in poultry seasoning to coat. Take the apple mixture and stuff into the neck and body cavities. Tuck and secure each wing tip in the hole made under the wings; tuck and secure each leg in the hole made near the tail.
- Put the turkey on a rack set over a roasting pan. Evenly distribute and stuff the cold butter pieces beneath the loosened turkey skin.
- Roast for 3 1/2hrs in the preheated oven until an inserted instant-read thermometer in the thickest thigh part without touching the bone registers 70°C or 160°Fahrenheit. Check the turkey after 3hrs for doneness.
- Take the pan out of the oven then use aluminum foil to cover the turkey; press the foil lightly on the turkey. Let it sit for 40mins before slicing.

Nutrition Information

- Calories: 774 calories;
- Sodium: 305
- Total Carbohydrate: 6.1
- Cholesterol: 285
- Protein: 91.3
- Total Fat: 40.3

Chapter 7: Turkey Breast Recipes

***

893. Aidan Special

Serving: 1 | Prep: 10mins | Cook: 5mins | Ready in:

Ingredients

- 1 tablespoon butter, softened, or as needed
- 2 slices rye bread
- 4 slices Swiss cheese
- 2 ounces turkey breast, or more to taste
- 2 slices tomato
- 2 slices cooked bacon, or more to taste
- 1 ounce Russian salad dressing

Direction

- Set a large skillet over medium heat.
- Coat 1 side of each bread piece with butter. Arrange the slices into the skillet, butter-side down. Lay 2 Swiss cheese slices atop each bread slice. Cook them for 3-4 minutes, or until the cheese melts.
- In a separate skillet, cook slices of tomato and turkey over medium heat for 2-3 minutes, or until warmed.
- Layer 1 bread slice (it must be the bottom of the sandwich) with tomato, turkey, and bacon. Pour the Russian dressing over tomato layer. Place the second slice of bread on top to form a sandwich.

Nutrition Information

- Calories: 968 calories;
- Sodium: 1305
- Total Carbohydrate: 48
- Cholesterol: 191
- Protein: 58.1
- Total Fat: 60.4

894. Awesome Turkey Sandwich

Serving: 1 | Prep: 10mins | Cook: | Ready in:

Ingredients

- 2 slices whole wheat bread, toasted (optional)
- 1 tablespoon mayonnaise
- 2 teaspoons Dijon-style prepared mustard
- 3 slices smoked turkey breast
- 2 tablespoons guacamole
- 1/2 cup mixed salad greens
- 1/4 cup bean sprouts
- 1/4 avocado - peeled, pitted and sliced
- 3 ounces Colby-Monterey Jack cheese, sliced
- 2 slices tomato

Direction

- Spread over one slice of toast with mayonnaise, then spread over the other with the mustard. On one side, arrange the sliced turkey. Spread over the turkey with guacamole. Then pile on the cheese, avocado, bean sprouts and salad greens. Ending with the tomato slices, then top with the rest of the slice of toast.

Nutrition Information

- Calories: 804 calories;
- Sodium: 1988
- Total Carbohydrate: 41.4
- Cholesterol: 124
- Protein: 37.9
- Total Fat: 56.6

895. Bacon Wrapped Turkey Breast Stuffed With Spinach And Feta

Serving: 4 | Prep: 15mins | Cook: 35mins | Ready in:

Ingredients

- 1 large turkey breast
- 1/2 teaspoon dried oregano
- 1/2 teaspoon ground cumin
- salt and ground black pepper to taste
- 1 cup fresh spinach, or to taste
- 1/4 cup crumbled feta cheese
- 12 slices reduced-sodium bacon, or as needed

Direction

- Prepare the oven and set to 350°F or 175°C.
- Make a slice in the middle of the turkey breast and place it flat. Drizzle salt, cumin, oregano and pepper on the side of the turkey. Place a layer of spinach leaves on one of the turkey and top with feta cheese. Repeat the process of layering with feta cheese and spinach. Then, fold the other turkey breast half over the feta cheese to seal the filling. Take the bacon and wrap the whole turkey breast with it. Put the wrapped turkey in a baking dish and dash with salt and pepper.
- Let the turkey breast cook for about half an hour or until an instant read thermometer inserted into the center reads at least 165°F /74 degrees C or until no longer pink in the center and juices run clear.
- Turn the oven's broiler on and broil the wrapped turkey for 2 minutes per side until the bacon becomes crisp on each side. Let it cool for about ten minutes before cutting.

Nutrition Information

- Calories: 371 calories;
- Total Fat: 27.6
- Sodium: 688
- Total Carbohydrate: 1.4
- Cholesterol: 82
- Protein: 27.7

896. Baked Hawaiian Sandwiches

Serving: 24 | Prep: 30mins | Cook: 15mins | Ready in:

Ingredients

- 24 Hawaiian bread rolls (such as King's®), split
- 12 thin slices of honey-cured deli ham, halved
- 12 slices Swiss cheese, halved
- 12 thin slices deli smoked turkey, halved
- 12 thin slices provolone cheese, halved
- 1/2 cup butter
- 1/4 cup white sugar
- 1/4 cup dried onion flakes
- 2 tablespoons poppy seeds
- 1 tablespoon honey mustard

Direction

- Set a rack into the lower half of the oven then prepare the oven by preheating to 400°F (200°C).
- On a baking sheet, arrange bottom halves of Hawaiian rolls. Then put a half slice each of ham, provolone cheese, smoked turkey, and Swiss cheese onto every roll bottom. Put top halves on every bottom to form sandwiches.
- In a saucepan set on low heat, dissolve butter and mix in honey mustard, poppy seeds, dried onion flakes, and sugar for approximately 2 minutes, until mixture is smoothly blended, creamy, and the sugar is melted; then sweep on the tops of every sandwich.
- Place sandwiches on preheated oven at the lower rack and bake for approximately 15 minutes until tops become golden brown and fillings become hot.

Nutrition Information

- Calories: 426 calories;
- Protein: 23
- Total Fat: 11.4
- Sodium: 488
- Total Carbohydrate: 46.6
- Cholesterol: 78

897. Bourbon And Molasses Glazed Turkey Breast

Serving: 4 | Prep: 10mins | Cook: 45mins | Ready in:

Ingredients

- 1 cup bourbon whiskey (such as Maker's Mark®)
- 1/2 cup blackstrap molasses
- 1/4 cup brown sugar
- 1 tablespoon kosher salt
- 1 teaspoon hot pepper sauce (such as Tabasco®)
- 1 (2 pound) bone-in turkey breast

Direction

- In a saucepan, mix brown sugar, molasses and whiskey till brown sugar has dissolved. Set over moderate heat, simmer, and switch off heat; into mixture, mix hot pepper sauce and salt. Into a big bowl, put the marinade.
- Into the marinade, put the turkey breast, skin side facing down; allow to sit for an hour, flipping turkey breast over from time to time. Turn turkey onto a roasting pan. Leave the marinade for basting.
- Preheat an oven to 230°C or 450°F.
- In the prepped oven, let the turkey breast roast for 45 minutes till inserted meat thermometer into the chunkiest portion of meat registers 70°C or 160°F. Baste the turkey from time to time with leftover marinade. Let the turkey breast sit for 10 minutes prior to cutting.

Nutrition Information

- Calories: 580 calories;
- Total Fat: 1.5
- Sodium: 1570
- Total Carbohydrate: 44.2
- Cholesterol: 164
- Protein: 59.3

898. Cheater's Thanksgiving Turkey

Serving: 4 | Prep: 15mins | Cook: 25mins | Ready in:

Ingredients

- 2 cups dry bread stuffing mix
- 2 teaspoons garlic powder
- 2 teaspoons onion salt
- 1/4 cup all-purpose flour
- 1 egg
- 1/2 cup milk
- 4 (6 ounce) turkey breast cutlets
- 2 (.87 ounce) packages turkey gravy mix
- 2 cups cold water

Direction

- Preheat the oven to 190°C or 375°F.
- In a bowl, mash stuffing mix into crumbs; mix in onion salt and garlic powder. In a shallow bowl, put the flour. In another shallow bowl, whisk the milk and egg together.
- Dredge turkey cutlets in flour, then dip in egg mixture; softly press into crumbs to cover. Put breaded cutlets into a baking dish, 9x13-inch in size.
- In the prepped oven, allow to bake for 20 minutes till cutlets are not pink anymore on the inside and juices run clear.
- In a saucepan, mix water and dry gravy mix till smooth, set over moderate heat, and boil, mixing continuously. Lower the heat and allow to simmer for a minute. Put gravy on top of cutlets then serve.

Nutrition Information

- Calories: 698 calories;
- Sodium: 3025
- Total Carbohydrate: 93.9
- Cholesterol: 174
- Protein: 60.1
- Total Fat: 7

899. Cranberry Stuffed Turkey Breasts

Serving: 10 | Prep: 45mins | Cook: 1hours | Ready in:

Ingredients

- 1 (12 ounce) package herb-seasoned bread stuffing mix
- 2 skinless boneless turkey breasts
- 1 cup chopped pecans
- 2 (8 ounce) packages dried, sweetened cranberries
- 2 tablespoons olive oil
- 6 lettuce leaves
- 1/2 cup pecan halves

Direction

- Set the oven to 350°F (175°C) for preheating. Follow the package directions on how to prepare the stuffing. Put the stuffing aside to cool.
- Use a sharp knife to butterfly open the breast for it to lay flat. Position each breast between the 2 sheets of waxed paper. Use a mallet to flatten the breast. Pour the prepared stuffing to within 1/4-inch of the edges of the breasts. Sprinkle each breast with dried cranberries and chopped pecans, reserving some of cranberries for the garnish. Roll the breast up tightly like a jellyroll style, making sure to start rolling with the long end. Tuck the ends of the roll and tie the rolls in sections using the string, about 4 sections around the center and 1 section running the length of the roll so that the ends are tightly secured.
- Put olive oil in a large cast-iron skillet and heat it over medium-high heat. Brown all the sides of the rolls carefully.
- Place the uncovered skillet inside the oven. Let the rolls bake inside the preheated oven for 1 hour or until their internal temperature reaches 170°F (78°C) when measured using a meat thermometer. Don't let the rolls get overly dry.
- Let the rolls set for 15 minutes before taking the string away. Slice the rolls into 1/2-3/4-inch circles. Cut the other roll for a nice presentation and leave one roll whole. The stuffing will be spiraled into the meat. Decorate the slices nicely on a platter with a bed of curly lettuce. Garnish the serving platter with the reserved dried cranberries and the remaining half cup of the pecan halves.

Nutrition Information

- Calories: 369 calories;
- Sodium: 858
- Total Carbohydrate: 28
- Cholesterol: 34
- Protein: 23.2
- Total Fat: 18.4

900. Croissant Club Sandwich

Serving: 4 | Prep: 15mins | Cook: 5mins | Ready in:

Ingredients

- 2 avocados, peeled and pitted
- 1/2 teaspoon garlic salt
- 1/2 teaspoon lemon juice
- 1/4 teaspoon dried oregano
- 4 croissants, split
- 8 slices smoked deli turkey breast
- 4 slices Swiss cheese
- 8 slices cooked bacon

- 8 slices tomato
- 4 lettuce leaves
- 4 teaspoons spicy brown mustard, or to taste

Direction

- Preheat oven to 350°F (175°C).
- Use potato masher or a fork to mash avocado in a bowl. Stir in oregano, lemon juice, and garlic salt.
- On a work surface, arrange split croissants. On bottom half of each croissant, place 2 slices turkey. Layer 1 slice Swiss cheese and 2 bacon slices over. Place each croissant top over bacon layer. Place sandwiches on a baking sheet.
- Bake for approximately 5 to 7 minutes in the preheated oven until cheese is melted.
- Open each sandwich and place 2 tomato slices and 1 lettuce leaf on top. On each croissant top, spread lightly 1/4 the avocado mixture and 1 teaspoon mustard. Place each top back to each sandwich.

Nutrition Information

- Calories: 636 calories;
- Cholesterol: 100
- Protein: 29
- Total Fat: 41
- Sodium: 1725
- Total Carbohydrate: 41.4

901. Deep Fried Turkey Breast

Serving: 12 | Prep: 5mins | Cook: 25mins | Ready in:

Ingredients

- 2 tablespoons sea salt
- 1 tablespoon red pepper flakes
- 1 tablespoon freshly ground black pepper
- 1 tablespoon granulated garlic
- 1 tablespoon chili powder
- 1 (7 pound) turkey breast
- 2 gallons canola oil for frying

Direction

- In a plastic container with a matching lid, combine the red pepper flakes, chili powder, granulated garlic, sea salt, and black pepper. Seal the container with its lid and shake until the seasonings are well-combined.
- Rub the spice mixture all over the turkey breast until well-coated. Use an aluminum foil to wrap the breast; refrigerate for 24 hours.
- Get the breast from the refrigerator and allow it to stand at room temperature.
- Meanwhile, heat the oil in a pot with a lid (enough to hold the oil and breast to 325°F or 165°C).
- Add the breast into the hot oil. Cover the pot with its lid. Fry the turkey for 25 minutes until its juices run clear and the turkey is no longer pinkish in the center. Make sure that the inserted instant-read thermometer into the turkey's center should read at least 165°F (74°C).

Nutrition Information

- Calories: 1040 calories;
- Sodium: 1041
- Total Carbohydrate: 1.7
- Cholesterol: 190
- Protein: 76.5
- Total Fat: 79.7

902. Easy Turkey Stuffing Roll Ups

Serving: 4 | Prep: 15mins | Cook: 15mins | Ready in:

Ingredients

- 1 1/2 cups water
- 1/4 cup margarine
- 1 (6 ounce) package dry bread stuffing mix

- 8 slices deli turkey breast
- 1 (12 ounce) jar turkey gravy

Direction

- Boil margarine and water in a pot then put in stuffing mix. Put cover and take away from the heat. Allow to stand for 5 minutes until the stuffing is tender. Using a fork, fluff the mixture.
- Over every slice of turkey, scoop in about 1/2 cup of stuffing. Roll the turkey over the stuffing and organize the rolls in a microwave-safe container, with the seam-side facing bottom. Pour gravy on top of the rolls.
- For 5 minutes, with the microwave set on full power, heat until you see bubbles from the gravy.

Nutrition Information

- Calories: 378 calories;
- Total Fat: 16.6
- Sodium: 1866
- Total Carbohydrate: 39
- Cholesterol: 23
- Protein: 15.6

903. Green Chile Posole (Low Fat)

Serving: 8 | Prep: 15mins | Cook: 55mins | Ready in:

Ingredients

- 2 pounds turkey breast tenderloins
- non-stick cooking spray
- 2 (15.5 ounce) cans yellow hominy, drained
- 2 (7 ounce) cans salsa verde
- 1 (8 ounce) can chopped green chile peppers
- 1 (4 ounce) can diced jalapeno peppers (optional)
- salt and ground black pepper to taste

Direction

- Set the grill for moderate heat to preheat and coat the grate lightly with oil. Use cooking spray to coat turkey tenderloins slightly.
- On the grill, cook turkey for 5-7 minutes each side, until juices run clear and turkey is not pink in the center anymore. Take turkey away from the heat and let it rest about 10 minutes. Slice turkey into strips with 1/2 inch size.
- In a big stockpot, combine together jalapenos, green chiles, salsa verde, hominy and turkey, then bring the mixture to a boil. Lower heat to low and simmer for 45 minutes, until thickens. Use pepper and salt to season.

Nutrition Information

- Calories: 239 calories;
- Total Carbohydrate: 21.2
- Cholesterol: 82
- Protein: 31.7
- Total Fat: 1.9
- Sodium: 1027

904. Grilled Turkey Breast With Fresh Sage Leaves

Serving: 8 | Prep: 20mins | Cook: 30mins | Ready in:

Ingredients

- 3 tablespoons freshly squeezed lemon juice
- 3 tablespoons extra-virgin olive oil
- 28 leaves fresh sage
- 4 skinless, boneless turkey breast halves
- sea salt and freshly ground black pepper to taste
- 2 tablespoons extra-virgin olive oil
- 3 tablespoons unsalted butter
- 2 lemons, halved

Direction

- Combine 3 tablespoons olive oil, sage leaves, and lemon juice in a big container, mix them together and put the turkey breast halves into the mixture. Marinate the breasts at room temperature for 30 minutes and occasionally turn over the meat.
- Prepare the grill by preheating it to medium heat then coat the grate lightly with oil.
- Take the turkey breasts out of the marinade and set the marinade and sage leaves aside.
- Dash with sea salt and black pepper on both sides of the turkey.
- Cook the turkey breasts on the grill for about 30 minutes until grill marks appear, the inside of the meat is no longer pink and an instant-read meat thermometer reads at least 160° F (70° C) when inserted into the thickest part of the turkey breast. Flip over the turkey pieces after 15 minutes.
- Heat 2 tablespoons olive oil mixed with unsalted butter in a large pan on medium high-heat until hot and bubbles form, while the turkey is grilling. Add the marinate and the sage that you've set aside, into the oil and butter and continue cooking and stirring for 10 to 15 minutes until the marinade completely evaporates and the sage leaves are fried to crispiness.
- Move the grilled meat to a cutting board and add salt and black pepper, seasoning if you prefer; cut the turkey in diagonal thick slices and arrange the slices on a plate. Top the turkey slices with fried sage leaves and put lemon halves for garnish.

Nutrition Information

- Calories: 377 calories;
- Total Carbohydrate: 3.8
- Cholesterol: 168
- Protein: 57.1
- Total Fat: 14.3
- Sodium: 139

905. Hatch Chile Turkey Panini

Serving: 1 | Prep: 10mins | Cook: 10mins | Ready in:

Ingredients

- 8 ounces Dietz & Watson Hatch Chile Turkey
- 3 ounces Dietz & Watson Hatch Chile Cheese
- 2 slices white bread
- 1/2 cup wilted spinach
- 1/4 cup julienned red onion
- 2 shishito peppers
-

Direction

- Stack your ingredients like this: bread, the spinach, Dietz & Watson Hatch Chile Cheese, the Dietz & Watson Hatch Turkey, the red onions, and the bread. Press for five minutes in a panini press. On a preheated outdoor grill on medium heat, grill the shishito peppers one to two minutes each side or until the skin blisters. Serve the panini topped with grilled shishito peppers.

Nutrition Information

- Calories: 743 calories;
- Total Carbohydrate: 41.1
- Cholesterol: 207
- Total Fat: 28.4
- Protein: 75.6
- Sodium: 3054

906. Heavenly Turkey Soup

Serving: 8 | Prep: 10mins | Cook: 30mins | Ready in:

Ingredients

- 10 cups water
- 1 cup cubed turkey breast meat, with bone, divided

- 1 large onion, chopped
- 4 garlic cloves, crushed
- 1 tablespoon crushed red pepper flakes
- 1 tablespoon sea salt
- 3 cubes chicken bouillon
- 2 cups chopped broccoli
- 1 (10.75 ounce) can condensed cream of mushroom soup
- 1 cup chopped fresh asparagus
- 1 cup sliced red bell pepper
- 1 (1.8 ounce) tub instant dry lentil soup mix
- 1/2 cup bean sprouts

Direction

- In a big pot, place bouillon cubes, sea salt, pepper flakes, garlic, onion, turkey breast bone, and water, then set to boil. Decrease heat and simmer the broth for 20 minutes.
- Stir in instant soup mix, bell pepper, asparagus, turkey breast meat, cream of mushroom soup, and broccoli into the broth, then, bring the soup back to a simmer. Cook for 10 minutes and take out the breast bone. Ladle the soup into bowls and top them with bean sprouts.

Nutrition Information

- Calories: 106 calories;
- Total Fat: 3
- Sodium: 1431
- Total Carbohydrate: 13.1
- Cholesterol: 13
- Protein: 8.4

907. Herbed Slow Cooker Turkey Breast

Serving: 6 | Prep: 10mins | Cook: 4hours | Ready in:

Ingredients

- 1 (3 pound) bone-in turkey breast half
- 2 tablespoons butter, softened
- 1/4 cup whipped cream cheese spread with garden vegetables
- 1 tablespoon soy sauce
- 1 tablespoon minced fresh parsley
- 1/2 teaspoon dried basil
- 1/2 teaspoon dried sage
- 1/2 teaspoon dried thyme
- 1/4 teaspoon ground black pepper
- 1/4 teaspoon garlic powder

Direction

- Into a slow cooker, put the turkey breast. In a small bowl, mix garlic powder, black pepper, thyme, sage, basil, parsley, soy sauce, whipped cream cheese spread and butter till smooth. Brush the turkey breast with herb mixture. Put cover on slow cooker.
- Let cook till turkey is soft, 4 to 6 hours on High or 8 to 10 hours on Low.

Nutrition Information

- Calories: 324 calories;
- Cholesterol: 181
- Protein: 60
- Total Fat: 7.4
- Sodium: 312
- Total Carbohydrate: 0.9

908. Inside Out Pizza

Serving: 2 | Prep: 10mins | Cook: 2mins | Ready in:

Ingredients

- 2 6-inch flour tortillas
- 1/4 cup grated Cheddar cheese
- 1/4 cup shredded Mozzarella cheese
- 2 (1 ounce) slices cooked deli turkey breast
- 1 tablespoon pizza sauce
- 1 tablespoon chopped tomato (optional)
- 1 tablespoon sliced black olives (optional)

- 1 tablespoon chopped green bell pepper (optional)

Direction

- On a sheet of paper that can fit in a microwave, place a tortilla. Spread 2 tablespoons each of Mozzarella and Cheddar cheeses over the tortilla. Place turkey slices over the cheese. Spread 1 tablespoon of pizza sauce over the turkey and top with 1 tablespoon each of black olives, green peppers and tomatoes. Use the leftover Mozzarella and Cheddar cheeses to sprinkle and place the second tortilla over it. Put on a microwave-safe plate and use a sheet of wax paper to cover it.
- Cook in a microwave on high power for about 1 1/2 minutes until the cheese is melted. Cut into wedges after cooling for 2 minutes.

Nutrition Information

- Calories: 354 calories;
- Sodium: 1040
- Total Carbohydrate: 39.9
- Cholesterol: 35
- Protein: 17.7
- Total Fat: 13.5

909. Instant Pot® Frozen Turkey Breast

Serving: 6 | Prep: 15mins | Cook: 1hours10mins | Ready in:

Ingredients

- 2 tablespoons butter
- 1 onion, quartered
- 1 apple, cut into chunks
- 3 stalks celery, chopped
- 2 cups chicken broth
- 1 (.87 ounce) package turkey gravy mix
- Spice Rub:
- 2 teaspoons kosher salt
- 2 teaspoons dried thyme
- 2 teaspoons dried rosemary
- 1 teaspoon ground black pepper
- 1 teaspoon dried sage
- 1/2 teaspoon garlic powder
- 1 (3 pound) frozen boneless turkey breast (such as Butterball®)
- 1 cup water
- 1/2 cup quick-mixing flour (such as Wondra®)

Direction

- Set a multi-function cooker like Instant Pot® to Sauté mode. Melt butter in the cooker then sauté celery, apple, and onion. Cook for 5 minutes until the celery and onion are somewhat translucent. Pour broth in and stir to scrape the browned bits at the bottom of the pot. Stir in the gravy mix until well melted.
- In a small bowl, mix garlic powder, salt, sage, thyme, black pepper, rosemary, and kosher salt. Massage the spice mixture on the turkey breast.
- Place an iron tripod in the pot and put the seasoned turkey on it. Secure pot and lock lid. Set the timer to 50 minutes and turn to the pressure to high as specified in the cooker's manual. Let the pressure build for 10-15 minutes.
- Let the pressure release naturally for 10-40 minutes as specified in the cooker's manual.
- In a small bowl, combine the quick-mixing flour and water; mix slurry slowly until smooth.
- Uncover; move the turkey on a plate. Strain liquid and place it back in the pot. Set the cooker in Sauté mode; boil. Gradually mix in slurry until the liquid thickens to your liking. Chop the turkey and serve with the gravy.

Nutrition Information

- Calories: 496 calories;
- Total Fat: 19.2

- Sodium: 1339
- Total Carbohydrate: 19.3
- Cholesterol: 159
- Protein: 59.3

910. Instant Pot® Thanksgiving Dinner

Serving: 4 | Prep: 25mins | Cook: 47mins | Ready in:

Ingredients

- 4 sweet potatoes
- 2 tablespoons maple syrup
- salt to taste
- 1 turkey breast
- 2 tablespoons barbeque dry rub (such as Charlie Vergos Rendezvous Famous Seasoning®)
- 1/2 cup butter, divided
- 1 cup chopped celery
- 1 small onion, chopped
- 3 cups crumbled cornbread
- 1/2 cup chopped pecans
- 2 slices crisp cooked bacon, cut into 1/2-inch pieces
- 1/2 teaspoon barbeque dry rub (such as Charlie Vergos Rendezvous Famous Seasoning®)
- 1 1/2 cups turkey stock

Direction

- Poke holes in a sweet potato using a fork; microwave for 8-10 minutes until tender on high. Set aside for 10 minutes until cool enough to hold; peel and mash in a bowl. Add maple syrup and salt then mix.
- Switch on an electric pressure cooker, like Instant Pot®, and place on "Sauté" mode. Rub barbeque seasoning on the turkey breast. Melt quarter cup butter in the cooker for 2 minutes then place in the turkey breast with the skin side down. Cook for 5 minutes until brown. Take off heat.
- On medium heat, melt the leftover quarter cup butter in a pan. Sauté onion and celery for 2 minutes until slightly soft; mix in bacon, pecans, and cornbread. Take off heat, add half teaspoon barbeque rub; mix gently.
- Make two rafts from sheets of aluminum foil. Punch holes in the first raft then fill it with cornbread mixture; place the mashed sweet potatoes in the second raft.
- Turn the turkey breast so its skin side is now up, put the raft with the cornbread mixture on top. Slowly pour stock on the dressing, the drips will make the turkey stay moist. Set the sweet potatoes raft on the dressing.
- Cover the pressure cooker, seal, and set it on the "Poultry" setting for half hour.
- Let the pressure escape naturally as specified in the manufacturer's instructions. Put aside for 5 minutes before cutting. Serve with the sweet potatoes and cornbread dressing.

Nutrition Information

- Calories: 770 calories;
- Protein: 40.2
- Total Fat: 40.3
- Sodium: 2706
- Total Carbohydrate: 62.7
- Cholesterol: 173

911. Instant Pot® Turkey Breast

Serving: 8 | Prep: 10mins | Cook: 33mins | Ready in:

Ingredients

- 1 (1 ounce) package onion soup mix
- 1 (6 pound) turkey breast, thawed
- 2 ribs celery, cut into large chunks
- 1 onion, cut into large chunks
- 1 cup chicken broth
- 2 tablespoons water
- 1 tablespoon cornstarch, or more as needed

Direction

- Rub onion soup mix all over turkey breast. Put turkey breast in the electric pressure cooker pot (like Instant Pot®). Add onion chunks and celery on top and around turkey breast then pour chicken broth all over it.
- Close and lock pressure cooker then select Poultry in the setting to bring to high/low according to manufacturer's directions. Cook for 30 minutes until juices run clear. Using the natural-release method, carefully release pressure for about 20 minutes. Place turkey breast to a serving platter and slice.
- Adjust electric pressure cooker setting to Sauté. Mix cornstarch in a bowl of water then add a bit of hot liquid from the pot. Mix well until cornstarch dissolves then pour mixture into the pot and blend well for about 3 minutes until thickened. Serve turkey along with this prepared gravy.

Nutrition Information

- Calories: 583 calories;
- Total Fat: 22.1
- Sodium: 630
- Total Carbohydrate: 5
- Cholesterol: 220
- Protein: 85.7

912. Jamaican Turkey Sandwich

Serving: 6 | Prep: 35mins | Cook: 6hours | Ready in:

Ingredients

- Pulled Turkey:
- 1/2 cup chopped celery
- 1/3 cup chopped green onion
- 1 (2 pound) skinless, boneless turkey breast, cut into 8 ounce chunks
- 1/2 cup juice from canned pineapple
- 1/4 cup sweet chile sauce
- 3 tablespoons distilled white vinegar
- 2 tablespoons water
- 1 tablespoon beef bouillon granules
- 2 teaspoons garlic powder
- 6 canned pineapple rings
- Coleslaw Topping:
- 1/4 cup mayonnaise
- 1 tablespoon lemon juice
- 2 tablespoons chopped fresh parsley
- 1/2 cup chopped onion
- 2 cups chopped cabbage
- 1 cup shredded Cheddar cheese
- salt and black pepper to taste
- 6 Kaiser rolls, split

Direction

- In the bottom of a slow cooker, sprinkle green onions and celery; top with turkey chunks. Mix together garlic powder, beef bouillon, water, vinegar, sweet chile sauce, and pineapple juice; pour over the turkey. On the turkey chunks, put pineapple rings.
- Cook on Low for 6-7 hours until the turkey is easy to pull apart.
- In the meantime, prepare the coleslaw: In a mixing bowl, combine onion, parsley, lemon juice, and mayonnaise. Add Cheddar cheese and cabbage, season with pepper and salt to taste. Put a cover on and chill in the fridge while the turkey is cooking.
- When the turkey is soft, use 2 forks to shred. On a Kaiser roll, stack a pineapple ring and some of the shredded turkey, put coleslaw on top and enjoy.

Nutrition Information

- Calories: 524 calories;
- Total Fat: 16.5
- Sodium: 808
- Total Carbohydrate: 42.8
- Cholesterol: 133
- Protein: 49.4

913. Jeanne's Slow Cooker Spaghetti Sauce

Serving: 12 | Prep: 20mins | Cook: 3hours20mins | Ready in:

Ingredients

- 1 (28 ounce) can crushed tomatoes
- 1 (28 ounce) can diced tomatoes
- 1 (6 ounce) can tomato paste
- 1 (10 ounce) can tomato sauce
- 1/2 pound turkey kielbasa, chopped
- 1/4 cup extra light olive oil
- 3 onions, chopped
- 6 yellow squash, diced
- 1 small green bell pepper, minced
- 3 cloves garlic, pressed
- 1/2 pound extra lean ground beef
- 1/2 pound extra-lean ground turkey breast
- 5 bay leaves
- 15 whole black peppercorns
- 1 1/2 teaspoons dried basil
- 1 teaspoon dried marjoram
- 2 teaspoons dried thyme
- 1/2 teaspoon dried oregano

Direction

- In a slow cooker, combine kielbasa, tomato sauce, tomato paste, diced tomatoes, and crushed tomatoes, then set the cooker to a high setting.
- In a big and deep skillet, heat olive oil over medium heat, then cook garlic, green pepper, squash and onions in oil until the onions become translucent. Move the vegetables to the slow cooker.
- In a big and deep pan, place ground turkey and ground beef, then cook over a medium-high heat until browned evenly. Drain and finely crumble, then transfer to the slow cooker. Season the meat with oregano, thyme, marjoram, basil, peppercorns, and bay leaves.
- Cook while covered on a high setting for two hours. Remove the lid and cook for 1 more hour.

Nutrition Information

- Calories: 212 calories;
- Protein: 14.1
- Total Fat: 9.5
- Sodium: 624
- Total Carbohydrate: 19.7
- Cholesterol: 38

914. Jill's Vegetable Chili

Serving: 6 | Prep: 15mins | Cook: 30mins | Ready in:

Ingredients

- 1 pound cubed turkey breast
- 1 cup minced onion
- 1 tablespoon minced garlic
- 2 teaspoons chili powder
- 1/2 teaspoon ground cumin
- 1/8 teaspoon ground cinnamon
- 1 (14.5 ounce) can peeled and diced tomatoes
- 1 (14 ounce) can chicken broth
- 1 (15 ounce) can kidney beans
- 1 (15 ounce) can pinto beans
- 1 (10 ounce) package frozen corn kernels

Direction

- In a large pot, cook turkey over medium heat until browned. Mix in onions. Cook, covered, for 5 mins.
- Stir in cinnamon, cumin, chili powder and garlic. Cook for a minute until fragrant. Put in the tomatoes. Boil. Stir in corn, pinto beans, kidney beans and broth. Return to a boil. Then lower the heat, simmer until heated thoroughly, or about 10 mins.

Nutrition Information

- Calories: 416 calories;
- Cholesterol: 51
- Protein: 33.3
- Total Fat: 7
- Sodium: 626
- Total Carbohydrate: 56.2

915. Karla's Nutty Turkey Cranwich

Serving: 1 | Prep: 10mins | Cook: | Ready in:

Ingredients

- 2 slices honey whole wheat bread, toasted
- 1 tablespoon mayonnaise
- 2 slices of smoked turkey breast
- 1 tablespoon whole berry cranberry sauce
- 1 tablespoon chopped walnuts
- 1 lettuce leaf

Direction

- Put mayonnaise on a side of every slice of toast. Put smoked turkey breast pieces on a slice of toast and put cranberry sauce on turkey; drizzle on walnuts. Garnish with a lettuce leaf and finish with the remaining toast making a sandwich.

Nutrition Information

- Calories: 341 calories;
- Sodium: 696
- Total Carbohydrate: 32.5
- Cholesterol: 17
- Protein: 13.9
- Total Fat: 18

916. Kickin' Turkey Club Wrap

Serving: 4 | Prep: 5mins | Cook: | Ready in:

Ingredients

- 4 (6 inch) flour tortillas
- 1/2 (8 ounce) tub PHILADELPHIA Spicy Jalapeno Cream Cheese Spread
- 4 lettuce leaves
- 8 slices OSCAR MAYER Deli Fresh Smoked Turkey Breast
- 4 slices OSCAR MAYER Bacon, cooked, drained
- 1 avocado, sliced
- 1/2 red pepper, sliced into thin strips

Direction

- Using cream cheese, spread on tortillas.
- Add the remaining ingredients on top, roll up.

Nutrition Information

917. Kids' Turkey And Cream Cheese Spread Bento Box

Serving: 2 | Prep: 45mins | Cook: | Ready in:

Ingredients

- Cream Cheese Penguins:
- 10 round carrot slices, 1/4-inch thick
- 10 jumbo pitted black olives
- 10 small pitted black olives
- 1/2 (8 ounce) package cream cheese, softened
- 10 toothpicks
- Party Vegetable Sandwich Spread:
- 2 tablespoons shredded carrot
- 2 teaspoons minced onion
- 2 teaspoons chopped pimento peppers
- 2 teaspoons chopped celery

- 2 tablespoons cream cheese, softened
- 1 teaspoon lemon juice
- 3/4 teaspoon mayonnaise
- 1 pinch salt
- 1 green apple, sliced
- 1 red apple, sliced
- 1 tablespoon lemon juice
- 1/2 carrot, sliced into rounds
- 6 thin slices cucumber, sliced lengthwise into wide ribbons
- 6 slices tomato, cut in half
- 6 toothpicks
- 8 round crackers
- 1/2 cup grapes, divided
- 8 slices deli turkey breast

Direction

- On the side of each jumbo olive, cut a slit from the top to the bottom. Ease the olive slightly open to insert around 1 teaspoon of cream cheese, making a penguin belly.
- To shape the feet, cut a small triangle-shaped notch out of 9 carrot rounds; press into each small olive with 1 triangular piece to create the beak (trimming if needed).
- Through the existing holes, thread each jumbo olive lengthwise onto a toothpick. Secure the toothpick onto a carrot slice (the belly is lined up with the feet); put on top with a small olive (the beak will face forward). Arrange the penguins on a dish; chill until assembly.
- In a bowl, combine celery, pimento peppers, onion, and shredded carrot. In a separate bowl, mix salt, mayonnaise, 1 teaspoon lemon juice, and 2 tablespoons softened cream cheese; beat until fluffy. Fold the carrot mixture into the cream cheese, then mix well. Chill for at least 60 minutes before using.
- In a bowl, toss 1 tablespoon lemon juice, red apple slices, and green apple slices.
- Use vegetable cutters to cut carrot rounds into decorative shapes. Wrap in a wet paper towel and put in a plastic bag; chill until assembly.
- Blot the cucumber slices dry. Arrange at the end of a cucumber slice with 1 half-slice tomato; roll up together and use a toothpick to secure.
- In a bento box, place half the carrot shapes. In a small silicone baking cup, put 1/2 the sandwich spread and set 4 crackers in another cup. Place grapes, red apple slices, and 1/2 the green apple slices. Put in 3 cucumber-tomato rolls, 4 turkey slices, and 5 cream cheese penguins. Use the leftover ingredients to make a second bento box. Chill until they're ready to eat.

Nutrition Information

- Calories: 689 calories;
- Total Fat: 38.3
- Sodium: 2311
- Total Carbohydrate: 65.3
- Cholesterol: 124
- Protein: 28.5

918. Low Carb Bacon Lettuce Turkey Wraps

Serving: 4 | Prep: 10mins | Cook: | Ready in:

Ingredients

- 4 large lettuce leaves
- 1/4 cup mayonnaise
- 8 slices bacon
- 12 slices deli smoked turkey
- 4 slices Swiss cheese
- (8-inch) lengths of baking string

Direction

- Use paper towels to dry the lettuce leaves. Spread each leaf with 1 tbsp. of mayonnaise.
- Arrange the bacon between paper towels set on a microwave-safe plate. Heat it inside the microwave for 4-6 minutes, or until crispy.
- Place 3 turkey slices, 1 Swiss cheese slice, and 2 bacon slices on top of each lettuce. Roll each

lettuce up and use a length of baking string to tie each wrap.

Nutrition Information

- Calories: 395 calories;
- Protein: 30
- Total Fat: 27.7
- Sodium: 1381
- Total Carbohydrate: 6.1
- Cholesterol: 87

919. Mama H's Fooled You Fancy Slow Cooker Turkey Breast

Serving: 6 | Prep: 20mins | Cook: 5hours | Ready in:

Ingredients

- 1/2 bunch fresh flat-leaf parsley, divided
- 1/2 bunch dill, divided
- 1 clementine, peeled and segmented, divided
- 1 (2 1/2 to 3 pound) turkey breast
- 2 2/3 tablespoons dried onion flakes
- 1 1/2 teaspoons dried parsley
- 1 teaspoon ground turmeric
- 1 teaspoon onion powder
- 1/2 teaspoon salt, or to taste
- 1/2 teaspoon white sugar, or to taste
- 1/2 teaspoon celery seed
- 1/4 teaspoon ground black pepper
- 1 (16 ounce) can whole berry cranberry sauce

Direction

- Place into the bottom and slightly up the sides of a slow cooker with at least 1/2 fresh parsley and 1/2 dill. Top with sprinkled 1/2 the clementine section. Add turkey breast.
- In a mixing bowl, combine black pepper, celery seed, sugar, salt, onion powder, turmeric, dried parsley, and onion flakes and stir well. Liberally sprinkle the spice mixture over the turkey breast in the slow cooker.
- Ladle dollops of cranberry sauce all over the turkey breast and in every corner of the pot of the slow cooker. Add remaining dill and fresh parsley, and finally the remaining clementine sections. Cook for about 5 hours on low power until the center of turkey breast is no longer pink and juices run clear, checking the turkey after 4.5 hours to make sure it's not overcooked.

Nutrition Information

- Calories: 417 calories;
- Protein: 55.6
- Total Fat: 6.3
- Sodium: 316
- Total Carbohydrate: 32.4
- Cholesterol: 170

920. Maple Glazed Turkey Roast

Serving: 6 | Prep: 10mins | Cook: 1hours30mins | Ready in:

Ingredients

- 1 (3 pound) boneless turkey breast roast, thawed
- 1/2 cup pure maple syrup, or more as needed
- 1 teaspoon liquid smoke flavoring (optional)
- 1 teaspoon ground paprika
- 1/2 teaspoon salt
- 1/2 teaspoon pepper
- 1/2 teaspoon garlic powder
- 1/2 teaspoon onion powder
- 1/2 teaspoon dried crushed thyme
- 1 pinch cayenne pepper, or to taste

Direction

- Start preheating oven to 325°F (165°C).

- Discard plastic wrap and netting from turkey roast, if any, but retain on string netting. (Discard and remove any the gravy packet). Rinse turkey, using paper towels to pat dry.
- In a bowl, mix cayenne pepper, thyme, onion powder, garlic powder, pepper, salt, paprika, smoke flavoring and maple syrup together, stirring to combine well. Brush all over turkey roast with syrup mixture.
- In a roasting pan, put roast on a baking rack, the skin side facing up. Roast in prepared oven, until the meat thermometer registers 170°F (75°C) when inserted into middle of roast and the roast turns golden brown, basting occasionally. Roasting time is approximately 90 mins. Cover the roast with foil. Allow to stand 10 mins. Then remove string netting for slicing.

Nutrition Information

- Calories: 351 calories;
- Total Carbohydrate: 32.9
- Cholesterol: 120
- Protein: 40.1
- Total Fat: 5.9
- Sodium: 1734

921. Marinated Turkey Breast

Serving: 12 | Prep: 20mins | Cook: 30mins | Ready in:

Ingredients

- 2 cloves garlic, peeled and minced
- 1 tablespoon finely chopped fresh basil
- 1/2 teaspoon ground black pepper
- 2 (3 pound) boneless turkey breast halves
- 6 whole cloves
- 1/4 cup vegetable oil
- 1/4 cup soy sauce
- 2 tablespoons lemon juice
- 1 tablespoon brown sugar

Direction

- Combine the garlic, pepper, and basil in a small bowl then rub the mixture onto the turkey breasts. Put one clove each on the ends of the turkey breasts and on the center.
- Combine the vegetable oil, lemon juice, soy sauce and brown sugar and blend them together in a big shallow plate.
- Put the breasts on the plate and coat it with the mixture. Cover then keep marinated in the refrigerator for at least 4 hours.
- Prepare the grill by preheating it on high heat.
- Coat the grate lightly with grease. Remove the marinade and grill the turkey breasts. Close the lid of the grill and cook the breasts to an internal temperature of 170° F (68° C), about 15 minutes on each side.

Nutrition Information

- Calories: 317 calories;
- Sodium: 405
- Total Carbohydrate: 2.2
- Cholesterol: 164
- Protein: 59.8
- Total Fat: 6

922. Mushroom Turkey Roulade

Serving: 10 | Prep: 15mins | Cook: 1hours | Ready in:

Ingredients

- 1 tablespoon light butter
- 2 leeks, cleaned and sliced
- 1 stalk celery, sliced
- 1 carrot, peeled and sliced
- 2 cups sliced mushrooms
- 2 shallots, minced
- 2 teaspoons herbes de Provence
- 1 cup chicken stock
- 1 pinch salt and ground black pepper to taste

- 2 cups whole wheat bread crumbs, toasted
- 2 1/2 pounds turkey breast half
- 1/4 cup cranberry sauce, or to taste

Direction

- Start preheating the oven to 375°F (190°C).
- In a large skillet, melt butter over medium-high heat. Sauté carrot, celery and leeks about 3 mins. Put in mushrooms and sauté for 5-10 mins or until tender. Put in herbes de Provence and shallots; sauté for 2 mins or until fragrant. Add the chicken stock over the vegetable mixture. Simmer and season with pepper and salt.
- In a bowl, mix together vegetable mixture and breadcrumbs. Put the stuffing aside to cool.
- Cut turkey breast horizontally from 1 side through center to within 1/2-in. of other side. Then open 2 sides; spread out like an open book, pound to an even thickness. Place the stuffing down butterflied turkey center. Roll the turkey around the stuffing; use twine to secure. Put into the baking dish, wrap in aluminum foil.
- Cook the turkey breast for 45-60 mins or until juices run clear and middle is no longer pink. The instant-read thermometer should register at least 165°F (74°C) when inserted into the middle. Discard from oven. Let turkey rest 10 mins. Then remove twine and slice. Enjoy with the cranberry sauce.

Nutrition Information

- Calories: 315 calories;
- Total Carbohydrate: 19.3
- Cholesterol: 87
- Protein: 36
- Total Fat: 10.2
- Sodium: 339

923. Oat And Herb Encrusted Turkey

Serving: 2 | Prep: 15mins | Cook: 30mins | Ready in:

Ingredients

- 1/2 cup milk
- 3 tablespoons prepared brown mustard
- 1/2 cup quick cooking oats
- 1 tablespoon dried sage
- 1 tablespoon dried rosemary
- 2 (6 ounce) fillets turkey breast
- 1 (6 ounce) container fat-free plain yogurt
- 1 tablespoon whole grain mustard
- salt and ground black pepper to taste

Direction

- Set the oven to 350°F (175°C) for preheating. Coat the baking sheet with cooking spray lightly.
- Mix the prepared brown mustard and milk in a bowl. In another bowl, mix the rosemary, sage, and oats. Dredge each of the turkey breast first in the milk mixture, and then in the oat mixture until coated evenly.
- Bake the turkey inside the preheated oven for 30 minutes until the oats are crisp and the turkey's internal temperature reaches a minimum of 180°F (80°C).
- Combine the whole grain mustard and yogurt in a bowl. Season the mixture with salt and pepper. Drizzle mixture all over the cooked turkey or use it as a dipping sauce. Serve.

Nutrition Information

- Calories: 402 calories;
- Protein: 55.6
- Total Fat: 6.8
- Sodium: 574
- Total Carbohydrate: 27
- Cholesterol: 133

924. Orange, Tea, Bourbon Brined Paprika Butter Turkey

Serving: 12 | Prep: 15mins | Cook: 2hours | Ready in:

Ingredients

- Brine:
- 2 quarts water
- 5 oranges - juiced and zest cut off in large strips
- 2 cups kosher salt
- 1 cup white sugar
- 12 black tea bags
- 4 bay leaves
- 6 whole cloves
- 12 whole black peppercorns
- 1 cup bourbon whiskey
- 4 quarts cold water, or as needed
- 1 (8 pound) whole turkey breast
- Seasoned Butter:
- 2 tablespoons coriander seeds, crushed
- 1 tablespoon paprika
- 2 teaspoons cumin seeds, crushed
- 6 cloves garlic, crushed and chopped
- 6 tablespoons butter, softened

Direction

- Into a big soup pot, add 2 quarts of water and mix in bourbon, peppercorns, cloves, bay leaves, black tea bags, sugar, kosher salt and orange juice and zest. Boil, turn the heat to low, and allow to simmer for 10 minutes. Into brine, add 4 quarts of cold water and allow to cool. Soak the turkey breast in brine, putting in additional water if necessary to cover. Chill for 8 hours up to overnight.
- Preheat the oven to 175°C or 350°F. In oven, position oven rack to the lowest place.
- Take turkey out of marinade; throw away the marinade. Wash the turkey and use paper towels to pat it dry. In a bowl combine garlic, cumin seeds, paprika and coriander seeds into softened butter.
- Using fingers, loosen skin on turkey breast and scatter a quarter cup seasoned butter under the skin. Massage the leftover 2 tablespoons of seasoned butter on turkey breast. Onto a roasting rack, put the turkey breast and place the rack into roasting pan.
- In the prepped oven, roast for 2 hours till skin turns golden brown and an inserted instant-read meat thermometer into the chunkiest part of breast registers 75°C or 165°F. Turn onto a chopping board and allow the turkey breast to sit for half an hour prior to slicing.

Nutrition Information

- Calories: 508 calories;
- Total Fat: 15.2
- Sodium: 16286
- Total Carbohydrate: 19.1
- Cholesterol: 126
- Protein: 58.9

925. Quick Turkey Peppers

Serving: 4 | Prep: 10mins | Cook: 10mins | Ready in:

Ingredients

- 2 red bell peppers
- 4 slices cooked turkey breast
- 1/3 cup finely chopped onion
- 4 teaspoons pesto
- 1 small head broccoli, separated into florets
- 1 1/2 cups shredded Colby-Monterey Jack cheese
- 4 teaspoons grated Parmesan cheese

Direction

- Start preheating the oven to 400°F (200°C).
- Cut peppers lengthwise by half. Discard the stem, seeds and pulp. Arrange on a baking sheet, the cut-side facing up. Lay one turkey slice inside per pepper. Evenly sprinkle turkey with the chopped onion. Drizzle one teaspoon of pesto inside per pepper half. Put a few

broccoli florets into per pepper. Then add the shredded Colby-Monterey Jack cheese to cover.
- Bake in prepared oven for 10 mins or until cheese has melted and peppers have heated through. Discard from the oven. Sprinkle one teaspoon of grated Parmesan cheese over each pepper.

Nutrition Information

- Calories: 316 calories;
- Total Fat: 19.9
- Sodium: 504
- Total Carbohydrate: 11.4
- Cholesterol: 76
- Protein: 24.3

926. Roasted Turkey Breast With Herbs

Serving: 12 | Prep: 10mins | Cook: 5hours | Ready in:

Ingredients

- 1 (8 pound) whole bone-in turkey breast with skin
- 1 1/2 cups chicken stock
- 6 tablespoons butter, melted
- 2 teaspoons chicken bouillon granules
- 1 teaspoon dried sage
- 1 teaspoon dried savory
- 1 teaspoon dried rosemary
- 1 teaspoon dried thyme

Direction

- Preheat the oven to 175°C or 350°F.
- Loosen skin from turkey breast meat.
- Into a big oven-safe pot or Dutch oven with a lid, put turkey breast and add chicken stock on meat. In a bowl, combine liquified butter with thyme, rosemary, savory, sage and chicken bouillon granules. Lift the loosened skin and put a bit more than 1/2 of butter-herb mixture beneath the skin. Put the rest of the herb mixture onto skin. Place cover on the pot.
- In the prepped oven, roast for 3 hours; turn the turkey breast over and roast for an hour longer; turn over once more and roast till juices run clear and an inserted instant-read meat thermometer into the chunkiest portion of breast without touching the bone registers 80°C or 180°F, an hour longer (in a total of 5 hours). With pan drippings, baste the turkey and allow to sit for 5 to 10 minutes prior to serving.

Nutrition Information

- Calories: 386 calories;
- Total Fat: 15
- Sodium: 1234
- Total Carbohydrate: 0.5
- Cholesterol: 126
- Protein: 58.6

927. Rotelle Pasta Salad

Serving: 5 | Prep: 20mins | Cook: 20mins | Ready in:

Ingredients

- 1 (8 ounce) package rotelle pasta
- 6 slices bacon
- 1 (16 ounce) package frozen mixed vegetables
- 1 cup Italian-style salad dressing
- 1 teaspoon yellow mustard
- 1 tablespoon seasoning salt
- 1/4 teaspoon black pepper
- 1/2 green bell pepper, chopped
- 3 ounces turkey breast, cut into bite size pieces
- 1 cup shredded Cheddar cheese

Direction

- Bring a large pot that contains lightly salted water to a boil. Put rotelle pasta in and cook

for 8 to 10 minutes or until pasta becomes al dente; drain off water.
- Cook bacon in a large, deep skillet over medium-high heat until becomes evenly brown. Drain off excess fat, crumble and set aside.
- Put the frozen vegetables in the microwave and cook for approximately 4 to 6 minutes, making sure they are still crispy; drain.
- Stir together pepper, seasoning salt, mustard, and Italian dressing in a big bowl. Combine 1/2 of the cheese, 1/2 of the bacon, turkey, bell pepper, mixed vegetables and pasta together; mix properly.
- Add remaining of bacon and cheese on top of salad. Cover salad and chill thoroughly before serving.

Nutrition Information

- Calories: 627 calories;
- Protein: 22.9
- Total Fat: 38
- Sodium: 1802
- Total Carbohydrate: 51.5
- Cholesterol: 58

928. Slow Cooker Bacon Ranch Beer Can Turkey

Serving: 8 | Prep: 15mins | Cook: 7hours | Ready in:

Ingredients

- cooking spray
- 1/4 cup butter, softened
- 1 (1 ounce) packet ranch dressing mix, divided
- 1 whole bone-in turkey breast, rinsed and patted dry
- 6 slices thick-cut bacon
- 1 cup light-colored beer

Direction

- Spray cooking spray over the inside of a big slow cooker.
- In a bowl, combine 1/2 the ranch dressing mix and butter until completely blended.
- Carefully loosen the skin of the turkey breast on each side and spread beneath the skin with the butter-ranch mixture. Place the turkey to the slow cooker with the skin-side turning up.
- Sprinkle the turkey breast with the leftover 1/2 ranch dressing mix. Evenly lay across the turkey the bacon strips. Pour the beer around the turkey breast.
- Cook in the slow cooker for 60 minutes on High. Lower the heat to Low and cook for 6-8 hours until the turkey is soft.

Nutrition Information

- Calories: 194 calories;
- Sodium: 472
- Total Carbohydrate: 3
- Cholesterol: 45
- Protein: 8.2
- Total Fat: 15.4

929. Slow Cooker Boneless Turkey Breast

Serving: 12 | Prep: 10mins | Cook: 8hours | Ready in:

Ingredients

- 1 (10 pound) boneless turkey breast
- 2 (1 ounce) packages dry onion soup mix
- 3/4 cup water
- 2 tablespoons garlic powder
- 2 tablespoons onion powder
- 1 tablespoon dried parsley
- 1 tablespoon seasoned salt (such as Season-All®)
- 1 tablespoon dried basil
- 1 tablespoon dried oregano

Direction

- Into a big slow cooker, put the turkey. In a bowl, mix water and onion soup mix and put mixture on top of turkey breast, scattering it out to equally cover the meat.
- In a bowl, mix oregano, basil, seasoned salt, parsley, onion powder and garlic powder till well blended; scatter seasonings on turkey breast.
- Allow to cook for 8 to 9 hours on Low till seasonings have flavored the meat and turkey is extremely soft. An inserted instant-read meat thermometer into the chunkiest portion of breast, without touching the bone, should register at a minimum of 75°C or 165°F.

Nutrition Information

- Calories: 468 calories;
- Protein: 99.7
- Total Fat: 2.6
- Sodium: 815
- Total Carbohydrate: 5.5
- Cholesterol: 273

930. Slow Cooker Cranberry Turkey Breast

Serving: 6 | Prep: 10mins | Cook: 7hours | Ready in:

Ingredients

- 1 (16 ounce) can cranberry sauce
- 1 (1 ounce) package dry onion soup mix
- 1/2 cup orange juice
- 1 (3 pound) boneless turkey breast

Direction

- In a bowl, put cranberry sauce, and crush. Stir in orange juice and onion soup mix together till the mixture is blended thoroughly.
- With cooking spray, coat the inside of slow cooker, and into the cooker, put breast of turkey. Add sauce ingredients on turkey breast. Turn cooker to Low, and allow to cook for 7 hours till turkey breast is really soft.

Nutrition Information

- Calories: 401 calories;
- Sodium: 537
- Total Carbohydrate: 34.1
- Cholesterol: 164
- Protein: 60
- Total Fat: 1.7

931. Slow Cooker Herbed Turkey Breast

Serving: 12 | Prep: 15mins | Cook: 6hours | Ready in:

Ingredients

- 1 (5 pound) boneless turkey breast
- salt and ground black pepper to taste
- 5 sprigs fresh rosemary, divided
- 5 sprigs fresh thyme, divided
- 1 white onion, chopped - divided
- 1/2 cup butter, sliced into pats
- 2 cups chopped fresh celery leaves
- 1/2 (750 milliliter) bottle white wine, or more to taste

Direction

- Wash turkey breast and using paper towels, pat it dry; scatter black pepper and salt over. Into turkey breast cavity, put butter slices, 1/4 cup chopped onion, 2 thyme sprigs and 2 rosemary sprigs.
- In a big slow cooker, put celery leaves, remaining white onion, and the rest of the thyme sprigs and rosemary. Set turkey breast on top of herbs and vegetables with surface side facing down. Into the cooker add white wine and put cover.
- Let cook on High for 6 hours till meat is soft and an inserted instant-read meat

thermometer into the chunkiest breast part of meat registers 75°C or 170°. Allow the turkey breast to sit for 15 minutes prior to cutting.

Nutrition Information

- Calories: 308 calories;
- Total Fat: 13.4
- Sodium: 726
- Total Carbohydrate: 2.4
- Cholesterol: 89
- Protein: 36.8

932. Slow Cooker Italian Turkey

Serving: 6 | Prep: 15mins | Cook: 8hours20mins | Ready in:

Ingredients

- 4 beef bouillon cubes
- 1 quart water, or as needed
- 1 skinless, boneless turkey breast half
- 1/4 cup white vinegar
- 1 medium onion, chopped
- 1 green bell pepper, seeded and cut into strips
- 2 cloves garlic, minced
- 1 teaspoon dried oregano
- 1 tablespoon Worcestershire sauce
- 1 (.75 ounce) packet brown gravy mix
- 1/2 cup water

Direction

- Place the beef bouillon cubes in a quart of water and dissolve them. Pour the dissolved cubes into the slow cooker. Put the turkey into the slow cooker and pour in more water to cover it, if necessary.
- Cover the slow cooker and cook it on low setting for 8-10 hours. Mix the green bell pepper, Worcestershire sauce, oregano, vinegar, garlic, and onion into the slow cooker two hours before the end of the cooking time.
- In a small bowl, blend the water and brown gravy mix. Pour it into the slow cooker; stir. Keep on cooking for 20 minutes.

Nutrition Information

- Calories: 117 calories;
- Sodium: 813
- Total Carbohydrate: 6.1
- Cholesterol: 52
- Protein: 20.1
- Total Fat: 1

933. Slow Cooker Mediterranean Roast Turkey Breast

Serving: 8 | Prep: 20mins | Cook: 7hours30mins | Ready in:

Ingredients

- 1 (4 pound) boneless turkey breast, trimmed
- 1/2 cup chicken broth, divided
- 2 tablespoons fresh lemon juice
- 2 cups chopped onion
- 1/2 cup pitted kalamata olives
- 1/2 cup oil-packed sun dried tomatoes, thinly sliced
- 1 teaspoon Greek seasoning (such as McCormick's®)
- 1/2 teaspoon salt
- 1/4 teaspoon fresh ground black pepper
- 3 tablespoons all-purpose flour

Direction

- In the crock of a slow cooker, put pepper, salt, Greek seasoning, sun-dried tomatoes, kalamata olives, onion, lemon juice, 1/4 cup chicken broth, and turkey breast. Put the lid on and cook for 7 hours on Low.

- In a small bowl, mix together flour and the leftover 1/4 cup chicken broth; stir until smooth. Mix into the slow cooker. Put the lid on and cook for another 30 minutes on Low.

Nutrition Information

- Calories: 333 calories;
- Total Fat: 4.7
- Sodium: 465
- Total Carbohydrate: 8.9
- Cholesterol: 164
- Protein: 60.6

934. Slow Cooker Thanksgiving Turkey

Serving: 12 | Prep: 15mins | Cook: 8hours | Ready in:

Ingredients

- 5 slices bacon
- 1 (5 1/2 pound) bone-in turkey breast, skin removed
- 1/2 teaspoon garlic pepper
- 1 (10.5 ounce) can turkey gravy
- 2 tablespoons all-purpose flour
- 1 tablespoon Worcestershire sauce
- 1 teaspoon dried sage

Direction

- In a skillet, put the bacon over moderately high heat and cook till equally brown. Brain and break up.
- With cooking spray, coat a slow cooker. In slow cooker, put the turkey. Add garlic pepper to season. Combine the sage, Worcestershire sauce, flour, gravy and bacon in a bowl. In slow cooker, add the mixture to the top of turkey.
- Put cover on slow cooker, and let turkey cook on Low for 8 hours.

Nutrition Information

- Calories: 382 calories;
- Sodium: 379
- Total Carbohydrate: 2.6
- Cholesterol: 139
- Protein: 54.2
- Total Fat: 15.6

935. Slow Cooker Turkey Breast With Dressing

Serving: 12 | Prep: 20mins | Cook: 4hours10mins | Ready in:

Ingredients

- 2 tablespoons butter
- 1 1/2 large yellow onions, diced
- 4 large celery ribs, diced - or more to taste
- 1 (8 ounce) package dry bread stuffing mix with seasoning packet
- 1 (16 ounce) can whole berry cranberry sauce
- 1/2 cup butter, melted
- 1/2 cup chicken broth
- 1/2 teaspoon salt
- 1 (7 pound) bone-in turkey breast with pop-up timer
- 1/2 teaspoon salt

Direction

- In a big skillet, melt 2 tablespoons butter over medium heat. In the hot butter, stir and cook celery and onions for 8 minutes until the onions turn translucent; take away from heat.
- In a 6-qt. slow cooker, put a plastic slow cooker liner. In the liner bag, put dry bread stuffing and sprinkle the bread with the contents of the seasoning packet. Mix 1/2 teaspoon salt, chicken broth, 1/2 cup melted butter, cranberry sauce, and the cooked celery and onions into the dressing mix, being careful to not tear the bag.

- Wash the turkey breast and tap with paper towels to dry; use 1/2 teaspoon salt to season the turkey breast. Push the dressing mixture to the edge of the cooker and put the turkey breast into the slow cooker, the pop-up timer turning up.
- Cook on High for 4-4 1/2 hours until the pop-up timer in the turkey breast has popped. Transfer the turkey breast to a cutting board and let rest before eating, about 10 minutes. Transfer the dressing to a serving bowl and enjoy next to the turkey.

Nutrition Information

- Calories: 512 calories;
- Cholesterol: 122
- Protein: 53.6
- Total Fat: 18.3
- Sodium: 1538
- Total Carbohydrate: 30.5

936. Slow Cooker Turkey Breast With Gravy

Serving: 8 | Prep: 10mins | Cook: 8hours | Ready in:

Ingredients

- 1 serving cooking spray
- 1 (3 pound) boneless turkey breast
- 1 (10.75 ounce) can cream of mushroom soup
- 1 (10.75 ounce) can Cheddar cheese soup

Direction

- With cooking spray, coat the inside of a slow cooker and put turkey breast into the cooker. Put Cheddar cheese soup and cream of mushroom soup, place a cover on cooker, and let cook for 8 hours on Low. If wished, cook for 4 hours on High.

Nutrition Information

- Calories: 347 calories;
- Total Fat: 14.8
- Sodium: 613
- Total Carbohydrate: 6.2
- Cholesterol: 111
- Protein: 43.8

937. Slow Cooker Turkey And White Bean Chili

Serving: 8 | Prep: 20mins | Cook: 4hours25mins | Ready in:

Ingredients

- 1 tablespoon vegetable oil
- 2 pounds boneless turkey breast
- 2 onions, chopped
- 4 cloves garlic, minced
- 1 (15 ounce) can cannellini (white) beans, drained
- 1 (29 ounce) can white hominy, drained
- 3 (14 ounce) cans low-sodium chicken broth
- 3 (15 ounce) cans cannellini (white) beans, drained
- 1/4 cup chopped fresh cilantro
- 1 1/2 tablespoons ground cumin
- 1 teaspoon Cajun seasoning
- 3 serrano chile peppers

Direction

- In a big skillet, heat vegetable oil on medium heat. Pan-fry turkey breast, 10 minutes per side, till meat isn't pink. Into a bowl, put turkey breast; cool. Use 2 forks to shred turkey. Put aside turkey meat. Cook garlic and onion in the same skillet on medium heat for 5 minutes till onion is translucent. Scrape garlic, onions and any drippings into bowl with turkey.
- Into slow cooker, put chicken broth, hominy and 1 can cannellini beans. Blend mixture with

an immersion blender till smooth. Put Cajun seasoning, cumin, cilantro, 3 more cans of cannellini beans, garlic, onions and shredded turkey into slow cooker. Mix to combine. Cut off serrano chili stems, wearing gloves. Split chiles. Use a spoon to scrape membranes and seeds from 2 chiles. Mince all 3 chiles. Remove membranes and seeds from all chiles for milder chili flavor. Mix serrano chiles into soup.
- Cover cooker. Cook for 4-6 hours on low setting or 2-3 hours on high setting.

Nutrition Information

- Calories: 427 calories;
- Total Fat: 4.7
- Sodium: 838
- Total Carbohydrate: 50.9
- Cholesterol: 84
- Protein: 42.3

938. Soy, Garlic, And Chile Zoodles

Serving: 4 | Prep: 25mins | Cook: 11mins | Ready in:

Ingredients

- 2 zucchini, sliced
- 1 tablespoon coconut oil
- 1 red chile pepper, minced and crushed
- 1 clove garlic, minced and crushed
- 1/2 pound turkey breast, cut into strips
- 1 1/2 cups chopped green beans
- 1 green bell pepper, chopped
- 3 tablespoons soy sauce

Direction

- Use a spiralizer to spiralize zucchini.
- In a frying pan, heat coconut oil on medium. Add garlic and chile pepper; stir and cook until aromatic, 3-5 minutes. Add the turkey; cook 4-5 minutes until turkey turns pale, flip once.
- To the pan, add bell pepper, soy sauce, and green beans. Cook until turkey is not pink in middle and the juices are clear, 2-3 minutes.
- Add the zucchini; stir constantly and cook until just tender, 2-3 minutes.

Nutrition Information

- Calories: 163 calories;
- Total Carbohydrate: 8.5
- Cholesterol: 36
- Protein: 16.9
- Total Fat: 7.3
- Sodium: 718

939. Stuffed Turkey London Broil

Serving: 8 | Prep: 15mins | Cook: 1hours45mins | Ready in:

Ingredients

- 1 (2 pound) skinless, boneless turkey breast half
- 1 (10 ounce) package frozen chopped spinach, thawed, drained and squeezed dry
- 2 cups cooked brown rice
- 2 tablespoons cream cheese, or as needed
- 2 tablespoons toasted pine nuts, or to taste
- 1 pinch ground allspice, or to taste
- 1 pinch salt and ground black pepper to taste
- 2 tablespoons butter, cut into thin slices

Direction

- Preheat oven to 165°C/325°F. Prepare a 9 x 13-inch baking dish coated with grease.
- On the thick side of the turkey breast, make a deep pocket by slicing horizontally one deep cut using a sharp knife.

- Combine black pepper, salt, allspice, pine nuts, cream cheese, brown rice, and spinach; mix until combined thoroughly. Add a bit more cream cheese as needed if the stuffing does not hold together.
- On the baking dish, stuff the pockets of the turkey breast with the rice mixture and close the turkey breast with skewers. Pat thin dabs of butter on top of the turkey. Use aluminum foil to wrap and cover the baking dish.
- Bake for 1 hour, until the stuffing is heated and the turkey is not pink anymore. Remove from the oven, unwrap aluminum foil, and return turkey to the oven and bake for 45 more minutes, until browned thoroughly. Occasionally baste the turkey with the juices on the pan. Pierce an instant-read thermometer in the stuffing of the thickest part of the breast, it should read 75°C/165°F. Slice turkey across the grain. Serve.

Nutrition Information

- Calories: 249 calories;
- Total Carbohydrate: 13.5
- Cholesterol: 93
- Protein: 32.9
- Total Fat: 6.6
- Sodium: 109

940. Sweet And Spicy Turkey Sandwich

Serving: 1 | Prep: 5mins | Cook: 10mins | Ready in:

Ingredients

- 2 slices (1/2 inch thick) hearty country bread
- 4 slices roasted turkey breast
- 1 slice pepperjack cheese
- 2 teaspoons butter
- 4 teaspoons strawberry preserves

Direction

- Set a small skillet on medium heat. Use a teaspoon of butter to coat one side of each of the bread slices. In the skillet, arrange one slice with the butter side down. Add cheese slices and turkey on top. Top with the second slice of bread with the butter side up.
- Flip and brown the other side of the sandwich once the first side turns golden brown until the cheese starts to melt, or for 3-5 minutes on each side.
- Transfer the sandwich onto a plate and arrange the strawberry preserves on top or serve preserves on the side.

Nutrition Information

- Calories: 434 calories;
- Total Fat: 16.3
- Sodium: 1817
- Total Carbohydrate: 47.1
- Cholesterol: 83
- Protein: 25.5

941. Tender Breaded Turkey Cutlets

Serving: 4 | Prep: 10mins | Cook: 15mins | Ready in:

Ingredients

- 1 cup Italian seasoned dry bread crumbs
- 1/4 cup grated Parmesan cheese
- 4 turkey breast cutlets, 1/4 inch thick
- 1/2 cup fat free sour cream
- 1 tablespoon extra virgin olive oil

Direction

- In a shallow dish, mix the cheese and bread crumbs. Spread sour cream on both sides of the turkey. Press the turkey into the bread crumb mixture until coated.
- Put oil in a skillet and heat it over medium heat. Cook the turkey in the skillet for 5-7

minutes per side until cooked through and lightly browned.

Nutrition Information

- Calories: 397 calories;
- Total Fat: 7.9
- Sodium: 750
- Total Carbohydrate: 24.8
- Cholesterol: 134
- Protein: 53.1

942. Tex Mex Turkey Soup

Serving: 6 | Prep: 10mins | Cook: 40mins | Ready in:

Ingredients

- 1 tablespoon olive oil
- 1/2 cup minced onion
- 3 cloves garlic, minced
- 2 teaspoons chili powder
- 1/2 teaspoon cumin
- 1/2 teaspoon oregano
- 4 cups water
- 1 (10.75 ounce) can condensed tomato soup
- 1 (28 ounce) can diced tomatoes
- 1 cup salsa
- 4 cups shredded cooked turkey
- 1 tablespoon dried parsley
- 3 chicken bouillon cubes
- 1 (14 ounce) can black beans, rinsed, drained
- 2 cups frozen corn
- 1/2 cup sour cream
- 1/4 cup chopped fresh cilantro
- Toppings:
- 6 cups corn tortilla chips
- 3/4 cup chopped green onion
- 1 cup shredded Cheddar-Monterey Jack cheese blend
- 1/2 cup chopped fresh cilantro
- 1/2 cup sour cream

Direction

- Use a large saucepan to heat olive oil on a medium heat and add the minced onions, and cook for 4 minutes until they start to soften. Add oregano, cumin, chili powder, and garlic, then cook while stirring for 1 minute.
- Stir in bouillon cubes, parsley, shredded turkey, salsa, diced tomatoes, tomato soup, and water, then boil the soup. Reduce the heat and simmer for 5 minutes or until the bouillon cubes are dissolved. Add cilantro, sour cream, corn, and black beans, then simmer for 20 - 30 minutes.
- Serve the soup with sour cream, more cilantro, shredded cheese, chopped green onion, and crushed tortilla chips.

Nutrition Information

- Calories: 684 calories;
- Total Carbohydrate: 59.2
- Cholesterol: 112
- Protein: 45.7
- Total Fat: 30.5
- Sodium: 2036

943. Thanksgiving Won Tons

Serving: 20 | Prep: 30mins | Cook: 15mins | Ready in:

Ingredients

- 1 1/2 cups cooked turkey breast meat, shredded
- 2/3 cup dried cranberries
- 1/3 cup slivered almonds
- 1/2 cup cranberry sauce
- 1 (14 ounce) package wonton wrappers
- 1 quart vegetable oil for frying

Direction

- In a bowl, mix cranberry sauce, almonds, cranberries and turkey. In middle of every wonton wrapper, put 1 teaspoon of mixture.

Fold the wrapped over the filling and moisten edges. Use a fork to press edges to seal.
- In big skillet/deep fryer, heat oil.
- In hot oil, fry wontons till golden brown then drain on paper towels.

Nutrition Information

- Calories: 146 calories;
- Total Fat: 6
- Sodium: 120
- Total Carbohydrate: 17.8
- Cholesterol: 10
- Protein: 5.6

944. The Hot Brown

Serving: 4 | Prep: 20mins | Cook: 1hours10mins | Ready in:

Ingredients

- For the Turkey (Enough for 4 portions):
- 2 pounds boneless turkey breast with skin on
- 1 tablespoon kosher salt
- 1 teaspoon herbes de Provence
- 1 teaspoon oil
- 8 slices bacon
- 2 tablespoons salted butter
- 2 tablespoons all-purpose flour
- 2 cups heavy cream
- salt and freshly ground black pepper to taste
- 1 pinch cayenne pepper, or to taste
- 1/2 cup grated Pecorino Romano cheese
- 1 pinch freshly grated nutmeg
- For 4 Hot Browns:
- 8 slices white bread, toasted
- 12 slices tomato
- 8 tablespoons grated Pecorino Romano cheese, or to taste
- 1 pinch paprika, or to taste
- 4 teaspoons chopped Italian parsley, or to taste

Direction

- Preheat your oven to 350°F (175°C).
- Coat the flesh side of the turkey breast evenly with herbes de Provence and 1/2 of the kosher salt. Spread the leftover half of the kosher salt in the skin side of the turkey breast to taste. In a greased baking dish, put in the seasoned turkey, skin-side up.
- Put in the preheated oven and let it roast for 45-60 minutes until an inserted instant-read thermometer on the meat indicates 148°F (64°C).
- Cover the bottom of a baking sheet with aluminum foil and put in the bacon. Take the roasted turkey out from the oven and allow it to cool down.
- Put the bacon in the preheated oven and let it cook for 10-15 minutes until it is cooked halfway through.
- Put the butter in a pot and let it melt on medium heat. Add in the flour and mix until well-blended. Let the roux mixture cook while occasionally stirring it for 3 minutes until it smells similar to a cooked pie crust. Add in all the cream at once and whisk it. Let it cook for 5 minutes until the Mornay sauce has begun to boil and its consistency is thick. Switch off the heat right away.
- Put black pepper, cayenne pepper and salt into the Mornay sauce to taste. Add in 1/2 cup of Pecorino Romano cheese and mix until everything is well-blended. Put in the nutmeg and give it a quick mix.
- Slice the turkey into fat slices. Remove the turkey skin.
- Put the 2 sliced breads over each other and cut off the edges. Cut 1 of the bread slices into 2 triangles. Put a small baking dish on top of a sheet pan and arrange the bread in the baking dish. Put 3 turkey slices on top of the bread layer. Put 3 sliced tomatoes in between the slices of turkey. Pour 1/4 of the Mornay sauce evenly on top and sprinkle it with 2 tablespoons of Pecorino Romano cheese. Dust it off with paprika and place the half-cooked bacon across the very top. Do the same procedure with the rest of the ingredients thrice more.

- Place the oven rack around 6 inches away from the source of heat then preheat the broiler in your oven.
- Put in the preheated oven broiler and let it cook under the broiler for 5 minutes until the top turns nicely brown in color and the bacon is crispy. Put it on a plate lined with table napkin and garnish it with parsley.

Nutrition Information

- Calories: 1280 calories;
- Cholesterol: 400
- Protein: 88.7
- Total Fat: 85.4
- Sodium: 2841
- Total Carbohydrate: 36.6

945. Tunisian Slow Cooked Turkey Breast

Serving: 6 | Prep: 25mins | Cook: 3hours40mins | Ready in:

Ingredients

- 2 tablespoons all-purpose flour
- 1 teaspoon chipotle chili powder
- 1/2 teaspoon garlic powder
- 1/2 teaspoon ground cinnamon
- 1/2 teaspoon ground coriander
- 1/2 teaspoon salt
- 1/4 teaspoon ground black pepper
- 1 (4 pound) skinless, boneless turkey breast half
- 1 tablespoon olive oil
- 1 acorn squash, seeded and cut into quarters
- 3 large carrots, peeled and cut into 3 pieces
- 2 red onions, quartered
- 6 unpeeled garlic cloves

Direction

- In a large resealable plastic bag, combine black pepper, salt, coriander, cinnamon, garlic powder, chipotle chili powder, and flour. Shake until thoroughly combined. Place in the turkey breast, seal, shake until turkey is evenly coated with the spice mix.
- In a large skillet, heat oil over medium heat. Sear the seasoned turkey breast in the hot oil for 5 minutes per side until all sides are nicely browned, make sure that the meat will remain pink color inside.
- In the bottom of a large slow cooker, place some garlic cloves, red onions, carrots, and acorn squash quarters. Top the vegetables with the browned turkey breast. Cover cooker.
- Cook turkey breast for 3 1/2 to 4 hours on High or 7 to 8 hours on Low, until everything is tender. Transfer turkey breast to a platter and set aside to cool for 10 minutes before slicing.
- Peel garlic cloves and squash. Surround the turkey meat with the cooked vegetables. Spoon juices left in the slow cooker over turkey and vegetables. Serve.

Nutrition Information

- Calories: 455 calories;
- Cholesterol: 218
- Protein: 81.1
- Total Fat: 4.6
- Sodium: 365
- Total Carbohydrate: 19.2

946. Turkey Avocado Panini

Serving: 2 | Prep: 17mins | Cook: 8mins | Ready in:

Ingredients

- 1/2 ripe avocado
- 1/4 cup mayonnaise
- 2 ciabatta rolls
- 1 tablespoon olive oil, divided

- 2 slices provolone cheese
- 1 cup whole fresh spinach leaves, divided
- 1/4 pound thinly sliced mesquite smoked turkey breast
- 2 roasted red peppers, sliced into strips

Direction

- In a bowl, mash the mayonnaise and the avocado together until mixed thoroughly.
- Preheat the panini sandwich press.
- To prepare the sandwiches, divide in half the flat way the ciabatta rolls and then use olive oil to polish the bottom of every roll. Onto the panini press, put the bottoms of the rolls with the olive oil side facing down. On each sandwich, put a sliced roasted red pepper, a provolone cheese slice, half the chopped turkey breast, and half spinach leaves. On the cut surface of each top, lay half of the mixture of avocado and then put top of the roll onto the sandwich. Use olive oil to polish the top of the roll.
- Cover the panini press and then cook for about 5 to 8 minutes until bun is crisp and toasted, cheese has melted and has golden brown grill marks.

Nutrition Information

- Calories: 723 calories;
- Total Fat: 51.3
- Sodium: 1720
- Total Carbohydrate: 42.1
- Cholesterol: 62
- Protein: 25.3

947. Turkey Bacon Avocado Sandwich

Serving: 1 | Prep: 15mins | Cook: | Ready in:

Ingredients

- 1 tablespoon reduced-fat mayonnaise (optional)
- 2 slices bread, toasted
- 1 slice provolone cheese
- 4 thin slices deli turkey breast
- 4 slices precooked bacon, microwaved according to package directions
- 1/2 avocado - peeled, pitted, and thinly sliced
- 1 slice ripe tomato
- 1 leaf lettuce

Direction

- Put mayonnaise on one side of both slices of toasted bread then spread. Put lettuce, tomato, avocado, bacon, turkey and provolone cheese on top of bread slice. Put the remaining bread slice on top, cut in half and serve.

Nutrition Information

- Calories: 578 calories;
- Total Fat: 34.9
- Sodium: 1762
- Total Carbohydrate: 37.9
- Cholesterol: 67
- Protein: 30.8

948. Turkey Breast Roulade With Apple And Raisin Stuffing

Serving: 8 | Prep: 45mins | Cook: 1hours30mins | Ready in:

Ingredients

- 1 1/2 cups water
- 1/4 cup butter
- 1/3 cup raisins
- 1 (6 ounce) package low sodium stuffing mix (such as Stove Top® Lower Sodium Chicken Flavor)
- 1 tablespoon poultry seasoning
- 1 apple - peeled, cored, and chopped

- 1 (6 pound) whole bone-in turkey breast with skin
- salt and pepper to taste
- 1 tablespoon poultry seasoning

Direction

- In a saucepan, combine the butter, raisins, and water. Bring the mixture to a boil. Remove the mixture from the heat and mix in the stuffing mix. Cover the pan and allow the mixture to stand for 5 minutes until the stuffing mixture absorbs all the liquid. Stir in apple and 1 tbsp. of poultry seasoning lightly. Let the stuffing mixture cool.
- Set the oven to 350°F (175°C) for preheating. Position the rack into the roasting pan.
- Remove the turkey breast skin carefully in one piece without ripping the skin; put it aside. Slowly bone the turkey breast, keeping the meat in one piece. If necessary, remove the strip of the cartilage and gristle between the two breast halves. Pull outward two tenderloin sections from the main part of the breast, making sure to keep them attached so that the boneless turkey would expand into a piece of roughly square-shaped meat. Sprinkle salt, 1 tbsp. of poultry seasoning, and pepper inside the breast.
- Fill the inside of the breast meat piece with the stuffing mixture. Roll the stuffed breast firmly into a compact roll. Lay the reserved turkey skin out and position the stuffed roll on its middle. Pull the skin and roll it over the stuffed meat. Use cooking twine to tie the stuffed role together. Arrange the roll into the roasting rack, seam-side down.
- Roast the stuffed breast inside the preheated oven for 1 1/2-2 hours until the meat is no longer pink inside, the skin is golden brown, and the roll's temperature is 170°F (75°C) when measured in the meat's thickest part. Cover it with an aluminum foil to tent the roll. Let it stand for at least 10 minutes before discarding the twine and slicing the roll.

Nutrition Information

- Calories: 680 calories;
- Protein: 86.3
- Total Fat: 29.7
- Sodium: 299
- Total Carbohydrate: 12.7
- Cholesterol: 235

949. Turkey Breast With Gravy

Serving: 6 | Prep: 25mins | Cook: 2hours35mins | Ready in:

Ingredients

- 1 (6 pound) bone-in turkey breast
- cooking spray
- 1 onion, quartered
- 2 celery ribs, sliced
- 1/4 cup butter, cut into 1 tablespoon sized pieces
- 1 cup chicken broth
- 1/4 cup dry white wine
- 1 tablespoon lemon pepper
- 1 1/2 teaspoons garlic powder
- 1 1/2 teaspoons onion powder
- 1 teaspoon rubbed sage
- 1 teaspoon paprika
- 2 tablespoons all-purpose flour
- 1 cup water
- 1 cube chicken bouillon

Direction

- Preheat the oven to 160°C or 325°F.
- In a shallow baking pan, put the breast of turkey; with nonstick cooking spray, coat the outer of turkey. In breast cavity, insert the celery and onion; put butter among skin and meat. Into the base of pan, add white wine and chicken broth.
- In a small bowl, mix paprika, sage, onion powder, garlic powder and lemon pepper; massage the seasoning mix on turkey.

- In the preheated prepped oven, let bake for 2-1/2 to 3 hours till a meat thermometer registers 80°C or 175°F, basting every half an hour. Take turkey off and retain warmth. Into a cup, put the pan drippings and get rid of oil.
- In a saucepan, mix water and flour till smooth. Add in chicken bouillon and pan drippings. Boil over moderate heat, mixing often, and cook for 2 minutes till thickened. Cut the turkey and serve along with gravy.

Nutrition Information

- Calories: 642 calories;
- Sodium: 868
- Total Carbohydrate: 6.6
- Cholesterol: 349
- Protein: 120.1
- Total Fat: 10.9

950. Turkey Divan

Serving: 6 | Prep: 10mins | Cook: 50mins | Ready in:

Ingredients

- 2 (10 ounce) packages frozen broccoli spears
- 1/4 cup margarine
- 6 tablespoons all-purpose flour
- salt and ground black pepper to taste
- 2 cups chicken broth
- 1/2 cup heavy whipping cream
- 3 tablespoons white wine
- 3 cups cooked turkey breast, sliced
- 1/4 cup shredded Monterey Jack cheese

Direction

- In a saucepan, put broccoli and 4 cups of water. Boil; lower the heat; simmer with a cover for 5-8 minutes, or till tender. Drain.
- Set the oven at 350°F (175°C) and start preheating.
- In a saucepan over medium heat, melt margarine; mix in pepper, salt and flour, stir properly. Pour in chicken broth; cook while stirring for around 10 minutes, or till the sauce bubbles and thickens. Pour in wine and cream; stir till well combined.
- On the bottom of a 7x12-in. baking sheet, place broccoli. Spread half of the sauce over broccoli. Arrange sliced turkey on top. In the saucepan, mix Monterey Jack cheese into the remaining sauce. Transfer the cheese sauce over the turkey.
- Bake in the preheated oven for around 20 minutes, or till bubbly. Keep broiling for around 5 minutes, or till the cheese sauce turns golden.

Nutrition Information

- Calories: 331 calories;
- Total Fat: 20.1
- Sodium: 218
- Total Carbohydrate: 11.4
- Cholesterol: 85
- Protein: 25.6

951. Turkey Paupiettes With Apple Maple Stuffing

Serving: 4 | Prep: 20mins | Cook: 25mins | Ready in:

Ingredients

- 2 tablespoons extra virgin olive oil, divided
- 2 links apple maple chicken sausage, casings removed
- 1 small onion, diced
- 2 cloves garlic, minced
- 1 cup crusty bread cubes
- 4 teaspoons finely chopped fresh parsley
- 1/2 tablespoon finely chopped fresh sage
- 1 (1 1/2-pound) skinless, boneless turkey breast half, halved lengthwise and pounded to 1/2-inch thickness

- salt and ground black pepper to taste
- 1 cup turkey stock

Direction

- Put 1 tbsp. of olive oil in a nonstick skillet and heat it over medium-high heat. Stir in sausage and cook for 5-10 minutes, breaking it using the wooden spoon until crumbly and browned. Place the cooked sausage into a large bowl. Set the skillet back into the heat.
- Cook and stir garlic and onion into the hot skillet for 3-4 minutes until fragrant and softened. Once cooked, place them into the bowl with sausage.
- In a food processor, blend the bread cubes until finely ground. Pour the bread crumbs, sage, and parsley into the sausage mixture. Mix well until the stuffing is combined.
- Season the turkey breasts with salt and pepper. Spoon half of the stuffing mixture onto each of the breasts. Roll the turkey breasts around the stuffing, tucking the sides inside as you roll. Secure the rolls with twine. Season each of the rolls with salt and pepper.
- Set the oven to 350°F (175°C) for preheating.
- Put leftover 1 tbsp. of olive oil in a large oven-proof skillet and heat it over medium-high heat. Cook the turkey rolls in hot oil for 3-5 minutes per side until golden brown on every side.
- Pour the turkey stock into the skillet. Let the mixture boil while scraping off any browned bits at the bottom of the pan using the wooden spoon. Place the skillet into the oven.
- Let them cook inside the preheated oven for 10-12 minutes until the juices run clear and the rolls are no longer pink in the middle. An inserted instant-read thermometer into the center registers at least 165°F (74°C). Get the rolls from the oven and allow them to rest for 5 minutes. Cut the rolls into 1-inch slices.

Nutrition Information

- Calories: 374 calories;
- Total Fat: 13.7
- Sodium: 526
- Total Carbohydrate: 7.7
- Cholesterol: 175
- Protein: 52.1

952. Turkey Sandwiches With Cranberry Sauce

Serving: 4 | Prep: 15mins | Cook: 2mins | Ready in:

Ingredients

- 1 loaf French bread
- 4 tablespoons margarine
- 8 ounces sliced deli turkey meat
- 8 slices provolone cheese
- 8 slices precooked bacon
- 4 tablespoons mayonnaise
- 4 tablespoons jellied cranberry sauce
- 8 slices fresh tomatoes
- 4 lettuce leaves

Direction

- Preheat an oven broiler.
- Cut bread to 4 pieces; split lengthwise nearly all the way through for 4 sandwiches. On inside of every piece, spread margarine. Put, cut side up, on a baking sheet.
- Under the preheated broiler, toast bread for 1-2 minutes till lightly browned. Take pan out of oven.
- Layer 2 slices each of bacon, cheese and turkey on 4 bread pieces. Remove leftover 4 bread slices from baking sheet; keep for sandwich tops. Slightly cool bread; spread mayonnaise on cut side of every 4 top slices.
- Put bread with cheese and turkey under the broiler for 1 minute till cheese melts. Remove from the broiler; spread 1 tablespoon of cranberry sauce on each sandwich. Layer with lettuce and tomatoes. Put a top slice of bread on each half; serve.

Nutrition Information

- Calories: 1068 calories;
- Total Fat: 65.8
- Sodium: 3322
- Total Carbohydrate: 70.1
- Cholesterol: 128
- Protein: 49.5

953. Turkey Scallopini And Squash Ravioli With Cranberry Brown Butter

Serving: 8 | Prep: 10mins | Cook: | Ready in:

Ingredients

- 8 (4 ounce) portions boneless turkey breast
- 1/4 cup extra-virgin olive oil
- 1/4 cup all-purpose flour
- 2 eggs, beaten
- 2 cups Progresso® plain Panko crispy bread crumbs
- 8 tablespoons unsalted butter
- 1 (18 ounce) package frozen squash ravioli
- 1/4 cup chopped fresh sage
- 1 1/2 cups fresh cranberries
- 3 tablespoons dark molasses
- 1/4 cup balsamic vinegar
- 1 cup Progresso® chicken broth or reduced-sodium chicken broth
- Salt and pepper

Direction

- In a big pot, boil 4 quarts lightly salted water.
- Using a meat mallet, pound turkey breast pieces between two sheets of plastic wrap to an even quarter-inch thickness. Back of a frying pan can be used if meat mallet is not available. This can be done a day in advance and keep in the plastic wrap, folded on top of each other. Or a butcher can cut and pound the turkey on your behalf.
- In a big sauté pan, heat olive oil over medium-high heat. Coat the turkey pieces lightly with flour, and shake off the excess; dunk in beaten eggs and then roll in bread crumbs. Once oil is bubbling and hot, put turkey pieces. Avoid crowding the pan. Let brown for 2 to 3 minutes, then flip to cook the other side, for another 30 seconds to a minute. The turkey will cook really quickly and will dry out if overcooked. Once done, take off to a baking sheet or platter and retain warmth. Avoid washing the sauté pan.
- For the sauce, put butter to sauté pan over medium-high heat. At the same time, into the boiling water, drop the ravioli. Once butter starts to become light brown, put fresh sage. Mix for several seconds; then put cranberries, and sauté till skins start to burst. Put broth, balsamic vinegar and molasses, scraping base of the pan to get all the flavor of the turkey. Allow to simmer till cranberries are tender and the sauce coats the back of a spoon for about 12 to 15 minutes. Season with salt and pepper to taste. Ensure to taste sauce for seasoning prior to pouring it on top of the turkey.
- Try ravioli doneness in about 3 minutes, press edges of dough; it should be soft. Let it drain. Arrange quarter of the raviolis per serving on hot plates and layer 1 piece of turkey on top of the ravioli. Spoon sauce on tops.

Nutrition Information

- Calories: 724 calories;
- Sodium: 1451
- Total Carbohydrate: 69.1
- Cholesterol: 135
- Protein: 34.3
- Total Fat: 34.1

954. Turkey Taco Salad

Serving: 12 | Prep: 15mins | Cook: 20mins | Ready in:

Ingredients

- 1 pound extra-lean ground turkey breast
- 1 head iceberg lettuce - rinsed, dried, and chopped
- 6 green onions, chopped
- 1 (15 ounce) can kidney beans, drained and rinsed
- 2 cups shredded Cheddar cheese
- 1/2 cup diced dill pickles
- 1/2 cup sliced black olives
- 2 cups fat-free mayonnaise
- 1 teaspoon lemon juice
- 1 teaspoon white wine vinegar
- 3/4 cup taco sauce
- 1 (14.5 ounce) package low-fat baked tortilla chips

Direction

- In a big deep skillet, cook turkey with garlic salt over medium-high heat until completely cooked. Let it crumble and cool in one side.
- Combine olives, lettuce, cheese, turkey, pickles, kidney beans and green onions.
- Combine taco sauce, lemon juice, and mayonnaise and vinegar.
- Put the dressing into the salad then place in the refrigerator. Add in two cups of crumbled tortilla chips then serve. Embellish with whole chips then serve.

Nutrition Information

- Calories: 343 calories;
- Sodium: 980
- Total Carbohydrate: 46.2
- Cholesterol: 50
- Protein: 17.4
- Total Fat: 11.4

955. Turkey A La King Deluxe

Serving: 4 | Prep: 10mins | Cook: 20mins | Ready in:

Ingredients

- 1 (10.75 ounce) can condensed cream of chicken soup
- 1 (10.75 ounce) can water
- 1 teaspoon vegetable oil
- 1 (8 ounce) package sliced fresh mushrooms
- 1 small carrot, diced
- 1 cup shredded cooked turkey breast
- 1/2 teaspoon onion powder
- 1/2 teaspoon salt
- 1/2 teaspoon ground black pepper
- 1 bay leaf
- 1/3 cup dry sherry
- 1/4 cup half-and-half cream
- 1 teaspoon dried parsley flakes
- 2/3 cup frozen peas
- 1 tablespoon butter

Direction

- Into one soup can of water, mix cream of chicken soup in the bowl.
- In a big saucepan over moderate heat, heat the vegetable oil, mix in carrot and mushrooms, and cook and mix for 5 minutes till mushrooms begin to release their liquid and carrot starts to soften. To the pan, put the sherry, bay leaf, pepper, salt, onion powder and shredded turkey and cook, mixing, for an additional of 5 minutes to cook pan juices down and cook away alcohol from wine.
- On top of turkey mixture, put the soup and boil. Lower the heat and put frozen peas, parsley and half-and-half. Let simmer for 5 to 10 minutes to cook down sauce and heat peas completely. Get rid of bay leaf and mix in the butter just prior to serving.

Nutrition Information

- Calories: 241 calories;
- Total Fat: 12.2
- Sodium: 1004
- Total Carbohydrate: 16.2
- Cholesterol: 46
- Protein: 15.8

956. Turkey A La Matt

Serving: 6 | Prep: 15mins | Cook: 55mins | Ready in:

Ingredients

- 1 1/2 pounds turkey breast, cooked and cubed
- 2 carrots, diced
- 2 potatoes, peeled and cubed
- 1 cup frozen green peas
- 1 (4.5 ounce) can mushrooms, drained
- 1/2 cup pearl onions
- 1 (10.75 ounce) can condensed cream of chicken soup
- 1 (10.75 ounce) can condensed cream of mushroom soup
- 1 cup crushed saltine crackers

Direction

- Set the oven to 350°F (175°C) and start preheating.
- In a medium pot of boiling water over high heat, place turkey breasts. After about 5 minutes, add cubed potatoes and diced carrots to the pot; boil all for about 5 minutes more. Drain water; place vegetables in a medium bowl.
- Add mushroom soup, chicken soup, onions, mushrooms and peas to the bowl. Cube cooked turkey breasts; stir into the mixture. Combine well; transfer mixture to a 2-quart casserole dish and spread. Place coarsely crushed saltine crackers on top.
- Bake with a cover for 30-40 minutes at 350°F (175°C).

Nutrition Information

- Calories: 390 calories;
- Sodium: 984
- Total Carbohydrate: 36.6
- Cholesterol: 98
- Protein: 40.8
- Total Fat: 8.4

957. Turkey A La Oscar

Serving: 6 | Prep: 15mins | Cook: 15mins | Ready in:

Ingredients

- 2 (10 ounce) packages frozen cut asparagus
- 1/4 cup water
- 1 tablespoon margarine
- 6 (4 ounce) turkey breast cutlets
- 1/4 teaspoon crushed garlic
- 1/4 pound cooked shrimp - peeled and deveined
- 1 (1.25 ounce) envelope hollandaise sauce mix

Direction

- In a saucepan, put asparagus and water, and boil over moderate heat. Cook with a cover for 5 minutes. Uncover and let cook for a minute or two, till soft. Drain and reserve, yet retain warmth.
- In a skillet, liquify margarine over moderately high heat. Let the turkey cutlets cook for 2 to 3 minutes per side, or till not pink anymore on the inside and browned. Take turkey out of the pan and reserve.
- Into already heated skillet, put shrimp and garlic. Cook over moderately high heat for a minute or two, mixing continuously till shrimp is heated completely.
- Make hollandaise sauce following package instructions.
- On a plate, put each turkey cutlet. Place shrimp and asparagus on top. Scoop hollandaise sauce on top of everything.

Nutrition Information

- Calories: 230 calories;
- Cholesterol: 119

- Protein: 37.3
- Total Fat: 6.3
- Sodium: 363
- Total Carbohydrate: 6.4

958. Turkey And Avocado Panini

Serving: 2 | Prep: 10mins | Cook: 10mins | Ready in:

Ingredients

- 4 slices artisan bread such as ciabatta
- 2 teaspoons honey Dijon salad dressing
- 1/2 cup baby spinach leaves
- 1/4 pound sliced oven-roasted deli turkey breast
- 1/4 red onion, cut into strips
- 1 ripe avocado from Mexico, peeled, pitted and thickly sliced
- Salt and pepper to taste
- 1/4 cup crumbled soft goat cheese
- Non-stick cooking spray

Direction

- Put honey Dijon dressing on one side of the sandwiches and put baby spinach leaves on top. Put a layer of turkey breast and red onion on top of the spinach.
- Meanwhile, put avocado slices on the other half of the sandwich. Sprinkle salt and pepper for added taste. Sprinkle goat cheese on top of the avocado slices. Combine sandwiches together to close.
- Follow the instructions on the manufacturer's manual on how to preheat a Panini press. Apply cooking spray onto Panini press. Put sandwiches into the press then close. Cook bread for 5-8 minutes until crisp and toasted, with grill marks, while the cheese starts to melt.

Nutrition Information

- Calories: 469 calories;
- Total Fat: 23.8
- Sodium: 1250
- Total Carbohydrate: 45.5
- Cholesterol: 37
- Protein: 22.1

959. Turkey And Feta Grilled Sandwich

Serving: 1 | Prep: 5mins | Cook: 5mins | Ready in:

Ingredients

- 2 slices smoked deli turkey
- 2 slices wheat bread
- 2 leaves lettuce
- 1 1/2 tablespoons crumbled feta cheese
- 1 tablespoon Italian salad dressing
- 1 tablespoon butter

Direction

- Lay slices of turkey on top of a bread slice. Place lettuce and then feta cheese atop turkey. Smear one side of the second bread slice with Italian salad dressing; place on top of the other slice, dressing-side down.
- Melt butter over medium heat in a skillet. Cook sandwich in melted butter, approximately 2 minutes on each side, until evenly browned.

Nutrition Information

- Calories: 377 calories;
- Total Fat: 21.6
- Sodium: 1418
- Total Carbohydrate: 27.8
- Cholesterol: 66
- Protein: 18.9

960. Turkey And Stuffing Casserole

Serving: 5 | Prep: 20mins | Cook: 45mins | Ready in:

Ingredients

- 1 (14 ounce) package seasoned dry stuffing mix
- 1 teaspoon ground sage
- 1 cup chopped celery
- 1/2 cup chicken broth
- 1 (10.75 ounce) can condensed cream of celery soup
- 1 (10.75 ounce) can condensed cream of chicken soup
- 2 boneless, skinless turkey breasts - cooked and shredded
- 1/4 cup melted butter

Direction

- Turn oven to 425°F (220°C) to preheat.
- Combine chicken broth, celery, sage, and stuffing crumbs in a large mixing bowl and put to one side. Place chicken soup and celery soup into 2 individual bowls; pour 1/2 of a soup can of water into each bowl. Mix well and put to one side.
- Scatter 1/3 of the stuffing crumb mixture over the bottom of a lightly oiled 9x13-inch baking dish. Place 1/2 of the shredded turkey meat over crumb mixture; stream celery soup over turkey. Scatter another 1/3 of the stuffing crumb mixture; place the rest of the turkey over crumb mixture. Stream chicken soup mixture over turkey and top with the remaining stuffing crumb mixture. Drizzle top with melted butter; pack the entire mixture firmly into the baking dish.
- Bake for 20 to 30 minutes in the preheated oven.

Nutrition Information

- Calories: 807 calories;
- Sodium: 2523
- Total Carbohydrate: 66.7
- Cholesterol: 239
- Protein: 86.3
- Total Fat: 19.7

961. Wild Turkey Gumbo

Serving: 20 | Prep: 20mins | Cook: 1hours45mins | Ready in:

Ingredients

- 1 cup wild rice
- water to cover
- 2 teaspoons Celtic sea salt, divided
- 3 quarts chicken broth, divided
- 2 tablespoons coconut oil
- 3 cups cubed wild turkey breast, or more to taste
- 1 large onion, chopped
- 2 large carrots, quartered lengthwise and sliced
- 4 stalks celery, chopped
- 1 pound bag frozen okra
- 1 teaspoon white pepper
- 3/4 teaspoon freshly ground black pepper
- 3 tablespoons chopped jarred jalapeno peppers
- 1 teaspoon hot sauce (such as Texas Pete®)

Direction

- In a bowl put wild rice and enough water to cover it; soak for 4 hours to overnight. Drain the rice.
- In a stockpot mix together 1 teaspoon of salt and wild rice, add about 3 cups of chicken broth. Bring to a boil, set heat to medium-low, cover and let it simmer for about 30 to 40 minutes until rice is soft. In a big skillet over medium heat, heat coconut oil. In the hot oil cook and mix celery, carrots, onion, and turkey for 10 to 15 minutes until vegetables are slightly soft and turkey is cooked through. Add okra into turkey mixture and cook for 5

to 7 minutes until okra is thawed. Season with black pepper, white pepper, and 1 teaspoon of salt.
- In a slow cooker combine the remaining chicken stock, hot sauce, jalapeno peppers, turkey mixture, and wild rice. Set to high and cook for 1 hour.

Nutrition Information

- Calories: 482 calories;
- Total Fat: 10.6
- Sodium: 939
- Total Carbohydrate: 10
- Cholesterol: 248
- Protein: 81.7

Chapter 8: Turkey Leg Recipes

***

962. African Turkey Stew

Serving: 6 | Prep: 30mins | Cook: 1hours30mins | Ready in:

Ingredients

- 3 smoked turkey legs, cut into 1-inch thick pieces
- 4 chicken bouillon cubes
- 4 red bell peppers - cored, seeded, and cut into chunks
- 6 tomatoes, cut into chunks
- 1 onion, cut into chunks
- 4 habanero peppers, seeded and chopped (wear gloves)
- 1 tablespoon minced garlic
- 2 tablespoons tomato paste
- 1 cup vegetable oil
- salt to taste

Direction

- In a big saucepan, use water to barely cover turkey legs. Add bouillon cubes. Boil on medium heat. Cook for about 30 minutes until water has nearly evaporated. In a blender, blend tomato paste, garlic, habanero peppers, onion, tomatoes and red bell peppers until veggies are pureed. Be careful because habanero peppers are really hot. When handling peppers, don't touch your eyes.
- In a Dutch oven, heat vegetable oil on medium heat. Put blended mixture in oil. Lower heat. Simmer for about 30 minutes until sauce starts to fry and oil separates. Mix turkey into sauce. Simmer to merge flavors for 15-20 minutes. Season with salt to taste.

Nutrition Information

- Calories: 630 calories;
- Total Fat: 48.2
- Sodium: 1951
- Total Carbohydrate: 14.8
- Cholesterol: 97
- Protein: 34.8

963. Colin's Turkey Casserole

Serving: 6 | Prep: 25mins | Cook: 1hours50mins | Ready in:

Ingredients

- 1 tablespoon butter
- 1 tablespoon vegetable oil
- 1 large onion, sliced
- 1/2 green bell pepper, cut into chunks
- 1/2 red bell pepper, cut into chunks
- 1 2/3 pounds turkey leg meat, cut into 1-inch cubes
- 8 large whole fresh mushrooms

- 1 apple, cored and sliced
- 2 cloves garlic, crushed
- 1 cup dry white wine
- 1 sprig fresh thyme
- 1 sprig fresh oregano
- 1 sprig fresh parsley
- 1 sprig fresh sage
- salt and ground black pepper to taste

Direction

- Set oven to 350°F (175°C) to preheat.
- Heat vegetable oil and butter in a large skillet; sauté onion for about 5 minutes, stirring from time to time, until transparent. Add red and green peppers; sauté for 5 minutes longer, then remove vegetable mixture to a 2-quart baking dish using a slotted spoon. Sauté turkey meat in the heated oil left in the skillet for about 8 to 10 minutes until browned; arrange cooked turkey in the baking dish with vegetables. Stir garlic, apple, and mushrooms into vegetables and turkey. Pour in white wine. Tie sage, parsley, oregano, and sprigs of thyme into a little bundle with a small piece of kitchen twine; put the bundle into the baking dish. Scatter pepper and salt to season.
- Bake for 90 to 120 minutes in the preheated oven until turkey is tender; discard the herb buddle before serving.

Nutrition Information

- Calories: 309 calories;
- Total Fat: 9.2
- Sodium: 124
- Total Carbohydrate: 9.3
- Cholesterol: 155
- Protein: 38.5

964. Eva's Savory Turkey Legs

Serving: 4 | *Prep:* 30mins | *Cook:* 1hours | *Ready in:*

Ingredients

- 2 cups dry bread cubes
- 1 large stalk celery, minced
- 1/3 cup dried cranberries
- 1/4 cup chopped walnuts
- 1 small yellow onion, diced
- 1/4 teaspoon minced garlic
- 1/2 teaspoon ground sage
- 1/2 teaspoon dried marjoram
- 1/2 teaspoon salt
- 1/4 teaspoon pepper
- 1 egg
- 1/4 cup hot water
- 2 turkey legs
- 1 1/2 tablespoons butter

Direction

- Preheat the oven to 190°C or 375°F. On a medium baking sheet, put a big aluminum foil sheet.
- Combine the garlic, onion, walnuts, cranberries, celery and bread in a medium bowl. Add pepper, salt, marjoram and sage to season. Mix in egg and sufficient amount of hot water to dampen.
- On foil sheet, set the turkey legs, and add pepper and salt to season. Scoop bread mixture around legs, and dot butter over. Securely seal the foil around the bread mixture and legs.
- In the prepped oven, let bake for an hour, or till turkey leg meat has attained an inner temperature of 80°C or 180°F.

Nutrition Information

- Calories: 398 calories;
- Sodium: 592
- Total Carbohydrate: 20.6
- Cholesterol: 210
- Protein: 39.6
- Total Fat: 17.3

965. Fried Cabbage With Turkey

Serving: 4 | Prep: 10mins | Cook: 10mins | Ready in:

Ingredients

- 1/4 cup olive oil
- 1/2 smoked turkey leg, meat removed and chopped
- 1/4 yellow onion, sliced
- 1/2 cup chicken broth
- 1 whole cabbage, chopped
- 1 teaspoon salt
- 1 dash ground black pepper
- 1 dash togarashi (Japanese red pepper condiment)

Direction

- In a big skillet, heat olive oil over moderate heat. In hot oil, cook and mix turkey for 3 minutes till heated. Put in the onion; cook and mix for a minute till hot.
- Turn the heat to moderately low. Put chicken broth on turkey mixture; mix. Simmer the liquid and cook for 3 minutes, mixing from time to time.
- Mix cabbage with turkey mixture; add togarashi, pepper and salt to season; cook and mix for 2 to 3 minutes till cabbage has started to soften. Turn the heat to low, cover the skillet, and keep cooking for an additional of 2 to 3 minutes till cabbage is fully soft.

Nutrition Information

- Calories: 245 calories;
- Sodium: 766
- Total Carbohydrate: 14.9
- Cholesterol: 26
- Protein: 11.1
- Total Fat: 16.8

966. Grilled Turkey Legs

Serving: 6 | Prep: 25mins | Cook: 50mins | Ready in:

Ingredients

- 1 (2 liter) bottle lemon-lime flavored carbonated beverage
- 2 tablespoons sugar
- 2 tablespoons hot sauce
- 1 tablespoon crushed red pepper flakes
- 1 tablespoon black pepper
- 1 large sweet onion, sliced
- 4 turkey legs
- 2 tablespoons honey
- 1 tablespoon steak seasoning

Direction

- Brush the grill grate lightly with oil. Preheat grill on high heat. Make a mixture of lemon-lime flavored carbonated beverage, hot sauce, sugar, pepper, red pepper and onion in a big pot. Add in turkey legs and boil for thirty to forty-five minutes. Internal temperature of the turkey must be 180 degrees F (80 degrees C). Take out the onions from a pot and transfer in the prepared grill. Put the turkey legs on top of the onions. Sprinkle with steak seasoning and a drizzle of honey. Grill the turkey legs, wait for a brown crisp crust to form before turning, or about 20 minutes.

Nutrition Information

- Calories: 496 calories;
- Total Fat: 9.6
- Sodium: 759
- Total Carbohydrate: 53
- Cholesterol: 119
- Protein: 49.4

967. It's Way Better Than Thanksgiving Turkey Turkey

Serving: 3 | Prep: 30mins | Cook: 3hours45mins | Ready in:

Ingredients

- 1/2 cup extra-virgin olive oil
- 3 turkey legs, rinsed and patted dry
- salt and ground black pepper to taste
- 2 teaspoons dried thyme
- 6 sprigs fresh rosemary
- 3 tablespoons butter, cut into small chunks
- 1 1/2 tablespoons minced garlic
- 1/2 cup diced onion
- 1/2 tablespoon red cooking wine, or to taste
- 1/2 tablespoon brown sugar
- 2 tablespoons all-purpose flour
- 1 1/2 cups chicken stock
- 4 dashes browning sauce (such as Gravy Master®)

Direction

- Set the oven to 400°F (200°C) for preheating.
- Put olive oil in a roasting pan. Coat the turkey legs in oil, flipping all over a few times until well-coated. Sprinkle the legs with thyme, black pepper, and salt. Get the leaves from the 3 sprigs of rosemary and sprinkle it into the turkey legs. Position the remaining 3 sprigs of rosemary all around the legs in the oil. Arrange the butter pieces onto the legs and sprinkle them with garlic. Scatter the onion into the pan.
- Roast the legs inside the preheated oven for 1 1/2-2 hours, basting the legs every 20 minutes until the juices run clear and the skin of the turkey is browned. Adjust the heat to 300°F (150°C) and flip the legs over in the pan. Roast the legs for 1 hour while basting them every 20 minutes. Adjust again the heat to 200°F (95°C) and roast the legs for 1 more hour until the skin turns golden brown. Transfer the turkey legs into the serving platter.
- For the gravy, position the roasting pan with drippings and oil into the burner set on medium heat. Whisk in brown sugar and cooking wine, stirring well until the sugar is completely dissolved. Scrape up and dissolve all the browned flavor bits that are left at the bottom of the pan using the whisk. Stir in flour, little by little, and mix until the flour is incorporated smoothly into the mixture. Add the chicken stock and whisk frequently for 5 minutes until the gravy thickens and starts to simmer. Mix in gravy browning sauce. Simmer the gravy for 3-5 minutes. Serve the gravy together with the roasted turkey legs.

Nutrition Information

- Calories: 927 calories;
- Total Carbohydrate: 11.8
- Cholesterol: 209
- Protein: 74.2
- Total Fat: 63.2
- Sodium: 647

968. Meaty Potato Leek Soup

Serving: 12 | Prep: 20mins | Cook: 1hours15mins | Ready in:

Ingredients

- 2 smoked turkey legs
- 2 (48 fluid ounce) cans chicken broth
- 6 slices bacon, coarsely chopped
- 6 large russet potatoes, coarsely chopped
- 3 large leeks, sliced
- 1 teaspoon dried thyme leaves
- salt and pepper to taste
- 1 cup heavy cream

Direction

- In a large soup pot, place turkey legs, and stream in chicken stock. Bring to a boil, turn heat to medium-low, then simmer for 30 to 45 minutes until turkey meat starts to come off the bones. Take the turkey legs out of the pan; drain broth and set aside to reserve. Separate turkey meat from the tendons and bones, put to one side.

- In a soup pot over medium heat, add bacon; cook and stir sometimes for about 10 minutes until crispy and browned. Transfer bacon pieces to paper towels to drain; set aside. Retain about 2 tablespoons of bacon grease in the pot. Sauté leeks in the drippings for about 5 minutes over medium heat until tender and thawed but not brown. Add the reserved broth, black pepper, salt, thyme, and potato cubes into the pan. Lower heat, then simmer for about 20 minutes until potatoes are tender.
- Transfer the potato and leek mixture into a blender, filling the container no more than halfway full. Hold the lid tightly with a folded kitchen towel. Pulse a few times to make the soup moving before leaving it onto puree. Process the mixture in batches until no lumps remain; pour the pureed soup into a clean pot. Another way; puree the soup right in the pot using a stick blender.
- Add cream and mix well, then mix in the reserved turkey meat. Cook over medium-low heat until the soup is heated; add a few bacon pieces over the top of each portion.

Nutrition Information

- Calories: 398 calories;
- Total Fat: 18.2
- Sodium: 1656
- Total Carbohydrate: 40.6
- Cholesterol: 75
- Protein: 18.3

969. Old Man's Turkey Noodle Soup

Serving: 8 | Prep: 30mins | Cook: 2hours | Ready in:

Ingredients

- 3 turkey drumsticks
- 3 quarts water
- 2 large onions, chopped
- 4 carrots, chopped
- 3 stalks celery, chopped
- 4 cloves garlic, chopped
- 1 tablespoon salt
- 1/2 teaspoon ground black pepper
- 1/2 teaspoon ground dried sage
- 1/2 teaspoon dried thyme
- 1/2 teaspoon dried rosemary
- 1/2 teaspoon celery salt
- 2 cups uncooked egg noodles

Direction

- In a big soup pot, combine water with the turkey drumsticks, then boil. Stir in celery salt, rosemary, thyme, sage, black pepper, salt, garlic, celery, carrots, and onions. Lower the heat to simmer. Cook for 2 hours until the turkey meat becomes very tender. Remove the drumsticks from the pot and allow to cool. Once cool enough to be handled, strip the meat off the bones and tendons, then chop the meat up and return into the soup.
- Set a big pot of lightly salted water to come to a rolling boil, then cook egg noodles for 5 minutes until cooked through but still firm to chew. Drain. Scoop the noodles into soup bowls and fill with the turkey soup.

Nutrition Information

- Calories: 234 calories;
- Total Fat: 5.8
- Sodium: 1093
- Total Carbohydrate: 14.9
- Cholesterol: 75
- Protein: 29.5

970. Orangey Turkey Legs

Serving: 4 | Prep: 15mins | Cook: 1hours30mins | Ready in:

Ingredients

- 1 (11 ounce) can mandarin oranges, drained with liquid reserved
- 2 tablespoons distilled white vinegar
- 1 tablespoon brown sugar
- 1/4 cup vegetable oil
- 2 turkey drumsticks
- salt to taste

Direction

- Process the brown sugar, vinegar and orange segments in a food processor or blender. Put into a big resealable plastic bag, and add oil and reserved mandarin orange liquid. In the bag, put turkey drumsticks, close bag, and refrigerate to marinate for an hour.
- Preheat the oven to 190°C or 375°F. Line aluminum foil on a baking sheet.
- On baking sheet, put the marinated turkey drumsticks, and add salt to season.
- Put cover on and in the prepped oven, bake for half an hour. Uncover, and keep baking for an hour, basting frequently with the rest of orange mixture, to an inner temperature of 80°C or 180°F.

Nutrition Information

- Calories: 379 calories;
- Cholesterol: 89
- Protein: 36.8
- Total Fat: 20.5
- Sodium: 397
- Total Carbohydrate: 10.7

971. Pammy's Slow Cooker Beans

Serving: 10 | Prep: 15mins | Cook: 8hours | Ready in:

Ingredients

- 2 pounds dried pinto beans
- 8 cups water, or more if needed
- 1 small onion, chopped
- 2 teaspoons garlic powder
- 1/2 teaspoon onion powder
- 1 teaspoon ground black pepper
- 2 bay leaves
- 1 smoked turkey leg
- 1/3 cup olive oil

Direction

- Rinse and pick on the beans, then put in a big bowl. With cold water, fill the bowl, and let the beans submerge for 6 to 8 hours.
- Let drain and wash the beans, then put into slow cooker. Add in 8 cups water. Mix in bay leaves, black pepper, onion powder, garlic powder and onion. Into the cooker, put the turkey leg, place the cover, and allow to cook for 6 hours on Low setting. Mix in olive oil, and put additional water in case beans are starting to dry out; let cook for 2 hours longer till beans are really soft.

Nutrition Information

- Calories: 415 calories;
- Sodium: 728
- Total Carbohydrate: 56
- Cholesterol: 19
- Protein: 25.3
- Total Fat: 10.8

972. Pressure Cooked Black Eyed Peas With Smoked Turkey Leg

Serving: 10 | Prep: 10mins | Cook: 25mins | Ready in:

Ingredients

- 2 pounds dried black-eyed peas, sorted and rinsed
- 1 large smoked turkey leg
- 1 onion, chopped
- 2 cloves garlic, chopped, or to taste
- olive oil
- 1 teaspoon ground black pepper, or to taste

Direction

- In pressure cooker, add turkey leg and peas. Mix in peas, olive oil, garlic, pepper, onion, and enough water to cover. Let it simmer then secure the lid.
- Adjust the heat until the regulator rocks gently; cook for 15-20 minutes at high pressure. Relieve the pressure naturally for 5 or more minutes in accordance with the cooker's manual. Uncover and add water if necessary. Cover and cook for another 5-15 minutes until the beans become tender. Cool the cooker 5 minutes before removing the lid. Debone the turkey.

Nutrition Information

- Calories: 451 calories;
- Cholesterol: 61
- Protein: 45
- Total Fat: 5.6
- Sodium: 71
- Total Carbohydrate: 55.9

973. Roasted Barbecued Turkey Legs

Serving: 4 | Prep: 15mins | Cook: 30mins | Ready in:

Ingredients

- 4 smoked turkey legs
- 4 cups hot water
- 2 teaspoons chicken bouillon granules
- 2 cups barbeque sauce

Direction

- Position the turkey legs into the 4-qt pressure cooker that is set over medium-high heat. Cover the turkey with sufficient amount of water. Sprinkle it with chicken bouillon granules. Stir the mixture well until lightly dissolved. Cover the cooker with its lid and bring it up to full pressure. Let the mixture cook for 5 minutes.
- In the meantime, preheat the oven's broiler. Remove the cooker from the heat after the time is up on the turkey. To help release the pressure, run cold water on top of the cooker and open its lid. Position the turkey legs in a roasting pan or broiling pan.
- Broil for 10-15 minutes until the skin of the turkey legs is crispy and brown. Brush barbeque sauce all over the legs towards the end of the cooking time. Serve the turkey with the remaining sauce on its side.

Nutrition Information

- Calories: 602 calories;
- Sodium: 4764
- Total Carbohydrate: 56.3
- Cholesterol: 223
- Protein: 57.1
- Total Fat: 14.5

974. Roasted Potatoes And Smoked Turkey Legs

Serving: 8 | Prep: 25mins | Cook: 1hours35mins | Ready in:

Ingredients

- 2 tablespoons olive oil
- 6 potatoes, peeled and cut into small cubes
- 1 onion, coarsely chopped
- 3 cloves garlic, peeled and coarsely chopped
- 1 red chile pepper, seeded and finely chopped (optional)
- 2 uncooked, smoked turkey legs
- 1 (8 ounce) can diced tomatoes
- 1/2 head cabbage, thinly sliced
- 1 cup canned baked beans in tomato sauce
- 1 teaspoon smoked paprika
- 1 pinch salt and ground black pepper to taste

Direction

- Preheat the oven to 175 °C or 350 °F.
- In an oven-proof pot or a Dutch oven, heat the olive oil over medium heat. Put chili pepper, garlic, onion and potatoes; let cook and mix for 5 minutes till onion becomes translucent. Put legs of turkey over; put diced tomatoes on top. Put Dutch oven lid to cover.
- In the prepped oven, bake for 45 minutes till potatoes are soft. Roll turkey legs over to cover with tomato mixture. Into the pot, mix baked beans and cabbage; put pepper, salt and paprika to season. Put lid back.
- Keep baking for 45 minutes till turkey legs are soft. Pull off meat of turkey from bones and slice into bite-sized portions. Add into pot.

Nutrition Information

- Calories: 325 calories;
- Sodium: 248
- Total Carbohydrate: 42.1
- Cholesterol: 45
- Protein: 24.4
- Total Fat: 7.2

975. Roasted Turkey Legs

Serving: 3 | Prep: 15mins | Cook: 2hours | Ready in:

Ingredients

- 3 stalks celery stalks, cut in thirds
- 3 turkey legs
- 6 tablespoons butter
- salt to taste
- 1/2 cup water, or as needed

Direction

- Preheat an oven to 175°C or 350°F. Wash the legs of turkey and pat dry.
- Stand the turkey legs upright, like turkey were standing. Insert a knife downward into deep tissue, making 2 to 3 lengthy pockets. Push 1 piece of celery into every opening. Pull back the skin on legs, massage with butter, and add a bit of salt to season. Return the skin into place, massage with additional butter, and lightly season with salt. In roasting pan, set the legs.
- Allow to roast for 1 1/2 to 2 hours without a cover till legs turn golden brown and inner temperature reaches 82°C or 180°F when inserting a meat thermometer in. Put in additional water if necessary while roasting, and baste from time to time with butter or juices.

Nutrition Information

- Calories: 643 calories;
- Total Fat: 36.9
- Sodium: 399
- Total Carbohydrate: 1.2
- Cholesterol: 239
- Protein: 73.1

976. Slow Cooker Turkey Legs

Serving: 12 | Prep: 10mins | Cook: 7hours | Ready in:

Ingredients

- 6 turkey legs
- 3 teaspoons poultry seasoning, divided
- salt and ground black pepper to taste
- 6 12x16-inch squares of aluminum foil

Direction

- Rinse turkey legs, and shake off extra liquid. Scatter every turkey leg with approximately 1/2 teaspoon of the poultry seasoning, black pepper and salt to taste. Securely wrap leg with aluminum foil. Redo with the rest of legs.
- Into a slow cooker, put wrapped legs of turkey without any other ingredients or liquids. Turn cooker to Low, and cook for 7 to 8 hours till meat is really soft.

Nutrition Information

- Calories: 217 calories;
- Protein: 36.3
- Total Fat: 6.9
- Sodium: 102
- Total Carbohydrate: 0.2
- Cholesterol: 89

977. Slow Cooker Turkey And Potatoes

Serving: 6 | Prep: 20mins | Cook: 6hours | Ready in:

Ingredients

- 2 1/2 cups water
- 2 (10.75 ounce) cans condensed cream of chicken and mushroom soup
- 1 (10.75 ounce) can condensed cream of mushroom soup
- 1/2 cup chopped onion
- 1/4 cup chopped green bell pepper
- 1/4 cup chopped red bell pepper
- 3 large turkey legs
- 2 potatoes, cut into chunks
- salt to taste
- 1 pinch seasoned meat tenderizer
- ground black pepper to taste
- garlic powder to taste
- 2 cups uncooked long grain white rice
- 4 cups water

Direction

- In a big slow cooker, combine cream of mushroom soup, cream of chicken and mushroom soup, and water until smoothly blended, and stir in red bell pepper, green bell pepper, and onion. In the slow cooker, put turkey legs and pour the sauce to cover.
- Turn the slow cooker to High to cook, tossing sometimes, about 3 hours.
- Once the 3 hours have finished, mix in potatoes and season with garlic powder, black pepper, meat tenderizer, and salt. Cook on High for another 2 hours, tossing sometimes. Take the turkey legs out and slice the meat off the bones, cut the meat, and put back into the cooker. Cook in High for another 60 minutes.
- About 25 minutes before serving time, in a saucepan, boil water and rice over high heat. Lower the heat to medium-low; put a cover on and simmer for 20-25 minutes until the rice is soft and absorbs the liquid. Enjoy the sauce and turkey over the hot cooked rice.

Nutrition Information

- Calories: 655 calories;
- Total Fat: 17.7
- Sodium: 1275
- Total Carbohydrate: 74.6
- Cholesterol: 101
- Protein: 45.7

978. Slow Cooked Turkey Legs

Serving: 4 | Prep: 15mins | Cook: 7hours30mins | Ready in:

Ingredients

- 3 tablespoons poultry seasoning
- 1 1/2 teaspoons salt
- 1/2 teaspoon ground black pepper
- 4 turkey legs
- 1 cube vegetable bouillon
- 1 cup water

Direction

- In a bowl, combine pepper, salt, and poultry seasoning. Rub over the turkey legs. Chill in the fridge for 8 hours to overnight.
- In a bowl, put bouillon cube in water to dissolve. Pour into the slow cooker.
- Shape aluminum foil into a coil form with a height at least 1-inch. Line the bottom of the slow cooker with it. On the aluminum foil, put the turkey legs, above the liquid.
- Cook on Low for 7 1/2 hours until the meat begins to fall apart.

Nutrition Information

- Calories: 421 calories;
- Total Fat: 12.7
- Sodium: 1118
- Total Carbohydrate: 2
- Cholesterol: 304
- Protein: 70.6

979. Smoked Turkey Broth

Serving: 24 | Prep: | Cook: | Ready in:

Ingredients

- 2 smoked turkey legs
- 1 large red onion, cut in half
- 1 large Spanish onion, cut in half
- 1 large carrot, cut in thirds
- 1 large red bell pepper, seeded (optional)
- 1 tablespoon olive oil
- 7 quarts cold water
- 5 cloves garlic, lightly smashed
- 10 whole black peppercorns
- salt to taste
- 1 cup water

Direction

- Preheat the oven to 200º C (400º F).
- Use olive oil to sweep the turkey legs, red bell pepper, carrot, Spanish onion, and red onion; put into a roasting pan.
- Next, roast the turkey and vegetables in the preheated oven for about 15 minutes, until they turn brown.
- Over medium heat, pour 7 quarts water into a large stockpot. Add black peppercorns, garlic, and the roasted turkey and vegetables to the water and boil. Reduce the flame to a simmer.
- Heat the roasting pan over a stove burner (two burners, if it fits) till the drippings sizzle. Next, pour in 1 cup of water, scrape up and dissolve all the browned items from the roasting pan into the water. Then put the drippings mixture into the stock.
- Simmer for 6 hours, skimming occasionally and removing the foamy scum on the top of the broth. Filter the stock through a strainer, removing the greens and turkey (their flavor are all gone). Allow to cool and store in airtight containers. It can be frozen.

Nutrition Information

- Calories: 39 calories;
- Total Fat: 1.4
- Sodium: 23
- Total Carbohydrate: 2.3
- Cholesterol: 10
- Protein: 4.2

980. Smoked Turkey Leg Salad

Serving: 6 | Prep: 15mins | Cook: | Ready in:

Ingredients

- 1 pound smoked turkey leg meat, cooked and chopped
- 1 apple, diced
- 2/3 cup dried cranberries
- 1 cup Greek yogurt
- 1/2 cup mayonnaise
- 1 tablespoon hot pepper sauce (such as Frank's RedHot®)
- 1 tablespoon olive oil
- 1 tablespoon seafood seasoning (such as Old Bay®)
- 1 tablespoon dried minced onion
- 2 teaspoons salt
- 2 teaspoons ground black pepper

Direction

- In a large bowl, mix together cranberries, apple and turkey.
- In a bowl, combine salt, pepper, dried minced onion, seafood seasoning, oil, hot pepper sauce, mayonnaise and yogurt; stir well in order that all ingredients combined properly.
- Pour dressing over turkey mixture, toss to coat. Allow to chill until serving.

Nutrition Information

- Calories: 382 calories;
- Total Fat: 24
- Sodium: 1289
- Total Carbohydrate: 17.4
- Cholesterol: 72
- Protein: 24.6

981. Smoked Turkey Split Pea Soup

Serving: 8 | Prep: 25mins | Cook: 50mins | Ready in:

Ingredients

- 1 tablespoon olive oil
- 1 yellow onion, diced
- 2 cloves garlic, chopped
- 6 cups low-sodium beef broth
- 2 pounds dried split peas
- 1 carrot, peeled and diced
- 2 small potatoes, peeled and diced
- 2 tablespoons soy sauce
- 1 tablespoon dried basil
- 1 tablespoon coarsely ground black pepper
- 1 tablespoon dried parsley
- 2 teaspoons crushed red pepper flakes
- 1 teaspoon ground sage
- 1 teaspoon kosher salt
- 2 bay leaves
- 2 1/2 pounds smoked turkey legs
- 2 cups water, or as needed
- 2 1/2 tablespoons sour cream, for garnish

Direction

- In a large pot, heat the oil over medium-high heat. Cook the onion in the hot oil for about 5 minutes until transparent; mix in the garlic and cook for additional 30 seconds. Spread in the beef broth; add bay leaves, kosher salt, sage, red pepper flakes, parsley, black pepper, basil, soy sauce, potatoes, carrot, and split peas. In the pot, add the smoked turkey legs and cover the peas by 1-inch of water. Dip the turkey legs' meaty ends into the liquid. Allow to boil, decrease heat to medium-low, and simmer while covered for about 45 minutes, until the peas are tender.
- Take away the turkey legs from the soup then leave it aside to cool. As soon as cool enough to process, debone the meat and remove tendons, properly chop the turkey meat, then set it aside. Puree the soup to your desired smoothness with a stick blender. Combine the

turkey meat into the soup. Serve in bowls and put on top of each a dollop of sour cream.

Nutrition Information

- Calories: 641 calories;
- Sodium: 692
- Total Carbohydrate: 78.2
- Cholesterol: 74
- Protein: 61.2
- Total Fat: 9.8

982. Smoked Turkey Wild Rice Soup

Serving: 6 | Prep: 30mins | Cook: 2hours | Ready in:

Ingredients

- 2 smoked turkey legs
- 8 cups water
- 4 cubes chicken bouillon (such as Knorr®)
- 1 onion, quartered
- 2 stalks celery, chopped
- 1 small inner stalk of celery with leaves, chopped
- 1 cup baby carrots, sliced
- 2 cloves garlic, minced
- 2 bay leaves
- 1 tablespoon garlic powder
- 1 tablespoon onion powder
- 2 teaspoons ground black pepper
- 1 teaspoon dried thyme
- 1 teaspoon dried marjoram
- 1 teaspoon curry powder (optional)
- 1 cup uncooked wild rice
- 1 quart half-and-half

Direction

- Place curry powder, marjoram, thyme, black pepper, onion powder, garlic powder, bay leaves, garlic, carrots, celery, onion, bouillon cubes, water and turkey legs in a soup pot and bring to a boil. Lower the heat and let it simmer for 30 minutes.
- Mix in wild rice. Let the soup simmer for 1 hour. Remove the turkey leg and separate the meat from the tendons and bones. Chop the meat and return to soup. Pour in half-and-half and heat below simmer. Cook it on low heat for 30 minutes.
- Mix in the wild rice. For at least 1 hour, simmer the soup. Remove the turkey legs then strip from the bones and tendons. Return the meat into the soup after chopping it. Pour in half-and-half and let it heat to just below a simmer. Cook for about 30 more minutes on low heat.

Nutrition Information

- Calories: 478 calories;
- Cholesterol: 124
- Protein: 30.2
- Total Fat: 26.4
- Sodium: 1630
- Total Carbohydrate: 30.7

983. Split Pea Smoked Turkey Soup

Serving: 8 | Prep: 25mins | Cook: 4hours | Ready in:

Ingredients

- 1 pound dried split peas
- 5 cups water, or more if needed
- 3 pounds smoked turkey legs
- 3 cups chicken broth
- 1 1/2 cups chopped carrot
- 1 cup chopped celery
- 2 potatoes, peeled and chopped
- 1 onion, chopped
- 1/2 teaspoon garlic powder
- 1/2 teaspoon dried oregano
- 2 bay leaves

Direction

- In a slow cooker, combine bay leaves, oregano, garlic powder, onion, potatoes, celery, carrot, chicken broth, smoked turkey legs, water, and split peas. Cover and set the cooker on a high setting, then cook for 4-5 hours until the peas become tender and the soup thickens. To serve, discard the bay leaves.

Nutrition Information

- Calories: 613 calories;
- Total Fat: 17.5
- Sodium: 1740
- Total Carbohydrate: 49.1
- Cholesterol: 145
- Protein: 63.1

984. Stuffed Turkey Legs

Serving: 4 | Prep: 15mins | Cook: 45mins | Ready in:

Ingredients

- 4 turkey legs
- 1 cup olive oil
- 2 green bell peppers
- 1 large white onion
- 2 tablespoons salt
- 1 pinch ground black pepper
- 1 teaspoon dried oregano
- 2 tablespoons distilled white vinegar
- 5 slices bacon
- 2 tablespoons teriyaki sauce

Direction

- On the turkey legs, create a good number of slits vertically. Mix oregano, vinegar, teriyaki, pepper, salt and olive oil together in a small bowl. Put the turkey legs into this mixture. Leave them marinating in the bowl.
- Following the size of the slits on the legs, start chopping up bacon, green pepper and onion into little squares that can fit in them. Insert a piece of each of bacon, onion and pepper into every slit. At medium high heat, start browning the turkey legs. Adjust the heat temperature to a low level. After putting the cover on, leave it cooking for about 45 minutes until the meat begins to detach from their bones. Feel free to adjust the temperature by lowering it or adding more water into the skillet in cases where the leg seems to be drying out during the cooking process.

Nutrition Information

- Calories: 581 calories;
- Cholesterol: 191
- Protein: 78.4
- Total Fat: 24.3
- Sodium: 4307
- Total Carbohydrate: 8.2

985. Super Soup

Serving: 7 | Prep: 15mins | Cook: 1hours10mins | Ready in:

Ingredients

- 2 turkey legs
- 1 cup diced celery
- 1 1/2 cups diced potatoes
- 2 (10.75 ounce) cans condensed cream of chicken soup
- 1 pound processed cheese, cubed
- 1 cup diced carrots
- 1 cup diced onion
- 1 (16 ounce) package frozen chopped broccoli
- 4 cups water

Direction

- Cook turkey in boiling water until tender. Cut up turkey meat, and return to the turkey broth.

- Put in celery, carrots, potatoes, and onions. Boil until tender.
- Put in frozen vegetables; cook for 15 minutes longer.
- Whisk in cubed cheese and cream of chicken soup. Cook mixture over medium-low heat, stirring frequently, until cheese is melted.

Nutrition Information

- Calories: 472 calories;
- Protein: 37.1
- Total Fat: 25.2
- Sodium: 1505
- Total Carbohydrate: 24.6
- Cholesterol: 146

986. Super Easy Drumstick Casserole

Serving: 2 | Prep: 20mins | Cook: 8hours | Ready in:

Ingredients

- 1 turkey drumstick, skin removed
- 1 cup celeriac (celery root), chopped
- 1 cup diced rutabaga
- 1 cup Brussels sprouts
- 1 sweet potato, chopped
- 2 1/4 cups chicken stock

Direction

- In a slow cooker, mix chicken stock, sweet potato, Brussels sprouts, rutabaga, celeriac, and turkey. Adjust the slow cooker to Medium. Cook for 8 hours.

Nutrition Information

- Calories: 997 calories;
- Sodium: 2236
- Total Carbohydrate: 69.7
- Cholesterol: 130
- Protein: 47.7
- Total Fat: 59.6

987. Tam's Black Eye Peas

Serving: 15 | Prep: 20mins | Cook: 2hours10mins | Ready in:

Ingredients

- 1 smoked turkey leg
- 3 links hot beef link sausage, diced
- 1/4 cup finely chopped onion
- 1 tablespoon garlic salt
- 1 teaspoon ground black pepper
- 1 teaspoon seasoned salt
- 6 cups water, or as needed
- 3 (16 ounce) packages frozen black-eyed peas
- 1 teaspoon white sugar

Direction

- In a big soup pot, add seasoned salt, black pepper, garlic salt, onion, sausage, and smoked turkey leg; cover with water. Boil over medium heat. Decrease heat and simmer for about 1 hour until meat gets tender.
- Mix the black-eyed peas into the soup, cover 1 inch above peas by adding enough water. Allow to boil. Lower heat and simmer again for 1 hour more, until the peas are softened and start to separate.
- Debone turkey, remove the tendons, and discard the bones. Add sugar and simmer while stirring often for about 10 minutes, until the soup turns condensed and slightly creamy.

Nutrition Information

- Calories: 132 calories;
- Sodium: 946
- Total Carbohydrate: 13.4
- Cholesterol: 19
- Protein: 9.8

- Total Fat: 4.3

988. Tasty Collard Greens

Serving: 10 | Prep: 30mins | Cook: 2hours | Ready in:

Ingredients

- 1/4 cup olive oil
- 2 tablespoons minced garlic
- 5 cups chicken stock
- 1 smoked turkey drumstick
- 5 bunches collard greens - rinsed, trimmed and chopped
- salt and black pepper to taste
- 1 tablespoon crushed red pepper flakes (optional)

Direction

- In a big pot, heat olive oil on medium heat. Add garlic. Sauté gently until light brown. Put in chicken stock. Add turkey leg. Cover pot. Simmer for 30 minutes.
- Add collard greens to cooking pot. Increase heat to medium-high. Cook down greens for about 45 minutes, occasionally stirring.
- Lower heat to medium. Season using pepper and salt to taste. Keep cooking for 45-60 minutes until greens are dark green and tender. Drain greens, keeping liquid. Stir in red pepper flakes if you want. Use the liquid to rewarm leftovers.

Nutrition Information

- Calories: 142 calories;
- Total Fat: 7.9
- Sodium: 689
- Total Carbohydrate: 10.6
- Cholesterol: 23
- Protein: 9.6

989. Turkey BBQ Sandwiches

Serving: 6 | Prep: 20mins | Cook: 8hours | Ready in:

Ingredients

- 2 turkey legs without skin
- 1/2 cup firmly packed brown sugar
- 1/4 cup prepared yellow mustard
- 1 tablespoon liquid smoke flavoring
- 2 tablespoons ketchup
- 2 tablespoons apple cider vinegar
- 2 tablespoons hot pepper sauce
- 1 teaspoon salt
- 1 teaspoon coarse ground black pepper
- 1 teaspoon crushed red pepper flakes

Direction

- Use nonstick cooking spray to spray inside the slow cooker, then put in the turkey legs. Mix together red pepper flakes, black pepper, salt, hot pepper sauce, cider vinegar, ketchup, smoke flavoring, yellow mustard, and brown sugar in a bowl until the sugar dissolves, then pour mixture over the turkey legs.
- Cook, covered, in the cooker that is set on a low setting for 8-10 hours. Take out the turkey legs and separate the meat from the tendons and bones, then shred the meat. Place the meat back into the sauce to serve.

Nutrition Information

- Calories: 279 calories;
- Sodium: 779
- Total Carbohydrate: 20.3
- Cholesterol: 131
- Protein: 32.7
- Total Fat: 6.9

990. Turkey Corn Chowder

Serving: 8 | Prep: 20mins | Cook: 40mins | Ready in:

Ingredients

- 3 potatoes, peeled and diced
- 2 smoked turkey legs
- 1/4 cup butter
- 1 large onion, chopped
- 3 tablespoons all-purpose flour
- 1 (32 ounce) carton chicken broth
- 1 (16 ounce) package frozen corn
- 1 quart light cream
- salt and ground black pepper to taste

Direction

- Put the potatoes in a pot and add salted water enough to cover them. Bring this to a boil then lower the heat to medium-low. Cover the pot and simmer for about 20 minutes, until the potatoes are tender. Drain the water out and leave the potatoes to steam dry for 1 to 2 minutes. Separate the meat from the turkey legs, discard the bones and tendons. Chop the meat of the turkey and set it aside.
- In a soup pot, heat the butter over medium heat. Put the onion in the butter and cook for about 8 minutes, until the onion is translucent. Sprinkle the flour over the onion and butter while constantly stirring until the mixture forms into a paste. Fry the paste for about a minute then stir in the chicken broth, turkey meat, corn, and potatoes. Stir this mixture for about 5 minutes until it comes to a low boil and thickens. Slightly mash the vegetables and potatoes using a potato masher until the potatoes look rounded off. Add the cream to the soup and bring it again to a simmer, leaving it to cook for 5 minutes without boiling and with constant stirring. Add salt and black pepper to season.

Nutrition Information

- Calories: 462 calories;
- Cholesterol: 111
- Protein: 23.8
- Total Fat: 26
- Sodium: 677
- Total Carbohydrate: 35.3

991. Turkey Drumsticks Paprika

Serving: 4 | Prep: 10mins | Cook: 4hours20mins | Ready in:

Ingredients

- 1/4 cup Hungarian smoked paprika
- 1/4 cup olive oil
- 1 onion, chopped
- 1 pinch ground black pepper
- 4 turkey drumsticks
- 1 (10.75 ounce) can condensed cream of mushroom soup
- 1 cup white wine (optional)

Direction

- Preheat an oven to 165 °C or 325 °F. In a roasting pan, combine paprika and olive oil to create a paste. On the roasting pan, put on the lid or place aluminum foil to cover.
- In prepped oven, let paprika paste bake for about 15 minutes till aromatic. Into paprika mixture, mix pepper and onion; put in drumsticks of turkey, flipping to coat. Using aluminum foil or a lid, cover the roasting pan and put back to oven.
- Keep baking for 4 to 5 hours till turkey is very soft and meat falls apart from bone. Take out the bones, retaining meat in the pan, and mix in white wine and cream of mushroom soup. Let mixture simmer for approximately 5 minutes over medium heat till hot.

Nutrition Information

- Calories: 700 calories;
- Protein: 75.2
- Total Fat: 32.7
- Sodium: 703
- Total Carbohydrate: 13.3
- Cholesterol: 178

- Calories: 1644 calories;
- Total Fat: 124.4
- Sodium: 2951
- Total Carbohydrate: 46.7
- Cholesterol: 280
- Protein: 83

992. Turkey Drumsticks Perfecto

Serving: 3 | Prep: 10mins | Cook: 1hours45mins | Ready in:

Ingredients

- 3 small turkey drumsticks
- 1/4 cup salt
- water to cover
- 2 tablespoons butter, melted
- 1/4 teaspoon ground black pepper, or to taste
- 1 cup chicken broth

Direction

- In a big bowl, put the turkey drumsticks and cover with enough water. Into the water, mix the salt to melt.
- Refrigerate drumsticks to brine for 2 hours; drain. In clean water, wash the drumsticks and pat dry.
- Preheat an oven to 175°C or 350°F.
- Coat drumsticks by brushing butter over; add black pepper to season.
- Into a roasting pan, add the chicken broth. Into the broth, arrange the turkey legs. Put lid on roasting pan.
- In the prepped oven, bake for 1 hour 45 minutes to 2 hours till juices run clear and not pink anymore at the bone. An inserted instant-read thermometer into the chunkiest part of thigh, close to the bone should register 74°C or 165°F.

Nutrition Information

993. Turkey Vegetable Soup

Serving: 10 | Prep: 30mins | Cook: 1hours30mins | Ready in:

Ingredients

- 6 cups turkey pan drippings, fat skimmed
- 8 cups water
- 2 turkey legs
- 2 cloves garlic, crushed
- 1 bay leaf
- 1/2 teaspoon dried thyme
- ground black pepper to taste
- 1/4 cup all-purpose flour
- 1/2 cup milk
- 2 cups cubed cooked turkey
- 6 red potatoes, diced
- 1/2 onion, quartered and sliced
- 3 carrots, sliced
- 2 stalks celery, sliced

Direction

- Stir together black pepper, thyme, bay leaf, garlic, turkey legs, water, and turkey drippings in a big stockpot, then boil. Decrease the heat to a simmer and cover, then simmer for 30 minutes until the turkey meat falls off the bones. Remove the turkey legs and pick out the meat from the bones, then return into the soup.
- In a bowl, whisk together 1/2 cup milk and 1/4 cup flour until blended, then stir into the soup. Bring back to a simmer, stirring continuously, and cook for another 30 minutes until it thickens. Mix in celery, carrots, onions, red potatoes, and the cubed cooked turkey

meat, then simmer, covered, until the celery becomes tender, another 30 minutes.

Nutrition Information

- Calories: 194 calories;
- Sodium: 778
- Total Carbohydrate: 11
- Cholesterol: 61
- Protein: 25
- Total Fat: 4.9

994. Tuscan Smoked Turkey Bean Soup

Serving: 6 | Prep: 20mins | Cook: 4hours | Ready in:

Ingredients

- 1 pound dry white beans
- 2 smoked turkey legs
- 1/2 onion, diced
- 2 bay leaves
- 2 stalks celery, diced
- 4 large carrots, sliced
- 1 (14.5 ounce) can petite diced tomatoes, undrained
- 2 tablespoons Italian seasoning
- salt and ground black pepper to taste
- 2 tablespoons grated Parmesan cheese, divided

Direction

- In a large bowl, cover the beans with water. Use a cloth to cover the bowl and let the beans soak overnight. Let the beans drain; rinse.
- In a large soup pot, combine the turkey legs, bay leaves, onion, and soaked beans. Cover the mixture with water. Let it boil over medium heat. Adjust the heat to medium-low. Simmer the mixture for 3 hours. Remove and discard the bay leaves. Get the turkey legs from the broth and separate its meat from its bones. Place the meat back into the broth. Mix in diced tomatoes, salt, pepper, Italian seasoning, celery, and carrots. Simmer the mixture for 1 hour until the carrots and celery are tender. Distribute the soup in bowls. Sprinkle each bowl with 1 tsp. of Parmesan cheese. Serve.

Nutrition Information

- Calories: 454 calories;
- Sodium: 939
- Total Carbohydrate: 53.8
- Cholesterol: 66
- Protein: 40.1
- Total Fat: 8.8

Chapter 9: Turkey Brine Recipes

***

995. Apple Cider Turkey Brine

Serving: 12 | Prep: 5mins | Cook: 10mins | Ready in:

Ingredients

- 1 gallon water, or as needed, divided
- 2 cups apple cider
- 1 cup kosher salt
- 1 tablespoon fresh sage
- 1 tablespoon fresh rosemary
- 1 tablespoon fresh thyme
- 1 tablespoon black peppercorns
- 4 cups ice cubes

Direction

- Mix together peppercorns, thyme, rosemary, sage, kosher salt, apple cider and 4 cups water then boil in a big stockpot; mix and cook brine till salt just dissolves. Take off the heat; add the ice cubes.

Nutrition Information

- Calories: 24 calories;
- Total Fat: 0
- Sodium: 7608
- Total Carbohydrate: 5.9
- Cholesterol: 0
- Protein: 0.1

996. Grandma's Farmhouse Turkey Brine

Serving: 7 | Prep: 5mins | Cook: 20mins | Ready in:

Ingredients

- 2 cups kosher salt
- 3 tablespoons poultry seasoning
- 3 tablespoons onion powder
- 1 tablespoon black pepper
- 4 quarts vegetable broth
- 2 quarts water
- 3 cups cranberry juice

Direction

- Combine black pepper, onion powder, poultry seasoning, and salt in a large stockpot. Add cranberry juice, water, and vegetable stock; bring mixture to a boil. Turn heat down to medium-low and simmer for 20 minutes. Turn off the heat; allow mixture to cool to room temperature.
- To use, immerse turkey entirely into the cooled brine and marinate in the fridge for 12 to 16 hours. Drain and pat dry turkey before roasting as directed.

Nutrition Information

997. Incredible Turkey Brine

Serving: 1 | Prep: 10mins | Cook: | Ready in:

Ingredients

- 2 gallons water
- 1 1/4 cups kosher salt
- 1/3 cup light brown sugar
- 1/4 cup Worcestershire sauce
- 6 cloves garlic, chopped
- 4 sprigs fresh thyme
- 1 sprig fresh rosemary
- 1 tablespoon whole black peppercorns
- 1 1/2 teaspoons whole allspice berries (optional)
- 1 bay leaf

Direction

- In a big pot, mix together bay leaf, allspice berries, peppercorns, rosemary, thyme, garlic, Worcestershire sauce, brown sugar, salt and water together; boil. Put aside to cool fully prior to brining the turkey.

Nutrition Information

- Calories: 382 calories;
- Total Carbohydrate: 97.2
- Cholesterol: 0
- Protein: 2.1
- Total Fat: 0.6
- Sodium: 114785

998. Make Your Turkey Melt In Your Mouth Turkey Brine

Serving: 30 | Prep: 20mins | Cook: | Ready in:

Ingredients

- 9 (14.5 ounce) cans chicken broth
- 1 (64 fluid ounce) bottle apple juice
- 4 oranges, halved
- 7 stalks celery, cut into large chunks
- 3 onions, cut into large chunks
- 6 sprigs fresh rosemary
- 6 sprigs fresh thyme
- 4 bay leaves
- 2 fresh sage leaves
- 1/2 cup kosher salt
- 1/4 cup poultry seasoning
- 2 tablespoons ground black pepper

Direction

- Mix apple juice and chicken broth together in a food-safe container big enough to hold brine ingredients and a turkey. Add juice squeezed from orange halves into the broth mixture along with the spent orange halves; add sage leaves, bay leaves, thyme, rosemary, onion, and celery to the mixture. Mix black pepper, poultry seasoning, and salt into the liquid until dissolved.

Nutrition Information

- Calories: 44 calories;
- Sodium: 2050
- Total Carbohydrate: 9.3
- Cholesterol: 3
- Protein: 0.8
- Total Fat: 0.4

999. Salty And Sweet Cranberry Citrus Brine

Serving: 12 | Prep: 10mins | Cook: | Ready in:

Ingredients

- 1 cup kosher salt
- 1 (12 fluid ounce) can frozen orange juice concentrate
- 1 (12 fluid ounce) can frozen cranberry juice concentrate
- 1 gallon water
- 1/2 cup brown sugar
- 1 cinnamon stick
- 1 lemon, cut into wedges
- 1 orange, cut into wedges
- 1 red onion, cut into wedges
- 3 cloves garlic
- 4 bay leaves
- 1 tablespoon dried thyme leaves
- 1 tablespoon freshly ground black pepper

Direction

- Combine black pepper, thyme, bay leaves, garlic cloves, onion wedges, orange wedges, lemon wedges, cinnamon stick, brown sugar, water, cranberry juice concentrate, orange juice concentrate, and kosher salt in a large stockpot. Whisk until brown sugar and salt are dissolved. To use, put a whole turkey into the brine; chill, covered, 14 to 16 hours before roasting. Pour off used brine.

Nutrition Information

1000. Terrific Turkey Brine

Serving: 8 | Prep: 15mins | Cook: | Ready in:

Ingredients

- 1 gallon distilled water
- 1 (750 milliliter) bottle white wine
- 1 1/2 cups salt
- 2 orange, quartered
- 2 tablespoons dried rosemary

Direction

- Line a large food safe bag over the bottom of a large stockpot. Add salt, wine, and water to the bag, whisking to dissolve salt. Add juice squeezed from orange quarters; drop the used orange quarters into the pot. Stir in rosemary.
- To use, gently put defrosted turkey into the brine and seal the bag; chill in the fridge for a minimum of 5 hours before cooking.

Nutrition Information

1001. Turkey Brine

Serving: 15 | Prep: 5mins | Cook: 15mins | Ready in:

Ingredients

- 1 gallon vegetable broth
- 1 cup sea salt
- 1 tablespoon crushed dried rosemary
- 1 tablespoon dried sage
- 1 tablespoon dried thyme
- 1 tablespoon dried savory
- 1 gallon ice water

Direction

- Mix the savory, thyme, sage, rosemary, sea salt, and vegetable broth in a large stockpot. Bring to a boil, stirring frequently to make sure salt dissolves. Take away from the heat, and allow it to cool at room temperature.
- Once the broth mixture is cool, place it into a clean 5-gallon bucket. Mix in the ice water.
- Rinse and dry your turkey. Be sure you have taken off the innards. Add the turkey into the brine with the breast down. Be sure that the cavity gets filled. Keep the bucket in the refrigerator overnight.
- Take the turkey gently draining off the excess brine and pat dry. Get rid of excess brine.
- Cook the turkey as wished, setting the drippings aside for gravy. Remember that brined turkeys cook faster for 20-30 minutes so check the temperature gauge.

Nutrition Information

Index

A

Almond 7,11,214,425

Apple 3,4,6,7,11,12,13,14,21,35,95,187,214,415,460,483,538,540,564

Apricot 7,13,215,484

Artichoke 10,360

Asparagus 8,9,278,314

Avocado 5,10,14,112,361,537,538,545

B

Bacon 3,5,10,11,13,14,23,80,112,129,342,348,420,510,521,522,528,538

Baking 334

Barley 3,7,11,12,36,208,217,387,395,426,427,439,447,450

Basil 3,8,10,24,260,355,387

Beans 3,4,5,6,7,8,14,32,77,103,125,148,213,257,552

Beef 5,8,10,144,277,363

Beer 4,14,86,528

Berry 8,9,12,265,299,315,451

Black pepper 246

Bread 4,7,9,10,11,14,96,100,147,218,325,334,411,534

Brie 6,155,156,161

Broccoli 10,364

Broth 14,556

Brussels sprouts 560

Buns 10,71,76,354

Burger 3,4,5,6,8,10,17,20,23,24,26,29,31,35,40,43,45,54,55,57,59,60,64,66,67,71,76,83,92,99,100,105,107,112,119,130,131,133,144,147,149,150,153,155,157,164,169,185,280,365

Butter 3,4,6,7,8,9,14,28,87,148,159,188,191,198,203,204,218,238,242,314,316,486,517,526,542

C

Cabbage 3,9,10,12,14,16,316,365,428,549

Carrot 3,29,387,446

Cashew 5,7,10,12,111,219,367,429,442

Cauliflower 5,145

Cayenne pepper 454

Celery 387,446

Champ 7,220,502

Chard 495

Cheddar 26,30,39,42,43,44,47,48,49,53,61,66,67,69,80,87,89,90,91,92,93,96,97,98,99,110,114,121,127,128,130,134,137,143,144,145,147,148,149,156,163,164,186,188,191,195,196,199,204,205,209,211,309,310,333,348,354,363,370,392,516,517,519,527,532,535,543

Cheese 3,4,5,6,7,9,10,12,13,27,30,49,55,64,107,127,129,156,191,196,325,348,352,354,436,452,515,521

Chestnut 12,13,477,492

Chicken 3,6,7,9,10,11,12,31,76,139,190,191,199,202,230,316,376,387,390,412,446,456,538

Chickpea 5,103

Chipotle 3,5,33,80,130

Chorizo 4,6,79,157

Chutney 10,12,369,373,430

Cider 13,14,483,564

Cocktail 3,35

Cola 12,469

Coleslaw 519

Collar 14,561

Coriander 3,36

Couscous 6,177

Crab 9,317

Crackers 326

Cranberry 3,4,6,7,9,10,13,14,15,21,67,166,170,171,201,222,292,306,317,328,333,349,356,372,373,485,493,512,529,541,542,566

Cream 3,5,6,7,9,10,13,31,38,76,139,143,166,223,289,291,303,348,373,374,375,521

Croissant 8,13,252,512

Crostini 9,317

Crumble 44,63,133,166,201,208,210,223,238,248,277,316,320,323,328,330,332,333,337,340,343,345,346,353,372,380,390,403

Cumin 3,40

Curry 12,430

D

Dab 354

Dijon mustard 35,36,105,118,141,152,158,159,164,175,176,192,215,224,231,236,246,256,273,306,319,323,347,354,364,367,394,404,409,415,420,421,428,442,443,444,445,447,453

Dill 349,446

Dumplings 9,10,296,322,342,368

E

Egg 3,5,6,7,10,44,49,51,110,135,173,199,211,335,350,356

F

Fat 4,13,16,17,18,19,20,21,22,23,24,25,26,27,28,29,30,31,32,33,34,35,36,37,38,39,40,41,42,43,44,45,46,47,48,49,50,51,52,53,54,55,56,57,58,59,60,61,62,63,64,65,66,67,68,69,70,71,72,73,74,75,76,77,78,79,80,81,82,83,84,85,86,87,88,89,90,91,92,93,94,95,96,97,98,99,100,101,102,103,104,105,106,107,108,109,110,111,112,113,114,115,116,117,118,119,120,121,122,123,124,125,126,127,128,129,130,131,132,133,134,135,136,137,138,139,140,141,142,143,144,145,146,147,148,149,150,151,152,153,154,155,156,157,158,159,160,161,162,163,164,165,166,167,168,169,170,171,172,173,174,175,176,177,178,179,180,181,182,183,184,185,186,187,188,189,190,191,192,193,194,195,196,197,198,199,200,201,202,203,204,205,206,207,208,209,210,211,212,213,214,215,216,217,218,219,220,221,222,223,224,225,226,227,228,229,230,231,232,233,234,235,236,237,238,239,240,241,242,243,244,245,246,247,248,249,250,251,252,253,254,255,256,257,258,259,260,261,262,263,264,265,266,267,268,269,270,271,272,273,274,275,276,277,278,279,280,281,282,283,284,285,286,287,288,289,290,291,292,293,294,295,296,297,298,299,300,301,302,303,304,305,306,307,308,309,310,311,312,313,314,315,316,317,318,319,320,321,322,323,324,325,326,327,328,329,330,331,332,333,334,335,336,337,338,339,340,341,342,343,344,345,346,347,348,349,350,351,352,353,354,355,356,357,358,359,360,361,362,363,364,365,366,367,368,369,370,371,372,373,374,375,376,377,378,379,380,381,382,383,384,385,386,387,388,389,390,391,392,393,394,395,396,397,398,399,400,401,402,403,404,405,406,407,408,409,410,411,412,413,414,415,416,417,418,419,420,421,422,423,424,425,426,427,428,429,430,431,432,433,434,435,436,437,438,439,440,441,442,443,444,445,447,448,449,450,451,452,453,454,455,456,457,458,459,460,461,462,463,464,465,466,467,468,469,470,471,472,473,474,475,476,477,478,479,480,481,482,483,484,485,486,487,488,489,490,491,492,493,494,495,496,497,498,499,500,501,502,503,504,505,506,507,508,509,510,511,512,513,514,515,516,517,518,519,520,521,522,523,524,525,526,527,528,529,530,531,532,533,534,535,536,537,538,539,540,541,542,543,544,545,546,547,548,549,550,551,552,553,554,555,556,557,558,559,560,561,562,563,564,565,566

Feta 3,5,6,13,14,55,56,133,177,510,545

Flatbread 204

Focaccia 7,216

French bread 156,273,275,283,317,327,411,541

Fruit 6,10,11,12,191,374,382,383,432,449,475

G

Game 3,9,25,320

Garlic 3,4,7,8,14,36,60,76,85,171,208,225,226,240,287,387,436,446,488,503,533

Gin 7,12,226,432

Gorgonzola 5,112

Gouda 136

Grapes 12,442

Gravy 6,8,12,13,14,162,170,171,232,241,242,284,465,468,484,485,487,488,494,532,539,550

Guacamole 4,71,72

H

Ham 9,11,12,71,76,305,313,385,386,387,450

Heart 4,7,9,11,75,109,201,230,323,388,389,390

Herbs 14,387,527

Hominy 7,229

Honey 7,9,12,13,236,323,354,473,479,481

Horseradish 4,9,67,324

Hummus 10,352

I

Iceberg lettuce 263

J

Jam 7,13,195,519

Jerusalem artichoke 207

Jus 275,305,359,367,371,378,382,430,456,458

K

Kale 4,6,11,71,157,163,392,405

Kidney 5,125

L

Leek 3,14,36,550

Lemon 8,9,11,13,240,289,327,395,403,484

Lettuce 5,6,8,13,119,160,253,271,275,278,281,358,359,370,385,421,438,442,522

Lime 8,143,284,319

Ling 8,258,285

M

Macaroni 5,127

Mandarin 9,12,328,433,499

Mango 7,201

Maple syrup 311

Marsala wine 295

Mayonnaise 10,355

Meat 3,4,5,6,7,8,9,10,11,12,14,18,23,24,25,26,27,28,30,33,34,35,38,41,48,49,50,51,55,61,64,69,75,76,77,80,81,82,84,101,106,108,112,113,115,117,124,126,128,130,138,139,141,145,146,147,150,152,156,161,162,163,175,176,178,179,181,182,228,238,245,248,269,272,275,286,291,314,315,316,319,323,324,328,329,333,335,336,339,340,345,346,372,389,400,412,433,434,550

Melon 11,12,401,452

Mince 221,229,293,295,373,456,533

Molasses 13,511

Mozzarella 5,106,124,516,517

Muffins 3,7,28,196

Mushroom 3,5,6,7,8,9,10,13,22,23,31,38,107,133,137,139,160,163,189,196,201,248,249,273,284,287,303,304,307,325,356,524

Mustard 6,9,164,323

N

Nachos 6,9,10,180,330,338,351

Noodles 7,135,209

Nut

8,12,13,16,17,18,19,20,21,22,23,24,25,26,27,28,29,30,31,32,33,34,35,36,37,38,39,40,41,42,43,44,45,46,47,48,49,50,51,52,53,54,55,56,57,58,59,60,61,62,63,64,65,66,67,68,69,70,71,72,73,74,75,76,77,78,79,80,81,82,83,84,85,86,87,88,89,90,91,92,93,94,95,96,97,98,99,100,101,102,103,104,105,106,107,108,109,110,111,112,113,114,115,116,117,118,119,120,121,122,123,124,125,126,127,128,129,130,131,132,133,134,135,136,137,138,139,140,141,142,143,144,145,146,147,148,149,150,151,152,153,154,155,156,157,158,159,160,161,162,163,164,165,166,167,168,169,170,171,172,173,174,175,176,177,178,179,180,181,182,183,184,185,186,187,188,189,190,191,192,193,194,195,196,197,198,199,200,201,202,203,204,205,206,207,208,209,210,211,212,213,214,215,216,217,218,219,220,221,222,223,224,225,226,227,228,229,230,231,232,233,234,235,236,237,238,239,240,241,242,243,244,245,246,247,248,249,250,251,252,253,254,255,256,257,258,259,260,261,262,263,264,265,266,267,268,269,270,271,272,273,274,275,276,277,278,279,280,281,282,283,284,285,286,287,288,289,290,291,292,293,294,295,296,297,298,299,300,301,302,303,304,305,306,307,308,309,310,311,312,313,314,315,316,317,318,319,320,321,322,323,324,325,326,327,328,329,330,331,332,333,334,335,336,337,338,339,340,341,342,343,344,345,346,347,348,349,350,351,352,353,354,355,356,357,358,359,360,361,362,363,364,365,366,367,368,369,370,371,372,373,374,375,376,377,378,379,380,381,382,383,384,385,386,387,388,389,390,391,392,393,394,395,396,397,398,399,400,401,402,403,404,405,406,407,408,409,410,411,412,413,414,415,416,417,418,419,420,421,422,423,424,425,426,427,428,429,430,431,432,433,434,435,436,437,438,439,440,441,442,443,444,445,446,447,448,449,450,451,452,453,454,455,456,457,458,459,460,461,462,463,464,465,466,467,468,469,470,471,472,473,474,475,476,477,478,479,480,481,482,483,484,485,486,487,488,489,490,491,492,493,494,495,496,497,498,499,500,501,502,503,504,505,506,507,508,509,510,511,512,513,514,515,516,517,518,519,520,521,522,523,524,525,526,527,528,529,530,531,532,533,534,535,536,537,538,539,540,541,542,543,544,545,546,547,548,549,550,551,552,553,554,555,556,557,558,559,560,561,562,563,564,565,566,567

O

Oil 44,45,67,139,143,148,276,287,326,347,350,356,392,476,489

Okra 11,403

Onion 8,13,249,446,484

Orange 5,6,8,10,13,14,136,170,171,250,251,252,335,445,479,489,526,552

Oregano 387

Oyster 504

P

Pancakes 9,292

Paprika 14,488,503,526,562

Parmesan 6,22,31,35,48,62,63,64,65,73,75,81,90,91,93,101,102,108,126,138,139,145,146,153,154,155,164,168,169,176,182,189,190,193,194,195,196,197,198,203,204,206,207,211,212,218,223,228,234,237,238,239,249,250,262,264,279,280,283,284,285,286,287,289,292,293,295,298,309,310,314,320,321,326,334,343,354,357,359,383,388,390,394,397,398,400,404,410,412,436,440,443,453,454,455,526,527,534,564

Parsley 10,11,365,403,446

Pasta 5,6,7,8,9,10,11,12,14,109,142,157,165,197,198,206,261,288,367,368,380,383,386,390,397,406,436,437,447,452,527

Peach 5,112

Pear 11,12,404,442

Peas 7,14,193,553,560

Pecan 9,11,308,348,391,398,412

Pecorino 536

Peel 182,276,317,442,537

Penne 5,6,7,9,109,155,158,198,289

Pepper 3,4,5,6,7,8,9,10,11,14,18,31,37,56,72,76,85,136,137,177,198,205,220,233,254,264,309,314,320,334,352,357,387,420,422,446,466,488,503,526

Pesto 5,8,106,263

Pie 3,4,5,6,7,8,9,46,66,87,121,140,145,172,210,211,277,280,282,310,534

Pineapple 6,147

Pistachio 10,335

Pizza 6,7,8,9,10,11,13,168,204,224,254,255,321,325,327,331,334,337,357,393,397,516

Plum 315

Polenta 10,348

Pomegranate 10,13,336,493

Pork 235,307,308,309,379,380,412,415

Port 6,99,168

Potato 3,5,6,7,9,10,11,12,14,38,80,110,139,140,141,175,177,199,205,208,211,212,291,292,340,354,368,376,379,388,389,399,405,410,444,550,554,555

Poultry 10,379,488,518,519

Pulse 551

Pumpkin 3,5,8,10,42,114,124,142,261,361,364

Q

Quinoa 3,4,5,6,29,31,68,93,115,116,137,178,179

R

Raspberry 8,256

Rice 4,5,6,7,8,9,10,11,12,14,33,53,84,103,113,119,129,161,179,200,205,213,245,257,261,302,307,322,373,378,384,386,387,395,431,438,439,446,448,451,457,458,469,558

Risotto 9,299

Roast chicken 503

Roast turkey 499

Rosemary 5,6,7,8,11,12,13,117,155,225,260,409,474,496

S

Sage 7,8,13,198,243,488,514

Salad 3,4,7,10,11,12,14,41,65,89,102,219,358,359,360,361,363,364,366,367,368,369,371,372,373,374,376,377,378,380,382,383,384,385,386,388,390,391,392,394,397,400,401,404,405,407,409,410,414,415,419,420,421,425,429,430,432,433,436,437,438,440,441,442,443,444,445,447,449,450,452,453,458,459,527,542,557

Salami 10,360,366

Salsa 3,7,9,10,29,201,329,349

Salt 15,34,62,124,142,234,244,287,293,371,378,388,423,446,459,464,542,545,566

Sausage 3,4,5,6,7,8,9,10,11,12,21,78,79,95,117,171,186,187,188,190,191,193,194,196,197,198,199,200,201,202,203,204,205,206,207,208,209,210,211,213,223,235,238,257,261,267,294,307,308,309,325,332,335,340,379,380,390,392,393,394,396,398,405,406,408,410,411,412,413,415,422,443,444,454,504

Savory 4,11,13,14,75,412,420,488,548

Scallop 9,14,295,542

Sea salt 208

Seasoning 34,86,127,143,171,287,354,488,518

Sesame seeds 147

Shallot 9,13,299,484

Sherry 13,497

Soup 3,4,5,6,7,10,11,12,13,14,31,36,38,48,65,71,75,76,110,129,139,143,152,157,174,175,182,187,188,190,194,199,207,208,358,362,363,366,371,372,373,374,375,381,384,387,389,391,392,393,395,396,397,400,402,405,406,407,408,409,410,4

11,415,416,417,418,421,422,424,426,427,428,431,432,434, 436,437,439,443,444,446,447,448,449,450,451,453,454,459,469,515,535,550,551,557,558,559,563,564

Spaghetti 4,5,6,8,9,13,58,62,81,98,101,128,173,266,267,298,520

Spinach 3,4,5,6,7,8,10,11,13,29,43,64,133,159,173,211,212,269,270,342,367,397,510

Squash 3,4,5,6,7,9,10,11,14,28,87,98,120,148,159,182,186,188,198,294,298,360,420,542

Steak 6,9,53,127,170,171,287

Stew 4,6,8,9,14,60,68,82,163,255,261,279,282,294,296,547

Stock 31,76,387,426,446,469

Stuffing 3,4,8,9,10,11,12,13,14,21,63,265,270,276,277,298,305,308,376,379,398,399,412,451,457,466,471,477,492,505,507,513,538,540,546

Sugar 13,75,232,235,290,307,308,309,330,349,355,375,379,380,412,415,436,459,499

Swiss chard 208

T

Tabasco 52,85,86,105,133,511

Taco 3,4,5,6,7,8,9,10,14,29,41,48,65,69,70,89,92,102,103,110,143,144,173,174,181,204,263,272,290,354,542

Tangerine 12,461

Tarragon 5,11,143,382,421

Tea 10,14,286,355,526

Tequila 5,146

Teriyaki 5,6,147

Thai basil 88

Thyme 9,13,299,446,503

Tofu 4,61

Tomato 3,5,6,7,10,11,19,29,110,124,142,163,194,269,338,344,387,405,411,424,427,439,446

Tortellini 11,393,400,403

Turkey 1,3,4,5,6,7,8,9,10,11,12,13,14,15,16,17,18,19,20,21,22,23,24,26,27,28,29,30,31,32,33,35,38,39,40,41,42,43,44,45,46,47,48,49,51,53,54,55,56,57,60,61,64,65,66,67,68,69,70,71,74,75,76,77,79,80,81,82,83,84,86,87,88,89,92,93,94,95,96,97,99,100,101,103,104,105,106,107,108,110,111,112,114,115,116,117,118,119,121,122,123,124,125,127,128,129,130,131,132,133,134,136,137,138,139,140,141,142,143,144,145,147,148,149,150,151,152,153,154,155,156,157,158,159,160,161,162,163,164,165,166,167,168,169,170,171,172,173,174,175,176,177,178,179,180,181,183,184,185,186,191,192,193,197,199,201,203,204,205,208,209,210,211,212,214,215,216,218,219,220,221,222,223,225,226,227,228,229,230,231,232,233,234,235,236,237,238,239,240,241,242,243,244,245,246,247,248,249,250,251,252,256,257,258,259,260,262,263,264,265,267,268,269,270,272,273,274,275,276,277,278,279,280,281,282,283,284,285,286,287,288,289,290,291,292,293,294,295,296,297,298,299,300,301,302,303,304,305,306,307,308,309,311,312,314,315,317,319,323,326,328,335,336,338,340,341,342,344,345,346,347,348,349,350,351,352,353,354,355,356,358,360,361,362,363,364,367,368,369,371,372,373,374,375,377,378,381,382,383,385,386,387,391,392,395,401,404,407,409,412,414,415,416,418,420,421,422,423,424,425,426,427,428,429,430,431,432,433,434,435,436,437,438,439,440,441,442,443,444,445,446,447,448,449,450,451,452,453,455,457,458,459,460,461,462,463,464,465,466,467,468,469,470,471,472,473,474,475,476,477,478,479,480,481,482,483,484,485,486,487,488,489,490,492,493,494,495,496,497,498,499,500,501,502,503,505,506,507,508,509,510,511,512,513,514,515,516,517,518,519,521,522,523,524,525,526,527,528,529,530,531,532,533,534,535,536,537,538,539,540,541,542,543,544,545,546,547,548,549,

550,551,552,553,554,555,556,557,558,559,561,562,563,564,565,566,567

V

Vegetables 5,7,8,136,202,258

W

Worcestershire sauce 19,20,24,26,27,34,40,52,55,60,75,77,78,86,95,105,106,112,113,116,117,129,131,132,133,138,140,141,146,153,156,158,159,163,170,175,176,177,178,179,239,244,246,251,266,268,277,282,296,298,314,317,324,348,353,365,372,386,406,466,530,531,565

Wraps 4,5,6,7,8,9,13,96,119,129,160,217,227,253,293,522

Y

Yam 6,7,181,213

Z

Zest 6,9,12,143,185,311,459

L

lasagna 22,43,73,90,91,92,133,134,159,264,283

Conclusion

Thank you again for downloading this book!

I hope you enjoyed reading about my book!

If you enjoyed this book, please take the time to share your thoughts and post a review on Amazon. It'd be greatly appreciated!

Write me an honest review about the book – I truly value your opinion and thoughts and I will incorporate them into my next book, which is already underway.

Thank you!

If you have any questions, **feel free to contact at:** *author@tempehrecipes.com*

Carrie Milian

tempehrecipes.com

Made in United States
Troutdale, OR
04/15/2025